Genetic Hypertension

Hypertension génétique

Colloques **INSERM**
ISSN 0768-3154

Other *Colloques* published as co-editions by John Libbey Eurotext and INSERM

133 Cardiovascular and Respiratory Physiology in the Fetus and Neonate. *Physiologie Cardiovasculaire et Respiratoire du Fœtus et du Nouveau-né.*
Scientific Committee : P. Karlberg,
A. Minkowski, W. Oh and L. Stern;
Managing Editor : M. Monset-Couchard.
ISBN : John Libbey Eurotext 0 86196 086 6
INSERM 2 85598 282 0

134 Porphyrins and Porphyrias. *Porphyrines et Porphyries.*
Edited by Y. Nordmann.
ISBN : John Libbey Eurotext 0 86196 087 4
INSERM 2 85598 281 2

137 Neo-Adjuvant Chemotherapy. *Chimiothérapie Néo-Adjuvante.*
Edited by C. Jacquillat, M. Weil and D. Khayat.
ISBN : John Libbey Eurotext 0 86196 077 7
INSERM 2 85598 283 7

139 Hormones and Cell Regulation (10th European Symposium). *Hormones et Régulation Cellulaire (10ᵉ Symposium Européen).*
Edited by J. Nunez, J.E. Dumont and R.J.B. King.
ISBN : John Libbey Eurotext 0 86196 084 X
INSERM 2 85598 284 7

147 Modern Trends in Aging Research. *Nouvelles Perspectives de la Recherche sur le Vieillissement.*
Edited by Y. Courtois, B. Faucheux, B. Forette, D.L. Knook and J.A. Tréton.
ISBN : John Libbey Eurotext 0 86196 103 X
INSERM 2 85598 309 6

149 Binding Proteins of Steroid Hormones. *Protéines de liaison des Hormones Stéroïdes.*
Edited by M.G. Forest and M. Pugeat.
ISBN : John Libbey Eurotext 0 86196 125 0
INSERM 2 85598 310 X

151 Control and Management of Parturition. *La Maîtrise de la Parturition.*
Edited by C. Sureau, P. Blot, D. Cabrol, F. Cavaillé and G. Germain.
ISBN : John Libbey Eurotext 0 86196 096 3
INSERM 2 85598 311 8

Genetic Hypertension

Hypertension génétique

Proceedings of the **7th International Symposium on SHR and related studies** held in Lyon (France), Ecole Normale Supérieure, October 28-30, 1991.

Under the patronage of : Ministère de la Recherche et de la Technologie, Ministère délégué à la Santé, INSERM, CNRS (Département des Sciences de la Vie), Conseil Général du Rhône, Mairie de Lyon, Chambre de Commerce et d'Industrie de Lyon.

Edited by

Jean Sassard

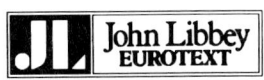

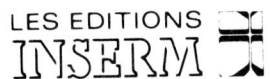

British Library Cataloguing in Publication Data

A catalogue record for this book
is available from the British Library

ISBN 0 86196 313-X
ISSN 0768-3154

First published in 1992 by

Editions John Libbey Eurotext
6 rue Blanche, 92120 Montrouge, France. (33) (1) 47 35 85 52
ISBN 0 86196 313 X

John Libbey and Company Ltd
13 Smiths Yard, Summerley Street, London SW18 4HR,
England.
(44) (81) 947 27 77

Institut National de la Santé et de la Recherche Médicale
101 rue de Tolbiac, 75654 Paris Cedex 13, France.
(33) (1) 44 23 60 00
ISBN 2 85 598 485 8

ISSN 0768-3154

© 1992 Colloques INSERM/John Libbey Eurotext Ltd,
All rights reserved
Unauthorized publication contravenes applicable laws

Préface

Comme tous les chercheurs s'intéressant à l'hypertension, au début des années 60, alors que je préparais une thèse sous la direction du Professeur Cier, j'ai été enthousiasmé par les travaux des Professeurs Okamoto, Aoki et Yamori au Japon et de Sir Horace Smirk en Nouvelle-Zélande. A cette époque, nous pensions impossible de pouvoir utiliser un jour les modèles d'hypertension génétique qu'ils développaient, c'est pourquoi les Docteurs Jeanne Dupont et Madeleine Vincent avec les Professeurs Alain Froment et Hugues Milon ont débuté la sélection du modèle lyonnais.

Grâce à ce modèle et grâce à leurs efforts, nous avons eu le privilège d'accueillir en 1991 le 7e symposium sur l'hypertension génétique à Lyon, après des centres de recherche renommés tels que Kyoto, Heidelberg et Iowa City.

Depuis le premier symposium (Kyoto 1971) un effort fantastique de recherche a été consacré aux mécanismes de l'hypertension génétique en utilisant les différents modèles disponibles et, principalement, les SHR d'origine japonaise. A l'évidence, cet effort a permis une amélioration considérable de nos connaissances sur les fonctions rénale et cardiaque, sur les mécanismes nerveux, endocriniens, paracrines et autocrines de régulation de la fonction des cellules contractiles... Malgré ces efforts, force est de reconnaître que la physiopathologie de l'hypertension reste très largement obscure, et nous mettons les plus grands espoirs dans les données qu'apporteront les expériences de génétique moléculaire. Toutefois, il semble maintenant parfaitement clair que la signification des résultats de biologie moléculaire doit être complétée par l'étude de systèmes plus intégrés et donc plus complexes. Ceci est valable pour tous les domaines de la science mais semble d'une importance toute particulière pour l'hypertension. En effet, il s'agit d'un symptôme qui touche une fonction soumise à de nombreux processus de régulation et dont les altérations relèvent d'un déterminisme polygénétique.

A cet égard, j'ai été spécialement heureux que les Professeurs Zech et Fontaine, précédent et actuel Président de l'Université Claude Bernard, aient présenté un diplôme de Docteur Honoris Causa aux

Professeurs F.M. Abboud et Y. Yamori qui, tous les deux, ont donné un remarquable exemple des liens étroits qui peuvent et doivent exister entre la biologie la plus fondamentale, l'expérimentation animale et la recherche clinique.

Nous avons été très sensibles à la confiance des Professeurs K. Okamoto et Y. Yamori qui ont suggéré que ce 7e symposium se tienne à Lyon et qui nous ont aidé dans son organisation. Malheureusement, notre joie a été tempérée par la tristesse ressentie lors du décès de notre ami et éminent collègue, le Professeur M.J. Brody, qui a organisé le 6e symposium à Iowa City. Nous espérons que sa veuve, Natalie, voudra bien accepter ces comptes rendus comme l'hommage de notre communauté scientifique à la mémoire de l'un de ses plus prestigieux et brillants représentants.

Rien n'eut été possible sans l'aide amicale des membres du Comité local d'Organisation. Ils ont eu pour moi des propriétés anxiolytiques remarquables, et j'aimerais adresser mes remerciements les plus chaleureux à M. Vincent, C. Barrès, D. Benzoni, C. Cerutti, G. Cuisinaud, C. Gharib, C. Julien et N. Rolland. Comme eux tous, je me suis senti profondément honoré lorsque le Professeur J.F. Cier, Doyen Honoraire des Facultés de Médecine et de Pharmacie, qui nous a initié à la recherche dans le domaine de l'hypertension a accepté d'être le Président Honoraire du symposium.

Je voudrais aussi remercier le bureau des Colloques de l'INSERM, dirigé par Madame Coadou, de même que Madame Krief, des éditions John Libbey Eurotext pour leur aide précieuse. Pour finir, il est clair que ce 7e symposium n'a pu se tenir que grâce aux dons généreux de nombreuses firmes pharmaceutiques françaises et étrangères. Je tiens à souligner que, dans cette circonstance comme dans beaucoup d'autres, leur soutien désintéressé montre la très profonde implication de cette industrie dans la recherche la plus fondamentale.

De même que lors des précédents symposiums et sûrement moins que lors de ceux qui le suivront, cette 7e réunion a permis de réunir les données les plus récentes obtenues à travers le monde par les chercheurs qui, grâce à des modèles animaux, se consacrent à l'étude des maladies cardiovasculaires génétiquement déterminées. Je souhaite que les résultats de leur recherche qui constituent le présent ouvrage puissent être utiles à notre communauté scientifique et contribuer à attirer de jeunes et talentueux chercheurs à un thème de recherche qui me semble à la fois très intéressant sur le plan intellectuel et potentiellement fort utile pour l'humanité.

Jean Sassard
Professeur de Physiologie
Faculté de Pharmacie de Lyon

Remerciements

- Laboratoires Servier
- Laboratoires Bristol-Myers Squibb, ICI-Pharma, Ipsen, Merck Sharp and Dohme-Chibret, Sandoz, Searle
- Institut Scientifique Roussel, Laboratoires Bayer, Boehringer-Ingelheim, Ciba-Geigy, Marion-Merrell Dow, Sanofi, Specia, UPSA, Société Lyonnaise de Banque
- Laboratoires Fournier, Parke Davis, Roche, Sterling-Winthrop

Avec l'aide généreuse des institutions suivantes : Conseil Général du Rhône, Institut National de la Santé et de la Recherche Médicale, Ecole Normale Supérieure de Lyon.

Comités

Comité international

Président d'Honneur : K. Okamoto (Japon)

Secrétaire général : Y. Yamori (Japon)

Membres d'Honneur : F.M. Bumpus (E.U.), A.E. Doyle (Australie), B. Folkow (Suède), F.O. Simpson (Nouvelle-Zélande), S. Spector (E.U.), H. Ueda (Japon), S. Undenfriend (E.U.).

Membres : D. Ben Ishay (Israël), G. Bianchi (Italie), M.J. Brody† (E.U.), E.D. Frohlich (E.U.), D. Ganten (Allemagne), M. Hallbäck (Suède), P. Hamet (Canada), S. Harrap (Australie), W. de Jong (France), E.M. Krieger (Brésil), W. Lovenberg (E.U.), Y. Masuyama (Japon), A. Millar (Nouvelle-Zélande), M. Mulvany (Danemark), T. Omae (Japon), Y.V. Postnov (Russie), J. Rapp (E.U.), M.P. Sambhi (E.U.), J. Sassard (France), D.F. Su (Chine populaire), H. Thurston (R.U.).

Conseils scientifiques

J. Atkinson (France), H. Brunner (Suisse), F. Bühler (Suisse), J. Chalmers (Australie), P. Corvol (France), G.F. DiBona (E.U.), J.L. Elghozi (France), A. Gairard (France), J.F. Giudicelli (France), J.L. Imbs (France), J. Ménard (France), P. Meyer (France), J.B. Michel (France), A. Mimran (France), J.L. Montastruc (France), P.F. Plouin (France), M. Safar (France), N. Samani (R.U.), J.C. Stoclet (France), T. Unger (Allemagne), M. Vallotton (Suisse), B. Waeber (Suisse).

Contents
Sommaire

V Préface
VII Remerciements
    Comités

ENDOTHELIAL FACTORS
FACTEURS ENDOTHÉLIAUX

3 **D.C. Junquéro, T. Scott-Burden, V.B. Schini, P.M. Vanhoutte**
The production of nitric oxide evoked by interleukin-1β in cultured aortic smooth muscle cells from spontaneously hypertensive rats is greater than that from normotensive rats

7 **B. Bucher, D. Paya, S. Ouedraogo, J.C. Stoclet**
Role of the L-arginine-NO-cyclic GMP pathway in the control of vascular tone

11 **L. El Fertak, B.I. Lévy, C. Pieddeloup, F. Barouki, M.E. Safar**
Role of endothelium in the mechanical response of the carotid arterial wall to calcium blockade in SHR and WKY rat

15 **K. Ikeda, Y. Nara, Y. Kobayashi, K. Hattori, Y. Yamori**
Age-related blood pressure lowering effect of dietary L-arginine in stroke-prone spontaneously hypertensive rats (SHRSP)

19 **I.N. Voynikova, T.I. Voynikov, Y. Yamanishi, N.A. Nicolov, A. Suzuki**
Vascular responses to some relaxants and cyclic nucleotide levels in SHRSP, with special reference to aging

23 **Y. Yamori, K. Ikeda, S. Mizushima, Y. Nara, M. Tagami**
Induction of malignant hypertension in stroke-prone spontaneously hypertensive rats (SHRSP)-treated with nitroarginine, an inhibitor of endothelium-derived relaxing factor (EDRF)

27   Z.Q. Zhang, C. Barrès, C. Julien
Nitric oxide synthesis and the control of blood pressure in sympathectomized rats

31   M.C. Mourlon-Le Grand, J. Benessiano, B.I. Lévy
Local hyperproduction of cGMP in carotid arteries from SHR is endothelium-dependent

35   H. Takahashi, S. Fukumitu, M. Nishimura, T. Nakanishi, T. Hasegawa, M. Yoshimura
Measurement of urinary excretions of nitrite and nitrate, and effects of inhibition of nitric oxide production on hemodynamics in SHR

39   F. Pourageaud, J.L. Freslon
Endothelium function in resistance and coronary arteries of spontaneously hypertensive compared to WKY rats: effects of nitro-L-arginine

43   H. Takeshita, M. Nishikibe, M. Yano, F. Ikemoto
Coronary vascular response to endothelin-1 in spontaneously hypertensive rats in relation to hypertension development

47   S. Sunano, K. Kaneko, K. Shimamura
Endothelium-dependent and -independent tension oscillation in aortae from SHRSP and WKY

51   Y. Kobayashi, K. Ikeda, K. Shinozuka, Y. Nara, Y. Yamori, K. Hattori
Endothelium-dependent and -independent vasodilations of stroke-prone spontaneously hypertensive rats with stroke

55   K. Yin, Z. Chu L.J. Beilin
Surprising changes in vascular reactivity *in vitro* in pregnant rats

NEURAL MECHANISMS
MÉCANISMES NERVEUX

61   H. Ohta, S.J. Lewis, W.T. Talman
Comparison of cardiovascular responses to stimulation of carotid sinus and aortic depressor nerves in rats

65   F. Ida, E.D. Moreira, V.L.L. Oliveira, E.M. Krieger
The magnitude of rapid resetting of the baroreceptors is attenuated in spontaneously hypertensive rats

69   N. Minami, G.A. Head
Effect of perindopril on the cardiac baroreflex in conscious spontaneously hypertensive (SHR) and stroke prone hypertensive rats (SHRSP)

73 A.U. Ferrari, A. Daffonchio, C. Franzelli
Interplay of sympathetic and parasympathetic mechanisms in the control of blood pressure variability in conscious, spontaneously-behaving SHR and WKY rats

77 W.C. Huang, P.S. Hsieh, J.S. Jin
Chronic hyperinsulinemia induces hypertension in rats

81 J. Bachmann, E. Ottens, W. Zidek
Cross circulation in spontaneously hypertensive rats. Evidence of a circulating hypertensive factor and effects of antihypertensive treatment

85 P.H.A. Eerdmans, H.A.J. Struyker-Boudier, J.G.R. De Mey
Effect of nerve stimulation on isolated mesenteric and intra-renal resistance arteries, SHR versus WKY

89 T. Ueyama, T. Hano, M. Hamada, I. Nishio, Y. Masuyama
Reduction of inhibitory effect of adrenergic transmission by nerve growth factor in the mesenteric vasculatures of spontaneously hypertensive rats

93 E. Thorin, C. Capdeville-Atkinson, J. Atkinson
Chronic treatment with captopril plus hydrochlorothiazide attenuates vascular noradrenergic transmission in the adult SHR

97 J.O. Habeck, J.M. Pequignot, M. Vincent, J. Sassard
The carotid and aortic bodies in the Lyon hypertensive rats

101 D.F. Su, X.B. Kong, Y. Cheng, L. Chen
Arterial baroreflex-blood pressure control in conscious hypertensive rats

105 A.U. Ferrari, A. Daffonchio, C. Franzelli, G. Mancia
Impairment of parasympathetic control of the heart in SHR is not due to reduced cardiac parasympathetic responsiveness

109 C.C. Lee, H. Ohta, W.T. Talman
Endothelin-1 microinjected into nucleus tractus solitarii of rat blocks arterial baroreflexes

113 M. van den Buuse, S. Itoh
Central injection of endothelin-1 augments baroreflex sensitivity in spontaneously hypertensive rats

117 D.R. Fior, D.T.O. Martins, C.J. Lindsey
Central kinin receptors in the spontaneously hypertensive rat and the pressor response to bradykinin

121 D.T.O. Martins, D.R. Fior, C.J. Lindsey
Increased sensitivity to the central pressor effect of bradykinin in hypertensive rats

125 M. van den Buuse, S. Sarhan, N. Seiler
A role of central GABA in the development of hypertension in the spontaneously hypertensive rat?

129 M. van den Buuse
Differential changes in central dopaminergic activity in the spontaneously hypertensive rat

133 D.T.W.M. van den Berg, E.R. De Kloet, B.J.A. Janssen
Central steroid receptor function in spontaneously hypertensive rats: effects of gluco- and mineralocorticoids

137 J. Shah, B.S. Jandhyala
Evaluation of the functional significance of Na^+-pump activity in the central nervous system of spontaneously hypertensive rats

141 W.C. Huang, J.S. Jin, C.Y. Chen, P.S. Hsieh
Exaggerated renal response to central angiotensin III in spontaneously hypertensive rats

145 S. Buisson, M. van den Buuse
The effect of MDL 73,005EF and putative $5-HT_{1A}$ receptor antagonists on the cardiovascular response to 8-OH-DPAT in conscious spontaneously hypertensive rats

149 D.F. Su, Y. Cheng, X.B. Kong, J. Yang
Effects of ketanserin on blood pressure, blood pressure variability and arterial baroreflex-blood pressure control in SHR

153 M. Heimburger, N. Pages, C. El Rawadi, M. Davy, C. Bohuon, Y. Cohen
Effect of ketanserin on catecholamines and NPY in peripheral tissues of normotensive (WKY) and spontaneously hypertensive rats (SHR)

157 F. Sannajust, M. Dubar, B. Jarrott
New evidence on the role of the spinal cord in the antihypertensive action of rilmenidine in conscious, unrestrained, spontaneously hypertensive rats

161 M.A. Mc Auley, I.M. Macrae, J.L. Reid
The involvement of cAMP in the central hemodynamic actions of neuropeptide-Y (NPY) and rilmenidine in the SHR

165 M. Abe, H. Yoshimoto, S. Matsuyama
Effect of bunazosin hydrochloride on blood pressure and retinal circulation in spontaneously hypertensive rat (SHR-SR)

169 **H. Ogawa, T. Tanaka, S. Sasagawa, S. Akai, T. Akai, M. Takahashi, M. Yamaguchi**
Enhanced emotional responses with aging in stroke-prone spontaneously hypertensive rats (SHRSP)

173 **H. Kawamura, M. Maki, K. Komatsu, K. Hara, K. Suzuki, S. Ito, W. Usui, T. Yasugi, M. Hatano**
Exaggerated renal vascular responses to different stresses in spontaneously hypertensive rats

177 **H.G. Spanos, R. Di Nicolantonio, S.L. Skinner**
Role of renin in the cardiovascular response to acute stress in conscious Sprague Dawley and spontaneously hypertensive rats

181 **J. Blanc, M.L. Grichois, M. Vincent, J. Sassard, J.L. Elghozi**
Spectral analysis of short-term oscillations in blood pressure and heart rate in hypertensive rats of the Lyon strain

185 **A. Daffonchio, C. Franzelli, M. DiRienzo, P. Castiglioni, A.J. Ramirez, G. Mancia, A.U. Ferrari**
Effects of sympathectomy on overall blood pressure variability and its spectral components in unanesthetized unrestrained rats

189 **M. Ducher, C. Cerutti, M.P. Gustin, C.Z. Paultre**
A new method to assess statistical dependence: application to the relationships between systolic blood pressure and heart rate

GROWTH FACTORS
FACTEURS DE CROISSANCE

195 **A.V. Chobanian** (invited lecture / *conférence plénière*)
Effects of hypertension on cellular growth of arterial tissue
Effets de l'hypertension sur la croissance cellulaire du tissu artériel

207 **J. Plouët, H. Moukadiri, L. Gouzi, B. Malavaud, M.M. Ruchoux**
Vasculotropin/VEGF hypersecretion by vascular smooth muscle cells from spontaneously hypertensive rats: a paracrine loop?

211 **A.W.A. Hahn, S. Regenass, T.J. Resink, F. Ferracin, F.R. Bühler**
Differential autocrine responses of SHR- and WKY-VSMC to stimulation with vasoactive peptides

215 **M.P. Sambhi, N. Swaminathan, H. Wang, H.M. Rong**
Upregulation of adrenal, renal and vascular growth factors in salt fed hypertensive Dahl rats

219 M. Hamada, E.L. Harris, J.A. Millar, F.O. Simpson, I. Nishio, Y. Masuyama
Flowcytometric analysis of cell cycle of cultured vascular smooth muscle cells from SHR and New Zealand GH rat

223 P. Guicheney, K. Soussan, R. Rota, E. Dausse
Dissociation of hypertension and genetically enhanced cell growth in skin fibroblasts of F2 hybrid SHR/WKY rats

227 N. Fukuda, J. Tremblay, P. Hamet
Participation of proteolysis and transforming growth factor $\beta 1$ activation in growth of cultured vascular smooth muscle cells from spontaneously hypertensive rats

HEART AND VESSELS
CŒUR ET VAISSEAUX

233 H.Y. Qiu, B. Valtier, H.A.J. Struyker-Boudier, B.I. Lévy
Mechanical and contractile properties of *in situ* isolated mesenteric artery in normotensive (WKY) and spontaneously hypertensive rats (SHR)

237 P.I. Korner, A. Bobik, C. Oddie, P. Friberg
Sympatho-adrenal system and development of cardiac and vascular amplifier properties in SHR

241 R. Tabei, M. Kondo, T. Miyazaki, T. Fujiwara, M. Terada, Y. Watanabe
Sympathetic hyperinnervation of the coronary artery in the stroke-prone spontaneously hypertensive rat

245 R.J. Summers, S. Fujimoto, H. Pak, D. Soukseun, P. Molenaar
Autoradiographic localization and quantitation of cardiac β-adrenoceptor subtypes in SHR

249 H. Nishimura, M. Ueyama, T. Oka, J. Kubota, H. Hanada, M. Suwa, K. Kawamura
Echocardiographic evaluation of left ventricular function and left ventricular hypertrophy in SHR

253 V. Mooser, A. Katopothis, S.B. Harrap, C.I. Johnston
Inhibition of cardiac ACE does not reduce left ventricular mass in salt-loaded spontaneously hypertensive rats

257 H. Ito, M. Torii, T. Suzuki
Myocardial vulnerability in cardiac hypertrophy : comparison of hypertensive and normotensive rat drug-induced myocardial changes

261 F. Boucher, S. Pucheu, C. Schatz, D. Guez, J. de Leiris
Cardioprotective effect of indapamide on experimental ischemia and reperfusion in rats

265 I. Drubaix, I. Berrebi-Bertrand, N. Kassis, Y. Leclercq, L.G. Lelièvre
Cardiac and aortic sarcolemmal Na^+/Ca^{2+} exchange and Ca^{2+}-ATPase activities in SHR and WKY

269 K. Kisters, E.R. Krefting, C. Spieker, U. Scholz, M. Tepel, K.H. Rahn, W. Zidek
Intracellular sodium ion content in vascular smooth muscle cells from normotensive and spontaneously hypertensive rats

273 H. Bouaziz, A. Benetos, B.I. Lévy, M. Safar
Arterial mechanical properties in Dahl sensitive rats

277 M.J. Black, J.F. Bertram, J.H. Campbell
Effect of angiotensin II on the number of smooth muscle cells in the SHR aorta

281 D. Hayoz, M. Niederberger, B. Rutschmann, H.R. Brunner, B. Waeber
Arterial wall distensibility in hypertensive rats

285 H.Y. Qiu, B. Valtier, C. Schatz, D. Guez, B.I. Lévy
Effects of indapamide on the mechanical properties of the mesenteric artery in spontaneously hypertensive rats (SHR)

289 N. Hirawa, S. Umemura, Y. Tokita, Y. Toya, K. Sugimoto, N. Takagi, Y. Kato, T. Ikeda, M. Ishii
The effects of a K^+ channel opener, BRL 38227, on blood pressure and vascular thromboxane A_2 generation in Dahl salt-sensitive rats

GENETICS
GÉNÉTIQUE

295 R. Di Nicolantonio, T. Imai, K. Ikeda, Y. Nara, A. Fukamizu, Y. Yamori, E. Soeda, K. Murakami
Polymerase chain reaction-based DNA fingerprinting in the spontaneously hypertensive rat : a new method of genetic analysis

297 T. Nabika, Y. Nara, K. Ikeda, M. Sawamura, J. Endo, Y. Yamori
Genetic analysis of the spontaneously hypertensive rat (SHR), Wistar-Kyoto rat (WKY) and their F2 generation using 26 human variable number of tandem repeats (VNTR) markers

301 N. Iwai, S. Chaki, T. Inagami
Identification of a hypertensinogenic gene in spontaneously hypertensive rats

305 P. Hamet, D. Kong, T. Hashimoto, Y.L. Sun, G. Corbeil, M. Pravenec, J. Kunes, P. Klir, V. Kren, J. Tremblay
Abnormal structure and expression of *hsp70* genes in hypertension

309 B. Bunnemann, S. Kimura, J.J. Mullins, F. Zimmermann, D. Ganten, M. Kaling
Correct expression of the transgene in the brain of hypertensive transgenic mice carrying the rat angiotensinogen gene

313 K. Lindpaintner, P. Hilbert, D. Ganten, M. Georges, M. Lathrop
Chromosomal mapping of genetic loci associated with hereditary hypertension in the rat

317 H.K. Bin Talib, V. Křen, J. Kuneš, M. Pravenec, J. Zicha
Red cell ion transport in genetic hypertension : recombinant inbred strain study

321 M.P. Printz, R. Casto, M.A. Spence, R. Cantor
Pattern of inheritance of the startle-induced heart rate response in the spontaneously hypertensive rat

325 Y. Nara, T. Nabika, K. Ikeda, M. Sawamura, Y. Yamori
Characterization of WKY, SHR and SHRSP substrains with fingerprint patterns

329 K. Matsumoto, T. Sakai, T. Yamada, T. Agui, Y. Nara, Y. Yamori, T. Natori
Genetic analysis for major histocompatibility complex in spontaneously hypertensive rat and its control strain

333 J. Kunes, M. Pravenec, V. Kren, P. Klir, D. Ganten, J.J. Mullins, J. Tremblay, P. Hamet
Search for genetic determinants of environmental susceptibility in hypertension : effect of heat, immobilization stress and endotoxin

337 R. Rota, C. Nazaret, M. Santarromana, J.G. Henrotte, R. Garay, P. Guicheney
Dissociation of hypertension and abnormal activation of [K^+,Cl^-] cotransport in SHR erythrocytes

341 S.B. Harrap, G.A. Mitchell, T.L. Norman
Is cardiovascular hypertrophy in young SHR the result of a recessive gene?

345 J. Peters, M. Sander, K. Münter, M.A. Lee, B. Djavidani, M. Bader, C. Maser-Gluth, P. Vescei, D. Ganten, J.J. Mullins
The role of adrenal renin in steroid metabolism and development of hypertension in transgenic rats TGR(mREN2)

349 E. Hackenthal, K. Münter, S. Fritsch
Kidney function and renin processing in transgenic rats (TGR mRen2-27)

353 J. Bachmann, U. Ganten, F. Zimmermann, J.J. Mullins, G. Stock, D. Ganten
Sexual dimorphism of blood pressure in transgenic rats TGR(mREN2)27 harboring the murine *Ren-2* gene

ANIMAL MODELS
MODÈLES ANIMAUX

359 M. Bader, R. Kreutz, J. Wagner, K. Zeh, M. Böhm, M. Paul, D. Ganten (invited lecture / *conférence plénière*)
Primary hypertension and the renin angiotensin system : from the laboratory experiment to clinical relevance
Hypertension essentielle et système rénine angiotensine : de l'expérience de laboratoire à la signification clinique

373 R.J. Koletsky, P. Ernsberger
Obese SHR (Koletsky rat) : a model for the interactions between hypertension and obesity

377 H. Ito, T. Suzuki, K. Okamoto
Pathophysiological characteristics of spontaneously hypertensive and hypercholesterolemic rats (hyper T-C rats)

381 M.E. Cooper, J.R. Rumble, R.C. O'Brien, T.J. Allen, G. Jerums, A.E. Doyle
Nephropathy in the diabetic SHR : the effects of perindopril and triple therapy

385 M. Bursztyn, D. Ben-Ishay, A. Gutman
Hyperinsulinemia and decreased muscle deoxyglucose uptake in SHR but not in secondary hypertension

389 G.F. DiBona, S.Y. Jones
Effect of acute NaCl depletion on NaCl sensitive hypertension in borderline hypertensive rats

393 Y. Ohta, T.A. Chikugo, K. Okamoto
The effect of certain antihypertensive drugs at several dose levels on hypertensive vascular lesions in M-SHRSP and SHRSP

- 397 S. Murakami, M. Yamashita, Y. Nara, Y. Yamori
  Taurine improves cholesterol metabolism in stroke-prone spontaneously hypertensive rats (SHRSP) fed on hypercholesterolemic (HC) diets

- 401 L. Carrier, K.R. Boheler, C. Wisnewsky, K. Schwartz
  Independent expressions of the sarcomeric α-actins in human and rat ventricles with development and aging : evidence of species dependent expressions

- 405 A.L. Markel
  Development of a new strain of rats with inherited stress-induced arterial hypertension

- 409 S. Kimura, H. Yoshimoto, S. Matsuyama
  Intraretinal newly formed vessel in experimental hypertensive rat

- 413 N. Saito, K. Noda, Y. Yamasaki, K. Matsubayashi, T. Okada, S. Nishiyama
  Cataracta in hypertensive rats

- 417 S. Tsuchikura, S. Fukuda, H. Iida, K. Ikeda, Y. Nara, Y. Yamori
  Effects of antihypertensive agents on osteoporosis in SHRSP

- 421 S. Fukuda, S. Tsuchikura, H. Iida, K. Ikeda, Y. Nara, Y. Yamori
  Further study on osteoporosis in SHRSP : quantitative analyses by bone histomorphometry and serum biochemical constituents related to bone

- 425 T. Sato, Y. Nara, Y. Kato, Y. Yamori
  Beneficial effect of alacepril on glucose metabolism in both non-diabetic and diabetic spontaneously hypertensive rats

- 429 E. Millanvoye-Van Brussel, J. Simon, M.A. Devynck, M. Freyss-Béguin
  Impairment of lipid metabolism in heart cell cultures from newborn spontaneously hypertensive rat

- 433 H. Ogawa, T. Tanaka, S. Sasagawa
  Age-related changes in activities of rate-limiting enzymes in lipid metabolism of stroke-prone spontaneously hypertensive rats

- 437 S.H. Azar, H. Hensleigh
  Reproductive characteristics are modulated by genetic and oviductal uterine milieu after one-cell embryo transfer in spontaneously hypertensive and normotensive rats

441 S.D. Gray, R.C. Carlsen, R. Atherley
Effect of hydralazine on the decline in force and fatigue resistance in skeletal muscles from spontaneously hypertensive rats

KIDNEY FUNCTION AND RENAL FACTORS
FACTEURS RÉNAUX

447 G. Bianchi, P. Ferrari (invited lecture / *conférence plénière*)
Renal factors involved in the pathogenesis of genetic forms of hypertension
Facteurs rénaux impliqués dans la pathogénie des formes génétiques d'hypertension

459 S. Kim, M. Hosoi, T. Takada, K. Yamamoto
Adrenal renin, angiotensinogen and angiotensin in stroke-prone spontaneously hypertensive rats

463 C.J. Chen, S.J. Vyas, J. Eichberg, R.E. Beach, M.F. Lokhandwala
Abolished DA-1 receptor-mediated inhibition of renal tubular Na^+, K^+-ATPase in spontaneously hypertensive rats

467 D.J. Campbell, A.C. Lawrence, A. Towrie, A. Kladis, A.J. Valentijn
Effect of converting enzyme inhibitor, perindopril, on angiotensin peptides in plasma and kidney of the rat

471 J.R. Haywood, P. Guerra
Hemodynamic and fluid and electrolyte changes associated with the development of one-kidney, figure-8 renal wrap hypertension during constant sodium intake

475 B. Michel, M. Grima, C. Welsch, C. Coquard, M. Barthelmebs, J.L. Imbs
Plasma and tissue angiotensin converting enzyme variability in Wistar Kyoto and spontaneously hypertensive rats

479 G. Dagher, C. Sauterey
H-pump and Na-H exchange in isolated single proximal tubule and cortical collecting duct of spontaneously hypertensive rats

483 S.R. Thomas, G. Dagher
A modeling study of alterations in transport processes along rat proximal tubule in hypertension : implications in solute reabsorption

487 Y. Liu, S. Umemura, N. Hirawa, Y. Toya, M. Kihara, T. Iwamoto, S. Hayashi, K. Takeda, S. Young, M. Ishii
Biphasic effects of an adenosine analogue on the cyclic AMP formation in isolated rat glomeruli

491 J.P. Valentin, S.A. Mazbar, M.H. Humphreys
Impaired natriuretic response to intermittent bilateral carotid artery traction in spontaneously hypertensive rats

495 B. Michel, M. Grima, C. Welsch, C. Coquard, M. Barthelmebs, J.L. Imbs
Effects of one hour and one week ramipril treatment on plasma and renal brush border angiotensin converting enzyme in the rat

499 F. Suzuki, A. Takahashi, K. Murakami, Y. Nakamura
Rat prorenin is activable at acidic pH

503 M. Kohzuki, B.Z. Chen, V. Mooser, K. Jandeleit, C.I. Johnston
Angiotensin converting enzyme in the spontaneously hypertensive rat

507 S.B. Harrap, A.E. Doyle
Long-term blood pressure effects of angiotensin in SHR are developmental stage-specific

511 B. Jover, K. Wahba, A. Mimran
Adaptation to sodium restriction in enalapril-treated spontaneously hypertensive rats

515 A. Tavares, D. Bossolan, M.T. Zanella, A.B. Ribeiro, O. Kohlmann Jr.
Chronic dopaminergic system impairment induces hypertension and hyperaldosteronism in rats

519 M. Barthelmebs, M. Grima, D. Stephan, J.L. Imbs
Renal dopamine excretion and vasodilatation in spontaneously hypertensive rats (SHR)

523 J.M. Lange, B.P. Brockway, M.F. Sylvestri
SHRsp response to high salt diet

527 R. Behm, H. Dewitz, H. Mewes
Hyperoxia alters salt intake in spontaneously hypertensive rats (SHR) but not in normotensive Wistar-Kyoto rats (WKY)

531 H. Morita, T. Matsuda, T. Horiba, K. Miyake, H. Yamanouchi, H. Ohyama, M. Hagiike, H. Hosomi, K. Ikeda, Y. Nara, Y. Yamori
Suppressed hepatointestinal reflex in spontaneously hypertensive rats

535 J.P. Dausse, J.F. Cloix, W. Qing, D. Ben-Ishay
Sabra salt-sensitive (SBH) rats are deleted in one α_2-adrenoceptor subtype in renal cortex when compared with Sabra salt-resistant (SBN)

539 P. Li, S.B. Penner, D.D. Smyth
Decreased alpha$_2$-adrenoceptor function in spontaneously hypertensive (SH) rats is secondary to an attenuated renal action of vasopressin

543 S. Fragman, M. Harnik, E. Peleg, N. Zamir, T. Rosenthal
The hypertensinogenic activity of 18,21-anhydroaldosterone in adrenalectomized rats

547 O. Chung, P. Rohmeiss, T. Schips, S. Rohmeiss, T. Unger
The acute antihypertensive action of cicletanine is mediated by muscarinic receptor stimulation

CALCIUM
CALCIUM

553 M.B. Anand-Srivastava, C. Thibault
Decreased expression of inhibitory guanine nucleotide regulatory proteins and adenylate cyclase activity in rat platelets in spontaneously hypertensive rats

557 S. Sunano, K. Moriyama, K. Shimamura
Ca-induced and IP3-induced Ca-release in vascular smooth muscle of SHRSP and WKY observed by Ca-indicator Fura 2

561 H. Ebata, Y. Houjoh, U. Ikeda, Y. Tsuruya, T. Natsume, K. Shimada
Altered calcium-dependent calcium release from intracellular sites of perfused heart in spontaneously hypertensive rats

565 B. Schüssler, W. Völker, K.H. Rahn, W. Zidek
Cytoplasmic free calcium concentration in isolated vascular smooth muscle cells from spontaneously hypertensive rats

569 M. David-Dufilho, E. Millanvoye-Van Brussel, M. Freyss-Béguin, C. Astarie, M.A. Devynck
Cytosolic Ca^{2+} and pH in cultured cardiac myocytes and fibroblasts from newborn hypertensive rats of the Okamoto strain

573 N. Thorin-Trescases, L. Oster, J. Atkinson, C. Capdeville-Atkinson
Chronic treatment with captopril plus hydrochlorothiazide and intracellular free calcium in the tail artery of the adult SHR

577 C. Burkard, M. Vincent, P. Ferrari, J. Sassard, A. Gairard
Parathyroid transplantation in Lyon and Milan rat strains : preliminary results on blood pressure

581 F. Pernot, M. Vincent, J. Sassard, A. Gairard
Differing blood pressure responses to dietary calcium between male and female LH, LN and LL rats

585 S. Chabanis, P. Duchambon, H. Banide, D. Auchère, A. Jardel, B. Lacour, T. Drüeke
Acute effect of Ca deprivation on duodenal CaBP, CaBP mRNA, Ca transport and plasma calcitriol levels in spontaneously hypertensive (SHR) and WKY control rats

589 L.M. Vianna, A.C.M. Paiva, T.B. Paiva
Treatment with vitamin D_3 reduces blood pressure of spontaneously hypertensive rats

CEREBRAL CIRCULATION
CIRCULATION CÉRÉBRALE

595 A. Nagaoka, T. Imamoto, M. Sekiguchi, K. Hirai, Y. Nagai, A. Shino
Manidipine, a new calcium antagonist, prevents the development and progression of cerebrovascular lesions in stroke-prone spontaneously hypertensive rats

599 K. Okamoto, Y. Ohta, T. Chikugo
The therapeutic effects of SQ 29,852 and manidipine on M-SHRSP and SHRSP with vascular lesions of brains and kidneys and other organs

603 M. Tagami, K. Yamagata, Y. Nara, Y. Yamori
Examination of astrocytic functions in stroke-prone SHR applying co-culture techniques

607 L. Bray-des Boscs, I. Lartaud, J. Atkinson, C. Capdeville-Atkinson
Acute administration of antihypertensive drugs produces different effects on cerebral blood flow in awake spontaneously hypertensive rats

611 Author index
Index des auteurs

Endothelial factors

Facteurs endothéliaux

The production of nitric oxide evoked by interleukin-1β in cultured aortic smooth muscle cells from spontaneously hypertensive rats is greater than that from normotensive rats

Didier C. Junquéro, Timothy Scott-Burden, Valérie B. Schini and Paul M. Vanhoutte

Center for Experimental Therapeutics, Baylor College of Medicine, Houston, Texas 77030, USA

Nitric oxide (NO), produced by the conversion of L-arginine into L-citrulline by the NO synthases, relaxes vascular smooth muscle by activating cytosolic guanylate cyclase (Moncada *et al.*, 1991). Vascular endothelial cells (Palmer *et al.*, 1987), brain cells (Bredt *et al.*, 1991) possess the constitutive type of NO synthase, whereas the subtype of enzyme present in vascular smooth muscle (Busse & Mülsch, 1990; Schini *et al.*, 1991) must be induced by cytokines. Impaired endothelium-dependent relaxations (Vanhoutte & Lüscher, 1990) and increased sensitivity of aortic smooth muscle cells to mitogens (Scott-Burden *et al.*, 1989) characterize the vascular wall of hypertensive (SHR) compared to normotensive rats (WKY). The purpose of this study was to determine whether interleukin-1ß (IL-1ß) stimulates the production of NO in SHR and WKY rats to the same extent.

METHODS

This study was performed with three isolates of cultured aortic smooth muscle cells from age-matched (20 weeks old) SHR and WKY male rats (Scott-Burden *et al.*, 1989). After phenotypic characterization (first subculture), cells were used for experimentations between the 6th and 15th passage. They were seeded either onto Cytodex 3 microcarrier beads or in 12 well multiwell plates. Once confluent, the monolayers were incubated in serum-free medium for 24 to 72 hours with IL-1ß (0.1-100 U/ml) or its vehicle (phosphate buffered saline). Aortic rings without endothelium from Wistar rats were used as bioassay tissues, and superfused with the perfusate from columns containing microcarrier beads covered with confluent cells (Schini *et al.*, 1991). The biological activity of the perfusates was assessed once donor and detector tissues had been equilibrated [in the presence of indomethacin (10^{-5}M)] for at least 45 minutes. The production of nitrite was estimated by colorimetry [Green *et al.*, 1982]. Concentrations were determined relative to a standard curve of sodium nitrite. The total number of cells present in each experiment was determined at the end by enzymatic dispersion.

Results are expressed as means ± standard error of the mean (SEM) and n represents the number of experiments. Statistical analysis was performed by using Student's paired t test (two-tailed). P values less than 0.05 were considered statistically significant.

RESULTS AND DISCUSSION

The perfusate from columns of microcarrier beads covered with cultured smooth muscle cells (SHR) treated with IL-1ß elicited relaxations of the contracted bioassay rings. Treatment of the cells with nitro-L-arginine (10^{-4}M), or treatment of the superfused bioassay tissues with methylene blue (10^{-5}M) inhibited the relaxation. The subsequent addition of L-arginine but not D-arginine ($10^{-4}-10^{-3}$M) restored the blockade evoked by nitro-L-arginine (Fig. 1). Perfusates from vehicle-treated cells, methylene blue and arginine analogs did not affect the tension of the bioassay tissues (data not shown).

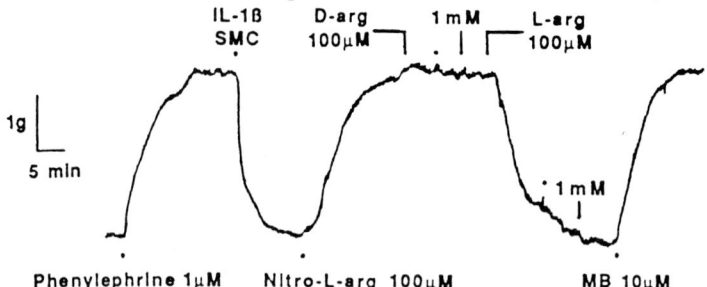

Figure 1 : Representative trace of experiments (n=3) showing the effects on nitro-L-arginine, D-arginine (D-arg), L-arginine (L-arg), methylene blue (MB) on the vasoactive properties of the perfusate from SHR smooth muscle cells (SMC) treated with IL-1ß (10 U/ml, 24 hours).

IL-1ß (0.1-100 U/ml) evoked a time- and concentration-dependent accumulation of nitrite in the culture media which was greater in smooth muscle cells from SHR rats (Fig.2).

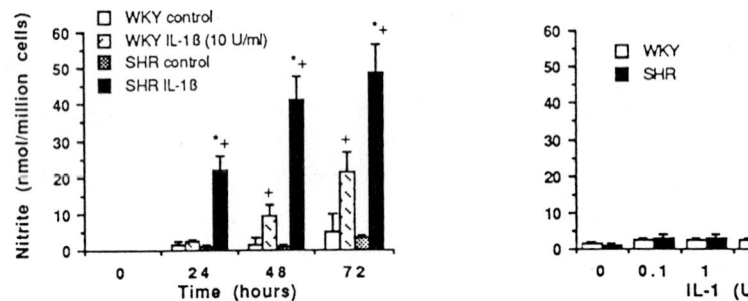

Figure 2 : Production of nitrite by cultured aortic smooth muscle cells from SHR and WKY rats: time-course and concentration-response to IL-1ß. Concentration-response curves to IL-1ß were performed after incubations for 48 hours. Values are means ± SEM (n=3, each experiment in triplicate). The cross and the asterisk denote significant differences from control and WKY cells, respectively.

The simultaneous treatment of cells with IL-1ß and cycloheximide abolished the production of nitrite in both strains after a 48 hours treatment period (Table 1). Lowering the L-arginine concentration to 10^{-4}M (it reached millimolar concentration in serum-free culture medium) significantly attenuated the production of nitrite evoked by the cytokine, a level which was further decreased in both cell types after incubation with IL-1ß plus nitro-L-arginine (Table 1).

	WKY		SHR	
	control	cyclo	control	cyclo
control	1.07±0.18	1.01±0.28	1.88±0.60	1.63±0.38
IL-1ß	12.99±3.21	1.74±0.30*	32.34±5.44	2.61±0.29*
When L-arginine concentration in culture medium was 10^{-4} M :				
	control	NLA	control	NLA
control	1.09±0.22	0.73±0.2	1.99±0.63	1.08±0.40
IL-1ß	5.97±1.49	2.38±0.36*	17.30±6.90	4.03±1.01*

Table 1 : Effects of cycloheximide (cyclo, 5 µg/ml) and nitro-L-arginine (NLA, 3×10^{-4}M) on the production of nitrite evoked by IL-1ß (10 U/ml) after 48 hours of treatment. Values are means ± SEM (n=3, each experiment in triplicate) expressed in nmol/million cells. The asterisk denotes significant differences from control.

These data demonstrate that IL-1ß induces the production of a non-prostanoid substance(s) by cultured smooth muscle cells which relaxes vascular smooth muscle by activating soluble guanylate cyclase. This relaxing factor is related to the metabolism of L-arginine, is accumulated as nitrite in the incubation media, and thus resembles NO. The production of NO by smooth muscle cells requires the stimulation by the cytokine, a lag period and protein synthesis, suggesting that the inducible NO synthase is involved. The findings demonstrate that aortic smooth muscle cells from both normotensive (WKY) and hypertensive rats (SHR) express the L-arginine NO pathway, the cells from the SHR responding more (three-fold) to IL-1ß than those from WKY rats. These quantitative differences in NO production between both strains may reflect differences in the induction process by the cytokine, or differential modulation of the L-arginine NO pathway by growth factors.

REFERENCES

Bredt, S.D., Hwang, P.M., Glatt, C.E., Lowenstein, C., Reed, R.R. & Snyder, S.H.S. (1991): Cloned and expressed nitric oxide synthase structurally resembles cytochrome P-450 reductase. *Nature* 351, 714-718.

Busse, R. & Mülsch, A. (1990): Induction of nitric oxide synthase by cytokines in vascular smooth muscle cells. *FEBS Lett.* 275, 87-90.

Green, L.C., Wagner, D.A., Glogowski, J., Skipper, P.L., Wishnok, J.S. & Tannenbaum, S.R. (1982): Analysis of nitrate, nitrite, and [^{15}N] nitrate in biological fluids. *Anal. Biochem.* 126, 131-138.

Moncada, S., Palmer, R.M.J. & Higgs E.A. (1991): Nitric oxide: physiology, pathophysiology, and pharmacology. *Pharmacol. Rev.* 43, 109-142.

Palmer, R.M.J., Ferrige, A.G. & Moncada, S. (1987): Nitric oxide release accounts for the biological activity of endothelium-derived relaxing factor. *Nature* 333, 524-526.

Schini, V.B., Junquero, D.C., Scott-Burden, T. & Vanhoutte, P.M. (1991): Interleukin-1ß induces the production of an L-arginine-derived relaxing factor from cultured smooth muscle cells from rat aorta. *Biochem. Biophys. Res. Commun.* 176, 114-121.

Scott-Burden, T., Resink, T.J., Baur, U., Bürgin, M. & Bühler, F.R. (1989): Epidermal growth factor responsiveness in smooth muscle cells from hypertensive and normotensive rat. *Hypertension* 13, 295-304.

Vanhoutte, P.M. & Lüscher, T.F. (1990): Endothelium-dependent vasoconstriction. In *Endothelium-derived relaxing factors*, eds. G.M. Rubanyi & P.M. Vanhoutte, pp. 1-7. Basel: Karger.

Role of the L-arginine-NO-cyclic GMP pathway in the control of vascular tone

Bernard Bucher, Dominique Paya, Sylvin Ouedraogo and Jean-Claude Stoclet

Laboratoire de Pharmacologie Cellulaire et Moléculaire, URA CNRS 600, Université Louis Pasteur de Strasbourg, B.P. 24, 67400 Illkirch, France

Nitric oxide (NO) (Palmer et al., 1987; 1988) or a NO conjugated compound (Myers et al., 1990) produced from L-arginine in endothelial cells accounts for cyclic GMP accumulation and vascular smooth muscle cell relaxation elicited by the endothelium dependent relaxing factor discovered by Furchgott and Zawadzki (1980). Recently it has been suggested that NO may also play a role as an non-adrenergic non-cholinergic mediator (Toda et al., 1990; Tucker et al;, 1990), producing neurogenic vasodilatation in bovine mesenteric artery (Ahlner et al., 1991) and dog cerebral artery (Toda & Okamura, 1990). Furthermore, it has been reported that intraneuronal NO and cyclic GMP may also modulate noradrenaline release from sympathetic nerves in canine mesenteric and pulmonary arteries (Greenberg et al., 1991a,b). However, such a role of neuromediator or of modulator of noradrenaline release has not been found in some other tissues such as the mouse atria (Johnston et al., 1987).

In the current study, the possible role of the L-arginine-NO pathway and of cyclic GMP in regulating noradrenaline release and vasoconstriction produced by electrical field stimulation was investigated in the rat tail artery. The effects of an arginine analogue which inhibits NO production (N^G-nitro-L-arginine methyl ester, L-NAME), of L- and D-arginine and of the NO donor SIN-1 (Feelisch & Noack, 1987) were compared to those of 8-bromo-cyclic GMP and of drugs which inhibit either cyclic GMP breakdown (Zaprinast) or cyclic GMP production by guanylate cyclase (methylene blue).

Sympathetically innervated rat isolated tail artery was used (Bucher et al., 1988). The preparation was incubated in [^{3}H]noradrenaline in order to load the transmitter pools of perivascular nerve terminals with the labeled amine. Thereafter, electrical field stimulation (24 pulses at 0.4 Hz, 0.3 ms, 200 mA) led to [^{3}H]noradrenaline release and vasoconstriction. The presence of endothelium was assessed by scanning electron microscopy and its function was determined by the relaxing action of acetylcholine (1-10µM) in noradrenaline (0.3 µM) precontracted arteries.

L-NAME (30µM) did not modify noradrenaline release, but it increased vasoconstriction produced by field stimulation (Fig. 1) and by exogenous noradrenaline (1 mM) added to the bath. These effects of L-NAME were stereospecific since they were inhibited by L- but not D-arginine (1 mM). None of the other tested drugs (SIN-1, Zaprinast, methylene blue) significantly altered noradrenaline release, except 8-bromo-cyclic GMP which markedly increased [^{3}H]noradrenaline release concentration-dependently (3-300 µM). In spite of this effect, 8-bromo-cyclic GMP decreased field-induced vasoconstriction. Both Zaprinast (0.1-30 µM) and SIN-1 ((0.1-30 µM) induced concentration-dependent inhibition of field-stimulated vasoconstriction. The latter was inhibited by methylene blue (3 µM).

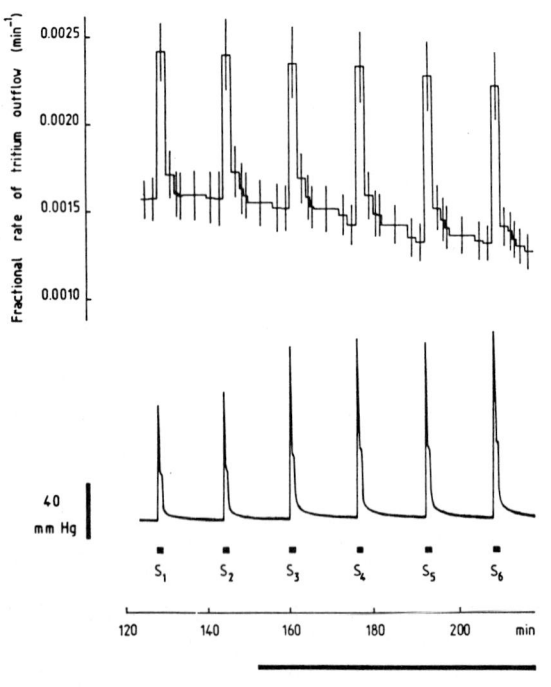

Fig.1. Effect of L-NAME 30 µM on stimulation-induced tritium outflow (upper panel) and vasoconstriction (lower panel) in the rat tail artery. Six periods of field stimulation (S_n : ■) were delivered at intervals of 16 min. L-NAME was infused for the period indicated by the horizontal line (from 8 min before S_3 until the end of the experiment). Means ± SEM from 6 arteries. The lower panel shows a representative tracing of the influence of L-NAME on vasoconstriction elicited by nerve stimulation.

The results confirm the observation that an NO-like substance derived from L-arginine inhibits vasoconstriction induced by neurally released as well as by exogenously applied noradrenaline in the rat tail artery (Vo et al., 1991). They further indicate that, in this vessel, the L-arginine-NO pathway acts through a postjunctional mechanism, since noradrenaline release was unaltered by drugs modifying either NO production (L-NAME, L-arginine, SIN-1) or cyclic GMP metabolism (Zaprinast, methylene blue). The discrepancy between these observations and the enhancing effect of 8-bromo-cyclic GMP could be caused either by a non specific action of the cyclic GMP analogue or by the absence of guanylate cyclase at the prejunctional level.

REFERENCES

Ahlner, J., Ljusegren, M.E., Grundström, N., and Axelsson, L. (1991): Role of nitric oxide and cyclic GMP as mediators of endothelium-independent neurogenic relaxation in bovine mesenteric artery. Circ. Res. 68: 756-762.

Bucher, B., Bettermann, R., Illes, P. (1988): Plasma concentration and vascular effect of β-endorphin in spontaneously hypertensive and Wistar-Kyoto rats. Naunyn Schmiedeberg's Arch. Pharmac. 335: 428-432.

Feelisch, M., and Noack, E. (1987): Correlation between nitric oxide formation during degradation of organic nitrates and activation of guanylate cyclase. Eur. J. Pharmacol. 139: 19-30.

Furchgott, R.F., and Zawadzki, J.V. (1980): The obligatory role of endothelial cells in the relaxation of arterial smooth muscle by acetylcholine. Nature 288: 373-376.

Greenberg, S.S., Cantor, E., Diecke, F.P.J., Peevy, K., and Tanaka, T.P. (1991a): Cyclic GMP modulates release of norepinephrine from adrenergic nerves innervating canine arteries. Am. J. Hypertens. 4: 173-176.

Greenberg, S.S., Peevy, K., and Tanaka, T.P. (1991b): Endothelium-derived and intraneuronal nitric oxide-dependent inhibition of norepinephrine efflux from sympathetic nerves by bradykinin. Am. J. Hypertens. 4: 464-467.

Johnston, H., Majewski H., and Musgrave, I.F. (1987): Involvement of cyclic nucleotides in prejunctional modulation of noradrenaline release in mouse atria. Br. J. Pharmacol. 91: 773-781.

Myers, P.R., Minor Jr, R.L., Guerra Jr, R., Bates, J.N., and Harsison, D.G. (1990): Vasorelaxant properties of the endothelium-derived relaxing factor more closely resemble S-nitrosocysteine than nitric oxide. Nature 345: 161-163.

Palmer, R.M.J., Ferrige, A.G., and Moncada, S. (1987): Nitric oxide release accounts for the biological activity of endothelium-derived relaxing factor. Nature 327: 524-526.

Palmer, R.M.J., Ashton, D.S., and Moncada, S. (1988): Vascular endothelial cells synthesize nitric oxide from L-arginine. Nature 333: 664-666.

Toda, N. and Okamura, T. (1990): Possible role of nitric oxide in transmitting information from vasodilator nerve to cerebroarterial muscle. Biochem. Biophys. Res. Commun. 170: 308-313.

Toda, N., Baba, H., and Okamura, T. (1990): Role of nitric oxide in non-adrenergic, non-cholinergic nerve-mediated relaxation in dog duodenal longitudinal strips. Japan. J. Pharmacol. 53: 281-284.

Tucker, J.F., Brave, S.R., Charalambous, L., Hobbs, A.J. and Gibson, A. (1990): L-N^G-nitro arginine inhibits non-adrenergic, non-cholinergic relaxations of guinea-pig isolated tracheal smooth muscle. Br. J. Pharmacol. 100: 663-664.

Role of endothelium in the mechanical response of the carotid arterial wall to calcium blockade in SHR and WKY rat

Lahcen El Fertak, Bernard I. Lévy, Christine Pieddeloup, Florence Barouki and Michel E. Safar

INSERM U.141, Hôpital Lariboisière, Paris, France

Summary

An experimental model allowing us to determine the volume-pressure relation of the "in situ" isolated carotid artery was used in spontaneously hypertensive (SHR, n=20) and normotensive control rats (WKY, n=20) before and after local incubation calcium-blockade by the diltiazem like substance TA-3090 (23µg/ml). The carotid compliance (CC, µl/mmHg . mm vessel) was calculated as the slope of the volume-pressure relationship at the operating arterial pressure.

With intact endothelium, calcium blockade induced in both strains a significant shift of the volume-pressure curve so that, at each given value of transmural pressure, volume was significantly higher after calcium blockade than under control conditions ($p<0.01$ in both WKY and SHR strains). In WKY rats, the static mechanical properties of the carotid wall (mean ±SD) were not significantly different after calcium blockade and after total abolition of the smooth muscle tone by potassium cyanide (KCN) poisoning (11.6±1.5 and 13.8±2.1 µl/mmHg . mm respectively). In contrast, in SHR, the carotid compliance measured after incubation with TA-3090 was significantly lower than that measured after KCN poisoning (8.1±1.1 vs 8.8±1.2 µl/mmHg . mm, $p<0.02$).

After removal of the endothelium, a significant shift of the volume-pressure curve toward the volume axis was observed in both strains. Consequently the carotid compliance was significantly increased by endothelium removal in WKY (from 8.5±2.5 to 10.5±1.6 µl/mmHg . mm , $p<0.01$) and SHR (from 6.9±1.6 to 7.8±0.3 µl/mmHg . mm, $p<0.001$). Local incubation with TA-3090 or KCN poisoning after endothelium removal did not induce further modifications of the volume-pressure relation neither in WKY nor in SHR.

Furthermore, in SHR and in WKY carotid arteries, the volume-pressure relation and the vessel compliance measured after incubation with TA-3090 were identical in the presence (11.6±1.5 and 8.1 ± 1.1 µl/mmHg . mm in WKY and SHR respectively) and without endothelium (11.9±1.8 and 8.0±0.7 µl/mmHg . mm in WKY and SHR respectively)

This study demonstrated that, in WKY and in SHR carotid arteries, acute calcium blockade with TA-3090 increases the compliance of the arterial wall independently of the endothelium integrity. Furthermore, our results suggest that part of the carotid compliance enhancement induced by calcium antagonist could be related to an antagonizing mechanism of the production of an endothelial constricting factor.

Introduction

In animal experiments, calcium has been shown to be important in endothelium-dependent relaxation of smooth muscle in several studies. It has been suggested that Ca^{++} plays a role in regulating either the production or release of endothelium derived relaxing factor (EDRF) (Peach et al. 1987, Singer et Peach 1982). Furthermore, smooth muscle response to Calcium channel antagonists could be a balance between their direct effects on smooth muscle and their contractile effects due to modulation of EDRF release (Williams et al. 1987).

In animal experiments, it has been shown that diltiazem significantly modified the arterial volume-pressure relation (Masafumi et al. 1989). In humans, Calcium-entry blockers are vasodilating drugs causing not only arteriolo-dilatation but also relaxation of large arteries (Brown 1985, Safar et al 1989). We have developed an experimental model allowing us to precisely measure the volume-pressure relation in the "in situ" localzed rat carotid artery (Levy et al. 1990) . The aim of this work was to test the direct effects of a Diltiazem derivative calcium-entry blocker on the compliance of the carotid artery in spontaneously hypertensive (SHR) and normotensive control Wistar Kyoto rats (WKY). These effects were assessed with intact endothelium and after endothelium removal of the studied carotid artery.

Methods :

These experiments were performed in 12-week-old SHR (n=20) and age-matched WKY rats (n=20) divided into three groups for each strain. The static mechanical properties of carotid arteries were studied in different conditions:

• Group 1 (10 WKY rats, 10 SHRs): under control conditions (E^+), after local incubation with Calcium entry blocker (E+TA3090; 0.023mg/ml), and then after total abolition of the smooth muscle tone (E+KCN; 1mg/ml).

• Group 2 (10 WKY rats, 10 SHRs): under control conditions (E^+), after mechanical removal of endothelium (E-), after local incubation with Calcium entry blocker (E-TA3090; 23µg/ml), and then after total abolition of the smooth muscle tone (E-KCN; 1mg/ml).

The volume-pressure relation of in situ localized carotid arteries was determined for transmural pressures varying between 50 and 225 mmHg. The carotid compliance (CC, µl/mmHg) was calculated as the slope ($\Delta V/\Delta P$) of the volume-pressure curves.

Statistical analysis : Results are expressed as mean ± SEM. A two-way analysis of variance (ANOVA) was performed and differences between groups were evaluated with the Newman-Keuls test. Differences were considered significant when $p<0.05$.

Results :

With intact endothelium :

Figure 1 shows the effects of local calcium blockade on the volume-pressure relations of SHRs and WKY rats. In both strains, calcium blockade induced a significant shift of the curves so that, at each given value of transmural pressure, volume was significantly higher after calcium blockade than under baseline conditions ($p<0.01$). In both strains, the curves obtained after KCN poisoning significantly differed from those obtained under control conditions ($p<0.001$). In WKY rats, there was no significant difference between volumes after calcium blockade and after KCN poisoning. In contrast, in SHRs, the volume-pressure curve was significantly higher after KCN than after TA-3090 ($p<0.02$).

With damaged endothelium :

Figure 2 shows the effects of TA3090 on the volume-pressure relationship before and after endothelium removal. In both strains, there were no differences between values obtained after calcium blockade in the presence or without endothelium.

Compliance of the carotid artery (CC) at the operating arterial pressure:

We defined the operating pressure as the mean arterial pressure of the animals, roughly 100 mmHg in WKY and 150 in SHR.

With intact endothelium: Under control conditions, CC was significantly smaller in SHR than in WKY ($p<0.001$), indicating stiffer carotid wall in SHR than in WKY. Local incubation with calcium blocker induced a significant increase in CC both in WKY and SHR ($p<0.01$ and $p<0.001$ respectively). Total abolition of vascular smooth muscle by KCN poisoning, after incubation with TA-3090, did not induce further increase in CC in WKY but induced a significant increased in CC in SHR ($p<0.02$).

After endothelium removal: Endothelium removal induced in both strains a significant increase of CC ($p<0.01$ in WKY and $p<0.001$ in SHR). Incubation with TA-3090 and KCN poisoning did not induce significant increases in CC both in WKY and in SHR. Furthermore, there were no differences between the CC values measured after incubation with calcium blocker with intact or after endothelium removal

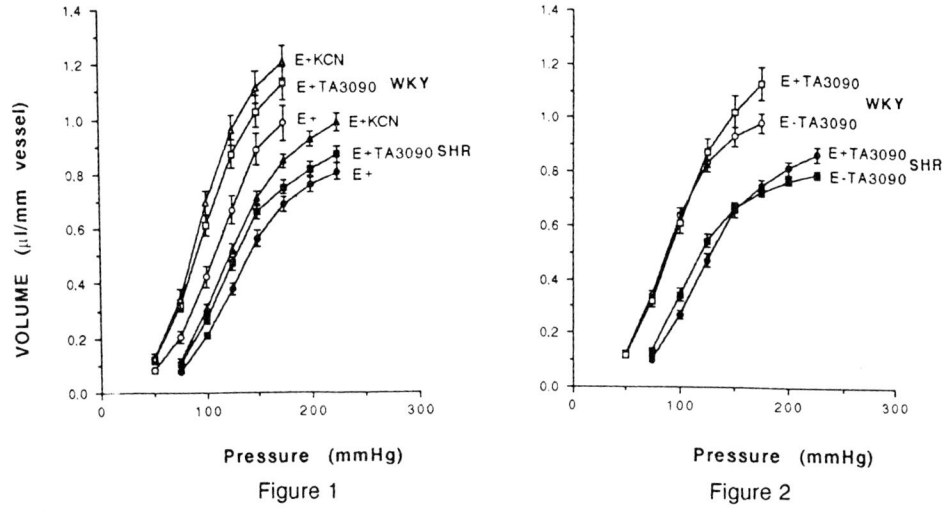

Figure 1

Figure 2

The main finding of the present study is that calcium blockade induced by TA-3090 at the dosage corresponding to the intravenous injection of 0.5mg/kg caused a shift of the volume-pressure curves toward higher values of carotid volume, both in WKY and SHRs. In WKY rats, there was no significant difference between the volume-pressure curves obtained after calcium blockade and after smooth muscle poisoning. In contrast, in SHRs, KCN induced a further shift of the volume-pressure curve compared to that obtained after calcium blockade, suggesting that, in SHRs, calcium influxes regulated only a part of the compliance reserve smooth muscle tone-dependent and that other neuro-humoral factors might be involved in the mechanisms influencing the carotid volume-pressure relationship.

In conclusion

The present study showed that calcium-blockade produced by local incubation with a diltiazem-like substance increases the carotid compliance in WKY and SHRs. The compliance increase was due to relaxation of arterial smooth muscle by direct and indirect mechanisms, the latter might involve endothelium vasoactive function. Furthermore, in SHRs, calcium influxes appear to regulate only a part of the compliance reserve smooth muscle tone dependent ; thus other neuro-humoral factors are likely involved in the control of the mechanical properties of the carotid arterial wall.

References

Brown BG. Response of normal and diseased epicardial coronary arteries to vasoactive drugs: quantitative arteriolo-graphic studies. Am J Cardiol 1985; 56: 23E-29E.
Levy BI, Benessiano J, Poitevin P, Safar ME. Endothelium dependent mechanical properties of the carotid artery in WKY and SHR: Role of ACE-inhibition. Circulation Res 1990; 66: 321-328
Levy BI, Poitevin P, Safar ME. Effects of alpha-1 blockade on arterial compliance in normotensive and hypertensive rats. Hypertension 1991; 17: 534-540.
Masafumi Y, Toshiaki F, Masuroni M, Michihiro K, Takafumi H, Shinya K, Toshiro M, Kazuhiro F, Masaharu O, Reizo K. Effect of diltiazem on aortic pressure-diameter relationship in dogs. Am J Physiol 1989; 256 (Heart Circ Physiol 25): H1580-H1587.
Peach MJ, Singer HA, Izzo NJ, Loeb AL. Role of calcium in endothelium-dependent relaxation of arterial smooth muscle. Am J Cardiol 1987; 59: 35A-43A.
Safar ME, Pannier B, Laurent S, London GM. Calcium-entry blockers and arterial compliance in hypertension. J of Cardiovascular Pharmacology 1989; 14 Suppl 10: S1-S6.
Singer HA, Peach MJ. Calcium- and endothelial- mediated vascular smooth muscle relaxation in rabbit aorta. Hypertension 1982; 4 suppl II: II-19-II-25.
Williams JS, Baik YH, Koch WJ, Schwartz A. A possible role for the endothelium in porcine coronary smooth muscle responses to dihydropyridine calcium modulators. J Pharmacol Exp Therap 1987; 241: 379-386.

Age-related blood pressure lowering effect of dietary L-arginine in stroke-prone spontaneously hypertensive rats (SHRSP)

Katsumi Ikeda [1], Yasuo Nara [1][2], Yuta Kobayashi [2], Keisuke Hattori [2] and Yukio Yamori [1][2]

Shimane Institute of Health Science [1], Department of Pathology [2] and Department of Pharmacology [2], Shimane Medical University, Izumo 693, Japan

SUMMARY

Chronic dietary L-arginine (1.74g/Kg bwt/day) when administered at an early age (9 weeks old) attenuated the development of hypertension in SHRSP, and the degree of attenuation diminished as SHRSP aged (up to 28 weeks old). Dietary N^G-nitro-L-arginine (NO2Arg) at the rate of 1.8 mg/Kg bwt/day for three days significantly increased the blood pressure in 9-week-old SHRSP, but not in 20-week-old SHRSP. The absolute increase in arterial blood pressure by NO2Arg infusion (7.8mg/Kg bwt; i.v.) was abolished by L-arginine infusion (500mg/Kg bwt;i.v.). Endothelium dependent relaxation (EDR) regulates blood pressure, and the EDR contribution to blood pressure regulation may be attenuated as the SHRSP ages.

INTRODUCTION

Previously, we documented the possibility that endothelium-dependent relaxation contributed to blood pressure regulation in adult rats (Kobayashi et al, 1991). Nitric oxide, one of the endothelium-derived relaxing factors, is formed from L-arginine by endothelial cells (Palmer et al, 1988). To study the effect of blood pressure on dietary L-arginine in SHRSP of different age groups, chronic L-arginine feeding on SHRSP was performed.

MATERIALS AND METHODS

SHRSPs at the age of 9 weeks were anesthetized with the inhalation of Halothane (Hoechst, Germany). The carotid artery was inserted with a polyethylene tube (PE 60, Clay Adams, U.S.A.), connected with a pressure transducer (P23XL-1, Nihon Koden, Japan) and arterial blood pressure was recorded on a polygraph. N^Gnitro-L-arginine (NO2Arg 7.8mg/Kg) which inhibited both endothelium dependent relaxation and synthesis of nitric oxide (Kobayashi et al 1990) and L-arginine (500mg/Kg) were administered as a infusion into the jugular vein. Forty-four of SHRSP(9,20 and 28 weeks of age) were divided into two groups. The experimental group obtained L-arginine at the rate of 1.74 g/Kg bwt/day through L-arginine-mixed commercial diet, while the control group received the regular commercial diet (Funabashi SP, Japan). Indirect blood pressure (Ikeda et al, 1991) and bodyweight were measured at regular intervals. NO2Arg was administered for three days in six of each of SHRSP at the age of 9 weeks and 20 weeks at the rate of 1.8 mg/Kg bwt/day through the NO2Arg mixed commercial diet.

RESULTS

NO2Arg(7.8mg/Kg bwt; i.v.) infusion in 9 weeks old SHRSP increased arterial blood pressure, while L-arginine (500mg/Kg bwt ; i.v.) infusion had no significant effect on blood pressure. But when L-arginine (500mg/kg bwt ; i.v.) was infused after pre-infusion with NO2Arg (7.8mg/kg bwt ; i.v.), it abolished the increase in blood pressure caused by NO2Arg(Figure 1).

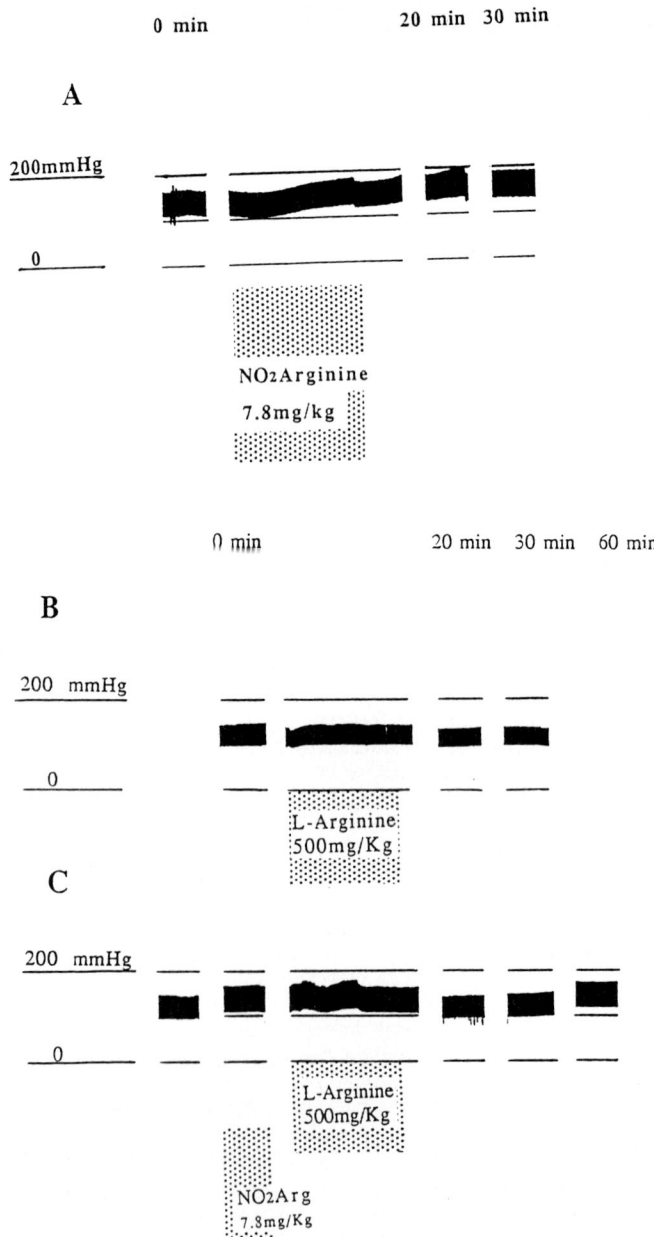

Figure 1.(A,B)The effects of NO2Arg (7.8 mg/Kg; i.v.)or L-arginine (500mg/Kg; i.v.)on blood pressure. (C) The effect of L-arginine (500mg/Kg;i.v.) on blood pressure pretreated with NO2Arg (7.8 mg/Kg; i.v.).

Significant and sustained lowering of blood pressure up to 28 weeks of age was observed in the 9-week old experimental group, and while in the 20 and 28-week old experimental group, the lowering blood pressure was insignificant. Figure 2 shows the development of blood pressure in the 9 and 20-week experimental groups.

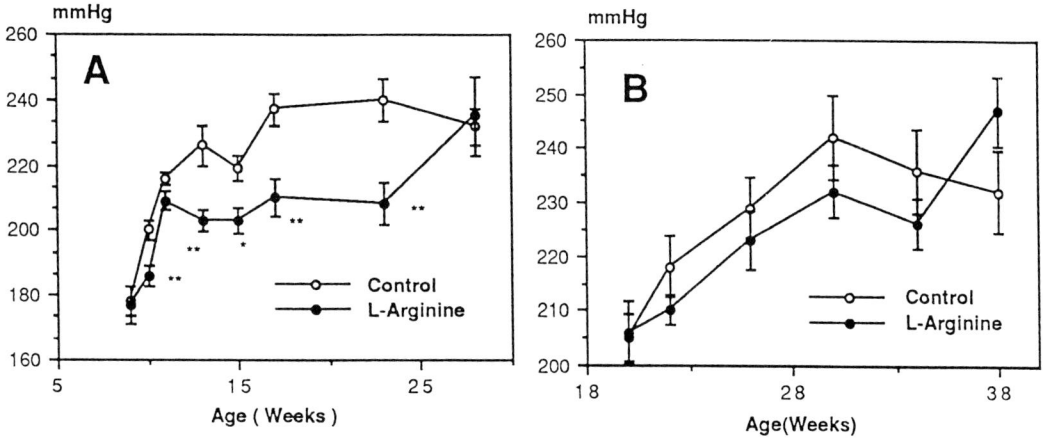

Figure 2. Blood pressure in SHRSP fed on L-arginine mixed diet starting at the age of 9(A) and 20 weeks(B). *: $p<0.05$, **: $p<0.01$

In a separate experiment in SHRSP, dietary NO2Arg administered at the rate of 1.8mg/Kg bwt/day for three days showed significant increase in blood pressure in the 9 weeks old experimental group, but not significasnt in the 20 weeks old experimental group(Table 1).

Table 1. Effect of dietary NO2Arg on blood pressure in 9 and 20-week-old SHRSP

	9-week-old SHRSP(n=6)		20-week-old SHRSP(n=6)	
	Before	3 days after	Before	3 days after
Blood pressure	180 ± 3	211 ± 5	223 ± 9	238 ± 2
Significance		$p<0.05$		n.s

DISCUSSION WITH CONCLUSION

The data on the effects of dietary L-arginine and NO2Arg on the blood pressure in different age-groups of SHRSP indicated that the dietary L-arginine at the rate of 1.74 g/Kg bwt/day could significantly decrease blood pressure in SHRSP, but the degree of response diminished with age. These data suggest that the contribution of the endothelium dependent relaxation to the blood pressure regulation attenuates with age in intact SHRSP.

REFERENCES

Ikeda,K., Nara,Y., and Yamori,Y. (1991) Indirect systolic and mean blood pressure by a new tail cuff method in spontaneously hypertensive rats. Laboratory animals. 25, 26-29.
Kobayashi,Y., and Hattori,K. (1990) Nitroarginine inhibit endothelium- derived relaxation. Jpn.J.Pharmacol. 52, 167-169.
Kobayashi,Y., Ikeda,K., Shinotsuka,K., Nara,Y., Yamori,Y., and Hattori,K.(1991) L-nitroarginine increased blood pressure in the rat. Clin.Exp.Physiol.Pharmacol. 18,397-399.
Palmer,R.M.J., Ashton,D.S., and Moncada,S.(1988) Vascular endotherial cells synthesize nitric oxide from L-arginine. Nature (Lond.) 333, 664-666.

Vascular responses to some relaxants and cyclic nucleotide levels in SHRSP, with special reference to aging

Irina N. Voynikova, Tencho I. Voynikov, Yukinori Yamanishi, Nicola A. Nicolov * and Aritomo Suzuki

*Department of Pharmacology, Kinki University School of Medicine, 589 Osaka-Sayama City, Japan; * Department of Pathophysiology, Medical Academy, 1431 Sofia, Bulgaria*

Cyclic nucleotides and the enzymes controlling their intracellular levels, cyclases and phosphodiesterases, are thought to play an important role in vascular smooth muscle function. Vascular relaxation is known to be connected with changes in the levels of cyclic nucleotides, and it was suggested that a defect in some steps of cyclic nucleotide systems can produce abnormal vascular responses (Triner et al., 1971; Amer, 1975). These can influence the changes in blood pressure levels which develop with age. Thus, we studied the relationship between the responses to some vascular relaxants and cyclic nucleotide levels to clarify the cause of hypertension with aging in SHRSP.

Materials and Methods. Male SHRSP and WKY at the age of 4, 12 and 24 weeks were used. Aortic rings, 3 mm in length, were contracted by 0.5 µM noradrenaline or 1 µM $PGF_2\alpha$ (approx. ED_{80}). When a plateau was reached, relaxants were added into the medium in a single dose method. Some rings were frozen in liquid nitrogen at the time of maximal relaxation and cyclic nucleotide levels were determined by radioimmunoassay, using New England Nuclear kits. Basal levels of cyclic nucleotides were measured as soon as possible after decapitation of animals.

Results. Blood pressure was found elevated in 4 week-old SHRSP, and with age its level increased significantly above that in WKY. Basal cAMP and cGMP levels tended to increase with age in both strains. Although there was not a definite distinction in cyclic nucleotide levels between SHRSP and WKY, cyclic AMP levels were slightly increased and cyclic GMP - slightly diminished in SHRSP compared with WKY (Table 1).

Table 1. Blood pressure (BP) and basal cyclic nucleotide levels in SHRSP and WKY

Age weeks	SHRSP			WKY		
	BP	cAMP	cGMP	BP	cAMP	cGMP
4	91±2	4.7±0.8	0.31±0.04	82±1	4.1±1.2	0.39±0.09
12	180±5*	5.9±1.3	0.33±0.03	126±5	4.9±1.1	0.47±0.08
24	195±8*	7.2±0.9	0.63±0.13	135±3	6.1±1.5	0.75±0.11

* $p<0.05$, compared to age-matched WKY

Isoproterenol increased cAMP level and inhibited $PGF_2\alpha$-induced contraction in a dose-dependent manner in both SHRSP and WKY rats at any of tested ages. These responses weakened with age, more noticeably in SHRSP than in WKY (Fig. 1).

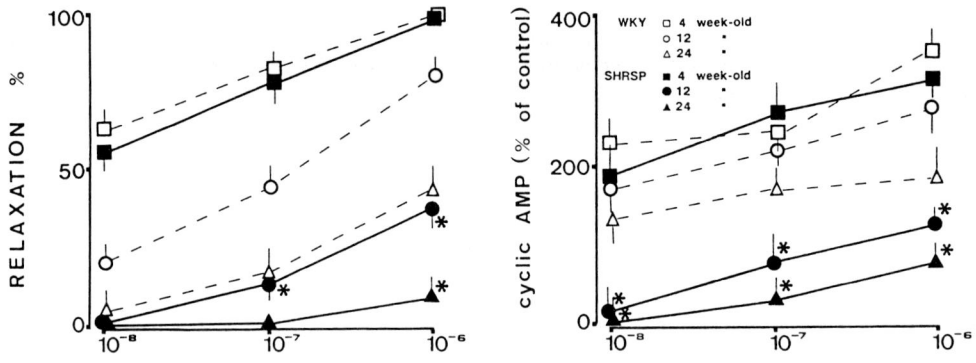

Fig. 1. Vascular relaxation and dose-response changes in cyclic AMP in response to Isoproterenol (M); * $p<0.05$, compared to age-matched WKY

Forskolin relaxed the vessels and increased cAMP levels in both strains, though these processes abated with age. The changes to forskolin in SHRSP were similar to those in the age-matched WKY. Papaverine and IBMX relaxed blood vessels and increased cAMP and cGMP levels in both strains. The levels of cAMP and cGMP rose with age in both SHRSP and WKY, whereas the relaxation responses followed just the opposite trend in both strains. The changes in SHRSP were not different from those in the age-matched WKY. Dibutyryl cAMP and cGMP produced relaxation in SHRSP and WKY alike, but the responses declined at the same rate, with age, in both strains. Vascular responses to ACh decreased with age in both strains. The decrease was more manifested in SHRSP: in older SHRSP the relaxation was transient, followed by strong contractions. However, there was no difference in the rise of cGMP levels by ACh between the age-matched SHRSP and WKY (Fig. 2).

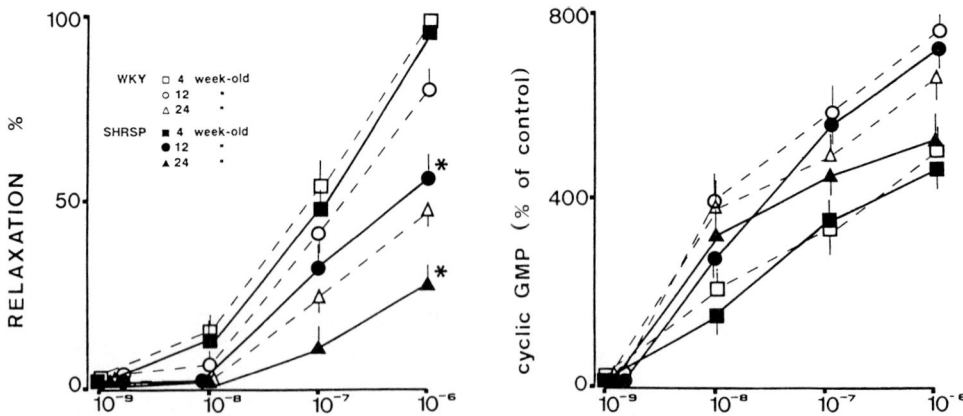

Fig. 2. Vascular relaxation and dose-response changes in cyclic GMP in response to Acetylcholine (M); * $p<0.05$, compared to age-matched WKY

The relaxation responses and the increases in cGMP levels by nitroprusside were endothelium-independent, and analogous in both strains.

Discussion. The relaxation responses to isoproterenol in the youngest SHRSP were quite similar to those in the age-matched WKY. Thus, the blunted cAMP production and impaired relaxation in older SHRSP (Sawyer & Docherty, 1987) appears to be secondary, perhaps due to a decrease in β-receptor numbers (Limas & Limas, 1979) and/or to a decreased activation of GTP-binding protein (Asano et al., 1988) caused by high blood pressure. Another possible explanation can be that the decrease in sensitivity to cAMP of the contractile protein in blood vessels from older SHRSP has an influence in part. However, the latter conception runs counter to the observed similarity in the relaxation responses to dibutyryl cAMP in older SHRSP and the age-matched WKY. On the other hand, results obtained with forskolin, papaverine and IBMX show that adenyl cyclase activity and phosphodiesterase activity change with age in both strains, but these changes are not affected by increased blood pressure (Donnelly, 1978). The relaxation responses to ACh declined with age in both strains, but this was more expressed in SHRSP than in WKY. In this case, the suggestion that the release of EDRF by ACh is reduced in older SHRSP can be denied by the fact that cGMP levels released by ACh in older SHRSP were not different from those in the age-matched WKY. Recently, it was reported that ACh releases EDCF (Luscher & Vanhoutte, 1986). In this study, the relaxation by ACh in older SHRSP was transient, and high concentrations of ACh produced small relaxation followed by a marked contraction. Thus, the reduced relaxation responses to ACh in older SHRSP can be partly due to the release of EDCF (Vanhoutte, 1989). The hypothesis that the sensitivity to cGMP of the contractile protein is reduced in older SHRSP contradicts the fact that nitroprusside-induced relaxation was parallel in both strains, and dibutyryl cGMP-induced relaxation in SHRSP was not different from that in the age-matched WKY.

These results suggest that the reduction in β-adrenoreceptor numbers and/or the decreased activation of GTP-binding protein are important in the elevation and maintenance of blood pressure, and that EDCF and/or EDRF also play an important role.

References:

Amer, M.S. (1975): Cyclic nucleotides in disease: on biochemical etiology of hypertension. Life Sci 17: 1021-1038.
Asano, M., Masuzawa, K., and Matsuda, T. (1988): Role of stimulatory GTP-binding protein (Gs) in reduced beta-adrenoceptor coupling in the femoral artery of spontaneously hypertensive rats. Br J Pharmacol 95: 241-251.
Donnelly, T.E. (1978): Lack of altered cyclic nucleotide phosphodiesterase activity in the aorta and heart of the spontaneously hypertensive rat. Biochim Biophys Acta 542: 245-252.
Limas, C., and Limas, C. (1979): Decreased number of beta-adrenergic receptors in hypertensive vessels. Biochim Biophys Acta 582: 533-536.
Luscher, T.F., and Vanhoutte, P.M. (1986): Endothelium-dependent contractions to acetylcholine in the aorta of the spontaneously hypertensive rat. Hypertension 8: 344-348.
Sawyer, R., and Docherty, J.R. (1987): Reduction with age in the relaxation to beta-adrenoceptor agonist and other vasodilators in rat aorta. Naunyn-Schmiedeberg's Arch Pharmacol 336: 60-63.
Triner, L., Nahas, G.G., Vullinernoz, Y., Overweg, N., Verosky, M., Nabif, D.V., and Ngai, S.H. (1971): Cyclic AMP and smooth muscle function. Ann NY Acad Sci 185: 458-476.
Vanhoutte, P.M. (1989): Endothelium and control of vascular function. Hypertension 13: 658-667.

Induction of malignant hypertension in stroke-prone spontaneously hypertensive rats (SHRSP)-treated with nitroarginine, an inhibitor of endothelium-derived relaxing factor (EDRF)

Yukio Yamori [1][2][3], Katsumi Ikeda [3], Shunsaku Mizushima [1][2][3], Yasuo Nara [1][2][3] and Motoki Tagami [3][4]

[1] Department of Pathology, Shimane Medical University, [2] WHO Collaborating Center for Research on Primary Prevention of Cardiovascular Diseases, [3] Shimane Institute of Health Sciences, Izumo 693, and [4] Department of Internal Medicine, Sanraku Hospital, Tokyo 101, Japan

Summary: Nitroarginine, an inhibitor of endothelium-derived relaxing factor (EDRF), 0.023% in a commercial diet was given to 8-week-old SHRSP, 8 in total, to investigate the role of EDRF at the incipient stage of hypertension. They developed severe hypertension over 200 mmHg with proteinuria on the 3rd day of the feeding thereafter and died all of stroke before the 15th day. Their major pathological findings were cerebral hemorrhage, hemorrhagic infarction and/or cerebral softening with arterionecrosis and thrombosis which were also observed in renal arteries and arterioles. These vascular lesions were electronmicroscopically demonstrated to be due to medial smooth muscle cell necrosis and degeneration and following thrombosis with platelet aggregation. Therefore, nitroarginine-fed young SHRSP could be a model for malignant hypertension and the impaired NO production may be a pathogenic mechanism of malignant hypertensive vascular lesions.

Nitric oxide (NO) is currently considered to be one of the endothelium-derived relaxing factor (EDRF) and formed from the guanidino nitrogen atom of L-arginine (Moncada, 1990). We previously reported L-arginine-rich diet was effective for preventing stroke in SHRSP before 300 days of age (Yamori et al., 1991) and the activity of L-arginine-NO pathway was reduced in the aged SHRSP as demonstrated by a lesser vasodilatory response to acetylcholine (Kobayashi et al., 1992). NO production from L-arginine may have a protective role against the development of severe hypertension and stroke in young SHRSP. On the other hand, Kobayashi et al. (1990, 1991) found nitroarginine was a useful inhibitor of L-arginine-NO pathway. Therefore, nitroarginine was dietary administered to evaluate the pathophysiological functional implication of L-arginine-NO pathway in the development of hypertension and stroke in young SHRSP.

MATERIALS AND METHODS

Male SHRSP/Izm, 18 in total which were bred and maintained at Shimane Institute of Health Sciences, were devided into 2 groups at the age of 8 weeks; one group of 10 rats were given a commercial stock (Funahashi SP) diet, while the other group of 8 rats was given the SP diet containing 0.023% of N^G-L-nitroarginine (Peptide Institute, Minoo, Japan). They were free to access to diet and water during the entire experiment. The systolic blood pressure was measured by a photoelectric oscillometric method (Ikeda et al., 1991). SHRSP which developed definite symptoms of stroke (Yamori et al., 1982) and were about to die were anesthetized for perfusion-fixation for histopathological and electronmicroscopical studies as described previously (Tagami et al., 1990).

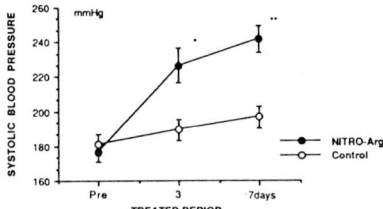

Fig. 1 Effect of nitroarginine (NITRO-Arg) on systolic blood pressure in 8-week-old SHRSP

Fig. 2 Effect of nitroarginine (NITRO-Arg) on urinary protein excretion in 8-week-old SHRSP

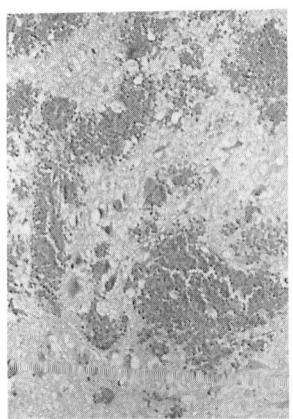

Fig. 3 Hemorrhagic infarction in nitroarginine-treated SHRSP

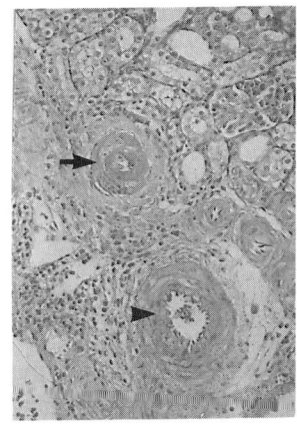

Fig. 4 Angionecrosis (arrow) and medial thickening (arrow head) in renal arteries of nitroarginine-treated SHRSP

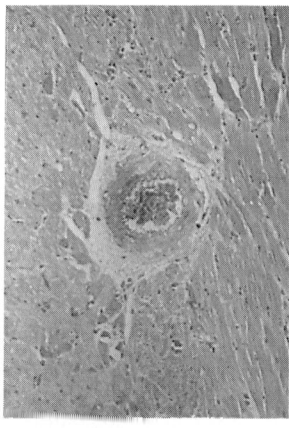

Fig. 5 Degeneration of cardiomyocytes in nitroarginine-treated SHRSP

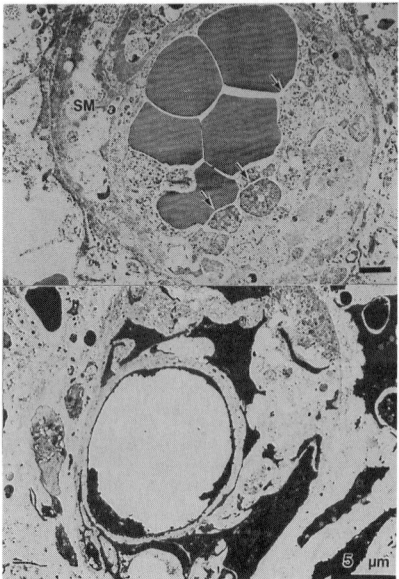

Fig. 6 Smooth muscle cell (SM) degeneration and necrosis with platelet (arrow) aggregation in a perforating artery of nitroarginine-treated SHRSP

Fig. 7 Smooth muscle cell degeneration and necrosis in a renal arteriol of nitroarginine-treated SHRSP

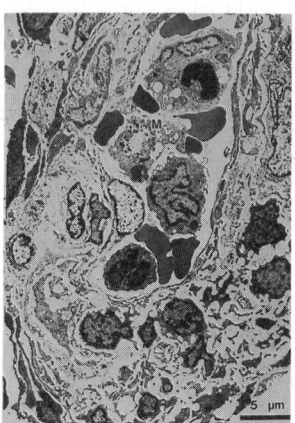

Fig. 8 Extensive medial degeneration with occlusion with macrophages (M) and platelets in a renal arteriols of nitroarginine-treated SHRSP

RESULTS

SHRSP fed on the nitroarginine containing diet developed from initial mild hypertensive level (177 ± 5 mmHg) quickly severe hypertension, 226 ± 10 and 241 ± 8 mmHg, respectively on the 3rd and 7th day of the feeding, while control SHRSP gradually developed moderate hypertension, 189 ± 6 and 196 ± 6 mmHg, respectively on the 3rd and 7th day of the feeding (Fig. 1). Urinalysis showed that protein excretion, electrophoretically proven as albumin, was significantly increased in the former group than in the control (Fig. 2).

The nitroarginine-administered SHRSP, all developed stroke to fall into the agonar stage from 6 to 15 days of the feeding (10 ± 1 days in average), but none of the control SHRSP developed stroke during this period. Macroscopically, hemorrhage and infarction in the brain were noted in 5 and 3 of these symptomatic SHRSP, respectively. Histopathological examination revealed hemorrhage in the brain section was mostly infiltrating, not expanding, and diagnosed as hemorrhagic infarction (Fig. 3).

Renal histology revealed angionecrosis (fibrinoid necrosis) in afferent arteriols and small arteries (Fig. 4), and wall-thinkening of these vessels with marked folding of internal elastic layers and inward bulging of endothelial cells, suggestive of severe vasoconstriction in the nitrosoarginine group. Cardiac histology with similar vascular changes and irregular staining of cardiomyocytes (Fig. 5) was suggestive of acute ischemic damages due to severe vasoconstriction.

Electron microscopic examination demonstrated marked medial smooth muscle cell degeneration and necrosis with endothelial cell degeneration and following platelet adhesion in perforating arteries of the brain (Fig. 6), and similar smooth muscle cell degeneration and atrophy without any endothelial changes (Fig. 7) as well as with some endothelial changes and occlusion due to thrombosis with macrophages and platelets (Fig. 8) in small renal arteries, indicating impaired NO production may accelerate thrombosis.

CONCLUSION WITH DISCUSSION

Dietary nitroarginine feeding in 8-week-old SHRSP successfully induced severe hypertension as well as marked vascular pathology similar to malignant hypertension within 3 to 7 days and stroke death within 15 days, indicating the importance of impaired NO production in the pathogenesis of malignant hypertensive vascular lesions.

REFERENCES

Ikeda, K., Nara, Y. and Yamori, Y. (1991): Indirect systolic and mean blood pressure determination by a new tail cuff method in spontaneously hypertensive rats. *Lab. Ani.* 25: 26-29.

Kobayashi, Y., Ikeda, K., Shinozuka, K., Nara, Y., Yamori, Y. and Hattori, K. (1991): Comparison of vasopressor effects of nitro arginine in stroke-prone spontaneously hypertensive rats and Wistar-Kyoto rats. *Clin. Exp. Physiol. Pharmacol.* 18: 599-604.

Kobayashi, Y., Ikeda, K., Nara, Y., Shinozuka, K., Hattori, K. and Yamori, Y. (1992): Endothelium-dependent relaxations of isolated ring preparations of the thoracic aorta of aged SHRSR. *Jpn. Heart J.* 33 (in press).

Moncada, S. (1990): The First Robert Furchgott Lecture: From endothelium- dependent relaxation to the L-arginine: NO pathway. *Blood Vessels* 27: 208-217.

Tagami, M., Nara, Y., Kubota, A., Fujino, H. and Yamori, Y. (1990): Ultrastructural changes in cerebral pericytes and astrocytes of stroke-prone spontaneously hypertensive rats. *Stroke* 21: 1064-1071.

Yamori, Y., Horie, R., Akiguchi, I., Kihara, M., Nara, Y. and Lovenberg, W. (1982): Symptomatological classification in the development of stroke in stroke-prone spontaneously hypertensive rats. *Jpn. Circ. J.* 46: 274-283.

Yamori, Y., Nara, Y., Ikeda, K., Mizushima, S., Sawamura, M and Horie, R. (1991): Protein intake and blood pressure reduction - experimental analysis on the mechanisms and epidemiological evidence in humans. *Clin. Exp. Hypertens.* A13: 442.

Nitric oxide synthesis and the control of blood pressure in sympathectomized rats

Zhi-Qi Zhang, Christian Barrès and Claude Julien

Département de Physiologie et Pharmacologie Clinique, URA CNRS 606, Faculté de Pharmacie, 8, avenue Rockefeller, 69008 Lyon, France

Previous studies from our laboratory have shown that the early chronic destruction of peripheral sympathetic nerves with guanethidine does not lower the mean arterial pressure (MAP) level but strongly increases its spontaneous variability in conscious rats (Julien et al., 1990). Preliminary experiments indicated that this enhanced lability of blood pressure was characterized by the spontaneous occurrence of hypotensive episodes associated with vasodilations in several regional circulations (Barrès et al., 1991).

Therefore, the aim of the present study was to evaluate the possible participation of the L-arginine - nitric oxide (NO) pathway in the mechanisms of the vasodilations in sympathectomized rats insofar as NO has been shown to exert a tonic vasodilatory influence in many vascular beds *in vivo* (Gardiner et al., 1990a).

Methods

Male offspring of Sprague-Dawley rats bred in the laboratory were used. Sympathectomy was produced by daily sc injections of guanethidine sulfate (Ciba-Geigy, Basel, Switzerland) between 1 and 13 weeks of age. Control rats were injected with the same volume of saline (2.5-5 µl/g of body weight). At 13 weeks of age, rats were anesthetized with a mixture of acepromazine (12 mg/kg ip) and ketamine (120 mg/kg ip). Doppler flow probes were then implanted for the measurement of blood flow velocity (Haywood et al., 1981) in the subdiaphragmatic aorta, superior mesenteric artery and distal aorta (hindquarters). After 10 days of recovery, the caudal artery and left femoral vein were cannulated under halothane anesthesia for MAP recording and iv injections, respectively. Twenty-four hours later, the cardiovascular parameters were recorded beat to beat in conscious unrestrained rats (Gustin et al., 1990). For each cardiac cycle, a computer calculated MAP, heart rate and indices of regional blood flows and vascular conductances (G as blood flow / MAP ratio). The means and variabilities (variation coefficient, VC) were calculated over 40-min periods, before and 5 min after administration of the NO synthesis inhibitor, N^G-nitro-L-arginine methyl ester (L-NAME, 20mg/kg iv). The pressor response to tyramine (500 µg/kg iv) was measured to assess the effectiveness of sympathectomy.

Statistical comparisons used the nonparametric Wilcoxon's test for paired and unpaired data.

Results

Tyramine induced pressor responses in control (ΔMAP = 52 ± 6 mmHg) but not in sympathectomized rats.

The 40-min average values of cardiovascular parameters recorded in conscious quiet rats before administration of L-NAME did not differ between control and sympathectomized rats. Sympathectomy significantly increased the variabilities of MAP, mesenteric blood flow, aortic and mesenteric conductances without changing the hindquarters blood flow and conductance variabilities (Table 1).

Table 1. Average values and variabilities of cardiovascular parameters recorded during 40 min in conscious 14 wk-old rats in baseline conditions.

		Controls			Sympathectomized	
	n	mean	VC (%)	n	mean	VC (%)
MAP (mmHg)	9	107±2	4.0±0.3	7	106±3	8.7±0.4 *
HR (beats/min)	8	399±8	4.0±0.4	7	384±12	4.9±0.7
AoBF (kHz)	6	5.1±0.9	6.2±0.5	6	5.4±0.7	7.5±0.8
HqBF (kHz)	7	3.0±0.8	13.8±0.7	6	2.6±0.3	14.6±1.5
MeBF (kHz)	8	5.1±0.7	9.1±0.5	6	4.7±0.7	15.6±3.4 *
AoG x 1000 (kHz/mmHg)	6	50±10	7.4±0.5	6	51±8	10.4±0.5 *
HqG x 1000 (kHz/mmHg)	7	28±7	15.0±0.8	6	25±3	17.6±1.5
MeG x 1000 (kHz/mmHg)	8	48±7	9.6±0.6	6	46±8	17.1±3.3 *

Values are means ± sem. VC : variation coefficient ; MAP : mean arterial pressure ; HR : heart rate ; AoBF : aortic blood flow ; HqBF : hindquarters blood flow ; MeBF : mesenteric blood flow ; AoG : aortic vascular conductance ; HqG : hindquarters conductance ; MeG : mesenteric conductance. * p < 0.05 vs. controls.

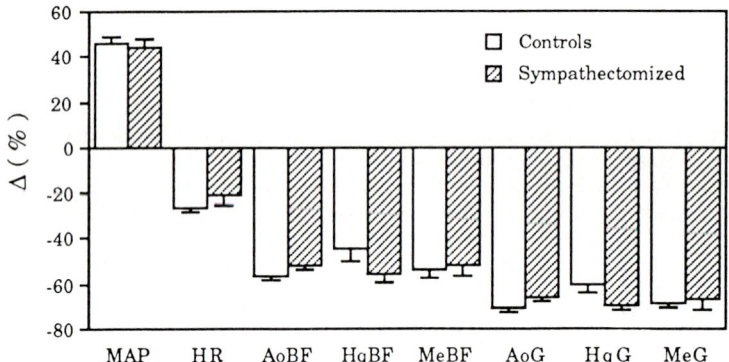

Fig. 1. Percent changes from baseline (Δ) in cardiovascular parameters after administration of L-NAME (20 mg/kg iv) in groups of conscious control and sympathectomized rats. Abbreviations and number of observations are same as in Table 1.

As indicated in Fig. 1, a single dose of L-NAME increased MAP by more than 40% in both control and sympathectomized rats. This pressor effect was associated with bradycardia and marked decreases in blood flows and vascular conductances which did not differ between the two groups of rats. L-NAME did not change blood pressure and hemodynamic variabilities in both control and sympathectomized rats, except for an increase (+61 ± 20 %, p < 0.05) in the hindquarters conductance variability of sympathectomized rats.

Discussion

In this study, conscious freely behaving rats with functional sympathetic denervation of the vessels, as evidenced by the disappearance of pressor responses to tyramine, did not show any change in the mean level of blood pressure but had a striking increase in the spontaneous MAP variability as compared with intact rats. This exaggerated blood pressure lability was associated with an increase in the variability of mesenteric conductance with no change in that of the hindquarters vascular bed, resulting in a significant increase in the variability of aortic conductance, which is the sum of vascular conductances of all regional circulations in the lower part of the body. These results point to an imbalance between regional hemodynamic changes after sympathectomy and suggest that the sympathetic nervous system may play an important role in reducing short-term hemodynamic variability.

Blockade of NO synthesis with L-NAME induced powerful pressor and vasoconstrictor effects which were identical in control and sympathectomized rats, which indicates that the basal synthesis and release of NO do not require integrity of the sympathetic vascular innervation. This conclusion is in agreement with the study by Fozard and Part (1991) in anesthetized rats and those of Gardiner *et al.* (1990b) and Wang and Pang (1991) in conscious rats, which have shown that ganglionic blockade does not attenuate the pressor effects of NO synthase blockers. In sympathectomized rats, L-NAME did not reduce MAP variability but increased the variability of hindquarters conductance, suggesting an increase in the relative amplitude of vasodilations which prevail in this particular bed.

In conclusion, the results of the present study suggest a major role for the sympathetic nervous system in the regulation of regional circulations, the loss of which in sympathectomized rats results in a marked instability of MAP. The vasodilatory component of MAP lability after sympathectomy does not appear to depend on an episodic release of NO synthesized by the L-arginine pathway. However, NO generates a powerful vasodilatory tone regardless of the presence of vascular sympathetic nerves.

Acknowledgements

This research was supported by the Institut National de la Santé et de la Recherche Médicale (Contrat de Recherche Externe 89-5001).

- Barrès C., Cantalupi I., Julien C. and Sassard J. Hemodynamic analysis of blood pressure lability after chronic sympathectomy in the conscious rat (Abstract). Fifth European Meeting on Hypertension, Milan, 7th - 10th June 1991.
- Fozard J. R. and Part M. L. Haemodynamic responses to N^G-monomethyl-L-arginine in spontaneously hypertensive and normotensive Wistar-Kyoto rats. *Br. J. Pharmacol.* 102: 823-826, 1991.
- Gardiner S. M., Compton A. F., Kemp P. A. and Bennett T. Regional and cardiac haemodynamic effects of N^G-nitro-L-arginine methyl ester in conscious, Long Evans rats. *Br. J. Pharmacol.*, 101: 625-631, 1990a.
- Gardiner S. M., Compton A. F., Kemp P. A. and Bennett T. Regional and cardiac haemodynamic responses to glyceryl trinitrate, acetylcholine, bradykinin and endothelin-1 in conscious rats: effects of N^G-nitro-L-arginine methyl ester. *Br. J. Pharmacol.*, 101: 632-639, 1990b.
- Gustin M. P., Cerutti C. and Paultre C. Z. Heterogeneous computer network for real-time hemodynamic signal processing. *Comput. Biol. Med.* 20: 205-215, 1990.
- Haywood J. R., Shaffer R. A., Fastenow C., Fink G. D. and Brody M. J. Regional blood flow measurement with pulsed Doppler flowmeter in conscious rat. *Am. J. Physiol.* 241 (*Heart Circ. Physiol.* 10): H273-H278, 1981.
- Julien C., Kandza P., Barrès C., Lo M., Cerutti C. and Sassard J. Effects of sympathectomy on blood pressure and its variability in conscious rats. *Am. J. Physiol.* 259 (*Heart Circ. Physiol.* 28): H1337-H1342, 1990.
- Wang Y. X. and Pang C. C. Y. Possible dependence of pressor and heart rate effects of N^G-nitro-L-arginine on autonomic nerve activity. *Br. J. Pharmacol.* 103: 2004-2008, 1991.

Local hyperproduction of cGMP in carotid arteries from SHR is endothelium-dependent

Marie-Christine Mourlon-Le Grand, Joëlle Benessiano and Bernard I. Lévy

INSERM U.141, Hôpital Lariboisière, Paris, France

INTRODUCTION:

Spontaneously hypertensive rats (SHR) have enhanced arterial smooth muscle tone compared to their normotensive control WKY rats. A simultaneous release of endothelium-derived relaxing factors (EDRFs) (inducing activation of the soluble fraction of guanylate cyclase (Forstermann et al.,1986)) and endothelium-derived constrictor factors (EDCFs) appears to be involved in the regulation of vascular tone (Lüscher & Vanhoutte, 1988). The relaxing function of endothelium is believed to be less effective in the SHR than in the WKY rat. Although cyclic GMP (cGMP) is involved in the control of smooth muscle relaxation, the relationship between vascular tone and cGMP metabolism in the SHR still remains unclear.
The aim of this work was to compared the cGMP pathway activity in WKY rats and SHRs. In both strains, the tissue cGMP content was measured in carotid arteries under basal conditions (with intact endothelium (E^+)), after inhibition of the soluble guanylate cyclase by methylene blue (MB) and after the mechanical removal of endothelium (E^-).

MATERIAL AND METHODS :

A) Material :

These experiments were performed in 16-week-old SHR (n=28; 359 ± 9 g) and age-matched WKY rats (n=28; 412 ± 9 g) divided into three groups for each strain. The carotid arteries were studied in different conditions:
- Group 1 (8 WKY rats, 8 SHR): under control conditions (E^+).
- Group 2 (10 WKY rats, 10 SHR): after local incubation with MB (10^{-5} M, 20 min).
- Group 3 (10 WKY rats, 10 SHR): after mechanical endothelium removal (E^-).

B) Methods :

Carotid arteries were carefully dissected, removed, frozen in liquid nitrogen and stored at -40°C. Frozen arteries were cut into strips and homogenized in 6% trichloroacetic acid; the samples were then centrifuged at 2000 g for 15 minutes at 4°C. Supernatant fractions were extracted with diethyl ether, lyophilized and assayed for cGMP content by radioimmunoassay (AMERSHAM kit) (Harper & Brooker, 1975) .

C) Statistical analysis :

Results are expressed as mean ± SE. A two-way analysis of variance (ANOVA) was performed and differences between groups were evaluated with the Newman-Keuls test (Zar, 1984). Differences were considered significant when p<0.05.

RESULTS :

Figure 1 shows cGMP levels (fmol/mg tissue) in the carotid artery in normotensive and hypertensive rats under control conditions (E^+), after mechanical stripping of endothelium (E^-) and after local incubation with methylene blue (MB).
There was a significantly higher cGMP content in the carotid arterial wall with intact endothelium in SHRs than in WKY rats (30.34 ± 3.69 vs 19.72 ± 2.28 fmol/mg tissue; p<0.02).
The deendothelialization of carotid arteries significantly decreased cGMP by 28% in WKY rats (p<0.02) and by 90% in SHRs (p<0.001). The decrease in cGMP content of carotid arteries after endothelium removal was significantly higher in SHRs than in WKY rats (p<0.001).
In MB-treated arteries, tissue cGMP content was similarly decreased in WKY rats and in SHRs by 88% (p<0.001) and 94% (p<0.001) respectively as compared to control values (E^+). The cGMP levels in E^- and MB-treated carotid arteries were significantly different in WKY rats (p<0.001) but not in SHRs.

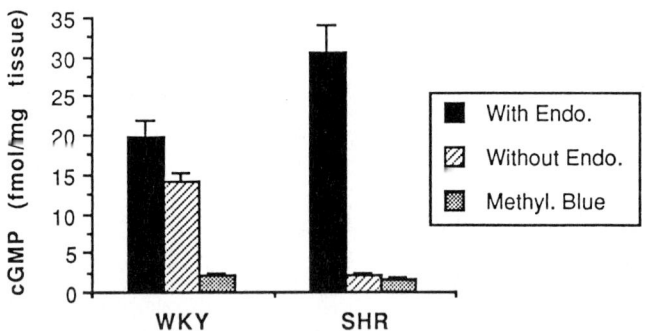

Fig 1: Cyclic GMP content (fmol/mg tissue, mean ± SE) in the carotid arterial wall from normotensive (WKY rats) and spontaneously hypertensive rats (SHR) under several experimental conditions.

DISCUSSION :

The present study reports the differences of the cGMP pathway in the SHR compared to the normotensive WKY rat. The specific effects of endothelium removal and inhibition of soluble guanylate cyclase were also investigated.
These results evidence that, despite a higher vasomotor tone in SHR, the tissue cGMP level was higher in SHR than in WKY rat, suggesting a more active cGMP pathway in the SHR. In agreement with these results, Amer et al. (1974) reported high arterial tissue cGMP content in the SHR. In contrast, Otsuka et al. (1988) reported lower aortic tissue cGMP content in DOCA-salt rats, aortic stenosis and renovascular hypertension than in their normotensive controls. The discrepancy between Otsuka's results and the present results could be attributed to differences in cGMP pathway activity in genetic and in secondary hypertension experimental models and/or to the different vessels studied.
Accumulation of tissue cGMP reported in this study in the SHR could be related 1) to an activation of cGMP synthesis due to the stimulation of guanylate cyclases (Goldberg & Haddox,

1977), 2) and/or to a decrease of cGMP hydrolysis due to cyclic nucleotide phosphodiesterase (PDE) decreased activity (Goldberg & Haddox, 1977; Weishaar, 1987; Harris et al., 1989).

Mechanical stripping allowed us to investigate the involvement of endothelium in the synthesis of tissue cGMP. Furthermore, methylene blue, an inhibitor of the soluble form of guanylate cyclase, was used to evaluate its relative contribution in the local production of cGMP. Under E$^-$ and MB conditions, a strong reduction of cGMP content was evidenced in the SHR. In contrast, tissue cGMP was slightly reduced in WKY rats only after removal of endothelium and dramatically decreased in MB conditions.
These results suggest that cGMP content in the carotid artery wall was predominantly dependent on the presence of the endothelium in SHRs but not in WKY rats. Similarly, Lüscher et al. (1988) reported normal EDRFs release associated with high EDCF activity in arteries from SHR. Conversely, in WKY rats, the slighter decrease in tissue cGMP after stripping of endothelium suggests that other non-endothelial mechanisms control the synthesis of cGMP (Wood et al., 1990; Taylor et al., 1991). Our data suggest that these mechanisms could be more active in WKY rat than in SHRs.

In conclusion, the present study shows that despite a higher vasomotor tone, the cGMP pathway is probably more active in the SHR than in the WKY rat. Our results evidence that the mechanism involved in cGMP synthesis regulation in the SHR is probably endothelium-dependent. However, this local hyperproduction of tissue cGMP does not seem sufficient to counteract the high vasomotor tone in the SHR. This may be interpreted as an insufficient endothelium-dependent compensatory relaxing phenomenon of local regulation against genetic constricting abnormalities.

REFERENCES:

Amer, S.M., Gomoll, A.W., Perhach, J.L., Hugh, J.R., Ferguson, C. & McKinney, G.R. (1974): Aberrations of cyclic nucleotide metabolism in the hearts and vessels of hypertensive rats. *Proc. Nat. Acad. Sci.* 71, 4930-4934.

Forstermann, J., Melsch, A., Bohme, E. & Busse, R. (1986): Stimulation of soluble guanylate cyclase by an acetylcholine-induced endothelium-derived factor from rabbit and canine arteries. *Circ. Res.* 58, 531-538.

Goldberg, N.D. & Haddox, M.K. (1977): Cyclic GMP metabolism and involvement in biological regulation. *Annu. Rev. Biochem.* 46, 823-896.

Harper, J.F. & Brooker, G. (1975): Fentomole sensitive radioimmunoassay for cyclic AMP and cyclic GMP after 2'0 acetylation by acetic anhydride in aqueous solution. *J. Cyclic Nucleotide Res.* 1, 207-218.

Harris, A.L., Lemp, B.M., Bentley, R.G., Perrone, M.H., Hamel, L.T. & Silver, P.J. (1989): Phosphodiesterase isozyme inhibition and the potentiation by zaprinast of endothelium-derived relaxing factor and guanylate cyclase stimulating agents in vascular smooth muscle. *J. Pharmacol. Exp. Ther.* 249, 394-400.

Luscher, T.F. & Vanhoutte, P.M. (1988): Hypertension and endothelium-dependent responses. In *Vasodilation*, ed. P.M. Vanhoutte, pp. 523-529, Raven Press, New York.

Otsuka, Y., DiPiero, A., Hirt, E., Brennaman, B. & Lockette, W. (1988): Vascular relaxation and cGMP in hypertension. *Am. J. Physiol.* 254, H163-H169.

Taylor, D.A., Bexis, S., Mano, M.T. & Head, R.J. (1991): Tonic endothelial cell (EC) constrictor activity is masked by nitric oxide generation in spontaneously hypertensive (SH) but not Wistar-Kyoto (WKY) rats. *Faseb J.* 5, A1422.

Weishaar, R.E. (1987): Multiple molecular forms of phosphodiesterase: An overview. *J. Cyclic Nucleotide Protein Phosphorylation Res.* 11, 463-472.

Wood, K.S., Buga, G.M., Byrns, R.E. & Ignarro, L.J. (1990): Vascular smooth muscle-derived relaxing factor (MDRF) and its close similarity to nitric oxide. *Biochem. Biophys. Res. Commun.* 170, 80-88.

Zar, J.H. (1984): Two-factor analysis of variance. In *Biostatistical Analysis*, pp 206-236, Englewood Cliffs, Prentice Hall, New Jersey.

Measurement of urinary excretions of nitrite and nitrate, and effects of inhibition of nitric oxide production on hemodynamics in SHR

Hakuo Takahashi [1], Shinji Fukumitu [2], Masato Nishimura [1], Tadashi Nakanishi [1], Takeshi Hasegawa [3] and Manabu Yoshimura [1]

Department of Clinical Laboratory and Medicine [1], Third Department of Medicine [2], Radioisotope Laboratory [3], Kyoto Prefectural University of Medicine, Kamikyo-ku, Kyoto 602, Japan

A potent vasorelaxing factor (EDRF) of the endothelium origin is thought to be nitric oxide (NO) produced from L-arginine (Palmer et al., 1988). L-N^G-monomethyl L-arginine (MMA) inhibits the production of NO (Moncada et al., 1989). NO is supposed to be degraded into nitrite (NO2) and nitrate (NO3) ions (Leaf et al. 1989). In order to determine whether or not EDRF is involved in the pathophysiology of spontaneous hypertension in rats, we measured urinary excretions of NO2 and NO3 ions with HPLC using 5 to 12-week-old SHR and WKY. Effects of inhibition of NO production with MMA on the hemodynamic parameters were also measured by using tracer microspheres with a reference sample method.

MATERIALS AND METHODS

MEASUREMENT OF NO2 AND NO3: Male SHR AND WKY (Charles River Japan) at from 5 to 12 weeks of age were housed in metabolic cages, and 24-hour urine was collected in containers with 5ml of 3N-HCl. The urine samples were stored in a freezer at -20 °C until the assay.
The sample was filtered through a membrane filter (Molcut II, Millipore Corp.). The filtrate was applied to an ion chromatography (IC-Pak A, Millipore Corp.), and eluted with phosphate buffer (0.02mM, pH 8.0).

EFFECTS OF L-N^G-MONOMETHYL L-ARGININE (MMA) ON REGIONAL BLOOD FLOW: Using 8 week-old male SHR and age-matched WKY, all experiments were performed under anesthesia with urethane (1.1 g/Kg, i.p.). Catheters were inserted into femoral artery and vein, and into the left cardiac ventricle through the right carotid artery. Blood pressure was recorded continuously during the experiments by connecting the femoral arterial catheter to a small volume displacement transducer, and pulse rate was calculated automatically with a tachometer. After recording blood pressure and heart rate for more than 10 minutes until the stabilization of these parameters, radioactive microspheres (15 µm in diameter, labeled with ^{57}Co and suspended in normal saline plus 0.01% Tween 80 (NEM-022A, New England Nuclear) were injected into the left ventricle, and the reference sample, 0.45ml was collected for 30 seconds from the femoral artery. Then, MMA, 15mg/Kg, or the vehicle was injected into the left ventricle in a volume of 10 µl, and followed by a 0.1ml of saline flush. Three minutes later, radioactive microspheres labeled with ^{51}Cr (NEM-025A) were injected similarly as the first isotope injection. Methods in detail are described elsewhere (Adachi et al., 1979).

DRUG INJECTIONS AND STATISTICS: L-N^G-monomethyl L-arginine was synthesized according to Nakajima et al. (1971). Data expressed as averages±SEM were analyzed using a t-test for comparing means of dependent or independent samples; differences at a 5% level ($p<0.05$) or less were considered significant.

RESULTS

URINARY EXCRETIONS OF NITRITE AND NITRATE: Urinary excretions of NO_2 decreased with age in both SHR and WKY. The difference between them was not significant. On the other hand, urinary levels of NO_3 were consistently lowered in SHR compared to those in WKY (Fig. 1).

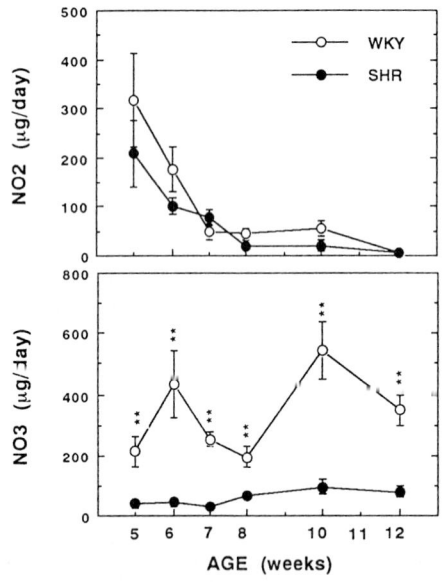
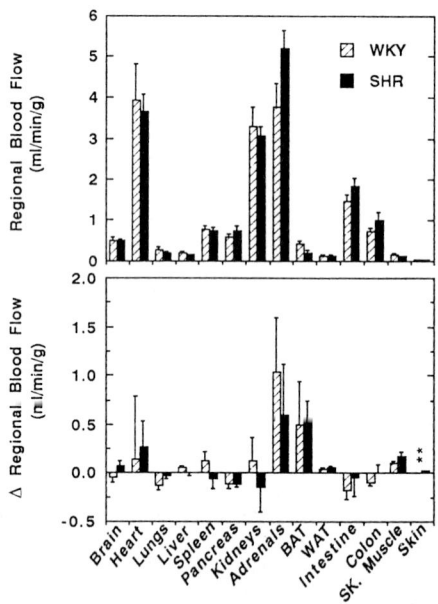

Fig. 1. Urinary excretions of nitrite (NO_2, upper panel) and nitrate (NO_3, lower panel) in WKY and SHR. Data are expressed as mean±SEM from 8 rats in each group. (**$p<0.01$ vs. SHR)

Fig. 2. Regional blood flow measured by using radioactive microspheres in 8-week old, male WKY and SHR (upper panel). Lower panel shows the effects of L-N^G-monomethyl L-arginine on the regional blood flow. Abbreviations: BAT=brown adipose tissue, WAT=white adipose tissue, SK.=skeletal (**$p<0.01$)

EFFECTS OF L-N^G-MONOMETHYL L-ARGININE (MMA) ON REGIONAL BLOOD FLOW: The magnitude of vasopressor responses to MMA was greater in SHR than in WKY ((at 3 minutes, +32±2 vs. +13±1mmHg). Heart rate, cardiac index and total peripheral resistance increased in all SHR rats, but increased in only 30-60% of WKY. However differences in the magnitude of responses between these two groups was not significant because of a large standard deviation of the data. MMA did not significantly change the regional blood flow in both rat groups except the skin;

MMA increased the blood flow more in SHR than in WKY only in the skin (Fig. 2).

CONCLUSION

Since NO is produced not only in the endothelial cells but also in the immune system such as macrophages (Stuehr et al., 1985) and comes from diets (Green et al., 1981), the urinary-excreted NO2 and NO3 may not directly reflect the amount of endothelial NO production. However, the marked reduction of NO3 in urine may indicate that the production of endothelial NO is at least partly reduced.

On the other hand, intraventricular injections of MMA increased mean arterial pressure more in SHR than in WKY. Thereby, the regional blood flow was not markedly influenced by MMA. This means that administration of MMA constricted arteries in almost all of organs and tissues; i.e., production of NO is suggested from the present results, to be distributed all the organs and tissues homogeneously. The augmented vasopressor responses could be attributed to augmented increases in cardiac output and vascular resistance with MMA in SHR.

These findings suggest that production of EDRF is decreased in SHR regardless of age. Since inhibition of NO production elicited augmented-vasopressor responses in SHR, deranged endothelial functions may have resulted in deficient production of EDRF and supersensitivity to the product, NO.

ACKNOWLEDGEMENTS

We are grateful to Dr. Teruo Nakajima, professor of Department of Psychiatry, Kyoto Prefectural University of Medicine, for his technical advises on the synthesis of MMA.

REFERENCES

Adachi, H., Hirano, S., Nakamura, M., Fujitani, S., Takahashi, H., Endo, N., Nakagawa, M., and Ijichi, H. (1979):Measurement of regional blood flow with radioactive microspheres in rats. J. Jpn. Coll. Angiol. 19:207-213.

Green, L.C., de Luzuriaga, K.R., Wagner, D.A., Rand, W., Istfan, N., Young V.R., and Tannenbaum, S.R. (1981): Nitrate biosynthesis in man. Proc. Natl. Acad. Sci. 78:7764-7768.

Leaf, C.D., Winshnok, J.S., and Tannenbaum, S.R. (1989):L-arginine is a precursor for nitrate biosynthesis in humans. Biochem. Biophys. Res. Comm. 163:1032-1037

Moncada, S., Palmer R.M.J., and Higgs E.A. (1989):The biological significance of nitric oxide formation from L-arginine. Biochem. Soc. Transact. 17:642-644

Nakajima, T., Matsuoka, Y., Kamimoto, Y. (1971): Isolation and identification of N^G-monomethyl, N^G, N^G-dimethyl- and N^G, N^G, N^G-trimethyl arginine from the hydrolysate of proteins of bovine brain. Biochim. Biophys. Acta 230:212-222

Palmer, R.M.J., Ashton, D.S., and Moncada, S. (1988): Vascular endothelial cells synthesize nitric oxide from L-arginine. Nature(Lond.) 333:664-666.

Stuehr, J.D., and Marletta, M.A. (1985): Mammalian nitrate biosynthesis: Mouse macrophages produce nitrite and nitrate in response to Escherichia coli lipopolysaccharide. Proc. Natl. Acad. Sci. 82:7738-7742.

Endothelium function in resistance and coronary arteries of spontaneously hypertensive compared to WKY rats: effects of nitro-L-arginine

F. Pourageaud and J.L. Freslon

Laboratoire de Pharmacodynamique, Faculté de Pharmacie, 3, place de la Victoire, 33076 Bordeaux Cedex, France

Introduction

Endothelial-derived relaxing factor (EDRF) was first proposed by Furchgott and Zawadzki (1980) as the substance involved in the acetylcholine-induced vasorelaxation. It has been pharmacologically characterized and chemically identified as nitric oxide (NO) or a related compound, which is synthesized by the endothelial cell (EC) from L-arginine and causes relaxation via stimulation of the soluble guanyl-cyclase of the smooth muscle cell.

In arteries of SHR's compared to their normotensive controls, the endothelium-dependent relaxation has been shown to be impaired in aortae (Lüscher and Vanhoutte, 1986), in mesenteric resistance and in cerebrals arteries (De Mey and Gray, 1985; Tesfamariam and Halpern, 1988). The aim of the present study was to determine if this impairment would also be present in SHR's coronary arteries compared in WKY rats. Thus, *in vitro* experiments were performed in coronaries taken from these two strains. Simultaneously, mesenteric arteries were used as controls. An inhibitor of the NO-synthetase, nitro-L-arginine (NOA), was used to test the basal or the acetylcholine-induced release of NO or NO-related compound by endothelial cells.

Methods

In vitro experiments were performed using mesenteric resistance arteries (MRA), left (LIC) and right (RIC) interventricular coronary arteries taken from 12 to 14 week-old SHR and age-matched WKY rats. After dissection, vessels were mounted on two stainless steel wires (diameter: 25 µm) in an isometric myograph allowing direct determination of the vessel wall force while the internal circumference was controlled (Mulvany and Halpern, 1977). The vessels were kept in oxygenated (5% CO_2 in O_2) physiological saline solution (PSS) with indomethacin (10 µM) to inhibit prostaglandins pathway.

The segments were submitted to a passive extension protocol and set up to a normalized internal diameter corresponding to 0.9 the diameter the vessel would have *in situ* when submitted to an internal pressure of 100 mm Hg (D_{100}).

The reactivity of each preparation was checked with K-PSS (NaCl exchanged for KCl on an equimolar basis). Concentration-effect curves were constructed by cumulative additions in the bath of either noradrenaline (NA, in MRA in the presence of cocaine, 3 µM) or serotonin (5-HT, in LIC and RIC). The EC_{50} (µM) expressed as concentration of mediator producing a 50% maximal response was determined for each artery. Acetylcholine (AC, 0.01-10 µM) was added similarly when contraction had reached a plateau in the presence of maximal concentrations of NA or 5-HT (10 µM for both). Maximal relaxations were expressed as % of maximal contractions.

Nitro-L-arginine (NOA, 100 µM) was used to inhibit either basal or AC-stimulated production of nitric oxide (NO) or NO-containing compound by endothelial cells. Results were obtained from 5 to 15 preparations in each group.

Results

D_{100} of MRA, expressed as µm, were slightly more important in WKY's compared to SHR's (278±8 vs 256±12, NS), but D_{100} of coronaries were smaller in WKY's compared to SHR's (RIC: 294±13 vs 361±14, p <0.01; LIC: 344±10 vs 355±18, NS). Sensitivities of arteries to NA or 5-HT were not significantly different in the two strains, but maximal contractile responses, expressed as mN/mm^2, tended to be lower in arteries of WKY's compared to those of SHR's (MRA : 37.0±1.9 vs 49.3±3.9, p <0,01; RIC: 13.5±2.6 vs 16.4±2,3, NS; LIC: 9.2±2.6 vs 9.4±1.1, NS).

In quiescent vessels, NOA induced a progressive rise in tension which was less rapid and less reversible in LIC and RIC compared to MRA and slightly more important in MRA and coronary of WKY's than in those of SHR's. Results are given in Table 1 and expressed as per cent of agonist maximal contraction.

	WKY	SHR
MRA	32 ± 9 (8)	11 ± 3 * (6)
RIC	98 ± 16 †† (5)	44 ± 5 **, ††† (11)
LIC	76 ± 10 ††† (5)	40 ± 8 *, †† (13)

Table 1
Contractions (% of agonist maximal contraction) induced by NOA.
Mean ± sem; ( ): number of arteries;
* p <0.05, ** p <0.01 : WKY compared to SHR;
†† p <0.01, ††† p <0.001, LIC and RIC compared to MRA.

These contractions provoked by NOA could be reversed by addition of L-arginine (100 µM) but not D-arginine (100 µM).

In precontracted mesenteric resistance arteries, maximal AC-induced relaxations, expressed as per cent of maximal contractions, were more important in arteries taken from WKY rats compared to those taken from SHR's : 62±7 (n=8) vs 27±8 (n=6), p< 0.01. In precontracted coronary arteries, the same phenomenon was observed, as shown in fig.1.

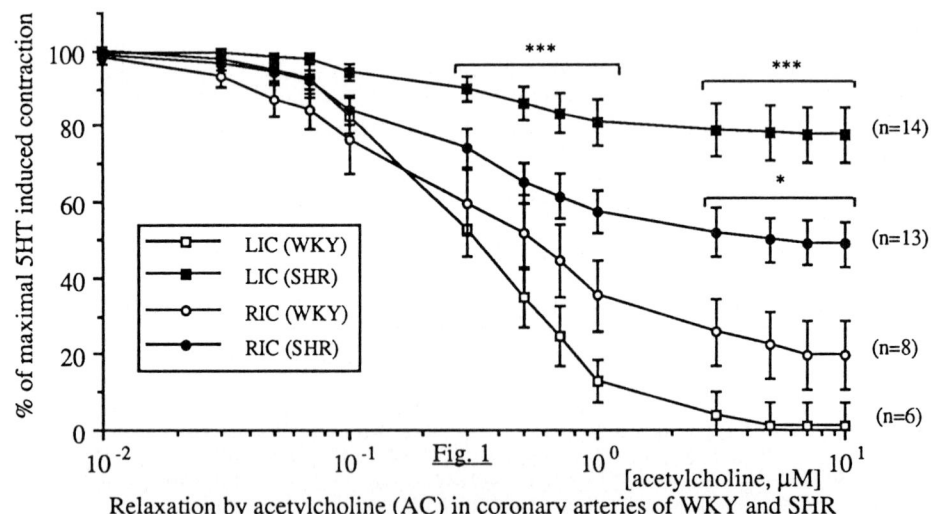

Fig. 1
Relaxation by acetylcholine (AC) in coronary arteries of WKY and SHR
(Mean ± sem; n: number of arteries; * p <0.05; *** p <0.001)

Maximal relaxations, expressed as per cent of maximal contractions induced by 5-HT, were : LIC : 99±6 vs 23±7, p<0.001; RIC : 80±9 vs 51 ± 6, p<0.05 for WKY and SHR's respectively.
After a 30-minute incubation period, NOA completely inhibited AC relaxation in all types of precontracted arteries.

This inhibition could be reversed by L-arginine (100 µM). Subsequent additions of sodium nitroprusside (10 µM) induced complete relaxations in the two groups.

Discussion

These results show:
1) that, in quiescent resistance and coronary arteries, NOA induces a contraction which appears to be due to the suppression of the synthesis and release of NO from the arginine pathway, since it was reversed by L- but not D-arginine.- This phenomenon was previously observed *in vitro* in aorta of WKY rats (Rees and coll.,1990) and *in vivo* in coronary vasculature of rabbit (Humphries et al.,1991). Regarding the magnitude of the contraction induced by NOA, our results suggest that this release is less important in MRA compared to LIC and RIC for both strains of rats, and less important in SHR's compared to WKY's for both type of arteries. However, considering the latter comparison, it cannot be ruled out from our data that a "normal" release of EDRF in the presence of an increased release of endothelium-derived contracting factors (EDCF's) could prevail in the vasculature of the SHR, as previously proposed (Lüscher, 1990).
2) that the inhibition of NO synthetase induces a complete inhibition of acetylcholine-induced relaxation. As a result of the stimulation of the muscarinic endothelial receptor, two factors are released : EDRF (NO) and probably an endothelium-derived hyperpolarizing factor, EDHF, which induces a relaxation of vascular smooth muscle secondary to an hyperpolarization (Chen et al., 1988). Since in our experiments no residual relaxation by acetylcholine was observed after incubation by NOA, it suggests that EDHF would not be involved or could be identical to EDRF, as previously postulated (Tare et al.,1990).
3) that the impaired relaxation by acetylcholine observed in large, in resistance and cerebral arteries of SHR's also prevails in the coronary vasculature of this strain. The complete relaxations of our preparations observed with sodium nitroprusside, which activate directly the guanylate cyclase, confirms that reactivity of smooth muscle was normal.

In conclusion, these results support the concept of a basal release of NO or NO-like compound by EC which seems to be reduced in both MRA and coronaries arteries of SHR's compared to their normotensive controls. In the latter strain, the reduced relaxation induced by acetylcholine appears to be due to a functional alteration of endothelium in the presence of a normal reactivity of smooth muscle cells.

References

Chen, G., Suzuki, H., Weston, A.H. (1988) : Acetylcholine releases endothelium-derived hyperpolarizing factor and EDRF from rat blood vessels. Br.J. Pharmacol., 95, 1165-74.
Demey, J.G., Gray, S. (1985): Endothelium-dependent reactivity in resistance vessels. Prog. Appl. Microcir., 8, 181-7.
Furchgott, R.F., Zawadzki, J.V. (1980): The obligatory role of endothelial cells in the relaxation of arterial smooth muscle by acetylcholine. Nature (Lond.), 288, 373-6.
Humphries, R.D., Nicol, A.K., Tomlinson, W., O'Connor, S.E. (1991): Coronary vasoconstriction in the conscious rabbit following intravenous infusion of nitro-L-arginine. Br.J. Pharmacol., 102, 565-6.
Lüscher, T.F., Vanhoutte, P.M. (1986) : Endothelium-dependent contractions to acetylcholine in the aorta of the spontaneously hypertensive rat. Hypertension, 8, 344-8.
Lüscher, T.F. (1990) : The endothelium : target and promoter of hypertension ? Hypertension, 15, 482-5.
Mulvany, M.J., Halpern, W. (1977): Contractile properties of small resistance vessels in spontaneously hypertensive and normotensive rats. Circ. Res., 41, 19-26.
Rees, R.D., Palmer, R.M.J., Schulz, H.F., Hodson, H.F., Moncada, S. (1990): Characterization of three inhibitors of endothelial nitric oxide synthase *in vitro* and *in vivo*. Br.J. Pharmacol., 101, 746-52.
Tare, M., Parkington, H.C., Coleman, H.A., Neild, T.O., Dusting, G.J. (1990): Hyperpolarisation and relaxation of arterial smooth muscle caused by nitric oxide derived from the endothelium. Nature, 346, 69-71.
Tesfamariam, B., Halpern,W. (1988): Endothelium-dependent and endothelium-independent vasodilation in resistance arteries from hypertensive rats. Hypertension, 11, 440-4.

Coronary vascular response to endothelin-1 in spontaneously hypertensive rats in relation to hypertension development

Hiroshi Takeshita, Masaru Nishikibe, Mitsuo Yano * and Fumihiko Ikemoto

*Pharmacology and * Biochemistry, Central Research Laboratories, Banyu Pharmaceutical Co., Ltd., Meguro, Tokyo 153, Japan*

1. Introduction
Endothelin, a potent endothelium-derived vasoconstrictor peptide, has been considered to be causally related to ischemic heart disease, mainly by its action of reducing coronary blood flow. (Watanabe et al. 1991). Hypertension is a known risk factor of ischemic heart disease, however, contribution of endothelin to the heart function in relation to hypertension has not been substantially evidenced. We describe herein the results of the coronary vasoconstrictive response to endothelin (ET-1) evaluated using the isolated perfused hearts of spontaneously hypertensive rats (SHR) and Wistar Kyoto rats (WKY).

2. Method
Hearts were obtained from male WKY and SHR (6-30W). Perfusion pressure (PP) was measured by modified Langendorff method. The heart was perfused by Krebs-Henseleit solution and PP was initially maintained at 35-45 mmHg. The change of PP was measured with a pressure transducer through the cannula inserted into aorta. Drugs were administered at a volume of 0.1 ml to the heart as bolus injections into the aortic cannula. Since the response to ET-1 is long-lasting, the magnitude of the response was determined in a cumulative manner. To elucidate the effect of nicardipine, the dose-response curve for ET-1 was calculated in the presence of nicardipine (10^{-8} M). To examine the effect of chronic antihypertensive treatments, coronary vascular responses to ET-1 and Bay K-8644 in isolated hearts from SHR were observed after the animals were orally administered with hydralazine (30 mg/kg/day) or enalapril (10 mg/kg/day) for consecutive 10 weeks. Systolic blood pressure (SBP) was measured every week by tail-cuff plethysmography. Furthermore, the effect of acute administration of enalapril (10 mg/kg, i.v.) on the response to ET-1 in SHR was examined. All values represent mean ± s.e. Data were analyzed by the Student's t-test or Neumann-Keuls test. A Difference was considered statistically significant when $p<0.05$.

3. Result & Discussion
The vasoconstrictive effect of ET-1, expressed as the increase in PP, was more potent than that of acetylcholine (Ach), vasopressin (VP) and angiotensin II (A II) in both WKY and SHR. As shown by pD_2 and maximum increasing response of PP (PPmax), the ET-1-induced vasoconstriction was significantly greater in SHR than in WKY, but for the other tested vasoconstrictors, there were subtle higher values in PPmax without significant difference in pD_2 in SHR (Table 1). Thus, the difference of response of the coronary vascular beds between SHR and WKY was most specific for ET-1, as compared with the other tested vasoconstrictors. In

the presence of nicardipine, the response curve for ET-1 was shifted to the right. The magnitude of the right-ward shift was greater in SHR than in WKY, resulting in the same magnitude of response to ET-1 in both strains; the values of pD_2 was 10.1±0.07 (N=5) for SHR and 9.8±0.24 (N=5) for WKY respectively. This suggests that the higher responsiveness of coronary vessels to ET-1 in SHR is attributed to the higher activity of dihydropyridine (DHP)-sensitive Ca^{2+} channels. In accordance with this contention, Bay K-8644 elicited a potent constrictive response in SHR; the values of pD_2 and maximum increasing response of PP afforded at a concentration of 10^{-9} M were 10.0±0.23 and 28.9±9.23 mmHg (N=13), respectively, but in WKY the maximum increase of PP at 10^{-9} M was only 7.7±1.88 mmHg (N=10). Similar result was reported by Tomobe et al (1991), who showed that the sensitivity of ET-1 in the aorta from 12-week-old SHR was greater than that from age-matched WKY. They considered that the altered sensitivity to ET-1 in the aorta from SHR can be explained by increased susceptibility for Ca^{2+} influx due to partial depolarization of the smooth muscle cells at the resting state. Indeed, they observed that, when the aortic strips from 12-week-old WKY rats were partially depolarized with high K^+-solution or ouabain, the vasoconstrictive effect of ET-1 became similar to that with the strips from SHR in a physiological solution. In our present study, therefore, the enhanced responses to ET-1 and Bay K-8644 in the coronary artery of SHR may also be explained by the same mechanism, involving the activation of DHP-sensitive Ca^{2+} channel.

Table 1 Coronary vasoconstrictive effects of ET-1, angiotensin II (AII), acetylcholine (Ach) and vasopressin (VP) in 15-week-old SHR and age-matched WKY.

	N	WKY pD_2	PPmax	N	SHR pD_2	PPmax
ET-1	5	10.6 ± 0.19	84.4 ± 4.30	5	11.8 ± 0.20*	141.2 ± 7.81*
A II	4	10.8 ± 0.23	25.0 ± 4.93	5	10.2 ± 0.14	35.6 ± 6.69
Ach	5	8.5 ± 0.05	50.0 ± 4.67	5	8.6 ± 0.04	58.0 ± 5.10
VP	5	10.6 ± 0.14	76.6 ± 5.64	5	10.6 ± 0.16	105.2 ± 3.23*

*Significantly different (P<0.05) from values in WKY.
pD_2: negative logarithm of the moles of drug required to produce 50 % of the maximum response.
PPmax: maximum increasing response of PP.

Table 2 Coronary vasoconstrictive effect of ET-1 and Bay K 8644 in 15-week-old SHR after chronic treatment with enalapril or hydralazine.

Drug	Dose (mg/kg/day)	N	ET-1 pD_2	N	Bay K-8644 pD_2
Control		4	11.5±0.04	14	10.0±0.23
Enalapril	10	7	10.2±0.23*	7	10.5±0.58
Hydralazine	30	4	11.4±0.31	7	10.1±0.19

*Significantly different (p<0.05) from control.

To assess the relationship between vascular reactivity to ET-1 and hypertension, the coronary vascular response to ET-1 was observed using SHR aged from 6 to 30 weeks old. Systolic blood pressure (SBP) in 6-week-old SHR did not differ from that of age-matched WKY; the values were 131.9±4.04 mmHg for WKY (N=6) and 139.7±4.81 mmHg for SHR (N=5). However, the SBP in SHR aged more than 15 weeks was significantly higher than that in age-matched WKY; for example, the SBP in 15-week-old SHR and age-matched WKY were 199.8±3.13 mmHg (N=5) and 140.6±2.37 mmHg (N=5), respectively. The increased response to ET-1 was observed in SHR aged more than 15 weeks, but not at 6 weeks ; the pD_2 values of 6-, 15- and 30-week-old SHR were 10.6±0.27 (N=5), 11.8±0.20 (N=5) and 11.6±0.66 (N=5), respectively. On the other hand, the vascular response to ET-1 was not significantly different between 6-, 15- and 30-week-old WKY; the pD_2 values were 10.4±0.24 (N=6), 10.6±0.19 (N=5) and 10.1±0.43 (N=3), respectively. This finding implies that the increasing vascular reactivity to ET-1 and the development of hypertension occur in a parallel manner. However, when SHR were chronically treated with antihypertensive drugs, enalapril and hydralazine, the increase in vascular response to ET-1 was prevented by enalapril, but not by hydralazine (Table 2), although these two drugs showed marked and almost equipotent antihypertensive activity; after completion of the treatments, the SBP were 129.0±3.81 mmHg (N=16) with hydralazine and 134.1±2.37 mmHg (N=16) with enalapril. Thus, the increasing reactivity to ET-1 in the coronary vascular beds of SHR is not the result solely from the development of high blood pressure.

It is unlikely that the effect of chronic treatment with enalapril to prevent the enhancement of vascular response to ET-1 is resulted from suppression of DHP-sensitive Ca^{2+} channel activity, since the coronary vascular response to Bay K-8644 was not affected by this treatment (Table 2). The coronary vascular response to ET-1 in SHR was not affected by a single dose of enalapril (10 mg/kg, i.v.) (the pD_2 values of SHR treated and untreated with enalapril were 11.2±0.25 (N=4) and 11.5±0.04 (N=4), respectively.). This result suggests that direct inhibition of ACE activity is not the reason for the decreased vascular response.

The mechanism by which enalapril prevented the enhancement of the vascular responsiveness to ET-1 remains unclear. However, an argument can be made for the possible contribution of renin-angiotensin system to this ET-1 specific vascular responsiveness. Yoshida et al (1990) recently reported the synergistic effect of chronic treatment with endothelin and A II to increase blood pressure in rats. The detail of this mechanism was not explained, however, in our study the sustained ACE inhibition might attenuate the synergistic effect by reducing the level of A II generated and acts locally. In conclusion, the coronary vascular response to ET-1 was significantly greater in SHR of more than 15-week-old than in age-matched WKY. The mechanism of the enhanced response may involve the activation of dihydropyridine sensitive Ca^{2+} channels and this mechanism may be at least partially modulated by renin-angiotensin-system.

5. Reference

Tomobe, Y. et al. (1991) Mechanisms of altered sensitivity to endothelin-1 between aortic smooth muscles of spontaneously hypertensive and wistar-kyoto rat. The Journal of Pharmacology and Experimental Therapeutics 257(2) 555-561.

Watanabe, T. et al. (1991) Contribution of endogenous endothelin to the extension of myocardial infarct size in rats. Circulation Research, 69, 370-377.

Yoshida, K et al (1990) Chronic synergistic effect of endothelin 1 and angiotensin II on blood pressure in conscious rats. Journal of Vascular Medicine and Biology, 2, 214 (abstract).

Endothelium-dependent and -independent tension oscillation in aortae from SHRSP and WKY

Satoru Sunano, Kyoko Kaneko and Keiichi Shimamura

Faculty of Pharmacy, Kinki University, Higashi-Osaka, and Research Institute of Hypertension, Kinki University, Osaka-Sayama, Japan

---

Arterial smooth muscles, especially those of larger arteries are known to be quiescent and exhibit no tension development or spontaneous contraction under a non-stimulated condition. Smooth muscles of arteries of hypertensive animal models on the other hand, often show spontaneous activities such as spontaneous elevation of tone and tension oscillations (Bruner et al., 1989; Sunano et al., 1991). In the blood vessels of normotensive animals, the tension oscillations of vascular smooth muscles are often endothelium-dependent and disappear when endothelium is removed (Garland, 1989). The present experiments were performed to investigate the differences of endothelium-dependent and -independent tension oscillation induced by noradrenaline or acetylcholine between the aortae from SHRSP and WKY.

METHODS

Ring preparations of aortae with or without endothelium from SHRSP and WKY were mounted in the organ baths filled with a modified Tyrode's solution and changes in tension were observed isometrically. In about one third of the preparations, endothelium was removed by rubbing the inner surface of the lumen with a small piece of soft rubber.

RESULTS AND DISCUSSION.

1) Blood pressure of animals
The blood pressure rose steeply with aging in SHRSP, reaching a plateau at ages between 14 to 16 weeks. The blood pressure at this age was 243 ± 3.5 mmHg (n = 20). The blood pressure of WKY also rose with aging but the elevation of the blood pressure was negligible when compared with that of SHRSP. It was 133 ± 0.9 mmHg (n = 20) at the age of 16 weeks.

2) Tension oscillation induced by noradrenaline
Aortic smooth muscle from 16 week old SHRSP often exhibited spontaneous tension oscillations including spontaneous twitch-like contractions even under a non-stimulated condition. The tension oscillation was inhibited by endothelium. In endothelium-removed preparations, low concentrations of noradrenaline induced the tension oscillations including twitch-like contractions.

The tension oscillation induced by noradrenaline was also depressed by endothelium. The tension oscillation of the aortic smooth muscle of SHRSP was abolished by the removal of Ca or by verapamil. These results indicate that the tension oscillation of the aortic smooth muscle is induced by a Ca influx through voltage-dependent Ca channels. Then, the grouped voltage-dependent Ca channels would be altered in the aortic smooth muscle of SHRSP, opening in a oscillating manner. In regard to this, the involvement of the oscillatory burst of the action potential in the initiation of the tension oscillation has been reported by Lamb and Webb (1989).

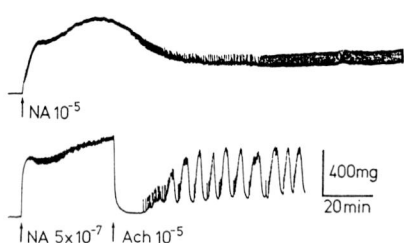

Fig. 1. Tension oscillation induced by noradrenaline and acetylcholine in endothelium-intact preparations from WKY. Upper : Noradrenaline of 10^{-5} M was applied. Lower : Acetylcholine (10^{-5} M) was applied to the preparation pre-contracted in the presence of 5×10^{-7} M noradrenaline. Note the tension oscillations during the contraction (upper) and during the relaxed state (lower).

In endothelium-intact preparations from WKY, on the other hand, a high concentration of noradrenaline induced the tension oscillation (Fig. 1). The results indicate that certain factor(s) released from endothelium is/are involved in the initiation of the tension oscillation. Then, lower rate of appearance of the endothelium-dependent tension oscillation in the preparation from SHRSP can be explained by the decreased function of the endothelium to release these factors. To support this, the decrease in the endothelium-dependent relaxation in the blood vessels of spontaneously hypertensive rats has been reported (Sunano, 1988; Shimamura et al., 1991).

3) Acetylcholine-induced tension oscillation
Application of acetylcholine to an endothelium-intact aorta precontracted in the presence of noradrenaline, induced a concentration-dependent relaxation in preparations from SHRSP and WKY. The relaxation was markedly impaired in the preparation from SHRSP. The application of acetylcholine also induced the tension oscillation including twitch-like contractions (Fig. 1). The tension oscillation induced by acetylcholine was more prominent in the preparation from WKY and nearly all preparations exhibited the oscillation, while it was less prominent in the preparation from SHRSP. The tension oscillation was endothelium-dependent and no tension oscillation was initiated by the application of acetylcholine in endothelium-removed preparation. It was negatively related to the age of the rats, being prominent in younger rats and less prominent in older rats. The effects of aging were more marked in the preparation from SHRSP. The tension oscillation was rarely observed in the preparation from aged SHRSP. These tension oscillations were abolished by the removal of extracellular Ca or by the application of verapamil.
Thus, it was demonstrated that the acetylcholine can also induce the tension oscillations by releasing certain factors. These tension oscillations are

thought to be initiated by the cyclical changes of the voltage-dependent Ca channel similarly to that induced by noradrenaline. Tension oscillation was more prominent when the endothelium-dependent relaxation was greater, suggesting that the tension oscillations are mediated by the release of endothelium-derived relaxing and/or hyperpolarizing factors. Since endothelium-dependent relaxation was impaired in the preparation from SHRSP (Sunano et al., 1988; Shimamura et al., 1991 and the results of the present experiment), the decreased tension oscillation in this preparation can be explained by the decreased release of factors which initiate the oscillation of the voltage-dependent Ca channels of the smooth muscle membrane. Endothelium-dependent tension and membrane potential oscillation have also been reported in other vascular smooth muscles (Garland, 1989).

CONCLUSION

Noradrenaline induced tension oscillations in the smooth muscle of rat aorta. The tension oscillation of the smooth muscle of the aorta from SHRSP was endothelium independent, while that from WKY was endothelium-dependent. Acetylcholine induced endothelium-dependent tension oscillation in both preparations. The endothelium-dependent tension oscillation was decreased while the endothelium-independent one increased in the aorta of SHRSP. The tension oscillation was extracellular Ca sensitive and blocked by Ca antagonist. It is suggested that the oscillatory opening of the voltage-dependent Ca channel is increased, while the release of oscillation-inducing factors are decreased in the aorta of SHRSP.

REFERENCES

Bruner, C.A., Webb, R.C. & Bohr, D.F. (1989): Vascular reactivity and membrane stabilizing effects of calcium in spontaneously hypertensive rats. In *Calcium in essential hypertension.* ed. K. Aoki and E.D. Frolich. E.D., pp. 275-306 Tokyo: Academic Press.

Garland, C.J. (1989): Influence of endothelium and α-adrenoceptor antagonists on response to noradrenaline in the rabbit basilar artery. *J. Physiol.* 418, 205-217.

Lamb, F.S. & Webb, R.C. (1989): Regenerative electrical activity and arteral contraction in hypertensive rats. *Hypertension* 13, 70-76.

Shimamura, K., Osugi, S., Moriyama, K. & Sunano, S. (1991) : Impairment and protection of endothelium-dependent relaxation in aortae of various strains of spontaneously hypertensive rats. *J. Cardiovasc. Pharmacol.* 17 (Suppl.3), S33-S36.

Sunano, S., Osugi, S. & Shimamura, K. (1988): Blood pressure and impairment of endothelium-dependent relaxation in spontaneously hypertensive rats. *Experientia* 45, 705-708.

Sunano, S., Osugi, S., Yamamoto, K. & Shimamura, K. (1991): Influence of the endothelium on the elevation of basal tension in aortae from various strains of spontaneously hypertensive rats. *J. Cardiovasc. Pharmacol.* 17 (Suppl.3), S137-S140.

Endothelium-dependent and -independent vasodilations of stroke-prone spontaneously hypertensive rats with stroke

Yuta Kobayashi, Katsumi Ikeda *, Kazumasa Shinozuka, Yasuo Nara **, Yukio Yamori ** and Keisuke Hattori

Departments of Pharmacology and Pathology **, Shimane Medical University and Shimane Institute of Health Science *, Izumo 693, Japan

SUMMARY: Endothelium-dependent and -independent vasodilations of the thoracic aorta ring strips of SHRSP with stroke and age-matched WKY male rats were compared. The relaxation of SHRSP strips by acetylcholine (1nM-10 μM) was concentration-dependent and the maximum relaxation was significantly smaller (about 40 percent) than that of WKY ($p < 0.01$). The relaxation of SHRSP by glyceryltrinitrate (10 μM) or verapamil (10 μM) was not significantly different from that of WKY. The relaxation of SHRSP by nitric oxide (NO), which was suggested as an endothelium-derived relaxing factor, was about 60 percent of that of WKY and the difference was significant ($p < 0.05$). These results indicate that the endothelium-dependent vasodilatory response was attenuated in SHRSP with stroke, although weak vasodilation still remained. The disturbance of diffusion of NO or enhancement of inactivation of NO in this model may have some contribution to this reduced response.

Acetylcholine (ACh)-induced relaxation of isolated arteries is endothelium-dependent and the relaxation is mediated through the release of endothelium-derived relaxing factor (EDRF) (Furchgott, 1984). The decline of the vasodilatory response to ACh in the isolated arteries of hypertensive model animals was observed (Cheng & Shibata, 1981; Kobayashi et al. 1991). The decline enhanced with the development of hypertension (Sunano et al., 1989) and it has been suggested that the attenuation is primarily due to the alternation of endothelium. Current studies suggested that at least one of EDRFs was nitric oxide (NO) or a related nitroso-compound and it was formed from L-arginine (Palmer et al., 1988). In the present study, endothelium-dependent and -independent vasodilations of SHRSP with stroke and age-matched WKY male rats were compared.

MATERIALS AND METHODS

Male SHRSP/Izm with stroke (n=6) and age-matched WKY/Izm rats (n=6), born and kept in Shimane Institute of Health Science, were compared. Ring strips of the thoracic aorta (2 mm width) were fixed vertically with stainless steel wires under a resting tension of 500 mg in a 20 ml organ-bath containing the Krebs-Henseleit buffer solution (Kobayashi, et al., 1991). Isometric tension changes were measured. The strips were contracted by prostaglandin $F_2\alpha$ ($PGF_2\alpha$; 10 μM) and then ACh (1nM-10μM), glyceryltrinitrate (GTN; 1nM-10 μM) or verapamil (1nM-10μM) was added cumulatively. The relaxation by NO (NO gas saturated solution; 0.5 percent in volume) was also studied. The relative relaxation of these agents to the maximum contraction induced by $PGF_2\alpha$ was calculated.

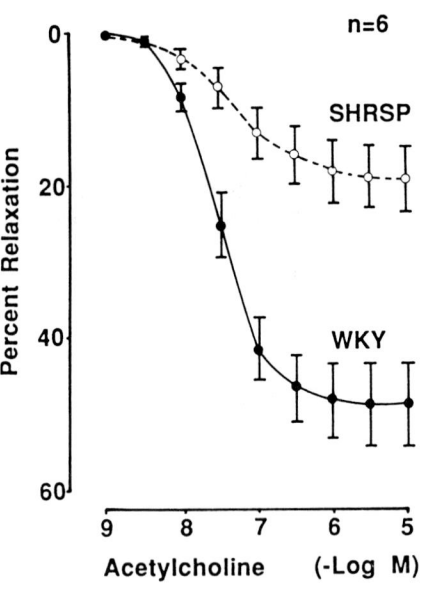

Fig. 1. Acetylcholine induced concentration-dependent vasodilatory responses of ring preparation of the thoracic aorta from SHRSP with stroke and WKY.
The preparation was contracted with 10 µM prostaglandin $F_2\alpha$ and the percent relaxation was obtained when the maximum contraction was taken as a 100 percent.

RESULTS

The relaxation of the strips of SHRSP with stroke by ACh was concentration-dependent and the maximum relaxation (10 µM) was about 40 percent of that of WKY and the difference was significant ($p<0.01$; Fig 1). The relaxation of SHRSP preparation by GTN was also concentration-dependent and it tended to decrease compared with WKY. The maximum relaxation of SHRSP preparation by GTN was about 90 percent of that of WKY, however, the difference was not significant (Fig. 2). The relaxation of SHRSP by verapamil was concentration-dependent and the concentra-

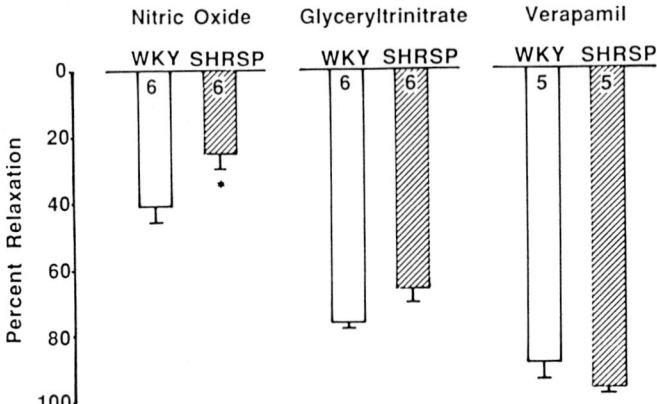

Fig. 2. Comparison of the maximum vasodilatory responses of ring preparation of the thoracic aorta of WKY and SHRSP with stroke to nitric oxide (saturated solution; 0.5 percent in volume), glyceryltrinitrate (10 µM) and verapamil (10 µM). Numbers in columns indicate the number of experiments.
* $p<0.05$ compared with the response of WKY preparation; t-test.

tion-response curve was not different from that of WKY. The maximum relaxation of SHRSP by NO was about 60 percent of that of WKY and the difference was significant ($p < 0.05$).

DISCUSSION

In the present study, the ACh-induced maximum relaxation of the thoracic aorta preparation of WKY was about 50 percent as the response decreased with aging (Kobayashi et al., 1992). ACh-induced relaxation was much smaller in the preparation of SHRSP with stroke compared with that of WKY. The decline of the response to ACh in the isolated blood vessels of hypertensive model animals agreed with the previous studies. In a separate study, one week of oral administration of nitroarginine, which inhibits endothelium-dependent relaxation and synthesis of NO (Kobayashi & Hattori, 1990; Mulsch & Busse, 1990), increased blood pressure of SHRSP (24 weeks of age) as well as WKY (Kobayashi et al., 1991). Weak response to ACh and NO was observed in the preparation of SHRSP with stroke in the present study. These results suggested that endothelium may have some contribution to blood pressure regulation in SHRSP. It has been considered that the alteration of endothelium caused the attenuation of the vasodilation responses in hypertensive model animals, however, the present results indicated further that not only endothelium-dependent relaxation but NO saturated solution-induced relaxation declined. NO-induced relaxation by GTN in the vascular smooth muscle cells (Chung & Fung, 1990) was not significantly affected in SHRSP with stroke. Reduction of the response to NO saturated solution may explained by disturbance of diffusion of NO or enhancement of inactivation of NO in this model.

In conclusion, the present results indicate that the endothelium-dependent vasorelaxation response was attenuated in SHRSP with stroke and the attenuation may not be only due to the alteration of endothelium.

Acknowledgements: This work was supported in part by a Grant-in-Aid for Scientific Research on Priority Areas from Ministry of Education, Science and Culture, Japan and a grant from the Takeda Medical Research Foundation, Japan.

REFERENCES

Cheng, J.B. & Shibata, S. (1981): Vascular relaxation in the spontaneously hypertensive rat. J. Cardiovasc. Pharmacol. 3, 1126-1140.

Chung, S.-J. & Fung, H.-L. (1990): Identification of the subcellular site for nitroglycerin metabolism to nitric oxide in bovine coronary smooth muscle cells. J. Pharmacol. Exp. Ther. 253, 614-619

Furchgott, R.F. (1984): The role of endothelium in the responses of vascular smooth muscle to drugs. Annu. Rev. Pharmacol. Toxicol. 24, 175-197.

Kobayashi, Y. and Hattori, K. (1990): Nitroarginine inhibits endothelium-derived relaxation. Jpn. J. Pharmacol. 52, 167-169.

Kobayashi, Y. Ikeda, K., Shinozuka, K., Nara, Y., Yamori, Y. & Hattori, K. (1991): Comparison of vasopressor effects of nitro arginine in stroke-prone spontaneously hypertensive rats and Wistar-Kyoto rats. Clin. Exp. Physiol. Pharmacol. 18, 599-604.

Kobayashi, Y. Ikeda, K., Nara, Y., Shinozuka, K., Hattori, K. & Yamori, Y. (1992): Endothelium-dependent relaxations of isolated ring preparations of the thoracic aorta of aged SHRSR. Jpn. Heart J. 33, (in press)

Mulsch, A. & Busse, R. (1990): N^G-nitro-L-arginine (N^5-(imino(nitroamino)methyl)-L-ornithine) inpairs endothelium-dependent dilations by inhibiting cytosolic nitric oxide synthesis from L-arginine. Naunyn-Schmiedberg's, Archives of Pharmacol. 341, 143-147.

Palmer, R.M.J., Rees, D.D., Ashton, D.S. & Moncada, S. (1988): L-arginine is the physiological precursor for the formation of nitric oxide in endothelium-dependent relaxation. Biochem. Biophys. Res. Commun. 153, 1251-1256

Sunano, S., Osugi, S. & Shimamura, K. (1989): Blood pressure and impairment of endothelium-dependent relaxation in spontaneously hypertensive rats. Experientia 45, 705-708.

Surprising changes in vascular reactivity *in vitro* in pregnant rats

Kingsley Yin, Zhuoming Chu and Lawrie-J Beilin *

University Department of Medicine, Royal Perth Hospital, Perth, WA 6000, Australia
* Author for correspondance

Summary

To examine possible mechanisms of diminished responses to pressor substances in pregnant rats, we have studied vascular reactivity of aortic rings and isolated perfused mesenteric resistance vessels of 13 day pregnant normotensive Wistar-Kyoto rats (WKY) and spontaneously hypertensive rats (SHR).

Systolic blood pressure (SBP) of pregnant WKY was 9 mmHg higher than non-pregnant controls (controls). SBP of pregnant SHR was similar to controls. Aortic rings from pregnant WKY and SHR showed respectively increased responses to noradrenaline (NA) compared to their controls between 30 nM to 30 uM. These increases were still evident in endothelium denuded preparations. Endothelium-dependent relaxations to acetylcholine (ACh) of rings from pregnant WKY were decreased compared to controls. There were no changes in vascular reactivity to NA, ACh and sodium nitroprusside (SNP) in perfused mesenteric resistance vessels.

These results demonstrate there is a difference in vascular reactivity changes in vitro during pregnancy compared with those previously reported in vivo.

Introduction

Diminished pressor responses to NA, angiotensin II (AII) and arginine vasopressin (AVP) have been observed in conscious pregnant rats (Paller et al 1984, Conrad et al 1986). This blunted response could be due to the changes in vascular reactivity. However, variable alterations in vascular reactivity during pregnancy have been reported. In vitro, some workers have claimed that during pregnancy vascular responses to NA to be decreased in perfused rat caudal arteries (Dogterom et al 1974), in aortic rings of guinea pigs (Harrison et al 1989), in rat mesenteric rings (Parent et al 1990), in the isolated perfused mesenteric beds and portal vein strips of rats (Massicotte et al 1987); while others have reported that reactivity to NA were increased in rat aortic rings (Jansakul et al 1989) and in mesenteric veins (Hohmann et al 1990).

Changes in vascular reactivity during pregnancy may be caused by an alteration in the vascular smooth muscle intrinsic constrictor property, and in the balance of endothelial production of dilatory factors such as endothelium-derived relaxing factor (EDRF) and vasoconstrictor products such as endothelin. In this study, we have further investigated the changes in vascular reactivity in aortic rings and isolated perfused mesenteric resistance vessels of normotensive and hypertensive pregnant rats.

Methods

Thirteen day pregnant and age matched non-pregnant (12 W) normotensive WKY and hypertensive SHR were used. SBP was taken by tail-cuff sphymomanometry. Animals were anaesthetized with 0.1 ml/100 g Nembutal (60 mg/ml) administered intraperitoneally. Aortic rings and isolated perfused mesenteric resistance vessels preparations were prepared as describe previously (Yin et al 1991).

Vascular reactivity: Aortic rings were allowed to equilibrate for 1h at 2g tension in Krebs solution, which was maintained at 37º C and bubbled continuously with carbogen (95% O_2, 5% CO_2). Some rings had endothelium removed by rubbing with a cotton probe. After a challenge with twice priming concentrations of 30uM NA, cumulative concentration-effect curves to ACh and SNP were constructed on rings precontracted with prostaglandin F2a to produce a tension of approximately 1.3g. Lastly, concentration-effect curves to NA were constructed. Mesenteric bed preparations were perfused with Krebs solution, which was maintained at 37º C and gassed continuously with carbogen (95% O_2, 5% CO_2) at a flow rate of 4ml/min. After 30 min equilibration the preparations were perfused with 5uM phenylephrine twice to ensure viability. Concentration-effect curves to ACh and SNP were constructed on the vessel beds preconstricted with phenylephrine. Then, concentration-dependent responses to NA were tested, and were repeated after removal of endothelium by perfusion with 0.05% Saponin for 90 seconds

Statistics: All data are express as mean + s.e.m.. The area under the curve was calculated and, using Students' unpaired t-test, p value of less than 0.05 was considered significant.

Results

Blood pressure: Systolic blood pressure (SBP) of pregnant WKY rats (131±3 mmHg; n=23) was higher than nonpregnant controls (122±2 mmHg; n=18:; P<0.05). SBP of pregnant SHR rats (199±2 mmHg, n=8) were similar to non-pregnant rats (197±4 mmHg, n=8).

Vascular reactivity: In Aortic rings the responses to NA were increased in the rings from either pregnant WKY or pregnant SHR rats compared to their non-pregnant controls between 30nM-30uM (P<0.05) (Fig 1). These increases were still evident in endothelium denuded preparations from normotensive WKY rats (P<0.05). In SHR rats, endothelium denuded rings still showed slightly higher NA responses than controls, although the difference was not significant. Endothelium-dependent relaxations to ACh of the rings (precontracted with $PGF_2\alpha$) from pregnant WKY rats were decreased compared to controls (Fig 2). In mesenteric beds there were no differences in responses to ACh, SNP and NA between pregnant and non-pregnant rats in either WKY or SHR rats (data not shown).

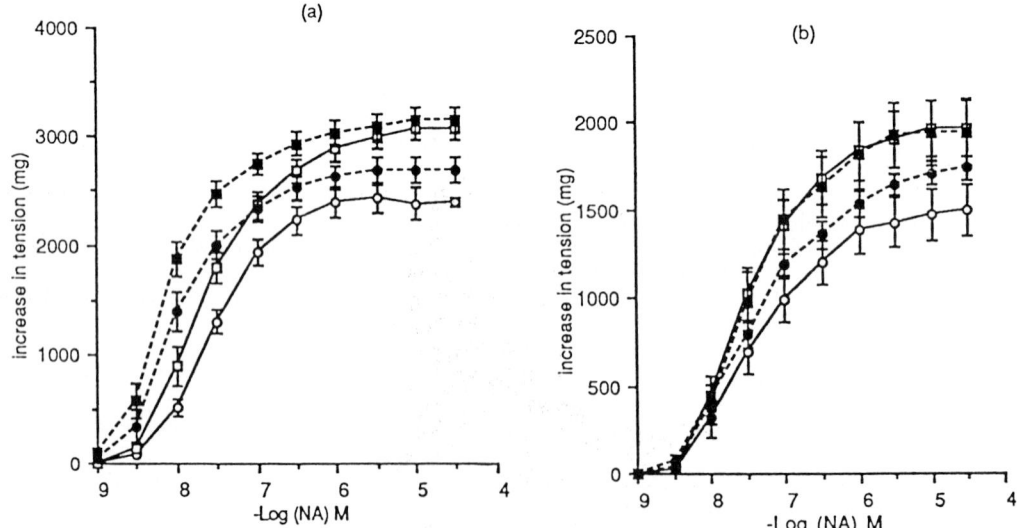

Fig. 1. (a) Cumulative concentration-effect curves in responses to NA of aortic rings from WKY rats. Intact rings from pregnant rats (—□—, n=10) and non-pregnant controls (—O—, n=12). Endothelium denuded rings from pregnant rats (--■--, n=8) and controls (--●--, n=11). (b) Concentration effect curves to NA were constructed on aortic rings from SHR rats. Aortic rings with endothelium from pregnant rats(—□—, n=8) and controls (—O—, n=8). Rings without endothelium from pregnant animals (--■--, n=5) and controls (--●-- , n=6).

Discussion

The present study confirmed previous reported that the vascular reactivity to NA was increased in aortic rings during pregnancy in the rats. This increase was still evident in endothelium denuded preparations (Jansakul et al 1989). It is not clear why reactivity to NA should be increased in vitro, but apparently decreased in vivo. This would suggested that the changes in vivo are dependent on a circulating vasoactive substance(s) and removal from this dilatory influence in vitro is associated with heightened reactivity.

In pregnant rats endothelium-dependent relaxations to ACh have been reported to be increased in aortic rings precontracted with U46619, and to be unchanged in rings preconstricted with NA or phenylephrine (Jansakul et al 1989). In contrast, our results indicated that ACh induced relaxations were decreased in the rings precontracted with $PGF_{2\alpha}$ from pregnant WKY rats while the rings from hypertensive SHR rats showed no differences in ACh responses between pregnant and controls. The mechanism by which endothelium-dependent relaxation to ACh is affected by the use of different preconstrictor substance still needs to be elucidated.

Our results demonstrated that there were no changes in vascular reactivity to NA in perfused mesenteric resistance vessels in 13 day pregnant rats. This contrasts with previous reports that sensitivity to NA is

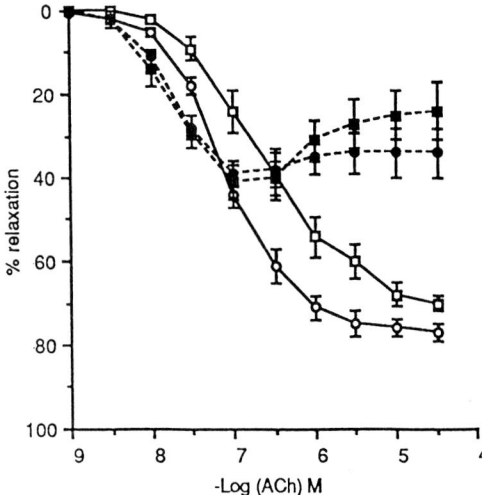

Fig.2. Endothelium-dependent relaxation to ACh of aortae from pregnant WKY rats (—□—, n=12) was significant decreased compared to controls (—O—, n=14, p<0.05). In contrast, ACh induced relaxation of aortae from pregnant SHR rats (--■--, n=8) was similar to controls (--●--, n=8)

decreased in isolated perfused mesenteric beds and mesenteric rings of 21 day pregnant rats (Massicotte et al 1987, Parent et al 1990). These could be due to the different term in pregnancy. Current work on in-situ blood perfused mesenteric bed of pregnant rats in our laboratory have showed that vascular reactivity to NA and AII were decreased in pregnant WKY rats (unpublished results). We speculate the surprising changes seen in vitro may be caused by removal from a circulating dilatory factor originating from the uterus or placenta.

References

Conrad, K.P. and Colpoys, M.C. (1986): Evidence against the hypothesis that prostaglandins are the vasodepressor agent of pregnancy. J. Clin. Invest. **77**: 236-245.

Dogterom, J and De Jong, W. (1974): Diminished pressor response to noradrenaline of perfused tail artery of pregnant rat. Eur. J. Pharmacol. **25**: 267-269.

Harrison, G.L. and Moore, L.G. (1989): Blunted vasoreactivity in pregnant guinea pigs is not restored by meclofenamate. Am. J. Obstet. Gynecol. **160**: 258-264.

Hohmann, M., Keve, T.M., Osol, G. and McLaughlin, M.K. (1990): Noradrenaline sensitivity of mesenteric veins in pregnant rats. Am. J. Physiol. **259**: R753-759.

Jansakul, C., Boura, A.L.A. and King, R.G. (1989): Constrictor and dilator responses of endothelium-intact and denuded aortae of pregnant rat. J. Aut. Pharmacol. **9**: 93-101.

Massicotte, G., St-Louis, J., Parent, A. and Schiffrin, E.L. (1987): Decreased in vitro responses to vasoconstrictors during gestation in normotensive and spontaneously hypertensive rats. Can. J. Physiol. Pharmacol. **65**: 2466-2471.

Paller, M.S. (1984): Mechanism of decreased pressor responses to ANG II, NE, and vasopressin in pregnant rat. Am. J. Physiol. **247**: H100-108.

Parent, A., Schiffrin, E.L. and Jean, S.-L. (1990): Role of the endothelium in adrenergic responses of mesenteric rings of pregnant rats. Am J Obstet Gynecol. **163**: 229-34.

Yin, K., Chu, Z.M. and Beilin, L.J. (1991): Blood pressure and vascular reactivity changes in spontaneously hypertensive rats fed fish oil. Br. J. Pharmacol. **102**: 991-997

This work was supported by the National Heart Foundation of Australia, the Royal Perth Hospital Research Foundation and the National Health & Medical Research Council of Australia.

Neural mechanisms
Mécanismes nerveux

Comparison of cardiovascular responses to stimulation of carotid sinus and aortic depressor nerves in rats

Hisashi Ohta, Stephen J. Lewis * and William T. Talman

Department of Neurology and Pharmacology *, The University of Iowa and VA Medical Center, Iowa City, IA 52242, USA

INTRODUCTION

Baroreceptors in the aortic arch and carotid sinus sense changes in arterial pressure and participate in maintaining cardiovascular homeostasis. Signals from these baroreceptors enter the central nervous system via the aortic depressor nerve (ADN), a branch of the vagus, and the carotid sinus nerve (CSN), a branch of the glossopharyngeal nerve. Both nerves terminate in the nucleus tractus solitarii (Ciriello, 1983; Kalia and Sullivan, 1982). Electrical stimulation of ADN often has been used to study baroreflex function in rats. Such stimulation produces cardiovascular responses similar to those seen with activation of the baroreflex (Kubo and Kihara, 1988; Sapru et. al., 1981). Although rats have frequently been used to study both the peripheral and central components of the baroreflex, no study has reported the cardiovascular responses to electrical stimulation of CSN in rats. Probably the absence of such reports is because the approach to the CSN in rat is technically difficult (McDonald, 1983a). The present study was, therefore, designed to stimulate CSN to evaluate its role in mediating the baroreflex in anesthetized rats.

METHODS AND MATERIALS

Ten male Sprague Dawley rats (Sasco, Omaha, NE) weighing 250-370g were used in these experiments. Under halothane anesthesia, the trachea was cannulated through the mouth and a femoral artery and vein were cannulated for recording arterial pressure and administering drugs respectively. Halothane was discontinued and anesthesia maintained with alpha-chloralose. Body temperature was maintained by heating lamp. The rat's head was fixed in a stereotaxic apparatus (David Kopf, Tujunga, CA), and the animal and stereotaxic apparatus were vertically rotated 70-80° to facilitate approaching the CSN and ADN from the lateral side of the neck.

Either the ADN or the CSN was stimulated in each rat. The nerves, carefully isolated from surrounding tissue, were placed over bipolar platinum-iridium electrodes and the connection covered with SilGel (Wacker, Munchen, Germany). Stimuli consisted of trains of positive, rectangular pulses delivered for 20 sec. (Other stimulation parameters are mentioned in results.) Inspiratory and expiratory movement of the chest, and thus respiratory rate, was measured by a force displacement transducer.

All data were expressed as mean ± S.E.M. Data were analyzed by repeated measures ANOVA with post hoc analysis done by t-test with Bonferroni's correction. p<0.05 was considered significant.

RESULTS

Cardiovascular Responses

Electrical stimulation of CSN in 6 rats increased respiratory rate and elicited initial pressor responses followed by depressor and bradycardiac responses. The depressor, bradycardiac responses were current (50-200 μA) and frequency (5-100 Hz) dependent. In 4 rats ADN stimulation elicited depressor, bradycardiac responses that also were current (50-200 μA) and frequency (2-50 Hz) dependent. However, the depressor (-18 ± 2 mmHg) and bradycardiac (-16 ± 2 bpm) responses to CSN stimulation were significantly different from those (-32 ± 4 mmHg and -48 ± 5 bpm) elicited by ADN stimulation at the same stimulus parameters (100 μA, 20 Hz, 2 msec).

When ipsilateral ADN was cut at least 30 min before stimulation of CSN, depressor and bradycardiac responses induced by activation of CSN were potentiated (-28 ± 2 mmHg and -23 ± 3 bpm vs. -37 ± 2 mmHg and -43 ± 6 bpm at 200 μA, 20 Hz, 2 msec). In contrast, cardiovascular responses induced by ADN stimulation were not affected by interruption of the CSN.

Respiratory Responses

Stimulation of CSN produced increases in respiratory rate during stimulation, even at low frequencies and intensities of stimulation that did not affect cardiovascular parameters. Stimulation of ADN produced no significant change in respiratory rate, but at high frequencies (50-100 Hz), respiratory depression tended to develop.

Removal of ipsilateral ADN tended to attenuate increases in respiratory rate induced by stimulation of CSN, but ablation of CSN did not affect the minimal changes in respiratory rate elicited by stimulation of ADN.

DISCUSSION

The present study demonstrates that stimulation of CSN elicits depressor and bradycardiac responses that are qualitatively similar, though of different magnitude, to those produced by ADN stimulation. Stimulation of CSN also produces transient pressor responses before the depressor response, and it increases respiratory rate during the entire period of stimulation. ADN stimulation does not significantly change respiratory rate, although high frequencies of stimulation tend to slightly decrease it. Anatomically ADN and CSN have both baro- and chemoreceptor afferents (Coleridge and Coleridge, 1979; McDonald, 1983a, 1983b), however as previously reported (Sapru and Krieger, 1977; Sapru et. al., 1981), the presence of functional chemoreceptor afferents in ADN was not supported by electrical stimulation of ADN. The present results suggest that depressor and bradycardiac responses induced by stimulation of CSN and ADN are due to activation of baroafferents and that transient pressor responses and increases in respiratory rate elicited by stimulation of CSN are due to activation of chemoreceptor afferents.

Denervation of ADN facilitates cardiovascular responses induced by activation of ipsilateral CSN but attenuates increases in respiratory rate. These results suggest that ADN and CSN have some interaction and that activity of ADN under normal conditions tends to inhibit CSN-mediated baroreflex responses and facilitate CSN-mediated chemoreflexes. It is known that activation of chemoreceptor afferents inhibits the baroreflex. Thus, electrical stimulation of CSN, by activating chemoreceptor afferents within

CSN, may to some extent inhibit CSN contributions to baroreflex responses. Removal of ADN may overcome this inhibition by removing its augmenting influence on the CSN mediated chemoreflex. In addition removal of ADN may remove a negative influence on central neurons that receive afferents from both the ADN and CSN (Mifflin & Felder, 1988); or, at similar neurons, it may lead to receptor upregulation and denervation supersensitivity to CSN stimulation. At the moment, the actual mechanisms underlying facilitation of cardiovascular responses to stimulation of CSN by removal of ADN are not known.

In conclusion, we demonstrate that stimulation of CSN in rat produces activation of both the baro- and chemoreflex and that ADN and CSN interact.

REFERENCES

Ciriello, J. (1983): Brainstem projections of aortic baroreceptor afferent fibers in the rat. Neurosci. Lett. 36, 37-42.

Coleridge, J.C.G., and Coleridge, H.M. (1974): Chemoreflex regulation of the heart. In: Handbook of Physiology, Sect. 2: The Cardiovascular System, vol. 1, The Heart, edited by R.M. Berne, N. Sperelakis, and S.R. Geiger, Bethesda, Maryland. Am. Physiol. Soc. pp:653-676.

Kalia, M. and Sullivan, J.M. (1982): Brainstem projections of sensory and motor components of the vagus nerve in the rat. J. Comp. Neruol. 211, 248-264.

Kubo, T. and Kihara, M. (1988): Evidence of N-methyl-D-aspartate receptor-mediated modulation of the aortic baroreceptor reflex in the rat nucleus tractus solitarii. Neurosci. Lett. 87, 69-74.

McDonald, D.M. (1983a): Morphology of the rat carotid sinus nerve. I. Course, connections, dimensions and ultrastructure. J. Neurocytol. 12, 345-372.

McDonald, D.M. (1983b): Morphology of the rat carotid sinus nerve. II. Number and size of axons. J. Neurocytol. 12, 373-392.

Mifflin, S.W. and Felder, R.B. (1988): An intracellular study of time-dependent cardiovascular afferent interactions in nucleus tractus solitarius. J. Neurophysiol. 59:1798-1813.

Sapru, H.N., Gonzalez, E. and Krieger, A.J. (1981): Aortic nerve stimulation in the rat: Cardiovascular and respiratory responses. Brain Res. Bull. 6, 393-398.

Sapru, H.N. and Krieger, A.J. (1977): Carotid and aortic chemoreceptor function in the rat. J. Appl. Physiol. 42, 344-348.

The magnitude of rapid resetting of the baroreceptors is attenuated in spontaneously hypertensive rats

Fumio Ida, Edson D. Moreira, Vera L.L. Oliveira and Eduardo M. Krieger

Hypertension Unit, Heart Institute, Faculty of Medicine, University of São Paulo, São Paulo, Brazil

Several lines of evidence (see Krieger, 1989) indicate that, during onset and maintenance of hypertension in the rat, there are two distinct phases of baroreceptor resetting: phase 1, a rapid or acute resetting (i.e., a partial resetting of approximately 40% that reaches its maximum within the first few minutes and remains relatively constant up to 6 hours) and phase 2, a complete resetting (100%) when the displacement of the pressure threshold for activation of the baroreceptors matches the total pressure rise, which closely coincides with the 2 day period taken for the aorta to achieve maximal dilation. A resetting of 26% was already observed 2 minutes after onset of hypertension produced by phenylephrine infusion in rats in vivo and maximal resetting (43%) was observed after 20 minutes (Moreira et al, 1988). In renal hypertensive rats (RHR) the characteristics and extent of rapid resetting of baroreceptors, which were completely reset to operate at the hypertensive levels, were similar to those of the normotensive control rats (NCR) (Moreira et al 1990). The acute resetting of the entire baroreflex control of lumbar sympathetic activity was also normal in RHR (Heesch and Carey, 1987). Magnitude of rapid resetting in spontaneously hypertensive rats (SHR) was found to be equivalent to that of NCR in studies using an aortic arch-aortic nerve preparation in vitro (Andresen and Yang, 1989a). Since the ability of the baroreceptors to rapidly reset is regarded as a useful mechanism, providing the baroreceptors to operate around a floating set point, the present experiment was undertaken to study the extent of acute resetting in SHR in vivo, within the first 30 minutes of hypertension produced by phenylephrine infusion.

Direct MAP of 9 SHR and of 14 NCR measured in conscious state was 183±4 mmHg and 116±3mmHg, respectively. The level of pentobarbital anesthesia was adjusted to maintain the AP at the same values existing in conscious state before recording the first baroreceptor function curve at the control period. Thereafter, infusion of phenylephrine (2-4 μg/Kg/min) into the femoral vein was adjusted to produce a constant rise of approximately 40 mmHg in MAP during a 30-minute period. Measurements of the baroreceptor function curves were repeated 2, 5, 10, 20 and 30 minutes after the beginning of the pressure rise. Whole nerve activity of the aortic baroreceptors was measured during rapid (10-15 seconds) changes of pressure produced by withdrawal and infusion of blood into the femoral artery (for details see Moreira et al, 1990). Arterial pressure (carotid artery) and aortic baroreceptor activity were continuously monitored on an oscilloscope and recorded on a tape recorder to study the pressure-nerve activity relation on a beat-to-beat basis by computer. The extent of resetting was calculated by the ratio of mean threshold pressure changes divided by total mean pressure changes (Δ MAPth/ Δ MAP x 100).

In the NCR the extent of acute resetting was 26, 29, 32, 37 and 45% after 2, 5, 10 and 30 minutes of phenylephrine infusion, respectively. The extent of acute resetting during the additional 30 minute period of pressure rise in SHR was smaller than in NCR, in average it was only 55% (42, 58, 50, 73 and 51% after 2, 5, 10, 20 and 30 minutes, respectively). Data of Fig. 1 illustrated the smaller extent of acute resetting produced by phenylephrine infusion in SHR when compared with NCR and when compared with RHR, in which the extent and characteristics of acute resetting are similar to those of NCR, as previously described (Moreira et al 1990).

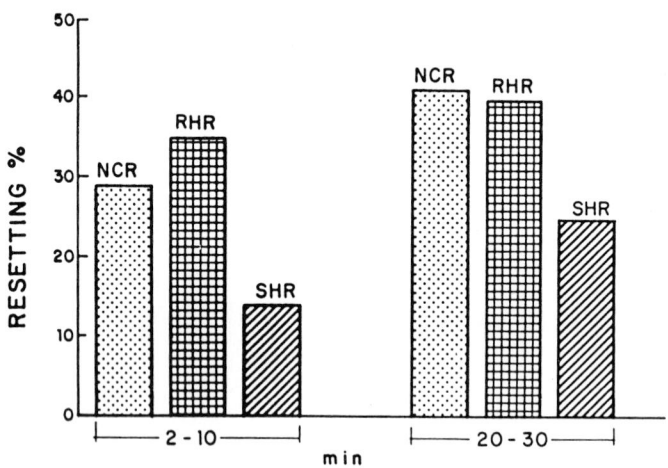

Figure 1. Attenuation in the extent (%) of rapid resetting of the aortic baroreceptor of spontaneously hypertensive rats (SHR) when compared to normotensive control rats (NCR) and renal hypertensive rats (RHR). MAP was increased by approximately 40 mmHg during 30 minutes by phenylephrine infusion. Average values after 2-10 and 20-30 minutes, respectively.

At the control period the systolic pressure threshold (146±15 mmHg) for activation of the baroreceptor in the SHR was slightly but not significantly different to the control diastolic pressure (159±12 mmHg), indicating that the baroreceptors were completely reset to operate at the hypertensive levels exhibited by the rats (see Krieger, 1989). Similar complete resetting was observed previously in the RHR (Moreira et al 1990). However, whereas in the RHR the extent and characteristics of acute resetting were similar to those of NCR in the SHR the extent was only half the magnitude of NCR. Rapid resetting in normotensive animals has been attributed to a slight viscoelastic relaxation of the arterial wall with progressive lengthening of viscoses elements that results in decreased force exerted on the baroreceptors (Coleridge et al 1984). Ionic alteration and alteration of the receptor ending itself has been also suggested as responsible for rapid resetting (Andresen and Yang, 1989b; Chapleau et al, 1989 and Korner, 1989). According to Andresen and Yang (1989a) the fact that the magnitude of acute resetting is equivalent for baroreceptors of rats with a wide range of aortic distensibilities favors a nonmechanical explanation for the process of rapid resetting. We found that conscious unrestrained RHR, which exhibited normal rapid resetting, had also normal dynamic distensibility of the aorta in spite of the fact that the aorta was 20% larger and pulsation was twice as great as in NCR (Michelini and Krieger, 1981). Further studies are necessary to correlate the stress/strain relationship of the aorta in freely moving SHR with the degree of acute resetting presently observed. Finally it should be mentioned that the attenuation in the extent of acute resetting of the baroreceptors of SHR may impair its ability to buffer the AP fluctuations in short-term changes of AP.

REFERENCES

Andresen, M.C. & Yang, M. (1989a): Rapid baroreceptor resetting is unaltered by chronic hypertension in rats. Am. J. Physiol. 1989; 256(Heart Circ Physiol), H-1228-H-1235
Andresen, M. C. & Yang, M. (1989b): Arterial baroreceptor resetting contributions of chronic and acute processes. Clin. Exp. Pharmacol. Physiol. 15 (Suppl), 19-30.

Chapleau, M. W.; Hajduczok, G. & Abboud, F. M. (1989): Peripheral and central mechanisms of baroreflex resetting. *Clin. Exp. Pharmacol. Physiol.* 15 (Suppl), 31-43.

Coleridge, H. M.; Coleridge, J. C. G.; Poore, E. R.; Roberts, H. M. & Schultz, H. D. (1984): Aortic wall properties and baroreceptor behavior at normal arterial pressure and in acute hypertensive resetting in dogs. *J. Physiol.* 350, 309-326.

Heesch, C. M. & Carey, L. A. (1987): Acute resetting of arterial baroreflexes in hypertensive rats. *Am. J. Physiol.* 253 (*Heart Circ. Physiol.* 22), H-974-H-979.

Korner, P. I. (1989): Baroreceptor resetting and other determinants of baroreflex properties in hypertension. *Clin. Exp. Pharmacol. Physiol.* 15 (Suppl), 45-64.

Krieger, E. M. (1989): Arterial baroreceptor resetting in hypertension. *Clin. Exp. Pharmacol. Physiol.* 15 (Suppl), 3-17.

Michelini, L. C. & Krieger, E. M. (1981): Mechanoelastic properties of the aorta in chronically hypertensive conscious rats. *Hypertension 3* (Suppl II), II-177-II-182.

Moreira, E. D.; Ida, F. & Krieger, E. M. (1988): Characteristics and extent of rapid aortic baroreceptor resetting in rat. *Am. J. Med. Sci.* 295, 335-340.

Moreira, E. D.; Ida, F.; Oliveira, V. L. L. & Krieger, E. M. (1990): Rapid resetting of the baroreceptors in renal hypertensive rats. *Hypertension* 15 (Suppl I), I-40-I-44.

Acknowledgments:

Research supported by grants from Conselho Nacional de Desenvolvimento Científico e Tecnológico (CNPq), Fundação de Amparo à Pesquisa do Estado de São Paulo (FAPESP) and Fundação E.J. Zerbini.

Effect of perindopril on the cardiac baroreflex in conscious spontaneously hypertensive (SHR) and stroke prone hypertensive rats (SHRSP)

Naoyoshi Minami and Geoffrey A. Head

Baker Medical Research Institute, Prahran, Victoria, 3181, Australia

SUMMARY

The present study examined the effect of 6 weeks of antihypertensive therapy with the ACE inhibitor perindopril on the baroreceptor control of heart rate in adult spontaneously hypertensive rats (SHR), stroke prone hypertensive rats (SHRSP) and normotensive Wistar Kyoto (WKY) rats. Steady state sigmoidal mean arterial pressure (MAP)–heart rate (HR) reflex curves were obtained for each conscious rat by injection of pressor and depressor agents before and after i.v. atenolol (= vagal component). MAP in SHR and SHRSP was 40% and 50% higher respectively than that of WKY while left ventricle to body weight ratio (LV/BW) was 24% and 40% greater. The vagal HR range of the MAP–HR baroreflex of SHR and SHRSP was 40% less than that of WKY. Perindopril–treated SHR were normotensive with little cardiac hypertrophy remaining. Vagal HR range was increased to be within 13% of WKY. In SHRSP, perindopril treatment was more effective in reducing cardiac hypertrophy than MAP (LV/BW 11% and MAP 28% greater than WKY). Nevertheless, the increase in the vagal HR range was only slightly less than that observed in treated SHR (19% less than WKY). These results show that treatment of adult SHR with perindopril reversed hypertension and cardiac hypertrophy and virtually restored baroreflex function. The findings with SHRSP suggest that reversal of cardiac hypertrophy was important for restoring the cardiac vagal baroreflex responsiveness.

INTRODUCTION

It is well established that hypertension results in resetting and a reduction in slope of the baroreceptor–heart rate reflex (Korner 1989). Using the steady state technique we have found that the reduced gain in SHR was due to a reduction in the HR range rather than a change in the curvature of the MAP–HR relationship (Head & Adams 1988). This was due to a lesser bradycardic plateau in response to a rise in MAP. The cardiac sympathetic response in SHR was similar to WKY suggesting that the major deficit lay in the vagal component of the reflex, namely a reduced vagal HR range. Cheng et al (1989) found that lifetime treatment of SHR with a converting enzyme inhibitor restored cardiac baroreflex function of SHR. The purpose of the present study was to examine whether a relatively short 6 week antihypertensive treatment with the ACE inhibitor perindopril of SHR and SHRSP could reverse these changes in the cardiac baroreflex. We were also interested in whether there was any relationship between the changes to the baroreceptor heart rate reflex and the reduction in cardiac hypertrophy.

METHODS

Age- and weight-matched male WKY, SHR and SHRSP were non-treated or treated with perindopril (3 mg/kg per day) in the drinking water from 14 to 20 weeks of age. At 21 weeks, i.e. 1 week after stopping treatment, all rats were implanted with arterial and venous catheters. Experiments were performed in conscious animals 1 week later. MAP was measured by a Statham transducer and HR was determined from a period meter. Steady-state MAP-HR curves were produced by intravenous injections of methoxamine and nitroprusside (Head & McCarty 1987). The vagal component was assessed in the presence of atenolol. The steady-state changes in MAP and the HR were fitted to a sigmoidal logistic equation. The LV/BW (mg:g) was determined at the end of the study. Data was analysed by 1 way analysis of variance with comparisons determined by orthogonal partitioning of between treatment sums of squares.

RESULTS

MAP of SHRSP was 11 mmHg higher than that of SHR ($P<0.001$) which was 46 mmHg higher than that of WKY (115 ± 3 mmHg in WKY, $P<0.001$). In addition the HR of the hypertensive rats was higher than WKY, particularly that of SHR (340 ± 11 in SHR, 286 ± 9 in WKY, $P<0.001$). LV/BW was +24% and +40% higher in SHR and SHRSP respectively compared to the value of 2.2 ± 0.1 mg/g in WKY. Baroreflex curves of hypertensive strains were located to the right of the WKY, in line with the higher basal MAP. The vagal HR range of the MAP-HR baroreflex of SHR and SHRSP were both 40% less than that of WKY due to lesser bradycardia in response to a rise in pressure (127, 77 and 75 b/min in WKY, SHR and SHRSP respectively, SEM = 9, F 1,39 = 18, d.f. = 39, $P<0.001$). Gain of the vagal curves was also reduced as a result of the diminished range in the hypertensive animals (−2.0, −1.3 and −1.0 b/min/mmHg in WKY, SHR and SHRSP respectively, SEM = 0.18, F 1,39 = 16, d.f. = 39, $P<0.001$).
Perindopril reduced basal blood pressure in SHR by 40 mmHg ($p<0.001$) but only by 25 mmHg in SHRSP ($P<0.01$). There was also a 20 mmHg reduction in MAP in WKY ($P<0.05$). LV/BW of SHR was reduced from 124% to 102% of WKY ($p<0.001$) and that of SHRSP from 140% to 111% of WKY. Perindopril did not affect the LV/BW ratio of WKY. In all cases perindopril shifted the baroreflex curves left ward in accordance with the effects on MAP. In addition vagal heart rate range increased in SHR from 61% to 87% of the WKY value and in SHRSP from 60% to 82% of WKY ($P<0.05$). Treatment abolished the differences between gain of the WKY and the hypertensive strains. There were no significant effects of perindopril on the vagal baroreflex gain or HR range of the WKY.

DISCUSSION

The main finding of the current study was that treatment of adult hypertensive rats with perindopril for a relatively short 6 week period markedly improved the baroreceptor-heart rate reflex properties. While the HR range was still somewhat less than that of WKY, the gain (slope) of the vagal component of the baroreflex was similar to that of the WKY. A small improvement in the cardiac baroreflex gain was observed with 3 weeks of urapidil treatment in SHR (Kobrin et al 1986) but otherwise treatments have been for very long periods and in young animals (Cheng et al 1989, Howe 1989). We believe that this is the first study that has examined the baroreflex after a considerable withdrawal period so as to eliminate any acute effects of the drug on the baroreflex itself. Thus we could be confident that the changes to the baroreflex were a consequence of the earlier antihypertensive treatment rather than an acute pharmacological effect of the drug itself.
From the present results it can be seen that the improvement in the baroreflex was not simply related to the lowering of blood pressure, but was more closely related to the reduction in cardiac hypertrophy. In treated SHRSP the increase in the vagal HR range was only slightly less than that observed in treated SHR (38% compared to 43 %) for about half the reduction in MAP (14% compared to 25%). By contrast there was a similar reduction in cardiac

hypertrophy of 17% in SHR and 21% in SHRSP. Another interesting point that emerges from the effects of perindopril in SHRSP was that the cardiac hypertrophy appears to be more readily reversed than the hypertension. In conclusion these results show that treatment of adult SHR with perindopril reversed hypertension and cardiac hypertrophy and virtually restored cardiac baroreflex function. The findings with SHRSP suggest an important role of cardiac hypertrophy in this process.

REFERENCES

Cheng, S.W.T., Swords, B.H., Kirk, K.A. & Berecek, K.H., (1989): Baroreflex function in lifetime–captopril–treated spontaneously hypertensive rats. *Hypertension* 13, 63–69.

Head, G.A. & Adams, M.A., (1988): Time course of changes in baroreceptor reflex control of heart rate in conscious SHR and WKY: Contribution of the cardiac vagus and sympathetic nerves. *Clin. Exp. Pharmacol. Physiol.* 15, 289–292.

Head, G.A. & McCarty, R., (1987): Vagal and sympathetic components of the heart rate range and gain of the baroreceptor–heart rate reflex in conscious rats. *J. Auton. Nerv. Syst.* 21, 203–213.

Howe, P., (1989): Effects of chronic enalapril treatment on plasma catecholamines, vasopressor sensitivity and baroreflex function in stroke–prone spontaneously hypertensive rats. In *Current Advances in ACE inhibition. Proceedings of an International Symposium.* ed. G.A. MacGregor & P.S. Sever, pp. 275–278. London: Churchill Livingstone.

Kobrin, I., Pegram, B.L. & Frohlich, E.D., (1986): Baroreflex control of heart rate after immediate and prolonged reduction with urapidil in conscious normotensive and spontaneously hypertensive rats. *Israel J. Med. Sci.*, 22, 438–441.

Korner, P.I., (1989): Baroreceptor resetting and other determinants of baroreflex properties in hypertension. *Clin. Exp. Physiol. Pharmacol.*, 15, 45–64.

ACKNOWLEDGEMENTS

This work was supported by a grant from the Servier Institute for International Research, France and by a block institute grant from the National Health and Medical Research Council of Australia.

Interplay of sympathetic and parasympathetic mechanisms in the control of blood pressure variability in conscious, spontaneously-behaving SHR and WKY rats

Alberto U. Ferrari, Anna Daffonchio and C. Franzelli

Centro di Fisiologia Clinica e Ipertensione, Semeiotica Medica e Clinica Medica, CNR, Università di Milano ed Ospedale Maggiore, Milano, Italy

Understanding of the autonomic mechanisms controlling blood pressure variability is incomplete: for example, the sympathetic nervous system is known to promote large blood pressure variations under mentally or physically stressful conditions (Mancia et al., 1983; Littler et al., 1978), but whether it also tends to enhance blood pressure variability in the absence of any excitatory stimuli is unknown. A further controversial point concerns the role of the parasympathetic system, which can also affect blood pressure variability by mediating rapid changes in heart rate and hence in cardiac output (Clement et al., 1984; Ferrari et al., 1987; Anderson et al., 1979). Finally, it is also not established whether and to what extent hypertension modifies blood pressure variability control. The aim of this study was therefore to assess the effects on blood pressure variability of interfering with sympathetic and parasympathetic influences in conscious undisturbed rats, the former influences being removed by means of chemical sympathectomy and the latter by cholinerigc blockade. The experiments were carried out in groups of normotensive Wistar-Kyoto rats as well as of spontaneously hypertensive rats.

METHODS

Injections of 6-hydroxydopamine (150 mg/kg i.p.) or vehicle alone were administered every 2-3 days for 1 week in a total of 41 Wistar-Kyoto and spontaneously hypertensive rats aged 10 to 12 weeks. Each animal was chronically instrumented by an arterial and a venous femoral catheter, which were periodically flushed by a 0.5% heparin solution. The rat was placed in a wide individual cage where it could freely move, explore, eat and drink, care being taken to minimize any environmental disturbances including noise. After a 24 hour recovery time, blood pressure was measured by connecting the arterial catheter to a Statham P23Dc transducer, heart rate being also recorded by tachographic conversion of the pulsatile pressure signal. Both variables were continuously displayed on an ink-writing Grass 7D polygraph (Quincy, MA, USA). Prior to the assessment of variability, the effectiveness of sympathectomy was evaluated from the pressor and tachycardic response to an iv bolus injection of tyramine, 100 ug/kg. After a 30 min interval the blood pressure signal was recorded continuously for 90 min and stored on a tape recorder (Racal Store 4, Southampton, UK) for subsequent computer analysis. A second blood pressure recording session was performed under vagal blockade by atropine, 0.75 mg/kg i.v. every 30 min. On each recording blood pressure variability was calculated via a beat-to-beat computer scanning procedure as the percent variation coefficient (standard deviation : mean x 100). The same technique was used to assess the variability of heart rate that was computed by reciprocating the pulse interval. Statistical comparisons were performed by the paired or unpaired t test complemented by the Bonferroni correction for multiple comparisons.

RESULTS

Baseline hemodynamic data. In sympathectomized rats the pressor and tachycardic responses to i.v. tyramine were reduced by at least 85% as compared to the control rats. The former animals had moderately lower mean arterial pressure than the latter, the difference reaching statistical significance in the Wistar-Kyoto (96.2±3.9 vs 118.8±3.0 mmHg, means±SEM, $p<0.05$) but not in the spontaneously hypertensive rats (120.7±4.6 vs 132.9±3.6 mmHg, p=ns). On the other hand, no significant sympathectomy-related changes in heart rate were observed. In both the Wistar-Kyoto and in the spontaneously hypertensive rats atropine injection failed to alter mean arterial pressure and significantly increased heart rate, the latter effect, however, being only observed in the control and not in the sympathectomized groups.

Blood pressure and heart rate variabilities. These data are summarized in Table 1 as percent variation coefficients: in both rat strains the variability of mean arterial pressure was much larger in the sympathectomized than in the control groups, whereas a concurrent sympathectomy-related increase in heart rate variability was observed in spontaneously hypertensive but not in Wistar-Kyoto rats. In both rat strains vagal blockade by atropine caused, as expected, a reduction in heart rate variability: the concurrent effects of vagal blockade on blood pressure variability consisted of insignificant changes in the control animals but of a further significant increase in the sympathectomized ones.

Table 1. Variation coefficients (means±SEM) of mean arterial pressure (VC-BP) and of heart rate (VC-HR) in conscious Wistar-Kyoto (WKY) and spontaneously hypertensive (SHR) rats pretreated with vehicle (Veh) or 6-hydroxydopamine (Sx) and examined in the basal condition (BAS) as well as after vagal blockade by atropine (ATR).

Rat Groups		Veh-WKY	Sx-WKY	Veh-SHR	Sx-SHR
VC-BP(%)	BAS	4.1±0.4	6.6±0.6*	3.6±0.2	6.7±0.8*
	ATR	4.5±0.4	9.7±0.7*#	3.9±0.2	8.6±1.0*#
VC-HR(%)	BAS	4.8±0.3	3.9±0.5	4.6±0.4	6.3±0.9&
	ATR	2.6±0.2#	2.7±0.4#	3.7±0.3	5.5±1.5&

[$p<0.05$: *, Sx vs Veh; #, ATR vs BAS; &, SHR vs WKY]

DISCUSSION

Our study provides new information on the way autonomic mechanisms operate and interact in the control of blood pressure variability. First, concerning the role of the sympathetic nervous system, our data suggest that this may be disparate according to different states of activation of the system: although a high sympathetic tone may contribute to enhance blood pressure variability, an opposite effect, namely a blood pressure stabilization, may take over under conditions of low sympathetic tone such as those of our undisturbed, spontaneously-behaving rats. Second, the further increase in blood pressure variability observed after cholinergic blockade indicates that also parasympathetic influences, presumably through the modulation of heart rate, have the potential to play a stabilizing role on blood pressure. This was well evident in the sympathectomized rats, although previous evidence suggests that this phenomenon can even occur in rats with an intact sympathetic nervous system (Ferrari et al., 1987): indeed, a trend in this direction was also observed in the vehicle-treated rats of the present study. The hemodynamic mechanisms underlying this phenomenon may relate to the ability of rapid, vagally-mediated changes in heart rate and hence in cardiac output to partially offset the blood pressure variations that would accompany the changes in total peripheral resistance. The latter may be particularly pronounced after sympathectomy, i.e. when an effective noradrenergic control of small resistance arterioles is lacking, but may also be sizeable in sympathetically intact, spontaneously-behaving individuals in relation to the moment-to-moment changes in regional vasomotor tone originating from humoral and/or metabolic factors. Third, no substantial differences in the way sympathetic and parasympathetic mechanisms control blood pressure variability were observed between Wistar-Kyoto and spontaneously hypertensive rats, further suggesting that in hypertension the moment-to-moment regulation of the cardiovascular system works normally although being "set" to maintain higher than normal blood pressure levels.

REFERENCES

Anderson DE, Yingling JE, Sagawa K. Minute-to-minute covariations in cardiovascular activity in conscious dogs (1979). Am J Physiol 236:H434-H439.

Clement DL, Jordaens LJ, Heindrickx P (1984). Influence of vagal nervous activity on blood pressure variability. J Hypertension 2(Suppl. 3):s391-s393.

Ferrari AU, Daffonchio A, Albergati F, Mancia G. Inverse relationship between heart rate and blood pressure variabilities in rats (1987). Hypertension 10:533-537.

Littler W, West MJ, Honour AJ, Sleight P (1978). The variability of arterial pressure. Am Heart J 95:180-186.

Mancia G, Ferrari A, Gregorini L, Parati G, Pomidossi G, Bertinieri G, Grassi G, Di Riezo M, Pedotti A and Zanchetti A (1983). Blood pressure and heart rate variabilities in normotensive and hypertensive human beings. Circ Res 53:96-104.

Chronic hyperinsulinemia induces hypertension in rats

Wann-Chu Huang, Po-Shiuan Hsieh and Jong-Shiaw Jin

Department of Physiology and Biophysics, National Defense Medical Center, Taipei, Taiwan, Republic of China

INTRODUCTION

Insulin resistance and/or hyperinsulinemia has been suggested to be intimately associated with the development of hypertension in humans and animals (Hwang et al., 1987; Reaven, 1990). However, the precise mechanism is unclear. Some studies demonstrated that insulin could stimulate renal reabsorption of sodium and sympathetic nervous system (DeFronzo et al., 1975; Baun, 1987; Landsberg, 1990). Thus acute hyperinsulinemia may exert a pressor effect by modification of plasma volume and/or sympathetic nerve activity. The current study was performed to evaluate if chronic hyperinsulinemia could increase blood pressure (BP), and if the kidney and sympathetic nervous system involve in the development of this form of hypertension.

MATERIALS AND METHODS

Male Sprague-Dawley rats initially weighing 250-300 g were housed individually in metabolism cage, fed control sodium diet (Teklad Labs, Madison, WI, USA) and allowed tap water <u>ad libitum</u>. A miniosmotic pump (No. 2002, Alza Corp., Palo Alto, CA, USA) filled with either porcine zinc insulin or vehicle was implanted subcutaneously. Food intake, water intake and urine output were measured daily and body weight was measured weekly. The systolic BP was measured twice a week by tail-cuff method (Hwang et al, 1989). Blood sampling and measurements of plasma insulin and glucose were similar to those described previously (Hwang et al., 1989). Seven newborn rats (1 week old) were sympathectomized chemically by intraperitoneally administering 50 µg/g guanethidine 5 times a week for 3 weeks before insulin treatment.

A separate group of neonatally chemical sympathectomized rats (n=7) and age-matched normal rats (n=5) were fed fructose-enriched diet containing 66% fructose, 12% fat, 22% protein, 4.9 g/kg sodium and 4.9 g/kg potassium (Teklad Labs, Madison, WI, USA) for 9 weeks. Body weight, BP and plasma insulin and glucose levels were measured as aforementioned. The sodium and potassium concentrations in plasma and urine samples were measured using a flame photometer

(Model 343, Instrumentation Lab., Lexington, MA, USA). The data were analyzed using Student's paired and un-paired t tests where applicable. Results are expressed as means±SE.

RESULTS

As illustrated in Fig. 1, infusion of insulin at either 1.5 or 3.0 mU/kg/min increased the systolic BP. In insulin-treated, sympathectomized group, the increase in BP delayed for 3 weeks. There were no significant differences in water intake, food intake, urine volume, urine sodium excretion, body weight gain and sodium accumulation between intact rats received insulin infusion (3 mU/kg/min) and vehicle treated, control rats. In insulin-infused (3 mU/kg/min) intact rats, plasma insulin increased from 34±5 µU/ml to 76±6, 59±6 and 77±21 µU/ml by the end of the first, third, and fifth week of insulin infusion, respectively. In vehicle-treated rats the insulin levels at the corresponding time period were 26±3, 38±4, 37±6 and 30±4 µU/ml, respectively (all p values <0.05). Plasma glucose did not alter significantly following insulin infusion and there were no significant differences in plasma glucose levels between control and insulin-infused rats throughout the experiment.

Fructose treatment for 3 weeks significantly increased BP and plasma insulin levels without significant change in plasma glucose concentrations in both groups (Table 1). By the 5th week of fructose feeding, however, the magnitude of increase in BP was significantly smaller in sympathectomized rats than in intact rats.

DISCUSSION

This study demonstrates that hyperinsulinemia achieved by either infusion of exogenous insulin or fructose feeding significantly increases BP. These observations support the suggestion that sustained increase in plasma insulin can induce hypertension in rats and human beings (Hwang et al., 1989; Reaven 1990).

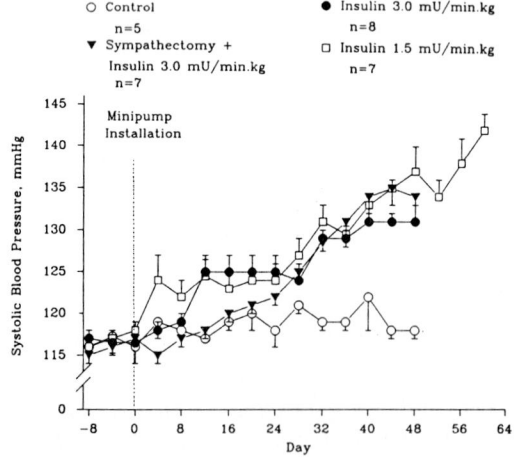

Fig. 1 Changes in blood pressure in normal and hyperinsulinemic rats with and without neonatally chemical sympathectomy.

Table 1. Effects of fructose feeding on the systolic blood pressure and plasma insulin and glucose levels in intact and neonatally chemical sympathectomized rats.

	Control	Fructose Feeding, Week				
		1	3	5	7	9
BP, mmHg						
N	117±1	118±1	124±1*	128±1*	137±2*	148±1*
S	117±1	118±1	123±1*	123±1*#	133±1*#	135±1*#
Insulin, μU/ml						
N	37±2	45±6	44±3*	103±35*	68±6*	61±6*
S	33±2	33±2	40±2*	68± 5*	61±7*	52±5*
Glucose, mg/dl						
N	144±4	55±3	147±4	141± 4	129±9	147±7
S	141±5	54±3	130±5	142± 2	124±4*	123±4*#

Abbreviations: N= normal rats (n=5); S= sympathectomized rats (n=7). BP= systolic blood pressure. * $p<0.05$ compared to control period; # $p<0.05$ compared to normal rats.

It has been suggested that acute hyperinsulinemia could enhance sympathetic nerve activity which might contribute to the elevation of BP (Landsberg 1990). In the present study, neonatally chemical sympathectomy delayed hyperinsulinemia-induced increase in BP for about 3 weeks. In fructose-fed rats, chemical sympathectomy also delayed the rise and reduced the magnitude of BP. These results suggest that activation of sympathetic nerve activity secondary to elevation of plasma insulin modulates but not mediates the pathogenesis of hyperinsulinemia-induced hypertension.

Despite increase in BP, the sodium accumulation in insulin-treated rats did not differ significantly from that of control rats. This suggests that the renal arterial pressure-excretion curve shifts to the right in insulin-treated rats. The hyperinsulinemia-associated right shift of the renal function curve may play a pivotal role in the development of hypertension. The potential pathophysiological mechanism warrants further investigation.

REFERENCES

Baum, M. (1987): Insulin stimulates volume absorption in the rabbit proximal convoluted tubule. J. Clin. Invest. 79, 1104-1109.
DeFronzo, R.A., Cooke, C., Andres, R., Faloona, G.R. and Davis, P.J. (1975): The effect of insulin on renal handling of sodium, potassium, calcium and phosphate in man. J. Clin. Invest. 55, 845-855.
Hwang, I.S., Huang, W.C., Wu, J.N., Shian, L.R. and Reaven, G.M. (1989): Effect of fructose-induced hypertension on the renin-angiotensin-aldosterone system and atrial natriuretic factor. Am. J. Hypertens. 2, 424-427.
Landsberg, L. (1990): Insulin resistance, energy balance and sympathetic nervous system activity. Clin. Exper. Hyper. - Theory and Practice. A12, 817-830.
Reaven, G.M. (1990): Insulin and hypertension. Clin. Exper. Hyper. -Theory and Practice. A12, 803-816.

Cross circulation in spontaneously hypertensive rats. Evidence of a circulating hypertensive factor and effects of antihypertensive treatment

Jürgen Bachmann, Elisabeth Ottens and Walter Zidek

Medizinische Universität-Poliklinik, Albert-Schweitzer-Strasse, 334400 Münster, Germany

INTRODUCTION

In spontaneously hypertensive rats parabiosis experiments demonstrated the transmission of hypertension (Dahl et al., 1969; Zidek et al., 1984; Greenberg et al., 1981). Furthermore, injection of hypertensive plasma or other blood components increased blood pressure in normotensive rats (Hirata et al., 1984; Wright & McCumbee, 1984; McCumbee & Wright, 1985). Therefore, it was tested by cross circulation between normotensive and spontaneously hypertensive rats, whether a circulating vasoconstrictor agent can be detected in the latter. Furthermore, the influence of various antihypertensive drugs on plasma levels of this factor were assessed.

METHODS

The experiments were performed in 66 male spontaneously hypertensive rats from the Münster strain. The age of the rats was 3 - 5 months, systolic blood pressure was 170-200 mm Hg. Wistar-Kyoto rats were used as normotensive controls. Cross circulation was performed between 30 untreated spontaneously hypertensive rats and the respective normotensive animals. The rats were anesthetized with 1,5 g/kg body weight urethane i.p. The common carotid artery and the external jugular vein of two rats were connected by a silastic tube, and vice versa. Then by a peristaltic pump blood was pumped in both directions at a rate of 3-5 ml/min. The tubes through which the blood was pumped were inserted into thick-walled silastic tubes with a larger diameter, so that different flow rates in both directions due to a different distension of the tubes by the blood pressure of either rat could be minimized. The tubing, which had a volume of 2,8 ml for each rat, was filled with saline prior to cross circulation. The rats were weighed continuously during the experiment with an electronic balance sensitive in the mg range. Thereby it was ensured that equal volumes were pumped in both directions, so that a net volume shift was avoided. The changes of weight during cross circulation were lower than 1 g. During the experiment mean arterial pressure was monitored by a Statham element every 10 min after stopping the peristaltic pump, using a plastic catheter inserted into the common carotid artery.

In groups of 6 spontaneously hypertensive rats the animals were treated with the antihypertensive drugs, nifedipine, furosemide, captopril, dihydralazine, propanolol and alpha methyldopa. With each drug systolic blood pressure was lowered to the range of 130 - 145 mm Hg (mg/kg body weight/d i.p.: alpha methyldopa 140, propranolol 5,4, furosemide 6, nifedipine 0,2, dihydralazine 7,5, captopril 6). The last dosis was applied 12 h prior to cross circulation to avoid a transfer of the drug from the spontaneously hypertensive to the normotensive rat. The treatment was maintained for 7-10 days. Cross circulation was performed 3-4 days after blood pressure had reached a steady state under treatment. Statistical significance of changes in mean arterial pressure was tested using Student's t-test.

RESULTS

Fig. 1A shows the changes of mean blood pressure in normotensive rats the circulations of which were connected to those of spontaneously hypertensive rats using a peristaltic pump. Blood pressure of the normotensive animals began to increase after about 10 min and further increased during the 30 min of cross circulation. After disconnection of the animals blood pressure in normotensive rats decreased again slowly, reaching baseline values after 1-1,5 h. When two normotensive animals were connected by this method, no rise in blood pressure could be detected. Initially a transient decrease in blood pressure was noted (Fig. 1A).

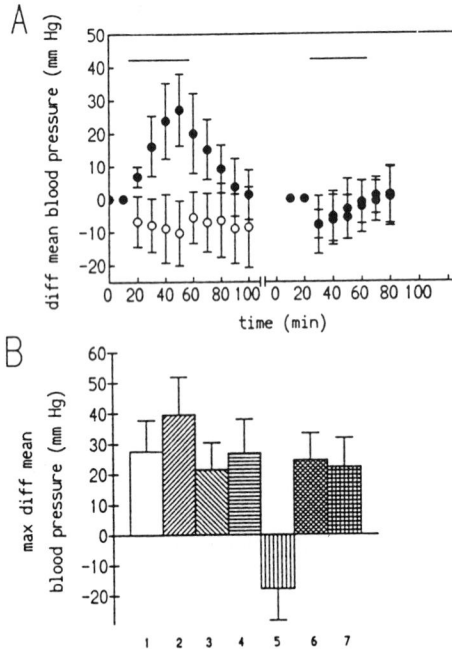

Fig. 1. Changes of mean arterial pressure during cross circulation (horizontal line). A: untreated spontaneously hypertensive rats (O) and normotensive (●) couples. B: maximal increase in mean arterial pressure of normotensive rats during cross circula-tion with spontaneously hypertensive rats, either untreated (1) or treated with nifedipine (2), furosemide (3), propranolol (4), alpha methyldopa (5), captopril (6), and dihydra-lazine (7). Mean values and standard deviations are noted.

Fig. 1B shows the effects of pretreatment with various antihypertensive drugs on the maximal increase in mean blood pressure in normotensive rats during cross circulation. The increase in blood pressure, which was elicited in the cross-circulated normotensive rats, did not change significantly, when the spontaneously hypertensive rats had been treated with propranolol, captopril, dihydralazine and furosemide. The increase in blood pressure of the normotensive rat during cross circulation was enhanced by pretreatment of the hypertensive animal with nifedipine and was suppressed after pretreatment with alpha methyldopa.

DISCUSSION

The results show that cross circulation between spontaneously hypertensive and normotensive rats induces an increase in blood pressure in the latter, suggesting that a circulating hypertensive factor exists in the spontaneously hypertensive rat.

With nifedipine, rather a tendency to an enhanced transmission of hypertension was observed, which may be explained by an increased secretion of the circulating factor to compensate for the fall in blood pressure. In a recent report on a circulating factor in essential hypertension, which increased cytosolic free Ca^{2+} in platelets, similar effects of nifedipine on this factor were found (Lindner et al., 1987). Incubation of platelets with ultrafiltrated plasms from essential hypertensives increased cytosolic free Ca^{2+} by a significant greater amount, when the patients were under treatment with nifedipine. This finding also suggests a stimulation of the hypertensive factor by nifedipine in man.

As to the origin of the hypertensive factor, earlier experiments pointed to an important role of kidneys and adrenals (Iwai et al., 1969; Knudsen et al., 1969). On the other hand, the results of this study suggest that the central nervous system plays an important role in the regulation of the hypertensive factor. Moreover, in hypothalamic tissue an inhibitor of the Na, K ATPase has been localized, although this does not necessarily indicate a vasopressor activity (Millett et al., 1986). The effect of alpha methyldopa on the transmission of hypertension could be explained by a blockade of the central nervous stimulatory action on the hypertensive factor. The decreased secretion of the hypertensive factor may either be related to the effects of alpha methyldopa on the central sympathetic nervous system or may represent an additional blood pressure lowering mechanism.

In summary, most of the tested antihypertensive drugs did not suppress the secretion of the hypertensive factor. Only alpha methyldopa prevented the transmission of hypertension by cross circulation. Further studies will have to show, whether this effect is common to all centrally acting antihypertensive drugs.

REFERENCES

Allen, J.M., Raine, A.E.G., Ledingham, J.G.G., Bloom, S.R. (1985) Neuropeptide Y: a novel renal peptide with vasoconstrictor and natriuretic activity. Clin. Sci. 68, 373-377.

Dahl, L.K., Knutsen, K.D. & Iwai, J. (1969): Humoral transmission of hypertension: Evidence from parabiosis. Circ. Res. 24/25, Suppl. I, 21-33.

Greenberg, S., Gaines, K. & Sweatt, D. (1981): Evidence for circulating factors as a cause of venous hypertrophy in spontaneously hypertensive rats. Am. J. Physiol. 241, H421-H430.

Hirata. Y, Tobian, L., Simon. G & Iwai, J. (1984): Hypertension-producing factor in serum of hypertensive Dahl salt-sensitive rats. Hypertension 6, 709-716.

Iwai, J., Knudsen, K.D., Dahl, L.K. & Tassinari, L. (1969): Effect of adrenalectomy on blood pressure in salt-fed, hypertension-prone rats: failure of hypertension to develop in absence of evidence of adrenal cortical tissue. J. Exp. Med. 129, 663-671.

Knudsen, K.D., Iwai, J., Heine, M., Leitl, G. & Dahl, L.K. (1969): Genetic influence on the development of renoprival hypertension in parabiotic rats. J. Exp. Med. 130, 1353-1365.

Lindner, A., Kenny, M. & Meacham, A.J. (1987): Effects of a circulating factor in patients with essential hypertension on intracellular free calcium in normal platelets. N. Engl. J. Med. 316, 509-513.

McCumbee, W.D. & Wright, G.L. (1985): Partial purification of a hypertensive substance from rat erythrocytes. Can. J. Physiol. Pharmacol. 63, 1321-1326.

Millett, J.A., Holland, S.M., Alaghband-Zadeh, J. & de Wardener H.E. (1986): Na-K-ATPase inhibiting and glucose-6-phosphate dehydrogenase-stimulating activity of plasma and hypothalamus of the Okamoto spontaneously hypertensive rat. J. Endocrinol. 108, 69-73.

Wright, G.L. & McCumbee, W.D. (1984): A hypertensive substance found in the blood of spontaneously hypertensive rats. Life Sci. 34, 1521-1528.

Zidek, W., Heckmann, U., Friemann, J., Losse, H. & Vetter, H. (1984): Role of kidney and adrenals in the humoral pathogenesis of primary hypertension. J. Hypertens. 2, suppl. 3, 515-517.

Effect of nerve stimulation on isolated mesenteric and intra-renal resistance arteries, SHR versus WKY

Pedro H.A. Eerdmans, Harry A.J. Struyker-Boudier and Jo G.R. De Mey

Department of Pharmacology, University of Limburg, P.O. Box 616, 6200 MD Maastricht, The Netherlands

INTRODUCTION

Sympathetic nerves play a key role in acute and long term regulation of vascular resistance. They also participate in the pathogenesis of hypertension. Sympatholytic interventions in young spontaneously hypertensive rats (SHR) prevent the development of hypertension and arterial structural changes [15,10]. Also in experimental models of secundary hypertension, sympathetic nerves play a role [10,4]. It is not clear to what extent this is indirect, i.e. mediated by hemodynamic variables, or when direct to which neurotransmitters or cotransmitters it can be attributed [10,1]. Compared to sympatholytic intervention less is known about the potential effects of more subtle interferences with sympathetic nerve activity to prevent or reverse arterial structural changes in hypertension.
Sympathetic nerve activity affects vascular beds to a different extent because of regional differences in (i) nerve density, (ii) prejunctional modulation, (iii) postjunctional effector responses and (iv) presence of non-adrenergic nerves [3,5,9].
We compared these aspects between mesenteric and intra-renal resistance-sized arteries of Wistar Kyoto (WKY) and Spontaneously Hypertensive rats of the Okamoto strain (SHR).

MATERIAL AND METHODS

Experiments were performed in resistance arteries isolated from 12 week old male WKY and SHR. Fourth to fifth-order side branches of the superior mesenteric artery (MrA) and interlobar renal arteries (RrA) were isolated and mounted in an myograph for measurement of isometric force development [11]. They were passively stretched to a diameter corresponding to 90 % of the diameter which the vessel would have when subjected to a transmural pressure of 100 mmHg [11]. This was in the range of 200 μm for MrA and 230 μm in RrA.
Electrical field stimulation (EFS) was applied by two platinum electrodes placed longitudinally across the vessel segment with a variable current, duration 2 msec, amplitude 85 mA and a frequency from 1 to 32 Hz [13,14]. Responses to EFS were expressed as % of the maximal response to exogenous noradrenaline (10 μM).

RESULTS

1. Postjunctional responses.
Vessels that had been pretreated with 6-hydroxydopamine did not respond to EFS but contracted in response to noradrenaline and phenylephrine. Compared to the MrA, the RrA were significantly more sensitive to phenylephrine. Mesenteric but not renal arteries that had been made to contract with 30 mM potassium responded to beta-receptor stimulation with concentration dependent relaxations [7]. In neither mesenteric nor renal vessels, the α_2-adrenoceptor agonists rilmenidine and BHT-933 altered basal tone. Postjunctional responses to α_1-,α_2- and ß-adrenoceptor stimulation did not differ between the WKY and SHR.

2. Electrical field stimulation.
EFS induced frequency dependent contractions in both mesenteric and renal resistance arteries, these were abolished by tetrodotoxin (0.1 µM). The maximal response to field stimulation averaged $45\pm9\%$ and $66\pm12\%$ (figure 1) for RrA and MrA of WKY and $71\pm4\%$ and $101\pm13\%$ for RrA and MrA of SHR. Differences between strains were statistically significant. After pretreatment with phenoxybenzamine (1 µM, 10 min) a small contractile effect of field stimulation (3%) persisted in MrA of SHR and WKY. This tiny response was abolished following 6-OHDA and by tetrodotoxin.

3. Prejunctional modulation
Cocaine (3 µM) and yohimbine (0.1 µM) increased responses to low (4 and 8 Hz) but not high frequency (32 Hz) stimulation in both types of vessels. Supersensitivity following blockade of neuronal reuptake and α2-adrenoceptors was, however, more marked in mesenteric (figure 1) than renal vessels. The increase in sensitivity did not differ between SHR and WKY.

4. Non-adrenergic nerves
In intrarenal vessels capsaicin, which depletes peptidergic nerves [8], did not affect contractile responses to Arg-vasopressin (30 nM). In mesenteric arteries, on the other hand, the sensory neuron selective agent potently (IC50=3.4 nM) and transiently abolished contractile responses to the peptide. Pretreatment with capsaicin (0.3 µM, 20 min) did not alter responses to noradrenaline but increased the sensitivity for the contractile effect of EFS in mesenteric resistance arteries but not in renal vessels. This increased sensitivity did not differ significantly between vessels of WKY and SHR.

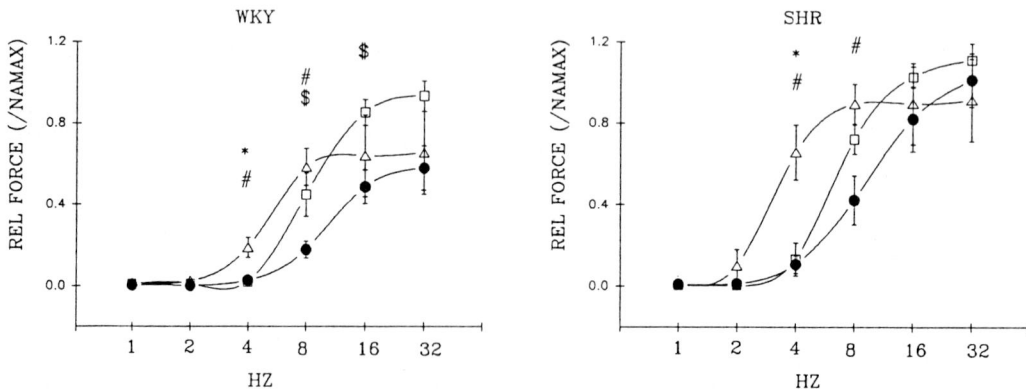

Figure 1. Frequency response curves of mesenteric resistance sized arteries of WKY (left) and SHR (right) in the absence (filled circle) or presence of cocaine (box) or cocaine and yohimbine (triangle). Data were expressed relative to the maximal responses to 10 µM noradrenaline and are shown as mean ± SEM. $ p<0.05 cocaine compared with control, # p<0.05 cocaine/yohimbine compared with control, * p<0.05 cocaine compared with cocaine/yohimbine.

DISCUSSION

Contractile responses to EFS were blocked by TTX and 6-OHDA indicating their sympathetic nervous origin. Responses were larger in mesenteric than renal resistance arteries and for both types, larger for SHR and WKY. We evaluated to what extent pre- and postjunctional phenomena contribute to this regional and interstrain difference.

All isolated vessels used, lacked postjunctional α_2-adrenergic responses [6]. β-adrenergic relaxing responses were present in the mesenteric but not in the renal vessels [7]. Renal vessels were, on the other hand, more sensitive to postjunctional α_1-adrenergic stimulation which accounts for most of the contractile responsiveness to EFS. No differences in postjunctional adrenergic responsiveness were observed between resistance arteries of WKY and SHR.

Blockade of neural re-uptake and α_2-adrenoceptors increased the responsiveness to low frequency EFS. This was more marked in mesenteric than renal vessels, but did not differ between vessels of SHR and WKY.

Provided that renal small artery smooth muscle can relax in response to calcitonin-gene-related-peptide and substance P, the observations with capsaicin indicate the absence and presence of vasodilator peptidergic nerves in renal and mesenteric resistance arteries, respectively. Depletion of these nerves, increased contractile responses to EFS in mesenteric but not renal vessels. Similar observations were obtained for WKY and SHR.

Taken together these observations indicate that although differences in postjunctional responsiveness, prejunctional modulation and presence of peptiderge nerves may contribute to regional differences in responsiveness to nerve stimulation, primarily differences in sympathetic nerve density underlie the differences between SHR and WKY. This adds complementary evidence to earlier observations [15].

REFERENCES.

1. Albino-Teixeira A, et al (1990): Purine agonists prevent trophic changes caused by sympathetic denervation. Eur J Pharmacol. 179, 141-149.
2. Angus JA, et al (1988):Role of alpha-adrenoceptors in constrictor responses of rat, guinea-pig and rabbit small arteries to neural activation. J. Physiol. Lond. 403, 495-510.
3. Bevan JA, et al (1980):Adrenergic regulation of vascular smooth muscle. In:Bohr DF, Somlyo AP, Sparks HV (eds) Handbook of physiology, Section 2, The cardiovascular system, Vol II, Vascular smooth muscle. Bethesda, MD. Am.Physiol. Soc. 515-566.
4. Bevan RD et al (1976):Hyperplasia of vascular smooth muscle in experimental hypertension in the rabbit. Circ Res. 38,58-62.
5. Bloom FE. (1988):Neurotransmitters: past, present and future directions. FASEB J 2, 32-41.
6. Eerdmans PHA et al, (in press):Sympathetic heterogeneity in mesenteric and renal resistance arteries. Elsevier's "International Congress Series"
7. Heesen BJ, De Mey JG, (1990):Effects of cyclic AMP-affecting agents on contractile reactivity of isolated mesenteric and renal arteries of the rat. Br. J. Pharmacol. 101, 859-864.
8. Holzer P, (1991):Capsaicin: cellular targets, mechanisms of action, and selectivity for thin sensory neurons. Pharmacological Reviews 43,2, 143-201.
9. Kawasaki H, et al (1988):Calcitonin in gene-related peptide acts as a novel vasodilator neurotramsmitter in mesenteric resistance vessels of the rat. Nature. 355, 164-167.
10. Lee RMKW, Smeda JS (1985): Primary versus secundary structural changes of the blood vessels in hypertension. Can J Physiol Pharmacol. 63, 392-401.
11. Mulvany MJ, Halpern W,(1977):Contractile properties of small arterial resistance vessels in spontaneously hypertensive and normotensive rats. Circ. Res. 41, 19-26.
12. Nilsson H, (1984):Different nerve responses in consecutive sections of the arterial system. Acta Physiol, Scand. 121, 353-361.
13. Nilson H, (1985):Adrenergic nervous control of resistance and capacitance vessels. Acta Physiol Scand. 124 (suppl 541), 1-34.
14. Nilsson H, et al (1986):Adrenergic innervation and neurogenic response in large and small arteries and veins from the rat. Acta Physiol. Scand. 126, 121-133.
15. Nyborg NCB et al (1986): Neonatal sympathetomy of normotensive WKY and SHR with 6-hydroxydopamine: effects on resistance vessel structure and sensitivity to calcium. J Hypert. 4, 455-465.

Reduction of inhibitory effect of adrenergic transmission by nerve growth factor in the mesenteric vasculatures of spontaneously hypertensive rats

Takashi Ueyama, Takuzo Hano, Masanori Hamada, Ichiro Nishio and Yoshiaki Masuyama

Division of Cardiology, Department of Medicine, Wakayama Medical College, Wakayama City, 640, Japan

Nerve growth factor(NGF) is a neurotrophic peptide for peripheral sympathetic neurons(Thoenen et al., 1980). There is a strong positive correlation between tissue NGF levels(Korshing et al.,1983), or NGF mRNA levels(Shelton et al., 1984) and the norepinephrine(NE) content, the latter being thought to reflect the density of sympathetic innervation. There is a considerable amount of data indicating that sympathetic innervation is greater in the vascular tissues of spontaneously hypertensive rats(SHR:Okamoto and Aoki) than in control Wistar-Kyoto rats(WKY)(Head, 1989). These data suggest that NGF contributes to the increased sympathetic nervous innervation of SHR tissues. In fact, Donohue et al.(1989) and ourselves (1991, a) have shown that the NGF levels are increased in young SHR tissues. The sympathetic nervous system is not only structurally, but also functionally, enhanced in young SHR. Hano et al.(1989) showed that the overflow of endogenous NE during the stimulation of peri-arterial nerves of the mesenteric artery in 7-week-old SHR was significantly greater compared with that in age-matched WKY, whereas the overflow in 13-week-old SHR was no longer increased. Recently, we(1991, b) have found that NGF has an inhibitory neuromodulatory effect on sympathetic nerve endings. These facts prompted us to consider that the neuromodulatory effect of NGF would be altered in the vascular tissue of SHR. To confirm this hypothesis, we investigated NE overflow from sympathetic nerve endings of SHR and WKY during electrical nerve stimulation in the presence of NGF.

We used 4-,12-week-old male SHR and age-matched groups of WKY. Systolic blood pressure was measured by the tail-cuff method(Ueda Corp. model UR-1000). NGF was purified as the 2.5S NGF sub-unit from mouse submandibular glands according to the method of Bocchini et al.(1969). The perfusion experiments were performed as previously reported(Hano et al., 1989). In short, we prepared mesenteric vasculatures by a modification of the method of Castelluci et al.(1981). The preparation was perfused with Krebs-Henseleit solution(pH 7.4, 37°C), saturated with 95% O_2 and 5% CO_2 mixture. A constant flow rate of 3 ml/min was maintained with a peristaltic pump(Tokyo Rikakikai:201, Tokyo). Peri-arterial nerve stimulation was performed with bipolar platinum electrodes around the proximal end of the mesenteric artery. The stimulation was applied by rectangular pulses of 5 msec duration at 10 Hz for 1 min. The perfusate through the mesenteric preparation was collected in a tube containing

10 mg EDTA for 3 min before(A) and after(B) nerve stimulation. NE in the perfusate was absorbed on alumina, extracted with 200 ul of 0.1N perchloric acid and assayed using high performance liquid chromatography with an electrochemical detector(Bioanalytical system LC-5, West Lafayette Indiana). We difined the NE overflow evoked by electrical nerve stimulation as the difference between the NE content of (A) and (B): This values were expressed as nanograms per gram of wet tissue weight for each preparation. NGF was added to the perfusion medium to achieve final concentrations of 0.1, 1.0 and 10 ng/ml. After NGF administration, a 9 min-period elapsed before the next electrical stimulation. Values were expressed as means ± SEM. Statistical significances were determined by Student's t-test. Differences of $p<0.05$ were considered to be significant.

The average weights of the animals at 4 and 12 weeks of age were $80.9 \pm 4.5g(n=8)$ and $312.0 \pm 2.2g(n=6)$ for SHR and $70.0 \pm 2.6g(n=8)$ and $318.5 \pm 2.9g(n=6)$ for WKY, respectively. The average systolic blood pressures of the animals at 4 and 12 weeks of age were 129 ± 3 mmHg and 185 ± 7 mmHg for SHR and 127 ± 3 mmHg and 156 ± 1 mmHg for WKY (4-week-old, SHR vs. WKY NS: 12-week-old, $p<0.01$)

Table 1. NE overflow and its percentage reduction in 4-week-old animals

	concentration of NGF (ng/ml)			
	0	0.1	1.0	10
WKY(n=7)	0.95±0.08	0.80±0.08 (-14.9±3.2 %)	0.66±0.06 (-29.9±5.1 %)	0.60±0.05 (-36.6±2.7 %)
SHR(n=7)	1.24±0.08	1.21±0.08** (-1.3±5.9 %*)	1.08±0.13** (-8.2±5.3 %**)	0.86±0.09** (-28.7±7.5 %)

NE overflow(ng/g wet wt.) / (percentage reduction)   mean±SEM, *$p<0.05$, **$p<0.01$

Table 2. NE overflow and its percentage reduction in 12-week-old animals.

	concentration of NGF (ng/ml)			
	0	0.1	1.0	10
WKY(n=6)	0.185±0.05	0.135±0.02 (-26.2±3.1 %)	0.11±0.04 (-40.2±7.0 %)	0.097±0.03 (-46.7±6.3 %)
SHR(n=6)	0.202±0.05	0.137±0.04 (-30.8±6.2 %)	0.118±0.04 (-40.0±7.6 %)	0.107±0.04 (-49.2±8.2 %)

NE overflow(ng/g wet wt.) / (percentage reduction)   mean±SEM, not significant.

Table 1 shows the effects of NGF on NE overflow by electrical nerve stimulation in 4-week-old animals and Table 2, in 12-week-old animals. NE overflow was inhibited by NGF dose-dependently in each animal. At 4 weeks of age, it was significantly greater in SHR than in WKY . Percentage reduction of NE overflow was significantly weaker in 4-week-old SHR. There was no significant difference in NE overflow and its percentage reduction between 12 week-old SHR and age-matched WKY . These data demonstrate that the inhibitory neuromodulatory effect of NGF is attenuated in young SHR. This finding confirms the enhanced NE release from sympathetic nerve endings in young SHR tissues, in spite of larger content of NGF in the tisssues. Interestingly, Zettler et al.(1991) showed that chronic administration of NGF to normotensive rats induced hypernoradrenergical nerve innervation, but it was not associated with the development of hypertension. One of the reasons to be considered might be that exogenously treated NGF inhibits NE release from sympathetic nerve endings and fails to increase vascular resistance. In conclusion, we think NGF is one of the essential, but not the only factor for the development of hypertension in SHR.

REFERENCES

Bocchini, V. and Angeletti, P.U.(1969): The nerve growth factor: purification as a 30,000-molecular-weight protein. Biochem. 64, 784-794.

Castellucci, A. et at.(1981): The rat mesenteric artery-intestinal loop preparation. Arzneimittelforsch Drug Res. 31, 54-58.

Donohue S.J. et al.(1989): Elevated nerve growth factor levels in young spontaneously hypertensive rats. Hypertension 14, 421-426.

Hano, T. and Rho, J.(1989): Norepinephrine overflow in perfused mesenteric arteries of spontaneously hypertensive rats. Hypertension 14, 44-53.

Head, R.J.(1989): Hypernoradrenergic innervation:Its relationship to functional and hyperplastic changes in the vasculature of the spontaneously hypertensive rats. Blood Vessels 26, 1-20

Korsching, S. and Thoenen, H.(1988): Developmental changes of nerve growth factor levels in sympathetic ganglia and their target organs. Dev. Biol. 126, 40-46

Shelton, D.L. and Reichardt, L.F.(1984): Expression of the beta-nerve growth factor gene correlated with the density of sympathetic innervation in effector organs. Proc. Natl. Acad. Sci. USA 81, 7951-7955

Thoenen, H. and Barde, Y.A. (1980): Physiology of nerve growth factor. Physiol. Rev. 60, 1284-1335.

Ueyama, T. et al.(1991): New role of nerve growth factor - an inhibitory neuromodulator of adrenergic transmission. Brain Res.(in press)

Ueyama, T. et al.(1991): Increased nerve growth factor levels in spontaneously hypertensive rats. J. Hypertension(in press)

Zettler, C. et al. (1991): Chronic nerve growth factor treatment of normotensive rats. Brain Res. 538, 251-262.

Chronic treatment with captopril plus hydrochlorothiazide attenuates vascular noradrenergic transmission in the adult SHR

Eric Thorin, Christine Capdeville-Atkinson and Jeffrey Atkinson

Laboratoire de Pharmacologie, Faculté de Pharmacie, 5, rue Albert Lebrun, 54000 Nancy, France

Several lines of evidence point to the involvement of the sympathetic nervous system in the antihypertensive effects of angiotensin I converting enzyme (ACE) inhibitors. Angiotensin II potentiates the vasoconstrictor responses to sympathetic stimulation by increasing noradrenaline release (Zimmerman, 1978) and blocking neuronal uptake of noradrenaline (Khairallah, 1971). Furthermore angiotensin II potentiates the post junctional vasoconstrictor effect of noradrenaline (Zimmerman, 1978). A corollary of these observations is that ACE inhibitors, such as captopril, attenuate sympathetic responses, at least *in vivo* (Atkinson et al., 1987). Thus the antihypertensive effect of ACE inhibitors may be partially dependent upon blockade of sympathetic pressor systems (for discussion see Brunner et al., 1990). Likewise diuretics appear to diminish vascular responsiveness to sympathetic stimulation (for discussion see Gifford, 1990). We investigated therefore whether changes in vascular noradrenergic transmission are correlated with drug-induced changes in blood pressure following treatment of adult SHR with captopril, hydrochlorothiazide or a combination of the two.

Forty-seven male SHR (IOPS SHR, Iffa-Credo, L'Arbresle, France, 3 months old, 240-260 g) were given specially prepared diets containing captopril, hydrochlorothiazide or a combination of the two for 10 weeks (Table 1). Systolic arterial pressure (mmHg) and heart rate (bpm) were measured in awake animals, using the tail cuff method, following prewarming.

Table 1. Body weight, systolic arterial pressure, heart rate (m ± SEM) and drug doses in SHR chronically treated with captopril, hydrochlorothiazide or a combination of the two for 10 weeks.

Group	n	Drug dose mg/kg per day	Beginning of treatment			End of treatment		
			Body weight (g)	Systolic arterial pressure (mmHg)	Heart rate (bpm)	Body weight (g)	Systolic arterial pressure (mm Hg)	Heart rate (bpm)
Controls	11	0	261 ± 5	190 ± 5	376 ± 8	363 ± 8	235 ± 8	431 ± 16
Captopril	12	41	257 ± 6	195 ± 5	419 ± 19	352 ± 8	191 ± 5*	465 ± 13
Hydrochlorothiazide	12	21	251 ± 3	196 ± 6	408 ± 7	325 ± 6*	227 ± 5	455 ± 19
Captopril + hydrochlorothiazide	12	44 + 22	259 ± 5	195 ± 5	423 ± 14	311 ± 5*	162 ± 6*	450 ± 12

* = $P < 0.05$ ANOVA/Scheffe test with controls.

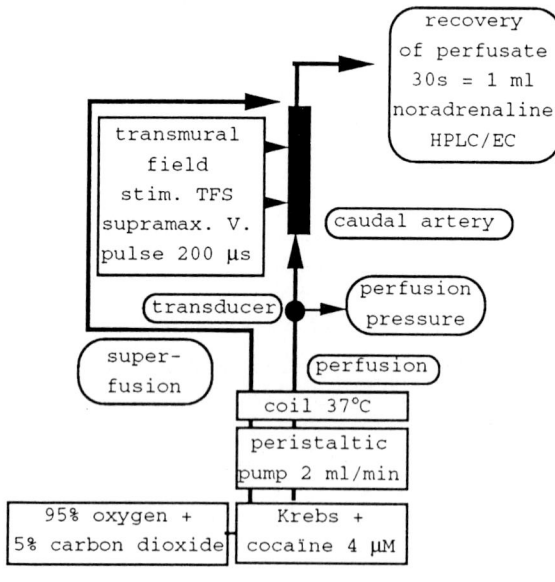

Fig. 1. Perfusion of the SHR caudal artery *in vitro*
Following 5 short TFS (1 Hz, 5s), perfusion pressure was recorded and the perfusate collected for determination of noradrenaline overflow before and during TFS (1 Hz for 30s, for further details see Fouda et al., 1987).

At the end of the 10 weeks' treatment period SHR were anesthetized with sodium pentobarbital (50 mg/kg, i.p.) and segments of the proximal portion of the caudal artery were removed (10 to 15 mm per segment). Segments were perfused and superfused, and stimulated with transmural field stimulation (TFS) as shown in Fig. 1 (see also Fouda et al., 1987).

Systolic arterial pressure (SAP) increased slightly in controls during the 10 weeks' period (Table 1). Captopril alone induced a minor fall in SAP but when combined with hydrochlorothiazide produced a pronounced fall in SAP (Table 1).

Basal and TFS-induced noradrenaline overflow were similar in all groups (Table 2). Basal perfusion pressure *in vitro* of the perfused caudal artery was lower in SHR treated with captopril or a combination of captopril plus hydrochlorothiazide. Increases in perfusion pressure following TFS were not significantly different. Noradrenaline transmission efficiency was significantly reduced in SHR treated with a combination of captopril and hydrochlorothiazide. There was a significant correlation between systolic arterial pressure (y) and noradrenaline transmission efficiency (x) recorded during TFS (y = 78 + 5.2 x, r = 0.97, P < 0.05) but not for basal (y = 133 + 3.2 x , r = 0.76, NS).

Table 2. Basal and TFS-induced noradrenaline overflow (pg/30s), perfusion pressure (mmHg) and noradrenaline transmission efficiency (mmHg/(pg/30s)) in adult SHR chronically treated with captopril (CAP), hydrochlorothiazide (HCTZ) or a combination of the two drugs (CAP/HCTZ)

Group	Basal mmHg	pg/30s	mmHg/(pg/30s)	TFS-induced ΔmmHg	pg/30s	ΔmmHg/(pg/30s)
controls	19.8±1.8	0.8±0.3	24±6	94.8±12.7	3.0±0.7	32±6
CAP	15.6±0.7*	0.7±0.1	23±3	87.2±5.7	4.2±0.7	21±2
HCTZ	16.3±0.8	0.5±0.1	33±3	77.3±7.0	2.9±0.6	27±4
CAP/HCTZ	15.1±0.4*	1.5±0.4	10±1*	75.2±9.0	4.3±0.6	17±2*

In conclusion these results suggest that attenuation of noradrenaline transmission efficiency plays a role in the antihypertensive effect of the combination of captopril plus hydrochlorothiazide.

The authors would like to acknowledge the financial assistance of Théraplix Laboratories, Paris and the helpful discussions with Joël Guillou from this laboratory.

REFERENCES

Atkinson, J., Sonnay, M., Sautel, M. and Fouda, A.K. (1987): Chronic treatment of the spontaneously hypertensive rat with captopril attenuates responses to noradrenaline in vivo but not in vitro. Naunyn-Schmiedeberg's Arch. Pharmacol. 335: 624-628.

Brunner, H., Waeber, B. and Nussberger, J. (1990): Angiotensin-converting enzyme inhibitors in arterial hypertension. In Cardiovascular Drug Therapy, ed. F.H. Messerli, pp. 732-760. Philadelphia: W.B. Saunders Company.

Fouda, A.K., Marazzi, A., Boillat, N., Sonnay, M., Guillain, H. and Atkinson, J. (1987): Changes in the vascular reactivity of the isolated tail arteries of spontaneous and renovascular hypertensive rats to endogenous and exogenous noradrenaline. Blood Vessels 24: 63-75.

Gifford, R.W. (1990): Diuretics in hypertension. In Cardiovascular Drug Therapy, ed. F.H. Messerli, pp. 298-309. Philadelphia: W.B. Saunders Company.

Khairallah, P.A., Darrila D., Papanicolaou, N., Glende, M. and Meyer, P. (1971): Effects of angiotensin infusion on catecholamine uptake and reactivity in blood vessels. Circ. Res. 28/29 : II-96 - II-106.

Zimmerman, B.G. (1978): Effects of angiotensin on adrenergic nerve endings. Fedn. Proc. 37: 199.

The carotid and aortic bodies in the Lyon hypertensive rats

Jörg-Olaf Habeck [1], Jean-Marc Pequignot [2], Madeleine Vincent [3] and Jean Sassard [3]

[1] Institute of Pathology, Städtische Kliniken, Chemnitz, Germany; [2] URA CNRS 1195, Faculté de Médecine, Lyon, France; [3] URA CNRS 606, Faculté de Pharmacie, Lyon, France

Whilst many recent studies have shown alterations in the morphology and function of the carotid body in arterial hypertension (Habeck, 1991) most of these studies have been performed in rats where different strains of animal alter the results obtained. A previous study of the Lyon strain of spontaneously hypertensive rats showed morphological and biochemical abnormalities in the carotid body of adult animals (Habeck et al., 1990).

The present investigation was undertaken for two main reasons: (1) to examine the influence of age upon the previous findings and, (2) to compare the morphological changes in the carotid body with those found in the aortic bodies which have a minor chemoreceptor role in the rat.

MATERIAL AND METHODS

Ninety five male rats (32 LH rats, 31 LN rats and 32 LL rats), all bred at the University of Lyon, were studied at ages of 1, 5 and 23 to 25 weeks. Systolic blood pressure (SBP) measurements were obtained using a tail cuff method in the two older groups. Both carotid bifurcations and the intrathoracic tissue except for the heart, lungs and thymus were removed immediately postmortem. The right carotid bifurcation and the thoracic tissue were fixed in buffered formalin and embedded in paraffin wax. Serial sections of 6 μm thickness were cut and stained with H.&E. The morphometric investigations of the carotid and aortic bodies were performed using techniques previously described (Habeck and Przebylski, 1989). The left carotid bodies were examined with high pressure liquid chromatography allied to electrochemical detection (HPLC-ED) for the assay of dopamine and norepinephrine (Pequignot et al., 1987). Variations between different groups of animals were assessed by Student's t test.

RESULTS

At 5 weeks of age no significant differences in SBP were seen between the three groups of animals whilst in the 23-25-week-old animals the LH rats showed higher blood pressure values.

A thickening of the walls of the small arteries within the carotid body was found in 10% of 5-week-old LH rats, and in 10% of LN rats and 60% of LH rats in the 23-25-week age group. These vascular alterations were small and did not obliterate the vascular lumen. Such changes were absent in the aortic bodies.

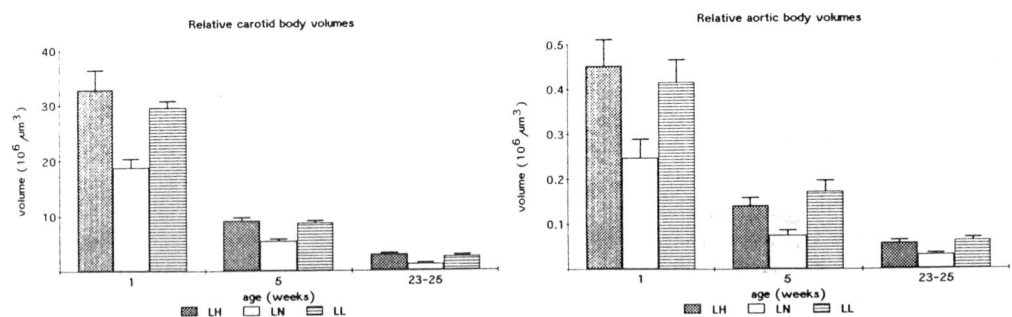

Figs. 1 and 2. Relative carotid (left) and aortic (right) body volumes in rats of the Lyon hypertensive strain.

In all age groups the LH and LL rats exhibited much larger carotid and aortic bodies than the LN rats (Figs. 1 and 2). Furthermore, in the latter, a smaller number of aortic bodies was detectable. The differences between LH and LL rats were not significant. No differences were noted between the three groups in respect of aortic body distribution.

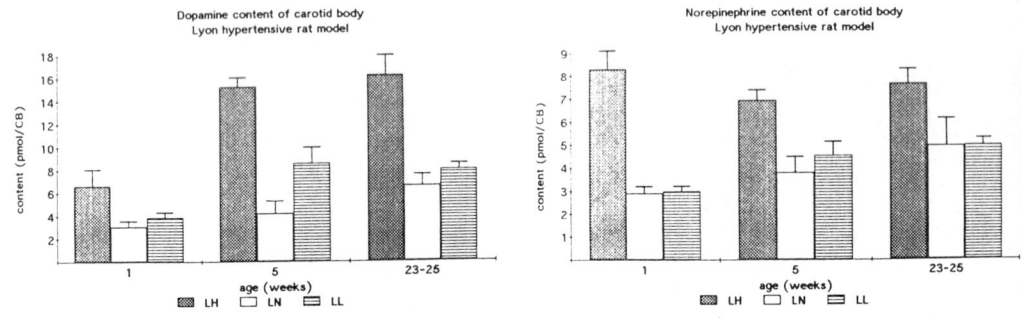

Figs. 3 and 4. Dopamine (left) and norepinephrine (right) content of the carotid body in rats of the Lyon hypertensive strain.

The LH rats exhibited in all age groups a higher dopamine and norepinephrine content in the carotid body than rats of the other both strains (Figs. 3 and 4).

DISCUSSION AND CONCLUSIONS

Spontaneously hypertensive rats of the OKAMOTO-AOKI strain (SHR) as well as of the New Zealand strain (GH) in the established phase of hypertension show hyperventilation under resting conditions and a reduced sensitivity to hypoxia. In both strains vascular alterations in the carotid bodies were seen.

An elevated norepinephrine content of carotid body was found only in SHR. However, the presence of increased dopamine levels in this strain of hypertensive rats has not be confirmed by all investigators. In contrast, in hypertensive New Zealand rats, a reduced norepinephrine and an unchanged dopamine content of the carotid body has been reported.

The SHR exhibited larger aortic bodies in all age groups, whereas the carotid body volume was only increased in the old animals as compared with WKY. In the GH no differences in carotid body volumes were observed (for review see Habeck, 1991).

The situation in the Lyon hypertensive model can be summarized:
(1) In LH rats an elevated norepinephrine and dopamine content is already observed in newborn rats, hence it is independent of an elevated blood pressure and likely an expression of a general disturbance of catecholamine metabolism in hypertensive disease.
(2) Differences in size of carotid and aortic bodies are strain-specific and independent of the blood pressure or intraglomic vascular pathology.
(3) There is only a small expression of intraglomic vascular alterations in LH rats. When comparing the findings in SHR it can be concluded that such changes are dependent upon blood pressure level.

Comparing the OKAMOTO-AOKI, the New Zealand and the Lyon strain there are different findings regarding the peripheral arterial chemoreceptors. Further functional studies in the Lyon strain and more morphological investigations in the other two strains are necessary, before final conclusions of the effects of hypertension upon function of peripheral arterial chemoreceptors are possible.

REFERENCES

Habeck, J.-O. (1991): Peripheral arterial chemoreceptors and hypertension. J. Auton. Nerv. Syst. 34: 1-8.

Habeck, J.-O., Pequignot, J.-M., Vincent, M., Sassard, J., and Huckstorf, C. (1990): The carotid bodies of the Lyon hypertensive rats. In Chemoreceptors and Chemoreceptor Reflexes, eds H. Acker, A. Trzebski, and R.G. ÒRegan, pp. 357-362, New York and London, Plenum Press.

Habeck, J.-O., and Przybylski, J. (1989): Carotid and aortic bodies in chronically anemic normotensive and spontaneously hypertensive rats. J. Auton. Nerv. Syst. 28: 219-226.

Pequignot, J.M., Cottet-Emard, J.M., Dalmaz, Y., and Peyrin, L. (1987): Dopamine and norepinephrine dynamics in rat carotid body during long-term hypoxia. J. Auton. Nerv. Syst. 21: 9-14.

Arterial baroreflex-blood pressure control in conscious hypertensive rats

Ding-Feng Su, Xian-Bo Kong, Yong Cheng and Li Chen

Department of Pharmacology, Second Military Medical University, Shanghai 200433, China

The role of the arterial baroreflex (ABR) in the regulation of cardiovascular activity has been a subject of considerable investigation. Most studies delineating the function of ABR have been performed in a variety of animal species and preparations, the majority of which have been anesthetized. Since general anesthesia is well known to affect the function of ABR, there is increasing interest in the role of ABR in the conscious state. In the last decade, several methods have been available for the measuring of ABR function in conscious freely moving rats. With these methods, many studies have confirmed that ABR−heart period control (ABR−HP) is impaired in hypertensive animals, including renovascular hypertensive rats (RVHR), SHR and LH (Jone et al., 1980; Struyker−Boudier et al., 1982; Su et al., 1986). But ABR−blood pressure control (ABR−BP) in conscious hypertensive rats is remained unclear due to the methodological limitation. Recently, we established a new method allowing to measure ABR−BP in freely moving rats. The main goal of the present investigation was to examine ABR−BP in conscious hypertensive rats.

MATERIAL AND METHODS

RVHR was prepared using male SD rats. All operative procedures were performed during ketamine anesthesia. 2K−1C hypertension was produced by placng a silver clip (0.2mm i.d.) on the left renal artery. Animals with systolic blood pressure (SBP) greater than 20 kPa (150 mmHg) at 3−4 weeks after clipping were selected as RVHR. Male SHR and WKY rats aged 15−20 weeks were used in this work.

Blood pressure was monitored by using a computerized technic (Su et al., 1986) with some modifications (Cheng et al., 1990). The ABR−BP was measured by comparing the pressor responses (in area, mmHg · sec) to angiotensin II (A II, 25ng / kg, iv) before (A1) and after (A2) blocking the baroreflex efferent pathway. We have: ABR−BP(%) = (A2−A1) / A2 × 100.
The blockade of baroreflex efferent pathway was performed by using guanethidine (10 mg / kg, iv, and a semi−dose was given 45 min late) and methyl−atropine (1 mg / kg, iv, 20 min after the second dose of guanethidine). For ABR−HP measurement, blood pressure was raised by a bolus injection of A II. The slope of the relationship between SBP and HP variations after A II was defined as ABR−HP (Su et al., 1986).

In blood pressure variability (BPV) study, BP was continuously monitored for 12h (2:00—14:00). BPV was expressed by the standard deviation of BP recorded during this period.

All data are expressed as means ± S.E. For comparisons between 2 groups, Student t test for unpaired data was used.

RESULTS

ABR-BP and BPV. In WKY rats (n = 13), a closed negative correlation was found between ABR-BP and BPV (r = 0.87, P < 0.01), but no significant correlation was found between ABR-HP and BPV (r = 0.17, P = 0.59).

ABR—BP and ABR—HP in hypertensive rats. As showed in Table 1, ABR—BP as well as ABR—HP was significantly lower in both SHR and RVHR compared with WKY rats.

Table 1. ABR—BP and ABR—HP in conscious hypertensive rats

	n	ABR—BP (%)	ABR—HP (msec / mmHg)
WKY	12	73 ± 3.1	1.04 ± 0.07
SHR	8	51 ± 4.3***	0.24 ± 0.05***
RVHR	8	59 ± 3.4**	0.44 ± 0.05***

**P < 0.01, ***P < 0.001, vs WKY rats.

The sympathetic and vagal components of ABR—BP. Component analysis was performed by blocking these two components separately. The results obtained in SHR and WKY rats were showed in Table 2.

Table 2. The sympathetic and vagal components of ABR—BP in SHR and WKY rats.

	n	Components of ABR — BP (%)		
		Sympathetic	Vagal	Total
WKY	8	68 ± 2.8	26 ± 4.6	73 ± 2.5
SHR	8	51 ± 1.4***	5 ± 5.0***	53 ± 1.8***

***P < 0.001, vs WKY rats.

DISCUSSION

The first contribution of the present paper is to provide an effective method for the ABR—BP measurement. It is logical to take the difference between the pressor responses to a vasoactive agent in two conditions, with and without buffering mechanism of baroreflex, as a quantitative measurement of ABR function. One can block ABR in three ways: sinoaortic denervation (SAD), deterioration of NTS and pharmacological blockade of the efferent pathway. The first two methods need unreversible surgery, so we chose the pharmacological method. In this method, the pressor responses were calculated in area under the SBP variation curve. Thuse, not only the magnitude of the BP change but also was the time taken for return to controlled level taken in consideration. It has been reported that, this return time was considerably prolonged in SAD dog (McRitchie et al., 1976). This method is also different from the conception of baroreflex "gain", which could be expressed as $(A2-A1)/A1$ if in a similar open–loop study.

The second contribution is to show, for the first time, a negative relationship between BPV and ABR–BP but not ABR–HP in one group rats (WKY). Therefore, it is not surprising that there was a poor relationship between BPV and baroreflex sensitivity (ABR–HP) in some previous studies. This finding gives an example revealing the value of this method.

The third contribution is the finding that ABR–BP is also impaired in hypertensive rats. Component analysis shows that ABR–BP is mainly determined by sympathetic system. The ratio of sympathetic component to vagal one is 2.6:1 in WKY and 10:1 in SHR. The lower ABR–BP in SHR is mainly due to the impairment of vagal component.

(The project supported by the National Natural Science Foundation of China, No 3880743)

REFERENCES

Cheng, Y., Zhang, H., Su, D.F., and Gu, K.m. (1990): Effects of ketanserin on blood pressure and blood pressure variability in conscious unrestrained rats. *J. Med. Coll. P.L.A. 5*, 389–393.

Jones, J.V., and Floras, J.S. (1980): Baroreflex sensitivity changes during the development of Goldblatt two–kidney one–clip hypertension in rats. *Clin. Sci. 59*, 347–352.

McRitchie, R.J., VATNER, S.F., Heyndrickx, G.R., and Braunwald, E. (1976): The role of arterial baroreceptors in the regulation of arterial pressure in conscious dogs. *Cir. Res. 39*, 666–670

Struyker–Boudier, H.A.J., Evenwel, R.t., Smits, J.F.M., and Van Essen, H. (1982): Baroreflex sensitivity during the development of spontaneous hypertension in rats. *Clin. Sci. 62*, 589–594.

Su, D.F., Cerutti, C., Barres, C., Vincent, M., and Sassard, J. (1986): Blood pressure and baroreflex sensitivity in conscious hypertensive rats of Lyon strain. *Am. J. Physiol. 252*, H1111–H1117.

Impairment of parasympathetic control of the heart in SHR is not due to reduced cardiac parasympathetic responsiveness

Alberto U. Ferrari, Anna Daffonchio, Cristina Franzelli and Giuseppe Mancia

Semeiotica Medica and Clinica Medica Generale, Centro Fisiologia Clinica e Ipertensione and CNR, Ospedale Maggiore, Università di Milano, Milano, Italy

Hypertensive individuals have impaired autonomic control of the heart (Mancia et al., 1978; Julius and Esler, 1975; Wei et al., 1983; Ferrari et al., 1991), but the mechanisms underlying this phenomenon are unclear. The reduction in the sympathetically-mediated responses is likely to depend on a cardiac adrenergic receptor hyporesponsiveness (Bertel et al., 1980; Sarugoca and Tarazi, 1981); on the other hand the hypothesis that a concurrent defect of cardiac muscarinic receptors is responsible for the reduced vagally-mediated responses has never been tested. This study was therefore designed to evaluate cardiac parasympathetic responsiveness in hypertension; the selected experimental model was the spontaneously hypertensive rat, in which the cardiac muscarinic receptors were pharmacologically activated via i.v. injections of metacholine.

METHODS

The experiments were carried out in spontaneously hypertensive rats and normotensive control Wistar-Kyoto rats purchased from Charles River Inc. (Calco, Italy) at the age of 11 to 12 weeks. Mean ($\pm$SEM) body weight at time of study was 283 ± 10 g in the hypertensive (n=8) and 289 ± 7 g (n=9) in the normotensive group. Under ketamine HCl anesthesia (80 mg/kg i.p., plus small supplements given as needed throughout the experimental protocol), polyethylene catheters were inserted into a femoral artery for blood pressure recording and into a femoral vein for drug administration. The neck was then opened via a ventral midline incision, and the vagal trunks were bilaterally isolated and sectioned.
Following a 30 min period of hemodynamic equilibration, graded i.v. bolus injections of metacholine were administered at the randomly sequenced doses of 1, 2, 4 and 8 ug/kg, with an interval of 3 to 5 min separating each injection from the following one. Blood pressure was measured by connecting the arterial catheter to a Statham P23Dc tranducer; heart rate was obtained beat-to-beat by tachographic conversion of the pulsatile blood pressure signal, all

data being continuously displayed on a Grass 7D ink-writing recorder. Since each injection was followed by a clearcut dose-dependent bradycardic response linear regressions lines of the peak reduction in heart rate to the dose of metacholine were obtained and the slope of the regression line was taken as the measure of cardiac parasympathetic responsiveness. Statistical comparison of the slopes observed in hypertensive versus normotensive rats of the same age was performed by the Wilcoxon non-parametric rank test, with a p<0.05 being considered as statistically significant.

RESULTS

Baseline hemodynamics. The average values for mean arterial pressure observed before metacholine injection in the spontaneously hypertensive rats and in the control Wistar-Kyoto rats were respectively 172±9 and 132±5 mmHg (means±SEM, p<0.01). The corresponding average heart rate values were 370±12 and 393±14 b.min-1 (p=ns).

Cardiac parasympathetic responsiveness. Metacholine injection caused an immediate and short-lived bradycardic response and a more sustained blood pressure fall which started to fade after the heart rate change had largely disappeared. The blood pressure fall was similar in the two groups whereas the heart rate reduction was clearly larger in the hypertensive as compared with the normotensive group in response to all doses of metacholine: likewise, the calculated slopes were significantly steeper in the spontaneously hypertensive rats than in the control Wistar-Kyoto rats, amounting respectively to 18.8±3.5 and 13.1±4.4 b.min-1/ug.kg-1 (p<0.045).

DISCUSSION

At variance with the hypothesis outlined in the introduction, the major finding of our study was that in the spontaneously hypertensive rat cardiac parasympathetic responsiveness is not only unimpaired but is actually markedly enhanced. Thus the defective cardiac parasympathetic control known to characterize the hypertensive condition is not due to a reduced ability of the heart to respond to vagal stimuli and is more likely to depend on alterations in the neural (central?) portion of the system. An additional implication of our findings is that the alterations in cardiac autonomic control associated with hypertension are complex and opposite for the two major sets of receptors subserving the neural modulation, the known beta-adrenergic hyporesponsiveness coexisting with a parasympathetic hyperresponsiveness.
Although on an admittedly speculative basis we propose that such a peculiar pattern of autonomic receptor alterations may be secondary and reciprocal to sustained alterations in neural drive in hypertension: the cardiac beta-adrenoceptors would undergo a down-regulation to compensate for a chronically enhanced cardiac sympathetic activity; conversely, the cardiac muscarinic receptors would undergo an up-regulation to compensate for a chronically diminished cardiac vagal activity. Experimental evidence compatible with this proposed model is indeed available for the hypertension-

related alterations in the cardiac sympathetic (Woodckock et al., 1979; Wallin and Sundlof, 1979) and, although to a more limited and indirect extent, the cardiac parasympathetic system (Julius and Esler, 1975; Wei et al.,1983).

Whatever the underlying mechanisms may be, a muscarinic hyperresponsiveness of the heart in chronically high blood pressure may also have clinical implications: first of all, treatment of hypertensive patients by drugs endowed with vagomimetic properties such as digitalis glycosides (Chai et al., 1967) or converting enzyme inhibitors (Campbell et al., 1985) may favor the occurrence of excessive bradycardia. In addition, it may also be that in hypertensive subjects certain psychological or somatic stimuli (e.g. the sight of blood, the distention of a viscus, etc.) known to be accompanied by transient and marked elevations of vagal tone may bring about exaggerated cardioinhibitory reactions.

R E F E R E N C E S

Bertel O, Buhler FR, Kiowski W, Lutold BE. Decreased beta-adrenoceptor responsiveness as related to age, blood pressure and plasma catecholamines in patients with essential hypertension. Hypertension 1980, 2:130-138.

Campbell BC, Sturani A, Reid JL. Evidence of parasympathetic activity of the angiotensin converting enzyme inhibitor, captopril, in normotensive man. Cli Sci 1985, 68:49-56.

Chai CY, Wang HH, Hoffman BF, Wang SC. Mechanism of bradycardia induced by digitalis substances. Am J Physiol 1967, 212:26-34.

Ferrari AU, Daffonchio A, Franzelli C, Mancia G (1991). Potentiation of the baroreceptor-heart reflex by sympathectomy in conscious rats. Hypertension 18:230-235.

Julius S, Esler M. Autonomic nervous cardiovascular regulation in borderline hypertension. Am J Cardiol 1975, 36:685-696.

Mancia G, Ludbrook J, Ferrari A, Gregorini L, Zanchetti A. Baroreceptor reflexes in human hypertension. Circ Res 1978, 43:170-177.

Sarugoca M, Tarazi RC. Impaired cardiac contractile response to isoproterenol in SHR. Hypertension 1981, 3:380-385.

Wallin G, Sundlof G. A quantitative study of muscle sympathetic nerve activity in resting normotensive and hypertensive subjects. Hypertension 1979, 1:67-77.

Wei JY, Rowe JW, Kestenbaum AD, Ben-Haim S. Post-cough heart rate response: influence of age,sex and basal blood pressure. Am J Physiol 1983, 245:R18-R24.

Woodcock EA, Funder JW, Johnston CI. Decreased beta-adrenergic receptors in DOCA-salt and renal hypertensive rats. Circ Res 1979, 45:560-565.

Endothelin-1 microinjected into nuleus tractus solitarii of rat blocks arterial baroreflexes

Chong C. Lee, Hisashi Ohta and William T. Talman

Department of Neurology, VAMC and University of Iowa, Iowa City, IA 52242, USA

INTRODUCTION

Endothelin (Et) exists in three known isoforms (Et-1, Et-2, and Et-3). Recent immunohistochemical studies have shown that Et-1 is present within brain. It has been localized to specific brain regions including the nucleus tractus solitarii (NTS)(Kohzuki et al, 1991), the primary site of termination of baroreceptor and other visceral afferents. Variable changes in mean arterial pressure (MAP) and heart rate (HR) have been reported after administration of Et-3 into the cisterna magna adjacent to NTS, and intracisternal injections of Et-1 have been reported to block the baroreflex in anesthetized rats (Kuwaki et al, 1990). We hypothesized that the effects of Et on baroreflex are mediated by an action on neurons within NTS. Therefore, the purpose of this study was to investigate the cardiovascular effects elicited by microinjection of Et-1 into NTS and the possible mechanisms by which Et-1 expresses those effects.

METHODS

Sixty adult male Sprague-Dawley rats were instrumented for measurement of MAP and HR and intravenous injection of chemical agents. The anesthetized animals were placed in a stereotaxic frame, and the dorsal surface of the medulla was exposed through a limited occipital craniotomy. Multibarrel glass micropipettes were stereotaxically placed within NTS for unilateral or bilateral injection of solutions containing Et-1 (10 pmol/100 nl, 2 pmol/100 nl,and 1 pmol/100nl), glutamate (L-GLU; 250 pmol/25 nl), acetylcholine (ACh; 250 pmol/25 nl), and N-methyl-D-aspartate (NMDA; 1 pmol/20 nl). Injections were made by a pneumatic pump. All drugs were diluted in artificial cerebrospinal fluid, which alone had no effect on MAP, HR, or the baroreflex. Injection sites were marked at the end of each experiment with rhodamine beads or methylene blue and were confirmed histologically at post mortem exam. Injection sites outside the NTS ($\pm$ 1.5 mm lateral to the midline) were used as controls. Changes in cerebral blood flow (CBF) within NTS were measured in some animals by laser flowmetry employing a 0.8 mm probe that detects changes in flow in a 1 mm sphere of tissue.

The baroreflex was assessed by intravenous injection of various doses (.5 μg/kg-30 μg/kg) of phenylephrine (PE) and sodium nitroprusside (SNP). Reflex changes in HR resulting from changes in MAP were analyzed by a sigmoid-curve fitting program (Korner, 1989). Statistical analysis consisted of repeated measures ANOVA with confidence limits at $p < 0.05$.

RESULTS

Unilateral injection of 1 pmol/100 nl Et-1 produced inconsistent changes in HR and MAP. Bilateral injection of all concentrations elicited increases in HR and MAP. The hypertensive and tachycardiac responses persisted for 20-30 min. Injection of Et-1 adjacent to NTS did not elicit changes in HR or MAP.

The baroreflex assessed by intravenous injection of SNP and PE was significantly attenuated by microinjection of Et-1 into NTS. Bilateral injection of 10 pmol Et-1 reduced the gain and range (the range of MAP over which reflex HR changes occurred) of the baroreflex. The gain and range were -1.2 ± 0.4 and 58 ± 9 mmHg before Et-1 and -0.1 ± 0.4 and 13 ± 9 mmHg after Et-1. Bilateral injection of 2 pmol of Et-1 similarly decreased gain and range (before: -1.5 ± 0.2 and 55 ± 5 mmHg; after: -0.1 ± 0.2 and 13 ± 5 mmHg). Bilateral injection of 1 pmol Et-1 caused similar changes in gain and range (data not shown), but both parameters were also reduced after unilateral injection of 1 pmol Et-1 (before: -1.8 ± 0.3 and 71 ± 9 mmHg; after: -0.2 ± 0.3 and 20 ± 9 mmHg).

Microinjection of 1 pmol/100 nl ± 1.5 mm lateral to the midline, produced no significant change in either gain or range. The gain before and after Et-1 was -1.8 ± 0.3 and -1.5 ± 0.3 respectively; range before and after Et-1 was 58 ± 11 and 85 ± 11 mmHg respectively.

To determine if changes in cerebral blood flow may be responsible for the effects of Et-1 on the baroreflex, laser flowmetry was used to measure changes in flow in NTS before and after 1 pmol Et-1. Et-1 caused approximately a 45% reduction in local cerebral blood flow within 10 min of injection into NTS. Blood flow in NTS had not returned to baseline 30 min after injection.

Et-1 interaction with other putative neurotransmitters was also investigated. Specifically the effects of Et-1 on the actions of L-GLU, ACh, and NMDA on HR and MAP were tested in 4 rats per experiment. The bradycardiac and hypotensive effects of L-GLU, ACh, and NMDA when injected into NTS were abolished for at least 30 min by Et-1 (1 pmol/100nl) injected at the same site.

DISCUSSION

Previous experiments (Kuwaki et al, 1990) showed that intracisternal injection of 100 pmol Et-3 produced a triphasic response in MAP and blockade of the baroreflex. An initial increase of MAP was followed by a decrease that was, in turn, followed by a prolonged increase. Our study has demonstrated that blockade of the baroreflex by Et (specifically Et-1) may be caused by effects within NTS. It is evident that Et-1 injected into NTS suppresses function locally as demonstrated by blockade of the baroreflex and increases in MAP and HR. The observed effects of Et-1 on MAP and HR are similar to those following bilateral injection of the local anesthetic lidocaine into NTS. Furthermore, within 10 min of injection of Et-1 responses could no longer be elicited by injection of L-GLU, ACh, or NMDA. The mechanism of these effects is not known but Et may modify calcium currents (Nishimura et al, 1991) and thus may produce it effects through alterations in neuronal permeability to calcium and other ions.

The current study also suggests that local tissue hypoxia resulting from the significant decrease in cerebral blood flow following Et-1 injection may be responsible for the cardiovascular changes.

The attenuation of the baroreflex observed in this study is in conflict with another recent study that demonstrated sensitization of the baroreflex after injection of Et-1 into the cisterna magna of conscious rats (Itoh and Van den Buuse, 1991). However, the different effects may be the result of the different state of consciousness of the rats since effects of putative transmitters themselves may be profoundly altered by anesthesia. For example, L-GLU microinjected in NTS elicits pressor effects in conscious rats and depressor effects in the same rats when anesthetized (Machado and Bonagamba, 1991; Talman et al, 1980).

In summary, this study suggests that Et may act in NTS when injected into the cisterna magna and that the cardiovascular effects elicited by Et injected in or near the NTS may be the result of secondary effects of the agent on local blood flow. Although the neural effects studied here may thus be an indirect effect, Et may specifically bind in the brain and disturbances of such binding may be associated with altered blood pressure control (Gulati and Rebello, 1991).

REFERENCES

Gulati, A., and Rebello, S. (1991): Down-regulation of endothelin receptors in the ventrolateral medulla of spontaneously hypertensive rats. Life Sci. 48:1207-1215.

Itoh, S., and van den Buuse, M. (1991): Sensitization of baroreceptor reflex by central endothelin in conscious rats. Am. J. Physiol. 260:H1106-H1112.

Kohzuki, M., Chai, S.W., Paxinos, G., Karavas, A., Casley D.J., Johnston, C.I., and Mendelsohn, F.A.O. (1991): Localization and characterization of endothelin receptor binding sites in the rat brain visualized by *in vitro* autoradiography. Neuroscience 42:245-260.

Korner, P.I. (1989): Baroreceptor resetting and other determinants of baroreflex properties in hypertension. Clin. Exp. Pharmacol. Physiol. 15, Suppl:45-64.

Kuwaki, T., Koshiya, N., Takahashi, H., Terui, N., and Kumada, M. (1990): Modulatory effects of rat endothelin in central cardiovascular control in rats. Jap. J. Physiol. 40: 97-116.

Machado, B.H., Bonagamba, L.G.H. (1991): Microinjection of L-glutamate (L-GLU) into nucleus tractus solitarii (NTS) increases arterial pressure in conscious rats. FASEB J. 5:A743 (abstract).

Nishimura, T., Akasu, T., and Krier, J. (1991): Endothelin modulates calcium channel current in neurones of rabbit pelvic parasympathetic ganglia. Br. J. Pharmacol. 103:1242-1250.

Talman, WT., Perrone, M.H., and Reis, D.J. (1980): Evidence for L-glutamate as the neurotransmitter of baroreceptor afferent nerve fibers. Science 209:813-815.

Central injection of endothelin-1 augments baroreflex sensitivity in spontaneously hypertensive rats

M. van den Buuse and S. Itoh

Marion Merrell Dow Research Institute, 16, rue d'Ankara, B.P. 447/R9, 67009 Strasbourg, France

Endothelin-1 (ET-1) is a 21-amino acid peptide which may cause a marked rise in blood pressure upon intravenous administration (Yanagisawa et al., 1988; Le Monnier de Gouville et al., 1989). ET-1 and ET-1 mRNA is present in the central nervous system (Takahashi et al., 1990; Giaid et al., 1989; MacCumber et al., 1989) and receptors for ET-1 have been found in a number of brain regions, with highest density in the cerebellum and striatum (Jones et al., 1989; Koseki et al., 1989). Some authors have shown that relatively high doses of ET-1 injected intracerebroventricularly (i.c.v.) cause a marked increase of blood pressure in rats (Ouchi et al., 1989; Kuwaki et al., 1990). We have shown that lower doses of intracisternally (i.c.) injected ET-1 do not change blood pressure or heart rate, but induce a significant sensitization of the baroreceptor-heart rate reflex in conscious, normotensive rats (Itoh and Van den Buuse, 1991). Spontaneously hypertensive rats (SHR) show decreased baroreflex sensitivity (Struyker Boudier et al., 1982; Head and Adams, 1988). Moreover, in some regions of SHR brain ET-1 receptors were found to be down-regulated (Gulati and Rebello, 1991). The object of the present study was to investigate the effects of central administration of ET-1 on mean arterial pressure (MAP), heart rate (HR) and the baroreceptor-HR reflex in conscious SHR and Wistar-Kyoto rats (WKY).

Male SHR and WKY were provided with an i.c. cannula one week before and a femoral artery and a double jugular vein catheter two days before the experiment. Baroreceptor-HR reflex was measured by sigmoidal curve fitting of the MAP and HR reponses evoked by alternating injections of different doses of phenylephrine or nitroprusside (Head and McCarty, 1987; Itoh and Van den Buuse, 1991). From curves obtained in individual rats baroreflex parameters were derived before and after ET-1 injection (see table). Average baroreflex gain was derived as a function of the HR range and the curvature coefficient (gain = -2.56 x P2 x P3). From the group-means of the baroreflex parameters, a group baroreflex curve was constructed (see fig. 1).

Resting blood pressure and HR were significantly higher in SHR than in WKY. Moreover, SHR had a significantly lower baroreflex gain (sensitivity) and HR range when compared to WKY. The i.c. injection of 25 pmol/kg ET-1, but not of 2.5 pmol/kg (not shown), induced a significant increase in baroreflex gain, without an effect on resting MAP or HR. This effect was not significantly different between SHR and WKY and was associated with a significant increase in curvature coefficient (P3), without an effect on HR range (table I and fig. 1).

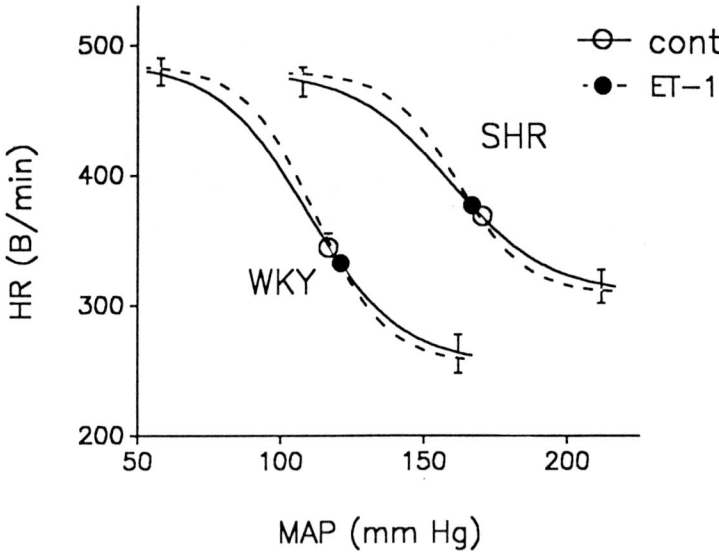

Figure 1: The effect of i.c. injection of 25 pmol/kg ET-1 on baroreceptor-heart rate reflex of SHR and WKY. Curves were generated by using the mean group-values obtained from the individual curves (see table I for data and statistics). Open and closed circles represent resting MAP and HR.

TABLE I: The effect of i.c. injection of 25 pmol/kg ET-1 on baroreflex parameters and blood pressure and heart rate of conscious SHR and WKY.

Strain/treatment Baroreflex parameters	SHR (n=7) control	SHR (n=7) ET-1	WKY (n=7) control	WKY (n=7) ET-1
Low HR plateau (P1, B/min)	309 ± 15*	309 ± 16*	255 ± 14	256 ± 11
HR range (P2, B/min)	171 ± 16*	170 ± 17*	232 ± 13	230 ± 12
Curvature (P3, mmHg^{-1})	0.06 ± 0.01	0.09 ± 0.01**	0.06 ± 0.01	0.08 ± 0.01**
BP50 (P4, mmHg)	159 ± 6*	162 ± 3*	110 ± 4	112 ± 3
Average gain (B/min/mmHg)	-2.11 ± 0.14*	-2.97 ± 0.27*,**	-3.06 ± 0.34	-3.90 ± 0.36**
Resting MAP (mmHg)	170 ± 4*	167 ± 3*	117 ± 2	121 ± 2
Resting HR (B/min)	369 ± 11*	377 ± 8*	345 ± 11	333 ± 5

(*) $P<0.05$ for strain difference; (**) $p<0.05$ for effect of ET-1 treatment. Data are mean ± S.E.M.

These results show that central injection of ET-1 caused a sensitization of the baroreceptor-heart rate reflex in SHR and WKY, as we have found previously in normotensive Wistar rats (Itoh and Van den Buuse, 1991). The effect of ET-1 was not different between SHR and WKY, suggesting it was mediated through a mechanism which is distinct from that underlying the difference in reflex sensitivity between SHR and WKY. Indeed, while the difference in baroreflex gain between SHR and WKY was caused by a difference in HR range, i.e. the maximum capacity of the heart to respond to changes in blood pressure, the effect of ET-1 on the baroreflex gain was mediated by an increase in the curvature, i.e. the steepness of the curve between the maxima (see fig. 1). The latter effect implies that for a given change in blood pressure ET-1 treated rats show a greater change in HR than controls. Further experiments have shown that in SHR and WKY treated with atropine, which blocks the action of the vagus, there was neither a strain difference in baroreflex sensitivity, nor an effect of i.c. administration of ET-1 (data not shown). This suggests that both the reduction of baroreflex gain and HR range in SHR vs. WKY, as well as the enhancing effect of ET-1 injection on baroreflex gain and curvature coefficient are mediated by the vagus nerve. The detailed analysis of the baroreceptor-HR reflex, as performed with the present method, allows the dissociation of these two mechanisms. It is concluded that central injection of ET-1 caused a significant increase of baroreflex sensitivity, but that this effect is not different between SHR and WKY.

REFERENCES

Giaid A., Gibson S.J., Ibrahim N.B.N., Legon S., Bloom S.R., Yanagisawa M., Masaki T., Varndell I.M. and Polak J.M. (1989): Endothelin 1, an endothelium-derived peptide, is expressed in neurons of the human spinal cord and dorsal root ganglia. *Proc. Nat. Acad. Sci. USA* 86: 7634-7638.

Gulati A. and Rebello S. (1991): Down-regulation of endothelin receptors in the ventrolateral medulla of spontaneously hypertensive rats. *Life Sci.* 48: 1207-1215.

Head G.A. and Adams M.A. (1988): Time course of changes in baroreceptor reflex control of heart rate in conscious SHR and WKY: contribution of the cardiac vagus and sympathetic nerves. *Clin. Exp. Pharmacol. Physiol.* 15: 289-292.

Head G.A. and McCarty R. (1987): Vagal and sympathetic components of the heart rate range and gain of the baroreceptor-heart rate reflex in conscious rats. *J. Auton. Nerv. Syst.* 21: 203-213.

Itoh S. and Van den Buuse M. (1991): Sensitization of baroreceptor reflex by central endothelin in conscious rats. *Am. J. Physiol.* 260: H1106-H1112.

Jones C.R., Hiley C.R., Pelton J.T. and Mohr M. (1989): Autoradiographic visualization of the binding sites for [^{125}I]endothelin in rat and human brain. *Neurosci. Lett.* 97: 276-279.

Koseki C., Imai M., Hirata Y., Yanagisawa M. and Masaki T. (1989): Autoradiographic distribution in rat tissues of binding sites for endothelin: a neuropeptide? *Am. J. Physiol.* 256: R858-R866.

Kuwaki T., Koshiya N., Takahashi H., Terui N. and Kumada M. (1990): Modulatory effects of rat endothelin on central cardiovascular control in rats. *Jap. J. Physiol.* 40: 97-116.

Le Monnier de Gouville A.C., Lippton H.L., Cavero I., Summer W.R. and Hyman A.L. (1989): Endothelin - A new family of endothelium-derived peptides with widespread biological properties. *Life Sci.* 45: 1499-1513.

MacCumber M.W., Ross C.A., Glaser B.M. and Snyder S.H. (1989): Endothelin: visualization of mRNAs by in situ hybridization provides evidence for local action. *Proc. Nat. Acad. Sci. USA* 86: 7285-7289.

Ouchi Y., Kim S., Souza A.C., Ijima S., Hattori A., Orimo H., Yoshizumi M., Kurihara H. and Yazaki Y (1989): Central effect of endothelin on blood pressure of conscious rats. *Am. J. Physiol.* 256: H1747-1751.

Struyker-Boudier H.A.J., Evenwel R.T., Smits J.F.M. and Van Essen H. (1982): Baroreceptor sensitivity during the development of spontaneous hypertension in rats. *Clin. Sci.* 62: 589-593.

Takahashi K., Ghatei M.A., Jones P.M., Murphy J.K., Lam H.C., O'Halloran D.J. and Bloom S.R. (1991): Immunoreactive endothelin, endothelin mRNA and endothelin receptors in human brain and pituitary gland: presence of immunoreacitve endothelin, endothelin messenger ribonucleic acid, and endothelin receptors. *J. Clin. Endocr. Metab.* 72: 693-699.

Yanagisawa M., Kurihara H., Kimura S., Tomobe Y., Kobayashi N., Mitsui Y., Yazaki Y., Goto K. and Masaki T. (1988): A novel potent vasoconstrictor peptide produced by vascular endothelial cells. *Nature* 332: 411-415.

Central kinin receptors in the spontaneously hypertensive rat and the pressor response to bradykinin

Debora R. Fior, Domingos T.O. Martins and Charles J. Lindsey

Department of Biophysics, Escola Paulista de Medicina, Caixa Postal 20.388, 04034 São Paulo, São Paulo, Brazil

The intracerebroventricular (icv) administration of bradykinin (Bk) causes an increase in the mean arterial pressure (MAP) of rats (Pearson et al. 1969) and other mammal species (Pearson et al. 1967; Graeff et al. 1969). This pressor response is mediated by kinin receptors in the medulla oblongata in or adjacent to the fourth cerebral ventricle (Lindsey et al. 1988, unpublished results). The receptors which mediate the central pressor response in the normotensive Wistar rat (NWR) are of the B_2 subtype (Lindsey et al., 1989). The spontaneously hypertensive rat (SHR) showed an increased sensitivity to the pressor action of icv administered kinins in comparison to normotensive Wistar rat (Lindsey et al., 1988). In order to gain insight on the mechanisms which underlie the increased sensitivity of the SHR on the central pressure effect the following experiments were examined: a) Effect of Bk injected into the IV ventricle of SHR and 1kidney 1clip (1K1C) renal hypertensive rat. b) Response to icv Bk in the SHR in the presence of kininase inhibitors c) "In vivo" pharmacological classification and characterization of the receptor which mediate the pressor response to Bk in the SHR.

METHODS

Adult female rats (200-230 g body weight) were anaesthetized with pentobarbitone and chloral hydrate and the cannula was placed in the fourth cerebral ventricle (11,0 mm antero-posterior (AP), 7,9 mm vertical and 0,0 mm lateral from bregma in SHR and 11,7 mm AP, 7.5 mm vertical and 0.0 mm lateral in NWR) and fixed to the skull by jeweller's screws embedded in dental acrylic cement. Following the intracerebroventricular surgery a polyethylene catheter was placed in the abdominal aorta through the left femoral artery. The other end of the catheter was slipped under the skin and exteriorized on the back of the animal. Two days after implantation of the cannula the effect of centrally administered bradykinin was examined in unanaesthetized and unrestrained animals. The kininase inhibitors N-[1 (RS)-carboxy-3 phenyl-propyl]-Ala-Ala-Phe-pAB (CPP-Ala-Ala-Phe-pAB 2.4 µmol and enalaprilat 0.6 µmol or the receptor antagonists D-Arg^9-Leu^8-Bk (DALBk 11 nmol) and D-Arg-[Hyp^3-Thi^{5,8}-D-Phe^7]-Bk

(DAHTDBK 0.08-0.8 nmol) were administered to the fourth cerebral ventricle prior to administration of Bk.

RESULTS AND DISCUSSION

Dose response curves for the pressor effect of bradykinin were obtained in NWR, SHR and 1 kidney 1 clip (1K1C) rats. The ED_{50} values obtained (table 1) showed that the SHR have an increased sensitivity to intracerebroventricular bradykinin when compared to NWR or renal hypertensive 1K1C rats. These results indicate that increased sensitivity of the SHR is not due to a direct effect of increased blood pressure since the renal hypertensive animals showed the same sensitivity in comparison to NWR.

Table 1. Pressor effect of bradykinin injected into the IV ventricle of NWR and 1K1C renal hypertensive rats.

GROUP	BLOOD PRESSURE (mmHg)	ED_{50} (pmol)	MAXIMAL EFFECT (mmHg)
CONTROLS	112 ± 12	22	31 ± 15
SHR	148 ± 16	3	31 ± 14
1K1C	149 ± 20	20	29 ± 10

The values represent the mean ± s.d. of at least 10 animals.

Kininase inhibitors were injected intracerebroventricularly in NWR and SHR in order to verify the contribution of kininase activity to the response to centrally administered bradykinin. Injection of a mixture of kininase inhibitors enalaprilat (0,6 µmol) and CPP-Ala-Ala-Phe-pAB (2,4 µmol) into the fourth ventricle 10 min before the administration of Bk, potentiated the effect of this peptide in the NWR and SHR (table 2). The SHR showed increased sensitivity to the central pressor effect of Bk in the presence of converting enzyme inhibitors which suggest that mechanisms other than decreased kininase activity may account for the increased sensitivity to the Bk in the SHR.

Table 2. Effect of kininase inhibitors enalaprilat (0.6 µmol) and CPP-Ala-Ala-Phe-pAB (2.4 µmol) on the pressor effect (MAP) of bradykinin injected into the IV ventricle of NWR and SHR.

	CONTROL MAP (mmHg)	KININASE INHIBITORS MAP (mmHg)
NWR (Bk 8 pmol)	4 ± 8	20 ± 13*
SHR (Bk 2 pmol)	12 ± 9	29 ± 9*

The values represent the mean ± s.d. of 20 animals.

In order to characterize the central kinin receptors which mediate the pressor response in the SHR selective agonist and antagonists of B_1 and B_2 receptors were used. The B_1 agonist (des-Arg^9-Bk) did not affect the Bk pressor action. The B_2 antagonist DAHTDBK antagonized the Bk pressor effect showing the kinin receptors which mediate the central pressor effect in the SHR as in the NWR are of the B_2 subtype. The B_2 antagonist DAHTDBk and interacted with the central kinin receptors in competitive and reversible manner and increasing concentration of the antagonist produced parallel displacement to the right in the Bk dose-response curves both in NWR and SHR. Schild plots from this data yielded linear plots (r = 0.98 and r = 0.99) with slope values close to the unity. The "in vivo" pA_2 estimated for the kinin receptors of the SHR was 10.66, 0.7 log units larger than the pA_2 value obtained for the kinin receptors in the NWR (figure 1). The difference of the pA_2 "in vivo" observed between the SHR and NWR suggest the existence of a difference in the central kinin receptors populations and the greater apparent affinity for the antagonist observed in the SHR could be related to the increased sensitivity observed in these animals to icv kinin agonists. However the determination of the pA_2 "in vivo" was carried out without control of the drug removal mechanisms and thus it is difficult to ascertain whether the pA_2 represents an increased affinity of the receptors or is a consequence of differences in peptidase activity.

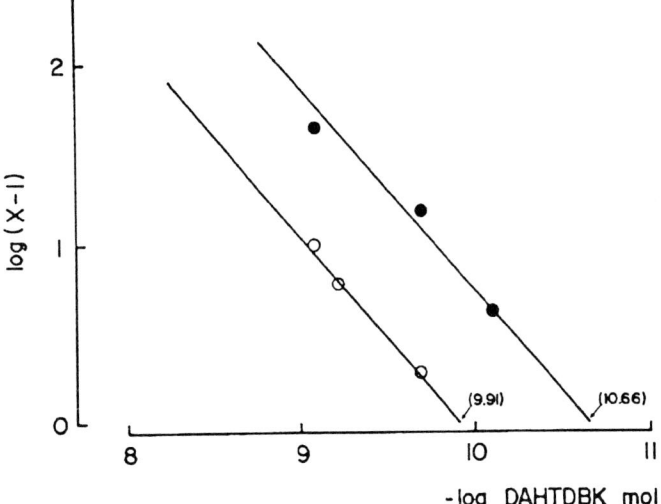

Fig 1. Schild plots obtained from log dose-response curves for the central pressor effect of bradykinin in the presence of different concentrations of the antagonist DAHTDBk in NWR ( ) or SHR ( ).

REFERENCES

Graeff, F.G., Pela, I.R. & Rocha e Silva, M (1969): Behavioral and somatic effects of bradykinin injected into cerebral ventricles of unanaesthetized rabbits. Br. J. Pharmacol. 37, 723-732.
Lindsey, C.J., Fujita, K. and Martins, D.T.O. (1988): The central pressor effect of bradykinin in normotensive and hypertensive rats. Hypertension 2, 126-129.
Lindsey, C.J., Nakaie, C.R. and Martins, D.T.O. (1989): Central nervous system kinin receptors and the hypertensive response mediated by bradykinin. Br. J. Pharmacol. 97, 763-768.
Pearson, L. and Lang, W.J. (1969). A comparison in concious and anaesthetized dogs of the effect on blood pressure of bradykinin, kallidin, eledoisin and kallikrein. Eur. J. Pharmacol. 2, 83-87.

Increased sensitivity to the central pressor effect of bradykinin in hypertensive rats

Domingos T.O. Martins [1], Debora R. Fior and Charles J. Lindsey

Department of Biophysics, Escola Paulista de Medicina, Caixa Postal 20.388, 04034 São Paulo, São Paulo, Brazil and [1] Universidade Federal de Mato Grosso, 78.000 Cuiabá, Mato Grosso, Brazil

Bradykinin causes an increase in blood pressure when injected into the cerebral ventricles of rats and other species (Pearson & Lang, 1967; Graeff et al., 1969). The pressor response to bradykinin is mediate by B2 receptors in both the normotensive Wistar (NWR) (Lindsey et al., 1989) and the spontaneously hypertensive rat (SHR) (Martins et al., 1991) which are localized in areas adjacent to the fourth cerebral ventricle (Lindsey et al., 1988, unpublished results). The SHR is more sensitive to the pressor effect of intracerebroventricularly administered bradykinin (Lindsey et al., 1988). The increased sensitivity of the SHR to centrally administered bradykinin has been related to a decreased kininase activity in these animals (Lindsey et al., 1988) and possibly to an increase of the affinity of the kinin receptors for the agonist (Martins et al., 1991). To investigate the participation of the central kininergic mechanisms on the regulation of blood pressure the pressor response to centrally administered bradykinin was examined in the NWR, the Wistar Kyoto (WKY), the SHR and in spontaneously hypertensive rats which did not develop hypertension (SHR*). Kininase inhibitors were also injected into the fourth cerebral ventricle of NWR and SHR in order to evaluate the functional significance of central kininergic mechanisms on blood pressure control.

METHODS

Adult female rats (200-230 g body weight) were anaesthetized with pentobarbitone and chloral hydrate and a cannula was placed in the fourth cerebral ventricle (11,0 mm antero-posterior (AP), 7.9 mm vertical and 0.0 mm lateral from bregma in SHR and 11.7 mm AP, 7.5 mm vertical and 0.0 mm lateral in NWR) and fixed to the skull by jeweller's screws embedded in dental acrylic cement. Following the intracerebroventricular (icv) surgery a polyethylene catheter was placed in the abdominal aorta through the left femoral artery. The other end of the catheter was slipped under the skin and exteriorized on the back of the animal. The animals were allowed to recover for two days. Dose-response curves were obtained by injecting different amounts of bradykinin in 1 µl of saline into the fourth cerebral ventricle and blood pressure was recorded in the unanaesthetized rats. The enzyme inhibitors enalaprilat (0.6 µmol) and CPP.Ala.Ala.Phe.pAB (2.4 µmol) were dissolved in 1 µl of saline for intraventricular injection.

RESULTS

The arterial pressure of the NWR was 112±8 mmHg, 105±8 in the WKY and 148±16 mmHg in the SHR. The SHR* group, with a mean arterial pressure of 129±11 mmHg, were SHR rats, selected from our breeding colony, which did not develop high blood pressure. Full dose-response curves for the central pressor response to bradykinin were obtained in the NWR, WKY, SHR and SHR*. In all groups of animals the mean maximal effect obtained was approximately 30 mmHg with the exception of the WKY where the maximal effect was significantly shorter (22 mmHg). The ED_{50} for the pressor effect was 22 pmol in NWR, 17 pmol in the WKY, 3 pmol in the SHR and 23 pmol in the SHR* (figure 1). Latency, measured as the time between the injection of bradykinin and the manifestation of the pressor effect was approximately 15 s in the NWR, WKY, and SHR*, and significantly shorter in the SHR (9 s). The administration of enalaprilat and CPP.Ala.Ala.Phe.pAB to the fourth ventricle did not alter blood pressure in the NWR, but in the SHR the association of kininase inhibitors induced a discreet but significant increase in arterial pressure between 7 and 12 min following administration (Table 1).

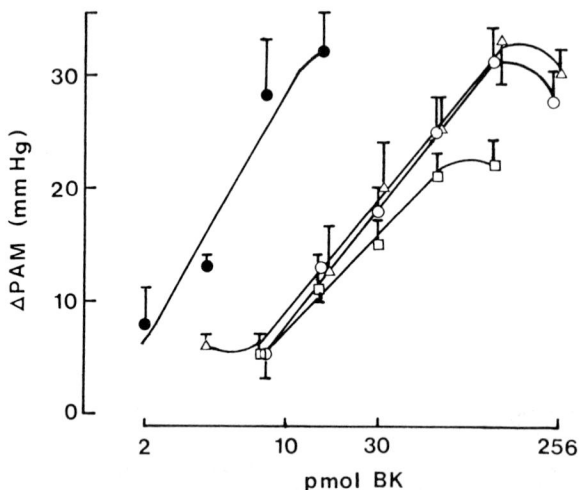

Fig. 1. Log dose-response curves for the pressor effect of bradykinin injected into the fourth cerebral ventricule of SHR (●), SHR* (△), NWR (○) and WKY (□). The curve for bradykinin in the SHR differed significantly (P < 0.001) from the others. Each point represents mean ± s.d. of at least 15 animals.

Table 1. Effect of a mixture of enalaprilat (0.6 μmol) and CPP.Ala.Ala.Phe.pAB (2.4 μmol) on the mean arterial pressure (MAP) of normotensive Wistar rats (NWR) and spontaneously hypertensive rats (SHR).

STRAIN	BLOOD PRESSURE (mmHg)	CONTROLS ΔMAP (mmHg)	INHIBITORS ΔMAP (mmHg)
NWR	100 ± 11	1 ± 2	3 ± 7
SHR	140 ± 13	2 ± 9	9 ± 11*

*Differs significantly from controls (P < 0.05, paired t test).
The values represent the mean ± s.d. of at least 10 animals.

DISCUSSION

The injection of bradykinin in the fourth cerebral ventricle of unanaesthetized rats produced an increase in arterial pressure. In the normotensive strains NWR and WKY the increase in arterial pressure was obtained with an ED_{50} of approximately 20 pmol and a latency of about 15 s. The mean maximal effect observed in the NWR was 30 mmHg and 22 mmHg in the WKY. The SHR with a mean arterial pressure of 150 mmHg were much more sensitive (ED_{50} = 3 pmol) to the pressor effect of bradykinin although the maximal effect was the same as in the NWR. Animals of the SHR strain which did not develop high blood pressure showed sensitivity to bradykinin similar to the normotensive strain. This result shows that the sensitivity to intracerebroventricular bradykinin is linked to the expression of high blood pressure in the SHR. At present however it is impossible to know whether or not the sensitivity to centrally administered bradykinin and high blood pressure represent a causal relationship. The increase in arterial pressure observed in the SHR following the administration of kininase inhibitors suggest that endogenous kinins may play a role in the central regulation of blood pressure. Enalaprilat is a specific inhibitor of angiotensin converting enzyme or kininase II and CPP.Ala.Ala.Phe.pAB inhibits metalloendopeptidase activity which degrades bradykinin (Macdermot et al., 1987) as well as other neuropeptides. The possibility that the pressor response is due to a reduction in the degradation of angiotensin II may be excluded since the simultaneous administration of enalaprilat interrupts angiotensin II generation.

The expression of high blood pressure in the SHR is related to an increased sensitivity to the pressor effect of centrally administered kinins. Endogenous kinins may play a role in the central regulation of blood pressure of the SHR.

REFERENCES

Lindsey, C.J., Fujita, K. and Martins, D.T.O. (1988): The central pressor effect of bradykinin in normotensive and hypertensive rats. *Hypertension* 2, 126-129.

Lindsey, C.J., Nakaie, C.R. and Martins, D.T.O. (1989): Central nervous system kinin receptors and the hypertensive response mediated by bradykinin. *Br. J. Pharmacol.* 97, 763-768.

Martins, D.T.O., Fior, D.R., Nakaie, C.R. and Lindsey, C.J. (1991): Kinin receptors of the central nervous system of spontaneously hypertensive rats related to the pressor response to bradykinin. *Br. J. Pharmacol.* 103, 1851-1856.

McDermott, J.R. Gibson, A.M. and Turner, J.D. (1987): Involvement of endopetidase 24.15 in the inactivation of bradykinin by rat brain slices. *Biochem. Biophys. Res. Commun.* 146, 154-158.

Pearson, L. & Lang, W.J. (1967): The nature of the pressor responses produced by bradykinin and kallidin. *Aust. J. Exp. Biol. Med. Sci.* 45, 35.

A role of central GABA in the development of hypertension in the spontaneously hypertensive rat ?

M. van den Buuse, S. Sarhan and N. Seiler

Marion Merrell Dow Research Institute, 16, rue d'Ankara, B.P. 447/R9, 67009 Strasbourg, France

The inhibitory neurotransmitter γ-aminobutyric acid (GABA) plays an important role in the central regulation of blood pressure (for references, see Gillis et al., 1984; Philippu et al., 1988). Central administration of GABA-agonists may cause a reduction of blood pressure and sympathetic nerve activity (Brennan et al., 1983; Sweet et al., 1979; Unger et al., 1984). In Spontaneously Hypertensive Rats (SHR) some authors have observed lower concentrations of GABA and GABA receptors in the hypothalamus (Czyzewska-Szafran and Wutkiewicz, 1983, Hambley et al., 1984) or medulla (Kubo et al., 1989). This suggests that SHR may have a deficient central GABA system and that this deficiency might play a role in the development of hypertension in these rats. However, other authors failed to observe differences in central levels of GABA and GABA receptors between SHR and WKY (Brennan et al., 1983; Thyagarajan et al., 1983; Tunnicliff et al., 1984). We therefore measured central GABA levels at different ages in the brain of SHR and WKY and investigated whether a long-term increase of brain GABA concentrations would influence the development of hypertension.

For the measurement of central GABA concentrations, SHR and WKY of 4 weeks or 10 weeks of age were decapitated and their brains were rapidly removed. Hypothalamus, medulla and rest of the brain were dissected on a cold plate and rapidly frozen in liquid nitrogen. GABA concentrations were measured in homogenates of these brain parts by a modification of a method previously used to determine central concentrations of vigabatrin (Schousboe et al. 1986). Table I shows the results. Although there were regional differences in the concentrations of GABA between different brain parts, there were no differences between the concentrations found in SHR and those found in WKY, either at 4 weeks of age or at 10 weeks of age.

TABLE I: Body weight (g) and brain concentration of GABA (μmol/g wet weight) of 4 and 10 weeks old SHR or WKY. Data are mean ± SEM of n=10 per group.

Strain/age	Body weight	Hypothalamus	Medulla	Rest of brain
SHR 4 weeks	87 ± 1	4.74 ± 0.10	1.67 ± 0.06	2.03 ± 0.01
WKY 4 weeks	98 ± 2	4.71 ± 0.08	1.58 ± 0.04	2.06 ± 0.02
SHR 10 weeks	285 ± 3	4.93 ± 0.08	1.49 ± 0.04	2.05 ± 0.02
WKY 10 weeks	264 ± 9	4.87 ± 0.07	1.43 ± 0.02	2.04 ± 0.02

TABLE II: Effect of six week treatment with 80 mg/kg/day vigabatrin on cardiovascular parameters in SHR and WKY. Data are mean ± SEM of n=6 rats per groups.

	SHR		WKY	
	water	vigabatrin	water	vigabatrin
Systolic blood pressure (mm Hg)	208 ± 4*	219 ± 7*	143 ± 4	139 ± 7
Mean arterial pressure (mm Hg)	161 ± 7*	176 ± 7*	128 ± 4	126 ± 3
Heart rate (B/min)	379 ± 15	392 ± 16*	355 ± 24	324 ± 16
Baroreflex sensitivity (B/min/mm Hg)	-3.7 ± 0.3	-3.2 ± 0.7	-4.5 ± 0.8	-4.2 ± 1.0
Baroreflex heart rate range (B/min)	150 ± 21*	146 ± 19*	228 ± 26	245 ± 37
Body weight (g)	308 ± 9	278 ± 7*,**	299 ± 5	302 ± 8

(*) $P<0.05$ for strain difference; (**) $P<0.05$ for effect of vigabatrin-treatment.

To test the effect of an increase in central GABA levels, three groups of ten SHR or WKY were given vigabatrin, an irreversible inhibitor of the GABA breakdown enzyme GABA-transaminase (Jung et al., 1977), in the drinking water. The concentration was adjusted such that the rats ingested 0, 40 or 80 mg/kg/day. The treatment started at the age of five weeks and was continued throughout the six week experiment. Systolic blood pressure and heart rate were measured regularly with a tail-cuff method. At the end of the treatment-period, the rats were provided with indwelling femoral and jugular catheters, to allow the direct measurement of blood pressure, heart rate and baroreflex sensitivity (Itoh and Van den Buuse, 1991).

Vigabatrin dose-dependently increased central GABA concentrations to a similar extent in SHR and WKY. Thus, in a subgroup measured after four weeks of treatment with 80 mg/kg/day, whole-brain GABA concentration was increased by 135% in SHR (4.2 µmol/g vs. 1.8 µmol/g in controls) and by 139% in WKY (4.6 µmol/g vs. 1.9 µmol/g in controls). No effect of either vigabatrin treatment was found on the development of hypertension in SHR or on blood pressure of WKY. Thus, after 2 and 4 weeks of treatment with 80 mg/kg/day (age 7 and 9 weeks) systolic blood pressure was 166 ± 6 and 210 ± 5 mm Hg in control SHR, 169 ± 3 and 217 ± 6 mm Hg in treated SHR, 140 ± 6 and 144 ± 4 mm Hg in control WKY and 141 ± 6 and 156 ± 3 mm Hg in treated WKY. Similarly, vigabatrin did not affect heart rate or body weight gain (not shown). After six weeks (age 11 weeks), the rats were cannulated in the femoral artery and jugular vein. Two days later, mean arterial pressure, heart rate and baroreflex responses to intravenous injections of phenylephrine and nitroprusside were measured. SHR had higher blood pressure and heart rate, but lower baroreflex sensitivity and baroreflex heart rate range when compared to WKY. However, treatment of the rats with vigabatrin did not significantly influence any of these parameters. A slight decrease in body weight in vigabatrin-treated SHR, but not WKY, was observed (table II).

Previously, Sasaki et al. (1990) showed a reduction of blood pressure of SHR treated chronically with valproic acid, a competitive inhibitor of GABA breakdown. Singewald et al. (1991) used vigabatrin treatment at a higher dose than those used in the present study. These authors reported a delay of the development of hypertension in the treated SHR. However, in both studies, there was also a significant decrease in body weight gain of the treated rats, so it remains to be shown whether the effect on blood pressure was mediated by the changes in central GABA levels or was the result of a more general inhibition of the development of the animals.

Our present results show that basal central concentrations of GABA are not different between SHR and WKY, either at the prehypertensive stage of development (4 weeks of age) or during the development phase of hypertension (10 weeks of age). Moreover, a marked increase in central GABA concentration during the development phase of spontaneous hypertension was not associated with any effect on blood pressure or on other cardiovascular parameters. Thus, it is concluded that central GABA systems probably do not play a major role in the development of hypertension in the SHR.

REFERENCES

Brennan T.J., Haywood J.R. and Ticku M.K. (1983): GABA receptor binding and hemodynamic responses to icv GABA in adult SHR. *Life Sci.* 33, 701-709.
Czyzewska-Szafran H. and Wutkiewicz M. (1983): Functional state of GABA-ergic system in spontaneously hypertensive rats. *Pol. J. Pharmacol. Pharm.* 35, 383-388.
Gillis R.A., Yamada K.A., DiMicco J.A., Williford D.J., Segal S.A., Hamosh P. and Norman W.P. (1984): Central γ-aminobutyric acid involvement in blood pressure control. *Fed. Proc.* 43, 32-38.
Hambley J.W., Johnston G.A.R. and Shaw J. (1985): Alterations in a hypothalamic GABA system in the SHR. *Neurochem. Int.* 6, 813-821.
Itoh S. and Van den Buuse M. (1991): Sensitization of baroreceptor reflex by central endothelin in conscious rats. *Am. J. Physiol.* 260, H1106-H1112.
Jung M.J., Lippert B., Metcalf M.W., Böhlen P. and Schechter P.J. (1977): γ-vinyl-GABA (4-amino-hex-5-enoic acid), a new selective inhibitor of GABA-T. *J. Neurochem.* 29, 797-802.
Kubo T., Kihara M. and Misu Y. (1989): Altered amino acid levels in brainstem regions of spontaneously hypertensive rats. *Clin. Exp. Hypert.* A11, 233-241.
Philippu A. (1988): Regulation of blood pressure by central neurotoransmitters and neuropeptides. *Rev. Physiol. Biochem. Pharm.* 111, 1-115.
Sasaki S., Nakata T., Kawasaki S., Hayashi J., Oguro M., Takeda K. and Nakagawa M. (1990): Chronic central GABAergic stimulation attenuates hypothalamic hyperreactivity and development of spontaneous hypertension in rats. *J. Cardiovasc. Pharmacol.* 15, 706-713.
Schousboe A., Larsson D.M. and Seiler N. (1986): Stereoselective uptake of the GABA-transaminase inhibitors gamma-vinyl-GABA and gamma-acetylenic-GABA into neurons and astrocytes. *Neurochem. Res.* 11, 1497-1505.
Singewald N., Pfitscher A. and Philippu A. (1991): Increase in brain GABA levels by vigabatrin delays the development of hypertension in spontaneously hypertensive rats. *Naunyn-Schmied. Arch. Pharmacol.* suppl. 343, R73.
Sweet C.S., Wenger H.C. and Gross D.M. (1979): Central antihypertensive properties of muscimol and related gamma-aminobutyric acid agonists and the interaction of muscimol with baroreceptor reflexes. *Can. J. Physiol. Pharmacol.* 57, 600-605.
Thyagarajan R., Brennan T. and Ticku M.K. (1983): GABA and benzodiazepine binding sites in spontaneously hypertensive rats. *Eur. J. Pharmacol.* 93, 127-136.
Tunnicliff G., Welborn K.L. and Head R.A. (1984): The GABA/benzodiazepine receptor complex in the nervous system of a hypertensive strain of rats. *Neurochem. Int.* 9, 1033-1038.
Unger T., Becker H., Dietz R., Ganten D., Lang R.E., Rettig R., Schömig A. and Schwab N.A. (1984): Antihypertensive effect of the GABA-receptor agonist muscimol in SHR: role of the sympathoadrenal axis. *Circ. Res.* 54, 30-37.

Differential changes in central dopaminergic activity in the spontaneously hypertensive rat

M. van den Buuse

Marion Merrell Dow Research Institute, 16, rue d'Ankara, B.P. 447/R9, 67009 Strasbourg, France

It was shown previously that depletion of central dopamine inhibits the development of hypertension in the spontaneously hypertensive rat (SHR). Thus, the intracerebroventricular (i.c.v.) injection of the catecholamine neurotoxin 6-hydroxydopamine (6-OHDA) in young, prehypertensive SHR inhibits the development of hypertension in these rats (Van den Buuse et al. 1984). This effect of 6-OHDA was shown to be due to the depletion of central dopamine (Van den Buuse et al. 1986a; 1986b). Subsequent studies showed that SHR display changes in central dopaminergic regulation when compared to normotensive wistar-Kyoto controls (WKY) (Van den Buuse and De Jong, 1989). The purpose of the present study was to further characterize alterations in central dopaminergic activity in SHR. The response of male, adult SHR and wistar-Kyoto rats (WKY) to different doses of the dopamine D-2 receptor antagonist sulpiride (1-125 mg/kg i.p.) was studied in a number of different functional tests (O'Connor and Brown, 1982; Rotrosen and Stanley, 1982).

Locomotor activity was measured with automated infrared-beam activity cages (n=6-8 per group). At 5 mg/kg sulpiride increased locomotor activity of SHR (1216 ± 156 photocell counts/30 min vs. 799 ± 75 counts in saline-treated SHR) but no effect was found in WKY (691 ± 50 counts in sulpiride-treated vs. 669 ± 107 counts in saline-treated WKY). At 125 mg/kg sulpiride markedly decreased locomotor activity of WKY (100 ± 41 counts), but there was no effect in SHR (892 ± 147 counts). These results could be interpreted to indicate that, with respect to locomotor activity, presynaptic dopamine D2 receptor mechanisms are upregulated in SHR, whereas postsynaptic D2 receptor mechanisms fail respond to sulpiride.

Serum prolactin concentrations were measured in trunk blood by radio-immunoassay. Sulpiride dose-dependently increased serum prolactin levels in both SHR and WKY, but the effect was significantly greater in SHR. Thus, the injection of 1 and 100 mg/kg sulpiride, 45 min before decapitation, in SHR increased prolactin concentration in the serum from 64 ± 14 to 153 ± 25 and 159 ± 23 ng/ml respectively (n=6-8 in all groups), while in WKY these doses increased prolactin concentration from 55 ± 8 to 103 ±12 and 123 ± 14 ng/ml respectively.

Salt-preference was measured in a two-bottle drinking test where one bottle contained 0.9% saline and the other normal tap water (Gilbert and Cooper, 1986). The rats were allowed to drink for one hour after a 23 hour water-deprivation period, and were subjected to one control test and, on the subsequent day, one test after treatment with sulpiride. Saline preference was calculated as the ratio of saline intake over total fluid intake. There were 12-14 rats per group. Sulpiride (100 mg/kg) increased salt-preference in WKY from 63 ± 7 % to 76 ± 6 %, but there was no significant effect in SHR (66 ± 5 % vs. 65 ± 6 % respectively). Lower doses of sulpiride had no effect. Total fluid intake was not influenced in either group by sulpiride.

Amphetamine-induced turning behaviour was measured in SHR and WKY with unilateral 6-OHDA lesions of the median forebrain bundle (Ungerstedt, 1971; Pycock, 1980). Amphetamine-induced turning was significantly inhibited by sulpiride in WKY, but not in SHR. The injection of 0.5 mg/kg amphetamine induced 180 ± 28 and 175 ± 38 turns/60 min in SHR and WKY, respectively (n=6 per group). After pretreatment with 100 mg/kg sulpiride these values were 111 ± 32 and 33 ± 19 turns/60 min. Lower doses of sulpiride did not significantly influence amphetamine-induced turning in either strain.

The concentrations of dopamine and its metabolites DOPAC and HVA three hours after injection of sulpiride (Tagliamonte *et al.* 1973) were measured by HPLC in homogenates of frontal cortex, striatum and hypothalamus. SHR showed a lower concentration of HVA in the frontal cortex when compared to WKY, but otherwise basal levels were similar in the two strains. Sulpiride dose-dependently increased the concentration of DOPAC and HVA, but not of dopamine. This lead to a significant increase in DOPAC/dopamine ratio and HVA/dopamine ratio, an index of dopamine turnover, which was similar in SHR and WKY (see table I for 100 mg/kg dose).

TABLE I: The effect of 100 mg/kg sulpiride on DOPAC/dopamine and HVA/dopamine ratio in different regions of the brain of SHR and WKY.

	DOPAC/dopamine ratio		HVA/dopamine ratio	
	Saline	Sulpiride	Saline	Sulpiride
Frontal cortex				
SHR	0.54 ± 0.09	1.34 ± 0.25*	0.34 ± 0.04	1.66 ± 0.35*
WKY	0.70 ± 0.09	1.36 ± 0.19*	0.56 ± 0.07	1.85 ± 0.38*
Striatum				
SHR	0.30 ± 0.04	0.88 ± 0.08*	0.14 ± 0.02	0.44 ± 0.06*
WKY	0.35 ± 0.02	0.75 ± 0.08*	0.14 ± 0.01	0.44 ± 0.05*
Hypothalamus				
SHR	0.57 ± 0.10	0.89 ± 0.13*	0.12 ± 0.01	0.24 ± 0.04*
WKY	0.61 ± 0.09	0.71 ± 0.09	0.13 ± 0.02	0.28 ± 0.03*

(*) $P<0.05$ for difference with saline-treated rats. Data are mean ± SEM of n=8 rats per group.

The binding of ^{125}I-sulpiride to brain sections was measured by autoradiography (Martres *et al.* 1985). No differences were observed in sulpiride binding between sections of SHR and of WKY. For example, in the caudate-putamen binding density was 102 ± 13 fmol/mg protein in SHR vs. 92 ± 5 fmol/mg protein in WKY (n=7).

These results show that SHR display differential changes in central dopamine D-2 receptor function when compared to WKY. In some tests (locomotor activity after high dose sulpiride, salt preference and turning behaviour) SHR show a markedly diminished response to sulpiride when compared to WKY. In other tests, however, SHR tended to show higher responses (locomotor activity after low doses, serum prolactin) or there was no difference between the strains (dopamine turnover, dopamine

D2 binding). These and previous results (Fuller et al. 1983; Linthorst et al. 1990; Van den Buuse and De Jong, 1989) might indicate that there are at least two different functional dopamine D2 receptor mechanisms, one of which is deficient in SHR, but the other of which is normal or upregulated in the SHR. The underlying neurochemical basis of these two mechanisms is unclear, but could relate to different dopamine D2 subtypes or different transduction mechanisms to which the D2 receptor is coupled. The differential changes in central dopamine D-2 function may play a role in the development of hypertension in SHR.

REFERENCES

Fuller R.W., Hemrick-Luecke S.K., Wong D.T., Pearson D., Threllkeld P.G. and Hynes M.D. (1983): Altered behavioural response to a D2 agonist, LY141865, in SHR exhibiting biochemical and endocrine responses similar to those in normotensive rats. *J. Pharmacol. Exp. Ther.* 227, 354-359.

Gilbert D.B. and Cooper S.J. (1986): Salt acceptance and preference tests distinguish between selective dopamine D-1 and D-2 receptor antagonists. *Neuropharmacol.* 25, 665-657.

Linthorst A.C.E., Van den Buuse M., De Jong W. and Versteeg D.H.G. (1990): Electrically stimulated [^{3}H]dopamine and [^{14}C]acetylcholine release from nucleus caudatus slices: differences between spontaneously hypertensive rats and Wistar-Kyoto rats. *Brain Res.* 509, 266-272.

Martres M.P., Bouthenet M.L., Sales N., Sokoloff P. and Schwartz J.C. (1985): Widespread distribution of brain dopamine receptors evidenced with [^{125}I]iodosulpiride, a higly selective ligand. *Science* 228, 752-755.

O'Connor S.E. and Brown R.A. (1982): The pharmacology of sulpiride - a dopamine receptor antagonist. *Gen. Pharmacol.* 13, 185-193.

Pycock C.J. (1980): Turning behaviour in animals. *Neuroscience* 5, 461-514.

Rotrosen J. and Stanley M. (1982): The benzamides: pharmacology, neurobiology and clinical aspects. New York: Raven Press.

Tagliamonte A., De Montis G., Olianas M., Vargiu L., Corsini G.U. and Gessa G.L. (1975): Selective increase of brain dopamine synthesis by sulpiride. *J. Neurochem.* 24, 707-710.

Ungerstedt U. (1971): Postsynaptic supersensitivity after 6-hydroxydopamine induced degeneration of the nigrostriatal system. *Acta Physiol. Scand.* (suppl) 367, 69-93.

Van den Buuse M., De Kloet E.R., Versteeg D.H.G. and De Jong W. (1984): Regional brain catecholamine levels and the development of hypertension in the spontaneously hypertensive rat: the effect of 6-hydroxydopamine. *Brain Res.* 301, 221-229.

Van den Buuse M., Versteeg D.H.G. and De Jong W. (1986a): Role of dopamine in the development of spontaneous hypertension. *Hypertension* 6, 899-905.

Van den Buuse M., Versteeg D.H.G. and De Jong W. (1986b): Brain dopamine depletion by lesions of the substantia nigra attenuates the development of hypertension in the spontaneously hypertensive rat. *Brain Res.* 368, 69-78.

Van den Buuse M. and De Jong W. (1989): Differential effects of dopaminergic drugs on open-field behaviour of spontaneously hypertensive rats and normotensive Wistar-Kyoto rats. *J. Pharmacol. Exp. Ther.* 248, 1189-1196.

Central steroid receptor function in spontaneously hypertensive rats: effects of gluco- and mineralocorticoids

Désirée T.W.M. van den Berg*, E. Ronald De Kloet* and Ben J.A. Janssen

*Department of Pharmacology, University of Limburg, Maastricht, and * Division of Medical Pharmacology, CPBS, Sylvius Laboratories, Leiden, The Netherlands*

INTRODUCTION

Adrenal steroids have been long associated with cardiovascular homeostasis. Besides peripheral actions of the corticosteroids recent studies have indicated the involvement of central corticosteroid receptor sites in blood pressure regulation as well. The brain contains mineralo- and glucocorticoids receptor sites (MR & GR respectively). Differentiation between MR and GR is based on their primary structure, neuroanatomical localization, steroid binding properties and function (De Kloet 1991). The MR localized in the circumventricular organs bind in vivo mainly aldosterone and display aldosterone-selective properties; the MR with corticosterone-selective properties is localized in the limbic system and has equal affinity for corticosterone and aldosterone. The GR, widespread throughout the brain found, bind corticosterone preferentially after exposure to stress as well as at the circadian peak (Reul and De Kloet 1985). In normotensive and adrenalectomized (ADX) rats, a single intracerebroventricular (icv) injection of an antagonist of the MR (RU28318) decreased the systolic blood pressure (SBP). A similar effect was detected after icv injection of the GR agonist RU28362 (Van den Berg et al 1990). Gomez-Sanchez showed that chronic icv infusion of aldosterone but not corticosterone for 14 days resulted in an increase in blood pressure in salt loaded uninephrectomized rats. Concomitant infusion of RU28318 blocked this hypertension (Gomez-Sanchez 1990-a, 1990-b). These data suggest that stimulation of the central aldo-selective MR may be involved in the induction and maintenance of hypertension. In the spontaneously hypertensive rats (SHR) the cardiovascular responses to stress are exaggerated and they exhibit increased (compared to WKY) circadian fluctuations in arterial blood pressure. The most profound changes in blood pressure and heart rate are found in the transition period from light to dark. During this wakening period, rat plasma corticosterone levels peak (De Boer et al 1987).
We hypothesized that SHR may have a genetically endogenous stimulated steroid receptor function which may contribute to the maintenance and greater variability of hypertension. We studied the effects following single icv injections of RU28318 and RU28362 on mean arterial pressure (MAP) and heart rate (HR) continuously in cannulated rats. Furthermore the effects of icv infusions of these steroids in the SHR were examined.

MATERIALS AND METHODS

Male SHR (12-16 weeks) were obtained from the inbred colonies of the central animal facilities of the University of Limburg. After surgery the rats were housed individually in a quiet room (21°C ± 2) lighted between 07.00 AM and 19.00 PM. Water and food were provided *ad libitum*. On day 0 the left femoral artery was cannulated and the rats were connected to equipment for computerized 24 h MAP/HR measurements as described by Janssen et al (1991). Permanent polyethylene cannulae for icv injections were implanted in the right lateral ventricle. At least 5 days after surgery, icv injections of 100 or 1000 ng of the steroids RU28318 and RU28362 or vehicle (2μl) were given between 10.00 and 10.30 AM . Steroids were dissolved in the vehicle solution (2% ethanol:saline). For chronic icv administration of the steroids the icv cannulae were connected via a polyethylene catheter to osmotic minipumps (ALZET, model 2002, ALZA corp, Palo Alto, CA, USA). The minipumps (infusion rate = $0.5\mu l/h$) were filled with steroid solutions and implanted subcutaneously on the back of the rat. The time of icv delivery of the steroids (5 ng/h or 100ng/h) was defined by the length of the connecting catheter filled with vehicle solution and was approximated between 06.00 and 10.00 AM on day 7.

RESULTS

Single icv injections of the vehicle or 100 ng of the steroids did not effect the MAP or HR. The single dose of 1000 ng of RU28318 induced, compared to the vehicle treatment, a slight but not significant suppression in nocturnal MAP at the day of the injection (Fig 1). The icv injection of 1000ng of RU28362 suppressed the increase in MAP during the darkphase for 2 days. Both injections did not influence HR. Chronic icv infusions of 5 or 100 ng/h of either steroid did not influence the circadian rhythm of MAP or HR in the SHR. Fig 2 shows the data of the 100 ng/h infusions. For each rat data obtained during icv infusion were averaged for 2-3 days of vehicle or steroid administration.

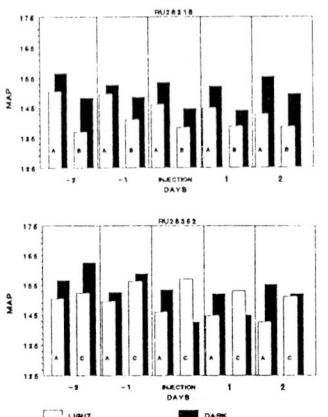
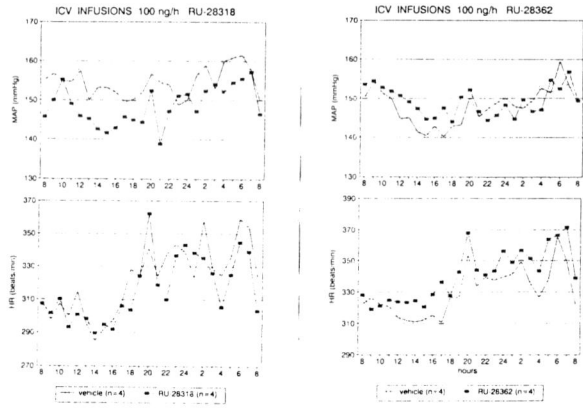

Fig 1: Effects of icv injections of 1000ng of the steroids on MAP. The average during the light period and the dark period is depicted in open en closed bars resp for A = vehicle treatment (n = 8), B = 1000ng RU28318 icv (n = 7), C = 1000ng RU28362 icv (n = 6).

Fig 2: Averged 24 h pattern of MAP during icv infusion of vehicle (open blocks) and steroids (closed blocks). For each rat data were averaged for 2-3 days of vehicle steroid administration.

DISCUSSION

The present data suggest that under basal conditions in SHR the central MR is not involved in the maintenance of the hypertensive state. Single icv injections of 1000 ng RU28318 induced minor changes in MAP. Previous results showed a hypotensive response of a 100 fold lower dose of RU28318 in normotensive and ADX-rats replaced with low doses of corticosterone, measured with the tail-cuff method (Van Den Berg et al 1990). Direct blood pressure measurements did not reveal this response (Van Den Berg et al, submitted). These results and those of chronic icv infusions by Gomez-Sanchez (1990) indicate that the central aldosterone-selective MR is involved in blood pressure regulation, although for such steroid mediated effects on blood pressure to occur a sensitized animal model appears to be a prerequisite. In the SHR icv injections of 1000ng RU28362 induced a slight suppression of the nocturnal rise in MAP for 2 days (Fig 1). However, the involvement of the central GR in MAP is less clear. Grunfeld (1990) stated that endogenous glucocorticoids do not play a significant role in the regulation of the blood pressure under basal conditions. The central GR is found widespread in neurons and glia cells. The occupancy of the GR fluctuates with the plasma corticosterone level and will be high during stress and at the circadian peak. The affinity of the synthetic glucocorticoid RU28362 for the GR is higher than of corticosterone. After icv injection of 100ng RU28362 in normotensive and ADX rats replaced with low doses of corticosterone we measured previously with the tail-cuff method a hypotensive response 24 and 48 h later (Van Den Berg et al 1990). The inhibition of the nocturnal rise in MAP we oberved in this study, is probably a result of a disturbed feedback mechanism of the central GR induced by the relative high dose of RU28362. Chronic icv infusions of the steroids did not exert any effect on the MAP or HR (Fig 2). According to the MR/GR balance hypothesis we suggest that due to (chronic) stimulation of the central GR or MR both receptor types will be influenced and induce a new MR/GR balance (De Kloet 1991).

In summary these data indicate that in SHR the central GR and MR do not play an important role in the maintenance of basal blood pressure.

REFERENCES

De Boer SF, Koopmans SJ, Slangen JL and Vand Der Grugten J (1987): Effects of fasting on plasma catecholamine, corticosterone and glucose concentrations under basal and stress conditions in individual rats. *Physiol. and Behav* 40:323-328.

De Kloet ER (1991): Brain corticosteroid receptor balance and homeostatic control. *Frontiers in Neuroendocr.* 12 (2): 95-164

Gomez-Sanchez EP, Fort KCM, Gomez Sanchez CE (1990-a): Intracerebroventricular infusion of RU28318 blocks aldosterone-salt hypertension. *Am J Physiol* 258:E489-491

Gomez-Sanchez EP, Venkatraman MT, Twhaites D and C Fort (1990-b) ICV infusion of corticosterone antagonizes icv-aldosterone hypertension. *AM J Physiol* 258:E649-E653

Grunfeld JP (1990) Glucocorticoids in blood pressure regulation. *Horm Res* 34:111-113

Janssen BJA, Thijssen CM and Struyker-Boudier HAJ (1991): Modification of circadian blood pressure and heart rate variability by five different antihypertensive agents in spontaneously hypertensive rats. *J of Cardiovascular Pharmacology* 17: 494-503

Reul JMHM & De Kloet ER (1985) Two receptor systems for corticosterone in rat brain: microdistribution and differential occupation.*Endocrinology* 117:2505-2512

Van Den Berg DTWM, Van Dijken HH, De Kloet ER, De Jong W (1990): Differential central effects of mineralocorticoid and glucocorticoid agonists and antagonists on blood pressure. *Endocrinology* 126:118-124.

Evaluation of the functional significance of Na⁺-pump activity in the central nervous system of spontaneously hypertensive rats

Jui Shah and Bhagavan S. Jandhyala

Department of Pharmacology, University of Houston, Houston, TX 77204-5515, USA

The relationship between membrane Na^+,K^+-ATPase activity and pathogenesis of hypertension in the spontaneously hypertensive rat (SHR) appears to be complex and has not been adequately clarified. Several studies in SHR have established that the Na^+-pump activity was enhanced in various tissues such as vascular smooth muscle, erythrocytes, etc. (Friedman, 1989; Wiley et al. 1980). In contrast, previous studies from our laboratories have demonstrated that stimulus induced sympathetic neurotransmitter overflow in perfused kidneys of SHR was significantly greater than that of Wistar-Kyoto rat (WKY) and this phenomena was due to diminished Na^+-pump activity in the sympathetic neurons of the SHR (Steenberg et al. 1988). Gheyouche et al. (1981) have found that ouabain binding sites were significantly lower in the heart and brain tissues of SHR when compared to age-matched controls.

Recently we have demonstrated that cerebroventricular administration (i.c.v.) potassium chloride solution produced concentration-dependent reductions in the arterial blood pressure and heart rate of anesthetized rats and these responses were significantly inhibited by prior i.c.v. administration of ouabain, a selective inhibitor of the Na^+-pump (Shah and Jandhyala, 1991). These observations revealed an important and inverse relationship between Na^+-pump activity in the circumventricular structures and central sympathetic discharge. Such a view is also consistent with the evidence that i.c.v. administration of adequate concentrations of ouabain markedly enhance sympathetic activity and arterial blood pressure (Jacomini et al. 1984).

One of the characteristics of SHR is exaggerated central sympathetic discharge, and mechanisms responsible for this phenomenon are not conclusive (Judy et al. 1976; Takeda and Buñag, 1978). Hence, the present studies are undertaken to determine whether alterations in the Na^+-pump activity in the brain would account for the enhanced sympathetic activity in SHR. The magnitude of the centrally-mediated hypotensive and bradycardic effects of KCl is considered a functional index for neuronal Na^+-pump activity.

METHODS

Eleven to twelve week old SHR and age matched WKY rats were used in these studies. Rats were anesthetized with Inactin® (100 mg/kg, i.p.) and arterial blood pressure and heart rate were monitored from a catheterized carotid artery. An 21g 'guide' cannula and a 30g injection cannula were introduced into a cerebrolateral ventricle. Various doses of KCl (0.375 to 1.25 μmol) were administered into the ventricles (i.c.v.) and corresponding changes in the blood pressure and heart rate were recorded, this was followed by a bolus injection of ouabain (1.0 mmol/l, i.c.v.). Responses to each dose of KCl were once again obtained 5 min after i.c.v. injection ouabain (0.1 mmol/l). Volume of any single injections was 5.0 μl. These procedures were described in detail in our previous publication (Shah & Jandhyala, 1991). Analysis of variance and Neuman-Keul's multiple range test were employed to evaluate the data.

RESULTS

Arterial blood pressures and heart rates (Mean ± SEM) of SHR and WKY are as follows.

Strain	Blood Pressure (mm Hg)		Heart Rate (b/min)	
	Before Ouabain	After Ouabain	Before Ouabain	After Ouabain
WKY	95.8±5.96*	96.0±8.19*	291.0±5.37*	317.5±22.81*
SHR	171.2±4.43	166.5±11.67	357.0±14.39	395.0±10.61

*indicate significantly different as compared to SHR. $p < 0.05$ (n=6 per group)

Cerebroventricular administration of KCl produced dose-dependent reductions in the blood pressure and heart rate. These variables returned to basal levels within 10 min. Alterations in the blood pressure are illustrated in Fig. 1. Depressor responses to i.c.v. KCl are significantly greater in SHR when compared to those of the WKY. After ouabain administration the differences between these two groups in their responsiveness to KCl, were completely eliminated. Although changes in the heart rate to KCl (which are not shown) are qualitatively similar, they are less consistent and not significantly different between the groups.

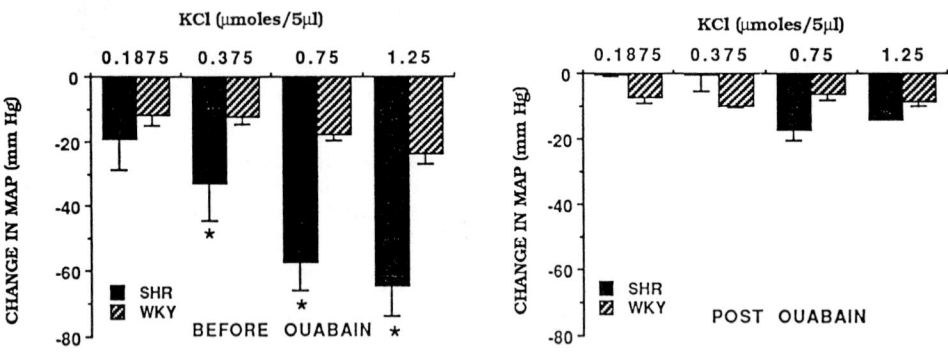

Fig 1. Reductions in the arterial blood pressure to i.c.v. KCl solutions in SHR (solid bars) and WKY (hatched bars). Left panel: before ouabain; right panel: after ouabain. Asterisk indicate that the responses are significantly different between the groups ($p < 0.05$; n=6 per group).

DISCUSSION

The doses of KCl employed in these studies, after being diluted in the natural cerebrospinal fluid (CSF), are estimated to raise CSF-K^+ levels by 1 to 6 mmol/l. These concentrations of KCl produced significant and dose-dependent reductions in the arterial pressure in SHR. These responses were significantly inhibited by ouabain, a selective inhibitor of the Na^+-pump. Therefore it follows that activation of the Na^+-pump in the circumventricular structures triggered in response to elevation of CSF-K^+ was involved in eliciting alterations in the arterial pressure. Stimulation of the Na^+-pump by K^+ enhances Na^+ and Ca^{2+} efflux from the neuronal cells which may have activated the sequence of events leading to reductions in sympathetic tone and arterial blood pressure (Shah and Jandhyala, 1991).

In the present studies the magnitude of the depressor responses to KCl are pronounced and significantly greater in SHR and ranged from 20-70 mmHg. In contrast, responses in WKY varied from 15-25 mm Hg only. Since ouabain essentially eliminated these differences it could be suggested that Na^+-pump activity in the central nervous system of SHR is significantly greater than that of WKY. However, prior to reaching any such conclusions, at least two alternative possibilities should be considered. One explanation could be that since the blood pressure of WKY is significantly lower than that of SHR, KCl could not produce similar hypotensive responses. In this context, it should be noted that in our previous study the average blood pressures of Sprague-Dawley rats (S-D) was about 120 mm Hg and significantly lower than that of SHR (170 mmHg); and yet the centrally-mediated hypotensive effects of KCl in S-D rats are comparable to that of SHR (Shah and Jandhyala, 1991). This observation would suggest that the difference in basal blood pressure by itself, may not be a primary factor. An alternative and more plausible explanation is that the central sympathetic tone is very low in WKY as compared to SHR and hence i.c.v. KCl could not futher lower sympathetic activity in WKY, even if the Na^+-pump activity in the CNS in the WKY is comparable to that of SHR. Therefore, the differences in the responsiveness of SHR and WKY to i.c.v. potassium chloride need not and may not be due to differences in central Na^+-pump activity. Such a view is also compatible with the observation that although Sprague-Dawley rats are normotensive central effects of KCl are comparable to that of SHR, suggesting that the neuronal Na^+-pump activity in SHR is similar to that of S-D rats, and only appears to be greater than that of WKY.

In conclusion, the results of this investigation do not support the hypothesis that enhanced central sympathetic discharge and high blood pressure in SHR are due to diminished Na^+-pump activity in the central circumventricular structures. Central mechanisms other than alterations in the neuronal Na^+-pump, would account for high sympathetic tone in SHR. These studies would also suggest that the central actions of K^+ may also contribute to the salutary effects of high K^+ diet in the hypertensive subjects (Fujita and Ando, 1984; Goto et al. 1981), especially if the high blood pressure is associated with increases in sympathetic neuronal activity.

REFERENCES

Friedman, S. M. (1979): Evidence for enhanced sodium transport in the tail artery of the spontaneously hypertensive rat. *Hypertension* **1**: 572-582.

Fujita, T. and Ando, K. (1984): Hemodyanmic and endocrine changes associated with potassium supplementation in sodium-loaded hypertensives. *Hypertension* **6**: 184-192.

Gheyouche, R., Uzan, A., Le Fur, G. and Corgier, M. (1981): Decrease in [^{3}H] ouabain binding sites in heart and brain from spontaneously hypertensive rats. *Experientia* **37**: 492-493.

Goto, A., Tobian, L. and Iwai, J. (1981): Potassium feeding reduces hyperactive central nervous system pressor responses in Dahl salt-sensitive rats. *Hypertension* **3** (suppl.1): I-128 -I-134.

Jacomini, L. C. L., Elghozi, J. L., Dagher, G., Devynck, M. A., and Meyer, P. (1984): Central hypertensive effects of ouabain in rats. *Arch. Int. Pharmacodyn. Ther.* **267**: 310-318.

Judy, W. V., Watanabe, A. M., Henry, D. P., Besch, H. R., Murphy, M. A., and Hockel, G. M. (1976): Sympathetic nerve activity: Role in the regulation of blood pressure in the spontaneously hypertensive rat. *Circ. Res.* (suppl. II) **38**: II21-II29.

Shah, J. and Jandhyala, B. S. (1991): Role of Na^+, K^+-ATPase in the centrally mediated hypotensive effects of potassium in anaestheized rats. *J. Hypertension* **9**: 167-170.

Steenberg, M. L., Lokhandwala, M. F. and Jandhyala, B. S. (1988): Abnormalities in sodium transport as the causative factor for enhanced norepinephrine overflow in the spontaneously hypertensive rat. *Clin. Exp. Pharmacol. Physiol.* A(**10**): 833-841.

Takeda, K. and Buñag, R. D. (1978): Sympathetic hyperactivity during hypothalamic stimulation in spontaneously hypertensive rats. *J. Clin. Invest.* **62**: 642-649.

Wiley, J. S. Hutchinson, J. S. Mendelsohn, F. A. O. and Doyle, A. E. (1980): Increased sodium permeability of erythrocytes in spontaneously hypertensive rats. *Clin. Exp. Pharmacol. Physiol.* **7**: 527-530.

Exaggerated renal response to central angiotensin III in spontaneously hypertensive rats

Wann-Chu Huang, Jong-Shiaw Jin, Chung-Yan Chen and Po-Shiuan Hsieh

Department of Physiology and Biophysics, National Defense Medical Center, Taipei, Taiwan, Republic of China

INTRODUCTION

The brain renin-angiotensin system (RAS) has been implicated in blood pressure (BP) and body fluid homeostasis. Recent studies demonstrated that angiotensin III (ANG III or des-Asp^1 ANG II) is one of the active components of the brain RAS and is as potent as ANG II in producing pressor, dipsogenic and renal effects in normal rats (Wright et al., 1985; Huang, 1991). In spontaneously hypertensive rats (SHR), the central RAS has been shown to be functionally hyperactive (Wright et al., 1986). The current study was thus conducted to compare the renal effect of intracerebroventricular (icv) injection of ANG III between SHR and WKY rats.

MATERIALS AND METHODS

Male SHR and WKY rats weighing 250-300 g were anesthetized by sodium pentobarbital (50 mg/kg, i.p.) and placed on a stereotaxic apparatus (David Kopf, CA, USA) for the right later ventricle cannulation with a sterile stainless steel cannula (26-gauge). Rats were fed a commercial rat chow and allowed tap water ad libitum for one week to recover from surgery.

For acute renal function experiments. Rats were anesthetized as aforementioned and placed on a thermostatically controlled table. Surgical preparations, blood pressure measurement, and renal clearance experiment procedures were similar to those described previously (Huang et al., 1988). Briefly, 2 µl of artificial cerebrospinal fluid (aCSF) was injected intracerebroventricularly and urine samples were collected. Each collection lasted for 20 minutes. After the control period, ANG III in 2 µl of aCSF was administered and urine samples were sequentially collected. When urine flow and blood pressure reached to the pre-drug level, the subsequent dose of ANG III was injected and urine collection was made. At the end of experiment, 2 µl of Evens blue was injected to validate the position of the cerebroventricular cannula. The concentrations of Inutest, paraaminohippuric acid (PAH), sodium and potassium in plasma and urine samples were determined as previously described (Huang et al., 1988). The data were analyzed using Student's paired and unpaired t-tests where applicable. Results are expressed as mean±SEM.

RESULTS

As shown in Table 1, icv injection of ANG III at 5 pmoles did not significantly change BP but significantly increased PAH and Inutest clearances and excretion rates of water, sodium and potassium in both SHR and WKY rats. Increase in ANG III dose to 50 pmoles slightly increased BP in WKY rats but not SHR, and further enhanced renal function in both groups. The augmented renal response to icv ANG III was completely blocked by prior icv administration of [Ile^7]-ANG III (100 nmoles).

The percentage increases in renal function in response to icv ANG III in SHR and WKY rats were compared in Fig. 1. ICV injection of ANG III at a smaller dose (5 pmoles) produced a significantly greater increase in renal function in SHR than in WKY rats. With a larger dose of ANG III (50 pmoles). A greater kaliuretic effect was noted in SHR.

Table 1. Blood pressure and renal function responses to central ANG III in SHR and WKY rats.

		WKY		SHR	
	ANG III	5	50	5	50 pmoles
MBP, mmHg	control	123±4	125±4	157±3	154±4
	ANG III	123±4	132±4*	161±4	158±5
C_{PAH}, ml/min	control	4.9±0.6	5.4±0.6	6.6±0.7	7.0±0.7
	ANG III	7.8±1.1*	8.8±1.2*	9.7±0.6*	10.5±0.7*
C_{IN}, ml/min	control	1.2±0.2	1.1±0.2	1.0±0.1	1.1±0.1
	ANG III	1.6±0.3*	1.8±0.3*	1.8±0.1*	1.9±0.1*
V, μl/min	control	7.7±1.1	7.4±1.2	7.4±1.1	7.6±0.6
	ANG III	17.2±3.8*	30.5±6.1*	27.1±5.7*	37.8±2.7*
$U_{Na}V$, μEq/min	control	0.8±0.3	0.6±0.3	0.9±0.3	0.9±0.1
	ANG III	2.2±1.1*	4.0±1.9*	3.7±0.6*	5.8±0.9*
U_KV, μEq/min	control	1.1±0.3	1.1±0.9	0.9±0.2	0.7±0.2
	ANG III	2.3±0.3*	2.7±0.3*	2.0±0.3*	3.3±0.6*

Abbreviations: MBP= mean blood pressure; C_{PAH}= PAH clearance; C_{IN}= Inutest clearance; V= urine flow; $U_{Na}V$= absolute sodium excretion; U_KV= absolute potassium excretion.   *$p<0.05$ vs control value. Rat number= 6.

DISCUSSION

The present study demonstrates that intracerebroventricular administration of ANG III produces significant increases in PAH and Inutest clearances, urine flow and excretions of sodium and potassium. These results indicate that the central ANG III is an active element of the RAS in the brain and that ANG III in the brain may be an important modulator in controlling blood pressure and body fluid balance in normal and hypertensive rats.

The most interesting observation in this study was that the magnitude of increase in renal effect of central ANG III was significantly greater in SHR than in WKY rats. The exaggerated diuretic and natriuretic response to icv ANG III in SHR occurred predominantly when a smaller dose of ANG III was injected, suggesting an increased renal sensitivity to central ANG III exists in SHR.

We previously demonstrated that icv injection of ANG III inhibited renal efferent nerve activity (Huang, 1991). The ANG-induced reduction in renal nerve activity may be responsible for the renal effect of icv ANG III observed in the present study. Furthermore, central ANG III-induced increase in renal function was inhibited by a specific ANG III antagonist, [Ile^7]-ANG III. This suggests that the enhanced renal response to central ANG III is resulted from an ANG III receptor mediated mechanism. Whether icv administered ANG III acts at the specific receptor site or at the common receptor shared with ANG II is still unclear and merits further investigation.

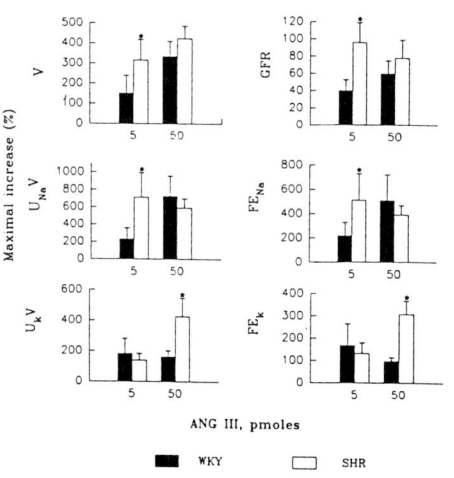

Fig. 1. Comparison of the maximal percentage increases in renal function response to icv administration of angiotensin III between SHR and WKY rats. V= urine flow; GFR= glomerular filtration rate (C_{IN}); $U_{Na}V$= absolute excretion of sodium; FE_{Na}= fractional excretion of sodium; U_kV= absolute excretion of potassium; FE_k= fractional excretion of potassium. *$p<0.05$ vs WKY rats.

REFERENCES

Huang, W.C. (1991): Renal hemodynamic and tubular effects of angiotensins II and III. Chinese J. Physiol. 34,121-138.

Huang, W.C., Tsai, L.M. & Wu, J.N. (1988): Effect of unilateral renal denervation on bilateral renal response to saline loading in anteroventral third ventricle-lesioned rats. Brain Res. 460, 83-93.

Wright, J.W., Morseth, S.L., Abhold, R.H. & Harding, J.W. (1985): Pressor action and dipsogenicity induced by angiotensin II and III in rats. Am. J. Physiol. 249,R514-R521.

Wright, J.W., Sullivan, M.J., Quirk, W.S., Batt, C.M. & Harding, J.W. (1986): Heightened pressor effect and dipsogenicity to intracerebroventricularly applied angiotensin II and III in spontaneously hypertensive rats. J. Hypert. 4(suppl. 6),S408-S411.

The effect of MDL 73,005EF and putative 5-HT$_{1A}$ receptor antagonists on the cardiovascular response to 8-OH-DPAT in conscious spontaneously hypertensive rats

S. Buisson and M. van den Buuse

Marion Merrell Dow Research Institute, 16, rue d'Ankara, B.P. 447 R/9, 67009 Strasbourg Cedex, France

Central 5-HT$_{1A}$ receptor activation plays a role in the control of cardiovascular function (Mir and Fozard, 1990). The 5-HT$_{1A}$ receptor subtype was principally characterized using 8-hydroxy-2-(di-n-propylamino)tetralin (8-OH-DPAT), a potent and selective 5-HT$_{1A}$ ligand (Middlemiss and Fozard, 1983). 8-OH-DPAT produces dose-related hypotension and bradycardia in normotensive and spontaneously hypertensive rats (SHR) (Fozard et al.,1987). At present, there are no selective antagonists described for 5-HT$_{1A}$ receptors. One problem is that many compounds developed are partial agonists. Although they appear to be 5-HT$_{1A}$ antagonists in some models, they reveal agonist properties in other models of investigations. MDL 73,005EF (8-[2-(2,3-dihydro-1,4-benzodioxin-2-yl-methylamino]-decane-7,9-dione methyl sulphonate) is a potent and selective ligand for the 5-HT$_{1A}$ site. This compound has been shown to exert anxiolytic effects (Moser et al., 1990). In behavioural, in vivo microdialysis and electrophysiological studies, MDL 73,005EF had been shown to possess both 5-HT$_{1A}$ receptor agonist and antagonist properties (Moser et al., 1990; Gartside et al.,1990; van den Hooff and Galvan, 1991; Sprouse, 1991). The actions of MDL 73,005EF on cardiovascular parameters have not yet been investigated. The present study was carried out to examine the effects of MDL 73,005EF on cardiovascular responses to the 5-HT$_{1A}$ agonists, 8-OH-DPAT and flesinoxan in conscious SHR and to compare these effects with a number of compounds with 5-HT$_{1A}$ receptor antagonist properties.

Conscious male SHR were used (weight range 250-300 g). Rats were anaesthetized with pentobarbital and polyethylene catheters were inserted into the right femoral artery and jugular vein. Experiments were performed at least two days after surgery. The rats were divided into two groups and they were pretreated with a single i.v or s.c. dose of either vehicle or putative 5-HT$_{1A}$ antagonists. The doses of various antagonists were chosen according to literature data. Fifteen or 30 min later 8-OH-DPAT (0.1 mg/kg) or flesinoxan (0.3 - 1 mg/kg) was injected. When antagonists were injected s.c., they were administered 1 hour before 8-OH-DPAT. Mean arterial pressure (MAP) and heart rate (HR) were then monitored continuously for 30 min. In preliminary studies, we found that 8-OH-DPAT induced a dose-dependent decrease in blood pressure and heart rate in SHR. The dose of 0.1 mg/kg of 8-OH-DPAT was chosen because this dose caused a maximal decrease in blood pressure (-27 ± 4 mm Hg) and HR (-57 B/min) with only a short period of behavioural side effects such as hyperactivity. In conscious Wistar Kyoto rats (WKY) this dose of 8-OH-DPAT decreased MAP and HR by -16 ± 3 mm Hg and -80 ± 6 B/min respectively, but the effect of 8-OH-DPAT was of longer duration in SHR. Control values for MAP and HR correspond to the values obtained immediately before each injection. The results are expressed as means ± S.E.M. Statistical analysis of the data was performed using an analysis of variance followed by Student's T-test.

The effects of MDL 73,005EF and of different 5-HT_{1A} antagonists against the cardiovascular actions of 8-OH-DPAT are summarized in table I. Low doses of MDL 73,005EF induced a transient decrease in MAP (maximal effect at 5 min after injection: 0.3 mg/kg -11 ± 4 mm Hg and at 1 mg/kg -12 ± 3 mm Hg). MAP returned to its initial level before the 8-OH-DPAT injection. MDL 73,005EF alone (0.1-1 mg/kg) had no effect on HR. Higher doses of MDL 73,005EF caused a significant and longlasting decrease in blood pressure and heart rate (not shown). MDL 73,005EF at 1 mg/kg significantly reduced both the hypotension (-83%) and the bradycardia (-82%) induced by 8-OH-DPAT, but no effects were seen with doses of 0.1 mg/kg and 0.3 mg/kg doses (table I). MDL 73,005EF at 1 mg/kg also reduced the hypotension induced by 0.3 mg/kg (-19 ± 4 mm Hg to -1 ± 3 mm Hg) or 1 mg/kg flesinoxan (-44 ± 3 to -21 ± 4 mm Hg). All the putative 5-HT_{1A} antagonists tested, with the exception of buspirone, reduced baseline MAP. BMY 7378 (1 mg/kg) caused a rapid but transient reduction in MAP. The peak effect occurred within 5 min after injection and MAP had a tendency to return to its initial level, but before 8-OH-DPAT injection MAP was still significantly reduced (-12 ± 2 mm Hg). (±)-Pindolol and NAN-190 (1 mg/kg) induced a large gradual decrease in baseline MAP, and before 8-OH-DPAT injection blood pressure was reduced by -11 ± 6 mm Hg and -29 ± 5 mm Hg respectively. The maximal effect of 8-OH-DPAT on MAP was significantly reduced by pretreatment with BMY 7378 (-59%), buspirone (-43%) and (±)-pindolol (- 48%) at 1 mg/kg. NAN-190 had no effect on the hypotension induced by 8-OH-DPAT. To rule out the possibility that the reduction in baseline blood pressure by BMY 7378 and (±)-pindolol might have influenced the response to 8-OH-DPAT, rats were pretreated i.v. with hydralazine, a peripherally acting vasodilator. At 0.3 mg/kg, hydralazine did not significantly alter the cardiovascular responses to 8-OH-DPAT (-25 ± 4 mm Hg to -20 ± 4 mm Hg) despite inducing a fall in baseline blood pressure (-23 ± 3 mm Hg).

TABLE I: Effect of pretreatment with MDL 73,005EF and putative 5-HT_{1A} antagonists on maximal blood pressure and HR responses to 8-OH-DPAT. (*) $P<0.05$ for difference with saline (n=6).

COMPOUNDS	mg/kg	MAP (mm Hg)		HR (B/min)	
		Saline	Antagonist	Saline	Antagonist
MDL 73,005EF	0.1	-24 ± 3	-19 ± 5	-56 ± 9	-26 ± 13
MDL 73,005EF	0.3	-24 ± 3	-20 ± 7	-56 ± 9	-59 ± 9
MDL 73,005EF	1	-24 ± 3	-4 ± 5*	-56 ± 9	-10 ± 18*
BUSPIRONE	1	-30 ± 3	-17 ± 3*	-61 ± 1	4 ± 8*
BMY 7378	1	-32 ± 7	-13 ± 2*	-46 ± 10	-35 ± 8
PINDOLOL (s.c.)	1	-25 ± 4	-13 ± 3*	-37 ± 4	-38 ± 13
NAN-190	1	-28 ± 4	-28 ± 4	-89 ± 8	-73 ± 17

The present study demonstrates a low dose of MDL 73,005EF, like buspirone, BMY 7378 and (±)-pindolol, displays antagonistic properties at 5-HT_{1A} receptors as it reduced the cardiovascular response to 8-OH-DPAT. MDL 73,005EF seems to be more potent compared to the other ligands. At 1 mg/kg it almost completely blocked the hypotensive and bradycardic response to 8-OH-DPAT, whereas the other compounds induced only partial inhibition. Although NAN-190 has been described as a useful 5-HT_{1A} antagonist (Glennon et al., 1988), in our study this compound had no effect on the blood pressure response to 8-OH-DPAT. Possibly the dose used (1 mg/kg) might have been too low as Glennon et al. (1988) showed a significant effect of NAN-190 in a dose range of 2-3.5 mg/kg. MDL 73,005EF induced a transient decrease in blood pressure per se, comparable to that observed with 8-OH-DPAT. Previous studies have also demonstrated that MDL 73,005EF acts as a mixed agonist/antagonist at central 5-HT$_{1A}$ receptors. The results of in vivo microdialysis and electrophysiological studies in the rat suggested that MDL 73,005EF acts as an agonist at dorsal raphe nucleus (presynaptic) 5-HT$_{1A}$ receptors and as antagonist at hippocampal (postsynaptic) 5-HT$_{1A}$ receptors (Gartside et al., 1990; van den Hooff et Galvan, 1991; Sprouse, 1991). It has been shown that pretreatment with a single dose of 8-OH-DPAT results in a rapid, marked and prolonged attenuation of 5-HT$_{1A}$ receptor-mediated hypothermia and hyperphagia (Larsson et al., 1990; Kennett et al., 1987; Beer et al., 1990). Recently, desensitization of 5-HT$_{1A}$ receptors also has been described by Mandal et al. (1991). In that study, 5-methyl-urapidil (1-300 µg/kg) was administered to anaesthetized cats and induced hypotension and bradycardia. The effects of 5-methyl-urapidil (300 µg/kg) were more than 2 times greater in naive animals than in animals that had been previously exposed to the drug. Similarly these animals were unresponsive to an i.v. dose of 8-OH-DPAT that normally produces large decreases in MAP and HR in naive animals. In conclusion, in the present study, a dose of MDL 73,005EF which did not markedly influence basal blood pressure by itself, inhibited the cardiovascular effects of 8-OH-DPAT. This effect may be explained by antagonist properties of MDL 73,005EF on 5-HT$_{1A}$ receptors, but desensitization of this receptor, as observed with 5-HT$_{1A}$ agonists, may also play a role.

REFERENCES

Beer, M., Kennett, G.A., and Curzon, G. (1990): A single dose of 8-OH-DPAT reduces raphe binding of [^{3}H]8-OH-DPAT and increases the effect of raphe stimulation of 5-HT metabolism. *Eur. J. Pharmacol.* 178, 179-187.

Fozard, J.R., Mir, A.K., and Middlemiss, D.N. (1987): The cardiovascular response to 8-hydroxy-2-(di-n-propylamino)tetralin (8-OH-DPAT) in the rat: site of action and pharmacological analysis. *J. Cardiovasc. Pharmacol.* 9, 328-347.

Gartside, S.E., Cowen, P.J., and Hjorth, S. (1990): Effects of MDL 73,005EF on central pre- and postsynaptic 5-HT$_{1A}$ receptor function in the rat in vivo. *Eur. J. Pharmacol.* 191, 391-400.

Glennon, R.A., Naiman, N.A., Pierson, M.E., Titeler, M., and Wiesberg, E. (1988): NAN-190: an arylpiperazine analog that antagonizes the stimulus effects of 5-HT$_{1A}$ agonist 8-hydroxy-2-(di-n-propylamino)tetralin (8-OH-DPAT). *Eur. J. Pharmacol.* 154, 339-341.

Kennett, G.A., Marcou, M., Dourish, C.T., and Curzon, G. (1987): Single administration of 5-HT$_{1A}$ agonists decreases 5-HT$_{1A}$ presynaptic, but not postsynaptic receptor-mediated responses: relationship to antidepressant-like action. *Eur. J. Pharmacol.* 138, 53-60.

Larsson, L.G., Renyi, L., Ross, S.B., Svensson, B., and Angeby-Moller, K. (1990): Differential effect on the responses of functional pre- and postsynaptic 5-HT$_{1A}$ receptors by repeated treatment of rats with the 5-HT$_{1A}$ receptor agonist 8-OH-DPAT. *Neuropharmacol.* 29, 85-91.

Mandal, A.K., Kellar, K.J., and Gillis, R.A. (1991): The role of serotonin-1A receptor activation and alpha-1 adrenoceptor blockade in the hypotensive effect of 5-methyl-urapidil. *J. Pharmacol. Exp. Ther.* 257, 861-869.

Middlemiss, D.N., and Fozard, J.R. (1983): 8-Hydroxy-2-(di-n-propylamino)tetralin discriminates between subtypes of the 5-HT$_1$ recognition site. *Eur. J. Pharmacol.* 90, 151-153.

Moser, P.C., Trickebank, M.D., Middlemiss, D.N., Mir, A.K., Hibert, M. F., and Fozard, J.R. (1990): Characterisation of MDL 73.005EF as a 5-HT$_{1A}$ selective ligand and its effects in animal models of anxiety: comparison with buspirone, 8-OH-DPAT and diazepam. *Br. J. Pharmacol.* 99, 343-349.

Sprouse, J.S. (1991) Inhibition of dorsal raphe cell firing by MDL 73005EF, a novel 5-HT$_{1A}$ receptor ligand. *Eur. J. Pharmacol.* 201, 163-169.

van den Hooff, P., and Galvan, M. (1991): Electrophysiology of the 5-HT$_{1A}$ ligand MDL 73005EF in the rat hippocampal slice. *Eur. J. Pharmacol.* 196, 291-298.

Effects of ketanserin on blood pressure, blood pressure variability and arterial baroreflex-blood pressure control in SHR

Din-Feng Su, Yong Cheng, Xian-Bo Kong and Jun Yang

Department of Pharmacology, Second Military Medical University, Shanghai 200433, China

Blood pressure variability (BPV) is a new concept arising from the development of techniques designed for continuous blood pressure monitoring in the last decade. It has been showed that BPV, now considered as a new parameter of cardiovascular activity, is positively related to the incidence and severity of target–organ damages in hypertensive patients (Parati et al., 1987). Ketanserin is a new antihypertensive agent with 5-HT_2 and $α_1$ receptor blocking actions. Many studies were performed on its antihypertensive effects, but no information available about its effect on BPV. Therefore, the effect of ketanserin on BPV is one subject of this work. Moreover, some studies showed that there was an interaction of ketanserin with the arterial baroreflex–heart period control (ABR–HP) in SHR (Smits et al., 1987). In the present study, the effect of ketanserin on the arterial baroreflex–blood pressure control (ABR–BP) was also investigated in SHR with a new method.

MATERIAL AND METHODS

Animal and drug. Male SHR and WKY rats from animal house of our Department were used at age of 18–22 weeks. They were housed in controlled conditions and received a standard rat chow and water *ad libitum*. Ketanserin was provided by JANSSEN Company (Belgium).

Blood pressure recording. The rats were anesthetized with a combination of ketamine (40 mg / kg) and diazepam (6 mg / kg). A polyethelene (PE) catheter (PE_{20}) was chronically placed into lower abdominal aorta via femoral artery for blood pressure measuring, and another catheter (PE_{50}) was inserted into a jugular vein for drug administration. Two days after the operation, the rats were placed in cylindrical cage. Blood pressure was recorded with a computerized technique (Su et al., 1986; Cheng et al., 1990). After at least 14-h habituation period, ketanserin (3 mg / kg) was administrered intravenously and blood pressure of rats was continuously monitored before and after ketanserin administration. In off-line analysis, the means and standard deviations of SBP, DBP and HP were calculated for 2 periods: 30 min pre–ketanserin and 30 min post–ketanserin. BPV was expressed by the standard deviation of blood pressure recorded during these periods.

ABR–BP Measurement. ABR–BP was measured by comparing the pressor responses (in area, mmHg · sec) to angiotensin II (A II, 25 ng / kg, iv) before (A1) and after (A2) blocking the baroreflex efferent pathway.

We have: ABR−BP (%) = (A2−A1) / A2 × 100

The blockade of baroreflex efferent pathway was performed by using guanethidine and methyl−atropine.

Brain slice study. In a separate *in vitro* study, the lower brainstem of the animal was removed and cut into coronal slices (500 μm). Two slices including the major part of the NTS area were transferred into the recording chamber. The slices were perfused with artificial cerebrospinal fluid. Glass micropipettes filled with 0.5 mol / L CH_3COONa were used for extracellular recording. Electrical signals were fed into an amplifier, displayed on an oscilloscope and processed with an IBM computer (histogram), then depicted by drawing instrument (Yang et al., 1991).

Statistical analysis. All results are expressed as means ± S.E. Student's *t* tests for paired data and for unpaired data were used for BPV study and ABR−BP study respectively.

RESULTS

Effects of ketanserin on blood pressure and BPV. As showed in Table 1, ketanserin decreased significantly SBP, DBP and systolic BPV (SBPV).

Table 1. Effects of ketanserin on blood pressure and BPV in conscious SHR (n = 14).

	Pre−ketanserin	Post−ketanserin
SBP(kPa)	26.7 ± 0.71	21.1 ± 0.64*
DBP(kPa)	20.5 ± 0.60	15.8 ± 0.56*
HP(msec)	16 5 ± 7.8	16 7 ± 9.1
SBPV(kPa)	1.3 ± 0.09	0.94 ± 0.04*
DBPV(kPa)	0.96 ± 0.04	0.85 ± 0.06*

* $P < 0.05$ *vs* pre−ketanserin

Effects of ketanserin on ABR−BP. ABR−BP is significantly ($P < 0.01$) higher in ketanserin−treated SHR (74.0 ± 2.5%, n = 11) than in control SHR (51.1 ± 4.3%, n = 8).

Effect of ketanserin on the spontaneous discharge of NTS neurons. Perfusing the slices with ketanserin, the spontaneous discharge of NTS neurons decreased (57.1%) or remained unchanged (42.9%). However, ketanserin potentiated the effect of NA on spontaneous discharge in 10 (of 21, 47.6%) neurons.

DISCUSSION

Ketanserin significantly lower blood pressure in hypertensive patients and in SHR, but not or only slightly in normotensives. In the present study, it was found that ketanserin not only decreased blood pressure but also decreased SBPV. As BPV is positively related to the incidence and severity of target−organ damages in hypertensive patients (Parati et al., 1987), it will be interesting to know if the inhibitory effect of ketanserin on BPV could play a substantial role in the prevention of the hypertensive target−organ damages apart from its antihypertensive effect.

Another finding of this work is that ketanserin enhanced ABR−BP in SHR. It is known that BPV increased after sinoaortic denervation (SAD) in rats. Thus, it is possible that the effect of ketanserin on ABR−BP may contribute to the decrease in BPV.

The enhanced ABR−BP could be a direct action of ketanserin on baroreflex arc or an effect secondary to the decrease in blood pressure. In the NTS slice study, ketanserin potentiated the excitatory effect of NE on the spontaneous discharge of NTS neurons. Therefore, it is suggested that the enhancement of ABR−BP is due at least in part to the direct action of ketanserin on NTS. It has been reported that ketanserin has a central sympathoinhibitory action (Yoshioka et al., 1988). According to the present findings, it seems that this inhibitory action may be mediated by baroreflex at NTS level.

(The project was supported by National Natural Science Foundation and National Educational Committee; We thank Dr. Schellekens K. for the donation of ketanserin).

REFERENCES

Cheng, Y., Zhang, H., Su, D.F., and Gu, K.M. (1990): Effects of ketanserin on blood pressure and blood pressure variability in conscious unrestrained rats. *J. Med. Coll. P.L.A. 5,* 389−393.

Parati, G., Pomidossi, G., Albini, F., Malaspina, D., and Mancia, G. (1987): Relationship of 24−hour blood pressure mean and variability to severity of target−organ damage in hypertension. *J. Hypertns. 5,* 93−98.

Smits, J.F.M., Van Essen. H., Tyssen, C.M., and Struyker−Boudier, H.A.J. (1987): Effects of ketanserin on hemodynamics and baroreflex effect in conscious spontaneously hypertensive rats. *J. Cardiovasc. Parmacol. 10,* 1−8

Su, D.F., Cerutti, C., Barres, C., Vincent, M., and Sassard, J. (1986): Blood pressure and baroreflex sensitivity in conscious hypertensive rats of Lyon strain. *Am. J. Physiol. 251,* H1111−H1117.

Yang, J., Bao, J., and Su, D.F. (1991): Effects of serotonin and noradrenaline on neuronal activities of the solitary tract nucleus and its alterations after ketanserin. *J. Med. Coll. P.L.A. 6,* 123−126.

Yoshioka, M., Machiko, M., Togashi, H., Minami, M., and Saito, H. (1988): Inhibitory effect of ketanserin on sympathetic nerve activity in rats. *Drugs. 36(Suppl),* 97−101.

Effect of ketanserin on catecholamines and NPY in peripheral tissues of normotensive (WKY) and spontaneously hypertensive rats (SHR)

Michèle Heimburger [1], Nicole Pages [2], Charles El Rawadi [1], Monique Davy [1], Claude Bohuon [3] and Yves Cohen [1]

[1] Laboratoire de Pharmacologie and [2] Laboratoire de Toxicologie, Faculté de Pharmacie, 92290 Châtenay-Malabry, [3] Laboratoire de Biologie Clinique, Institut Gustave Roussy, 94805, Villejuif, France

There are some functional and biochemical evidences that an hyperactivity of the sympathetic nervous system is involved in the pathogenesis of hypertension in the SHR (Judy et al, 1976). The consequence of this neural activation is an increase in plasma catecholamine concentrations as in sympathetically-innervated tissues catecholamine levels. In many peripheral organs, like blood vessels and heart NPY is present in sympathetic fibers where it is colocalized with noradrenaline (NA) in large dense core vesicles. Likewise, NPY is stored with adrenaline (A) in chromaffin cells of the adrenal medulla (Lundberg et al, 1990 ; Walker et al, 1991). Sympathetic nerve activation results in release of NPY. NPY participates in cardiovascular regulation by peripheral effects such as direct and indirect vasoconstrictor activities, and by prejunctional inhibition of stimulation-evoked NA output.

In the present study, we compared the catecholamine and NPY concentrations in caudal artery, atria and adrenal gland of adult WKY and SHR. Then we investigated the effect of ketanserin in these two strains. Ketanserin is a selective 5-HT$_2$ antagonist with a moderate α_1-adrenergic blocking activity, which has been described to promote the release of catecholamines (Leysen et al, 1990).

Methods

Male Wistar Kyoto (WKY) and spontaneously hypertensive (SHR) rats weighing 250-300 g were used. Two groups of each strain received by i.p. route saline or ketanserin (20 mg/kg). Two hours after injection, they were killed by decapitation and adrenals, atria and caudal artery were dissected out.

The tissues were homogenized in 1 ml ice-cold 0,4 M perchloric acid containing 0,1 % (w/v) Na$_2$ EDTA, Na$_2$S$_2$O$_5$ and cystein for NPY assay. Then homogenate was centrifuged (3500 g, 15 min 4°C) and the supernatants were stored at -80°C until monoamines determination.

NPY was assayed in the homogenate by means of an immunoradiometric assay using two anti-NPY monoclonal antibodies, the first one being tube coated, the other being ^{125}I labelled, as described in detail by Comoy et al (1989).

The results are presented as mean values ± S.E.M. Statistical analysis was performed using analysis of variance and LSD Fischer's test.

Results

The levels of NA in caudal artery and atria were the same in WKY and SHR. In adrenal gland, the NA level was higher in SHR than in WKY ($p < 0.05$) (table I).

Table I - Effect of ketanserin treatment on the NA and NPY contents in caudal artery, atria and adrenals of WKY and SHR.
C = control rats ; K = treated rats

CAUDAL ARTERY		WKY C	WKY K	SHR C	SHR K
NA	µMole/g	38 ± 1.2	20 ± 1.4*	38 ± 0.7	28 ± 0.4*
NPY	pMole/g	131 ± 5.4	109 ± 3.5	84 ± 3.4++	77 ± 3.4
ATRIA					
NA	nMole/g	11.9 ± 0.52	9.2 ± 0.71*	10.8 ± 0.71	9.0 ± 1.10
NPY	pMole/g	109 ± 5.6	115 ± 3.8	137 ± 7.2	132 ± 4.9
ADRENALS					
NA	µMole/g	0.81 ± 0.032	0.75 ± 0.015	1.13 ± 0.05+	1.04 ± 0.03
A	µMole/g	3.6 ± 0.02	3.6 ± 0.06	3.8 ± 0.12	3.1 ± 0.09
NPY	pMole/g	207 ± 6.4	183 ± 4.1	226 ± 6.2	197 ± 3.9

* $p < 0.05$ significant difference between C and K groups in the same strain
+ $p < 0.05$)   significant difference between the C groups of the two strains
++ $p < 0.01$)

The A values were the same in WKY and SHR adrenals.

NPY levels in caudal artery were lower in SHR than in WKY ($p < 0.01$), and there was no significant difference in atria and adrenals of the two strains.

Ketanserin significantly decreased the NA content in caudal artery of SHR and WKY and the level of NA in WKY atria ($p < 0.05$).

The same treatment did not affect NPY values in any of the tissues investigated.

Discussion

There is no relation between NA and NPY relative values in the tissues studied. Thus, the higher NA level in caudal artery is not associated with a larger NPY content. This finding is likely to correspond with a different localization of these two agents (Fried et al, 1985).

In SHR strain, the elevated sympathetic activity is observed in adrenals with a higher NA content than in WKY. However, no parallel increase in NPY level was observed. A parallel increase in plasma NA and NPY has been reported in hypertension in man (Edvinson et al, 1991) and in SHR (Howe et al, 1986) as an elevation in NPY in adrenal cells of phaeochromocytoma patients (Lundberg, 1986). It is likely that a correlation exists in adrenals between NPY and A rather than NPY and NA.

NPY in caudal artery of SHR is lower than in WKY. This could be interpreted as a modulatory role of this peptide on the perivascular sympathetic fibres activity in this strain whose vascular reactivity is increased.

Two hours after i.p. acute administration, ketanserin, as previously reported (Leysen, 1990), decreased catecholamines in caudal arteries and to a less extent in atria, but did not affect A and NA levels in adrenal medulla. However, NPY values did not vary significantly. Some agents which interfere with NA release were reported to affect in a similar extent the NPY release : reserpine (Franco-Cereceda et al., 1987), guanethidine (Benarroch et al., 1990), clonidine (Poncet et al., 1991). On the other hand, tyramine (Lundberg et al., 1989) or propranolol (Poncet et al., 1991) modified NA but not NPY concentrations. The lack of change in NPY levels observed in ketanserin treated rats could result from the mechanism of its releasing activity, given exocytosis in the chief pathway for NPY. Besides, sympathetic nerve activation results in release of NPY with a delayed time course versus NA overflow due to the characteristics and metabolic pathways of these two agents (Lundberg, 1990). In our experiments, the two hours delay after ketanserin injection could be quite long enough for NA but not for NPY depletion.

In conclusion, ketanserin is able to induce the release of NA from a sensitive pool in both caudal artery and atria from WKY and SHR rats, without any change in NPY levels. Thus, this study further suggests that NA and NPY release are not necessary linked.

REFERENCES

Benarroch, E.E., Schmelzer, J.D., Ward, K.K., Nelson, D.K., and Low, P.A. (1990) : Noradrenergic and neuropeptide Y mechanisms in guanethidine-sympathectomized rats. Am. J. Physiol. 259 : R371-R375.

Comoy, E., Legoc, E., Grouzmann, E., and Bohuon, C. (1989) : Neuropeptide Y et tumeurs neuro-endocriniennes. In Biologie Prospective, Comptes-rendus du 7ème Colloque de Pont-à-Mousson, eds M.M. Galteau, G. Siest and J. Henry p 471, John Libbey Eurotest, Paris.

Edvinson, L., Ekman, R., and Thulin, T. (1991) : Increased plasma levels of neuropeptide Y-like immunoreactivity and catecholamines in severe hypertension remain after treatment to normotension in man. Regulatory Peptides : 32 : 279-287.

Franco-Cereceda, A., Nagate, M., Svensson, T.H., and Lundberg, J.M. (1987) : Differential effects of clonidine and reserpine treatment on neuropeptide Y content in some sympathetically innervated tissues of the guinea-pig. Eur. J. Pharmacol. 142 : 267-273.

Fried, G., Terenius, L., Hökfelt, T. and Goldstein, N. (1985) : Evidence for differential localization of noradrenaline and neuropeptide Y in neural storage vesicles isolated from rat vas deferens. J. Neurosci. 5 : 450-458.

Howe, P.R.C., Rogers, P.F., Morris, M.J., Chalmers, J.P., and Smith, R.M. (1986) : Plasma catecholamines and neuropeptide-Y as indices of sympathetic nerve activity in normotensive and stroke-prone spontaneously hypertensive rats. J. Cardiovasc. Pharmacol. 8 : 1113-1121.

Judy, W.V., Watanabe, A.N., Henry, D.P., Besch, H.R., Murphy, W.R., and Hockel, G.M. (1976) : Sympathetic nerve activity : Role in regulation of blood pressure in the spontaneously hypertensive rat. Circ. Res. 38 : (suppl II) II21-II29.

Leysen, J.E., Wynants, J., Eens, A., and Janssen, P.A.J. (1990) : Reduction of a distinct pool of monoamines by ketanserin in peripheral tissues. In Cardiovascular pharmacology of 5-hydroxytryptamine, eds P.R. Saxena, D.I. Wallis, Wouters W. and Bevan P. pp 61-66. Kluwer Academic Netherlands.

Lundberg, J.M., Hemsen, A., Fried, G., Theodorsson-Norheim, E., and Lagercrantz, H. (1986) : High plasma levels of neuropeptide Y (NPY)-like immunoreactivity and catecholamines in newborn infants. Acta Physiol. Scand. 126 : 471-473.

Lundberg, J.M., Rudehill, A., Sollevi, A., and Hamberger, B. (1989) : Evidence for cotransmitter role of neuropeptide Y in pig spleen. Br. J. Pharmacol. 96 : 675-687.

Lundberg, J.M., Franco-Cereceda, A., Hemsen, A., Lacroix, J.S., and Pernow, J. (1990) : Pharmacology of noradrenaline and neuropeptide tyrosine (NPY)-mediated sympathetic cotrans mission. Fund. Clin. Pharmacol. 4 : 373-391.

Poncet, M.F., Damase-Michel, C., Valet, P., Tran, H.A., Montastruc, J.L., and Montastruc, P. (1991) : Clonidine but not propranolol decreases plasma neuropeptide Y (NPY) levels. Fund. Clin. Pharmacol. 5 : 473-480.

Walker, P., Grouzmann, E., Burnier, M., and Waeber, B. (1991) : The role of neuropeptide Y in cardiovascular regulation. TIPS 12 : 111-115.

New evidence on the role of the spinal cord in the antihypertensive action of rilmenidine in conscious, unrestrained, spontaneously hypertensive rats

Frédéric Sannajust, Michel Dubar * and Bevyn Jarrott

*Department of Medicine, Austin Hospital, Heidelberg, Victoria 3084, Australia and * I.R.I. Servier, 27, rue du Pont, 92202 Neuilly-sur-Seine, France*

INTRODUCTION

Rilmenidine is a new centrally acting anti-hypertensive agent with an oxazoline structure that belongs to the class of mixed alpha-2 adrenoceptor/imidazoline receptor agonists of which clonidine is the reference imidazoline. While the mechanism of the antihypertensive action of these drugs is thought to rely upon stimulation of postsynaptic adreno- or non-adrenoceptors (Laubie et al., 1985 ; Gomez et al., 1991) inducing a decrease in the peripheral sympathetic tone (Van Zwieten, 1988 ; Sannajust et al., 1990), rilmenidine presents more important differences in pharmacological profile to that of clonidine (Jarrott, 1988). These differences may be explained by the recent discovery of specific imidazoline receptors (Ernsberger et al., 1990) and recent extensive studies (Ernsberger et al., 1990 ; Gomez et al., 1991) suggesting the involvement of brainstem nuclei in their mechanism of action. However, little is known about the importance of the spinal cord and the contribution of spinal receptors in the antihypertensive effects of these drugs. Moreover, in previous experiments (Sannajust et al., 1990) we provided direct evidence that the sympathoinhibitory effect of rilmenidine could involve spinal or ganglionic sites of action. Therefore, this study was designed to: i) investigate the effects of intrathecal (i.th.) administration of rilmenidine on blood pressure (BP) and heart rate (HR) and, ii) compare the intracisternal (i.cist.) administration since there is evidence for potent antihypertensive effect of i.cist. clonidine in conscious spontaneously hypertensive rats (SHRs).

MATERIAL AND METHODS

Experiments were performed in 15 week old male SHRs (320-371g). Under anaesthesia, i.th. cannula were implanted in the Th8-Th10 segment of the thoracic spinal cord as described by Dib (1984), while i.cist. cannula were implanted into the cisterna magna by the technique of Bouman & Greidanus (1979). After a 5-day period of recovery, the animals were reanaesthetized and an arterial cannulae was inserted into the abdominal aorta via the femoral artery. Finally, after a 4-day recovery period, the animals were connected to a BP transducer and, mean arterial pressure (MAP) and HR were continuously recorded during 12 hours on a Grass Polygraph and displayed on a computer (MacIntosh IIsi with a Mac Adios II, A/D card). The animals were studied in 4 groups (n=6-7) which received by i.th. or i.cist. routes, in a volume of 10μl, increasing doses of rilmenidine (30-100-300μg/kg) or of clonidine (1-3-10μg/kg), successively at 11.00, 14.00 and 17.00hr. Each dose was preceded by an injection of artificial cerebrospinal fluid (CSF). Statistical analysis used Wilcoxon's signed rank test for paired differences, or Wilcoxon's unpaired test for comparison of two independent groups.

This work was supported by a grant from the NH&MRC / INSERM Exchange Fellowship (Australia-France) N°. 90/10698).

RESULTS

In *rilmenidine-treated SHRs*, the average basal (predrug) values (x ± sem) of MAP (139 ± 12 and 139 ± 12 mmHg) and HR (332±13 and 341 ± 21 bpm) for i.th. and i.cist.-treated groups respectively, were not strikingly different from those observed in *clonidine-treated SHRs* (147 ± 19 and 143 ± 13 mmHg) and (356 ± 14 and 336 ± 27 bpm) for i.th.and i.cist.-treated groups respectively. In addition, by i.th. or i.cist. route, artificial CSF did not modified MAP and HR of any animal. As shown in Fig.1, we observed that, 1) rilmenidine and clonidine administered i.th. or i.cist. exhibited potent antihypertensive and bradycardic effects, 2) rilmenidine induced more marked decreases in MAP by i.th. than i.cist. route, and in contrast, clonidine is more antihypertensive when given i.cist. than i.th. Regarding the time-course of the effects (data not shown) we observed that: - by i.cist. and i.th. routes, at the doses used rilmenidine and clonidine exerted no initial, short-lasting peripherally mediated pressor effect, nor reflex bradycardia, contrary to those previously observed when injected intravenously; - by i.cist. route, for each dose of rilmenidine or clonidine, HR always started to decrease before MAP. The maximal bradycardic response was obtained 15-20 min. before the maximal antihypertensive effect, and were quicker with clonidine than with rilmenidine, while by i.th. route, the maximal bradycardic and antihypertensive responses appeared at the same time (30-50 min. after injection).

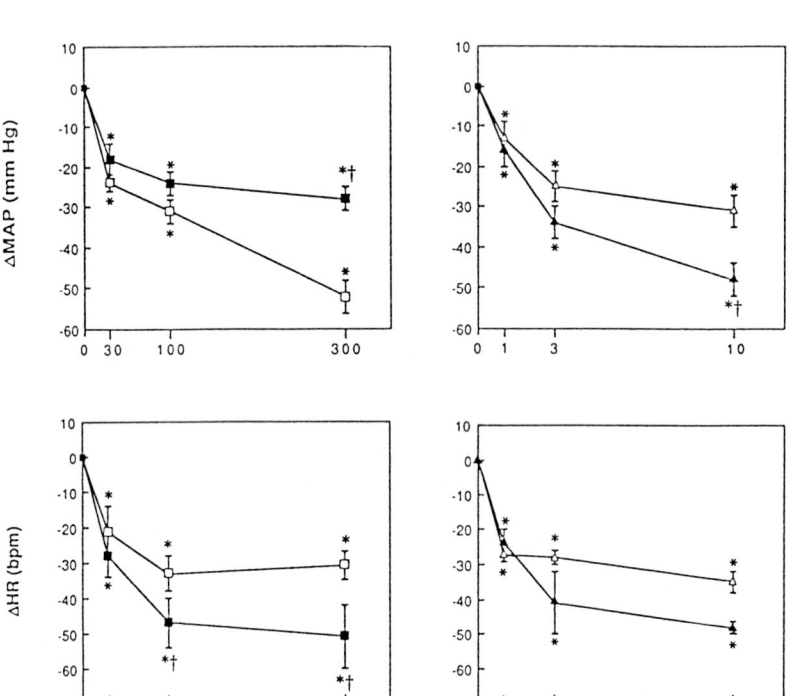

Fig.1 : Maximum decreases in mean arterial pressure (ΔMAP) and heart rate (ΔHR) after injection of rilmenidine by i.th. (□) or i.cist. (■) routes, or of clonidine by i.th. (△) or i.cist. (▲) routes, in groups of conscious SHRs (n=6-7 per group). * : P<0.01: significant differences from basal level (average of 20 min. prior injection); † : P<0.05: difference i.cist. vs i.th. cardiovascular responses.

DISCUSSION

The major findings of the present study was that: i) doses of rilmenidine injected at the Th9 level of the spinal cord of conscious freely moving SHRs produced more marked decreases in MAP than the same doses injected into the cisterna magna; ii) while rilmenidine acts more caudally via the thoracic spinal cord than clonidine, this suggests that the spinal cord plays an important role in the antihypertensive action of rilmenidine and, iii) a major part of the cardiovascular effects of clonidine seems to be mediated by brainstem or cervical structures. The fact that rilmenidine and clonidine administered i.th. or i.cist. produced a profound reduction in MAP and HR in conscious SHRs, showed that both drugs reached their sites of action by these two routes. Thus, in our conditions, we administered drugs at the Th9 level in order to avoid any supraspinal or peripheral diffusion and compare with the i.cist. route of administration. The antihypertensive and bradycardic actions of clonidine and rilmenidine following i.th. administration were not unexpected in view of their ability to inhibit the sympathetic outflow from the central nervous sytem (Van Zwieten, 1988), but surprisingly, and contrary to the study of Solomon et al. (1989), we observed that the antihypertensive effects of clonidine, as well as rilmenidine, were not associated with initial peripherally mediated pressor effects, nor reflex bradycardia. This data reveals that, in our experimental conditions and at the doses chosen, rilmenidine and clonidine are not rapidly redistributed systemically after i.th. injection. Moreover, the cardiovascular effects of i.th. rilmenidine or clonidine did not appeared to be due to retrograde diffusion of the drugs into supraspinal structures since we observed that the i.th. administration of a similar volume (10µl) of dye diffused only approximately 1.0 cm from the catheter tip. Therefore, it is likely that alpha-2 adrenoceptors or non-adreno receptors (i.e. imidazoline or gabaergic receptors) localized in the intermediolateral column of the thoracic spinal cord which has a role in modulating cardiovascular activities may be the primary site of rilmenidine-produced sympathoinhibitory effect. In addition, the comparison of the time-course of each equieffective dose revealed that, rilmenidine and clonidine could act on two distinct sites controlling BP and HR separately. All these data confirm that rilmenidine and clonidine might differ, not only in their adreno- or non-adrenoceptors affinities, but also in their sites of action. In conclusion, the findings of the present study indicate that contrary, or to a lesser degree than clonidine, the thoracic spinal cord may be one target for the antihypertensive action of rilmenidine in conscious freely moving SHRs.

REFERENCES

Bouman, H.J. and Greidanus, T.B. (1979) : A rapid and simple cannulation technique for repeating sampling of cerebrospinal fluid in freely moving rats. Brain Res. Bull., 4, 575-577.

Dib, B. (1984) : Intrathecal chronic catheterization in the rat. Pharmacol. Biochem. Behav., 20, 45-48.

Ernsberger, P., Giuliano, R., Willette, R.N. and Reis, D.J. (1990) : Role of imidazole receptors in the vasodepressor response to clonidine analogs in the rostral ventrolateral medulla. J. Pharmacol. Exp. Ther., 253, 1, 408-418.

Gomez, R.O., Ernsberger, P., Feinland, G. and Reis, D.J. (1991) : Rilmenidine lowers arterial pressure via imidazole receptors in brainstem C1 area. Eur. J. Pharmacol., 195, 181-191.

Jarrott, B. (1988) : Clonidine and related compounds. In Handbook of Hypertension, Vol. 11, Clinical Pharmacology of Antihypertensive Drugs,ed. A.E. Doyle,pp.125-186. Amsterdam : Elsevier.

Laubie, M., Poignant, J-C., Scuvée-Moreau, J., Dabiré, H., Dresse, A. and Schmitt, H. (1985) : Pharmacological properties of (N-dicyclopropylmethyl) amino-2 oxazoline (S3341), an alpha-2 adrenoceptor agonist. J. Pharmacol. (Paris), 16, 3 : 259-278.

Sannajust, F., Barrès, C., Koenig-Bérard, E. and Sassard, J. (1990) : Effect of rilmenidine on sympathetic nerve activity in conscious and anaesthetized spontaneously hypertensive rats. Eur. J. Pharmacol., 183, 2063.

Solomon, R.E., Brody, M.J. and Gebhart, G.F. (1989) : Pharmacological characterization of alpha adrenoceptors involved in the antinociceptive and cardiovascular effects of intrathecally administered clonidine. J. Pharmacol. Exp. Ther., 251, 27-38.

Van Zwieten, P.A. (1988) : Pharmacology of the alpha-2 adrenoceptor agonist Rilmenidine. Am. J. Cardiol., 61, 6D-14D.

The involvement of cAMP in the central hemodynamic actions of neuropeptide-Y (NPY) and rilmenidine in the SHR

Moira A. Mc Auley, Iseabail M. Macrae and John L. Reid

University of Glasgow, Department of Medicine and Therapeutics, Gardiner Institute, Western Infirmary, Glasgow, G21 3UW, UK

The imidazole rilmenidine is a novel centrally acting antihypertensive agent which differs from other established hypotensive agents in this class, including clonidine, in that it causes less of the undesirable side effects such as sedation and dry mouth (Beau et al 1988). This divergence has been suggested recently to be due to the action of rilmenidine on a novel class of receptor, the imidazoline preferring receptor (IPR; Bricca et al 1989). The IPR itself may be responsible for the hypotensive activity alone or alternatively alleviate the sedative effect of $alpha_2$-adrenoceptor stimulation. Several lines of evidence indicate that the former be the case, including the existence of an imidazoline-sensitive, catecholamine-insensitive population of binding sites in the brainstem and finding that the hypotensive potency of a number of centrally acting anti-hypertensive agents correlates with their in vitro binding affinity to the IPR and not $alpha_2$-adrenoceptor binding sites (Gomez et al 1991).

The initial aim of the present study was to determine the cardiovascular action of rilmenidine following intracisternal administration in the conscious spontaneously hypertensive rat (SHR). The second objective concerned the possible molecular mechanisms involved in mediating the central hypotensive actions and interactions of Rilmenidine. Modulation of medullary cAMP production was examined since this second messenger has been implicated in mediating the effects of $alpha_2$-adrenoceptor agonists. The central hypotensive effects of Neuropeptide Y (NPY) and known interactions between central NPY receptors and α_2 adrenoceptors, (influencing haemodynamic function) formed the basis of the third study aim. Possible functional interactions between rilmenidine and NPY were examined at both the haemodynamic and second messenger level.

Three to four month old male spontaneously hypertensive rats (SHR, Harlan Olac,UK) were used in the present study. Study 1: One week prior to the experimental day a 26 guage intracisternal guide cannula was stereotaxically implanted under the short acting anaesthetic methohexitone sodium (60 mg kg^{-1}; i.p.). On the study day the animals were reanaesthetised as above, the femoral artery and vein cannulated (PE-90), and exteriorised at the back of the neck. The animals were then placed in a jacket with tether and swivel to protect the cannulae and allow free movement of the animal. A period of two hours was allowed before commencement of the experiment. Arterial pressure was continuously monitored using a Statham pressure transducer connected to a Grass Polygraph with tachograph for direct heart rate recording. Rilmenidine, NPY, vehicle or a combination thereof was injected intracisternally, in order to maximize effect in the brainstem area, via a 31 guage injector (5 µl delivered 1 minute). Study 2: A separate group of rats were killed by decapitation, the brain removed and the medulla quickly dissected out on ice. Slices (500x500um) were cross-cut with a McIlwain tissue chopper, placed in separate glass tubes and incubated at 37^0C in a physiological buffer solution pH 7.4 containing (mM) 118 Na Cl, 5 KCl, 2.5 $CaCl_2$ 2 $KH_2PO_2, 2MgSO_4/7H_2O$, 25 $NaHCO_3$, 0.02 EDTA disodium salt and 11 glucose, gassed with 95% O_2/5% CO_2 for 30 minutes. The slices from two brains were pooled and transferred to buffer containing the phosphodiesterase inhibitor theophylline (1.08mg ml^{-1}) and the peptidase inhibitor bacitracin (0.1mg ml^{-1}) for a further 10 minutes. Rilmenidine, NPY, vehicle or a combination thereof were added for 5 minutes followed by the addition of forskolin (10^{-5} M) or vehicle for a further 10 minutes. The reaction was terminated and tissue cAMP released by boiling the sample at 100^0C for 4 minutes followed by homogenisation. Samples were taken for protein determination by the method of Lowry et al (1951). Tissue debris was removed by centrifugation (2800g / 15mins / 4^0C) and duplicate samples taken for cAMP determination using a sensitive radioimmunoassay (Amersham).

Intracisternal injection of rilmenidine (25,75,225,µg kg^{-1}) produced a dose-dependent fall in blood pressure and heart rate in the conscious SHR rat. The maximum hypotension and bradycardia which occurred between 30-45 minutes, were as follows: -19mmHg, -43 beats min^{-1} at 25ug kg^{-1}; -37mmHg, -56 beats min^{-1} at 75µg kg^{-1}; -56mmHg, -98 beats min^{-1} at 225µg kg^{-1}. NPY (1.7,5,15 µg kg^{-1}) injected via this route also elicited a reduction in blood pressure and heart rate. The nadir for both parameters occurred between 30-45 minutes and were as follows: -13 mmHg, -28 beats min^{-1} at 1.7µg kg^{-1}; -20 mmHg, -39 beats min^{-1}, at 5µg kg^{-1}, -26 mmHg, -50 beats min^{-1} at 15µg kg^{-1}.

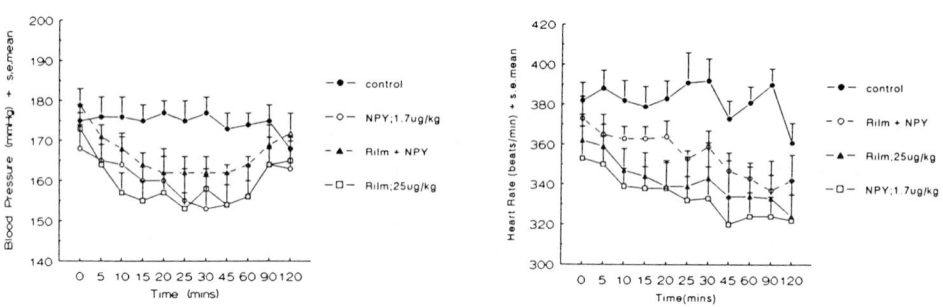

Fig. 1. Effect of NPY or rilmenidine alone or in combination on blood pressure and heart rate in the conscious SHR. Data are expressed as mean ± s.e.mean.

Submaximal doses of rilmenidine were then coadministered intracisternally in the SHR to examine possible interactions between these agents and their respective receptors. As depicted in figure 1 combined administration resulted in a hypotension and bradycardia which were less than individual responses and significantly less than the sum of the individual responses indicating the existence of a negative interaction between the receptors responsible for mediating the haemodynamic actions of these agents.

The involvement of cAMP in the haemodynamic actions of NPY was suggested by a significant dose-dependent reduction in forskolin-stimulated cAMP levels (e.g. basal, 2.9 $\pm$ 0.4; forskolin, 7.0 $\pm$ 0.7; forskolin + 10^{-6}M NPY, 5.5 $\pm$ 0.3 pmols. mg^{-1} protein). Rilmenidine itself had no effect on forskolin-stimulated cAMP levels (e.g. basal, 2.8 $\pm$ 0.4; forskolin, 5.9 $\pm$ 0.4; forskolin + 10^{-6}M rilmenidine, 5.9 $\pm$ 0.7). However, when co-administered with NPY, rilmenidine abolished the NPY evoked decrease in cAMP indicating an antagonistic interaction at the second messenger level (e.g. basal, 4.4 $\pm$ 0.4; forskolin, 7.9 + 0.3; forskolin + NPY + rilmenidine (both 10^{-6}M), 7.3 $\pm$ 0.4).

The results of the present study demonstrate that rilmenidine reduces blood pressure and heart rate in a dose-dependent manner following intracisternal administration in the SHR rat, thus confirming the central antihypertensive properties of this agent. The higher selectivity of rilmenidine for IPR's compared to $alpha_2$-adrenoceptors suggests that the observed hypotension and bradycardia may be mediated via IPR's which are known to be located in the brainstem (Bricca et al 1989; Gomez et al 1991). The significant fall in blood pressure and heart rate evoked by NPY as well as the antagonistic effect between this peptide and rilmenidine, with regard to their hypotensive and bradycardic properties, suggests an interaction between their respective receptors and a further system that may be modulated in the treatment of hypertension. It would appear that cAMP is involved in the interaction between these agents since the reduction in stimulated cAMP levels produced by NPY is attenuated in the presence of rilmenidine.

REFERENCES

Beau, B., Mahieux, F., Paraire, M., Laurin, S., Brisgand, B. and Vitou, P. (1988) Efficacy and safety of rilmenidine for arterial hypertension. Am. J. Cardiol. 61:95D-102D.

Bricca, G., Dontenwill, M., Molines, A., Feldman, J., Tribrica, E., Belcourt, A., and Bousquet, P. (1989) Rilmenidine selectivity for imidazoline receptors in human brain. Eur. J. Pharmacol. 163:373-377.

Gomez, R.E., Ernsberger, P., Feinland, G., and Reis, D.J. (1991) Rilmenidine lowers arterial blood pressure via imidazole receptors in brainstem C1 area. Eur. J. Pharmacol. 195:181-191.

Lowry, O.H., Roxbrough, N.J., Farr, A.L. and Randal, F.R.J. (1951) Protein measurement with the folin phenol reagent. J. Biol. Chem. 193:265-275.

The authors would like to acknowledge the support of the British Heart Foundation and the Institute de Recherches Internationales Servier, Neuilly sur Seine, France.

Effect of bunazosin hydrochloride on blood pressure and retinal circulation in spontaneously hypertensive rat (SHR-SR)

Momoko Abe, Hiroshi Yoshimoto and Shuichi Matsuyama

Department of Ophthalmology, Hirosaki University School of Medicine, 5 Zaifu-cho, Hirosaki 036, Japan

It is well known that peripheral resisthance induced by contraction or narrowing of the arteriole is one of the most important factors causing systemic hypertension and sustained hypertension induces arteriolar sclerosis with irreversible narrowing. It is also known that ophthalmoscopic examination is useful for the detection of hypertensive changes and differentiation of arteriolar contraction (hypertonic or functional narrowing) from arteriolar sclerosis (arteiolosclerotic or organic narrowing) (Irinoda et al., 1970).

In this report, the hypotensive effect of bunazosin hydrochloride (BN), an $alpha_1$ – blocker which dilates peripheral vessels by its selective blockage of the postsynaptic adrenoreceptor (Igarashi et al., 1982 ; Kawasaki et al., 1981 ; Shoji, 1981), was studied in connection with the change in the caliber of the retinal arteriole using rats (Okamoto and Aoki, 1963).

Animals used were 13 younger stroke – resistant SHR – SR (YSHR – SR) with age of 3 months, 14 elder SHR – SR with age over 12 months (ESHR – SR), and age – matched normotenisive Wistar – Kyoto rat (11 YWKY and 7 EWKY) whose blood pressure was estimated without anaesthesia prior to the experiment (Table 1).

Table 1. Age and blood pressure in the animals used (mean ± SD).

Animals	Number	Age in monhs	Age in weeks	Blood pressure without anaesthesia (mmHg)
YSHR – SR	13	3	15.0 ± 2.2	251.2 ± 11.2
ESHR – SR	14	12	58.6 ± 12.3	248.2 ± 23.1
YWKY	11	3	13.7 ± 1.0	131.3 ± 8.2
EWKY	7	12	55.7 ± 10.2	133.8 ± 3.8

Table 2. Changes of blood pressure in SHR-SR and WKY rats under ketamine anaesthesia before and after intravenous injection of bunazosin hydrochloride 0.5mg/kg (mean ± SD).

Animals	Blood pressure		reduction after BN
	Before BN	after BN	
YSHR-SR	243.5 ± 23.4	156.9 ± 35.4	86.6 ± 28.4
ESHR-SR	230.2 ± 23.9	184.4 ± 38.8 **	45.7 ± 38.2 *
YWKY	130.1 ± 10.2	101.1 ± 13.0 **	29.0 ± 16.1 **
EWKY	134.4 ± 4.3	114.0 ± 27.9	20.4 ± 26.8 **

* significant vs younger SHR-SP ($0.001 < p < 0.01$)
** significant vs younger SHR-SR ($p < 0.001$)

Table 3. The effect of intravenously injected bunazosin hydrochloride 0.5 mg/kg on the caliber of the retinal arteriole, shown with vasodilation ratio vs. the caliber before the administration (mean ± SD).

Animals	number	Time after BN administration				
		1 min.	2 min.	5 min.	10 min.	15 min.
YSHR-SR	13	1.20 ± 0.12	1.28 ± 0.24	1.27 ± 0.20	1.32 ± 0.19	1.29 ± 0.18 *
ESHR-SR	14	1.03 ± 0.07	1.03 ± 0.06	1.02 ± 0.05	1.04 ± 0.09	1.01 ± 0.04 **
YWKY	11	1.05 ± 0.08	1.07 ± 0.01	1.08 ± 0.09	1.05 ± 0.07	1.03 ± 0.06 **
EWKY	7	1.07 ± 0.06	1.13 ± 0.07	1.10 ± 0.09	1.13 ± 0.12	1.11 ± 0.12 **

* $p < 0.001$, ** $0.01 < p < 0.005$, before vs after BN
NS : not significant

During the experiment, all animals were anaesthetized by intravenous injection of ketamine hydrochloride 20-30 mg/kg body weight.
Blood pressure was measured by tail cuff plethysmographic method.
Retinal arterioles were documented by color photography before and after intravenous administration of BN 0.5 mg/kg. The caliber of the retinal arteriole was measured on the print of fundus photograph with micrometer. The change of the caliber of the rerinal arteriole and blood pressure before and after BN injection were evaluated by vasodilation ratio and blood pressure reduction ratio, respectively calicualted as follows and Students t-test was used.

Vasodilation ratio = DA after BN injection／DA before BN injection,
BP reduction ratio = (BP an - BP after BN injection)／BP an.
DA : diameter of the retinal arteriole, BN : bunazosin hydrochloride, BP : blood pressure,
BP an : blood pressure under anaesthesia.

Blood pressure was 243.5 mmHg in YSHR-SR, 230.2 mmHg in ESHR-SR, 130.1 mmHg in YWKY and 134.4 mmHg in EWKY before BN administration while it was 156.9 mmHg, 184.4mmHg, 101.1 mmHg and 114.0 mmHg, respectively, after BN administration. The fall of blood pressure after BN administration was significant in the rats of 3 groups except

ESHR – SR (Table 2). The retinal arterioles dilated significantly in YSHR – SR ($p < 0.01$), YWKY ($p < 0.05$) and EWKY ($0.01 < p < 0.05$), 15 – 20 min. after BN administration. No significant dilatation was seen in ESHR – SR (Table 3). In SHR – SR, correlation between blood pressure reduction ratio and vasodilation ratio was significant ($Y = 0.9028 \pm 0.7383X$, $r = 0.5515$, $0.005 < p < 0.01$). In WKY rats, however, no correlation was found ($Y = 1.1405 - 0.3423X$, $r = -0.5126$, $p < 0.05$).

Histopathologic changes of retinal arteriole in SHR could be classified into 3 Stages ; hypertrophic stage, regressive stage and necrotic stage, and ophthalmoscopic change of diffuse narrowing of retinal arteriole, arteriolar caliber irregularities of slight grade and marked caliber irregularities with tortuosity and retinal oedema corresponded to each stages, respectively (Yoshimoto and Takahashi, 1977). Electron microscopic features in hypertrophic stage was protrusion of endothelial cells into the vascular lumen, probably due to contraction of medial smooth muscle cells and those in necrotic stage were narrowing of the lumen due to marked thickening of degenerated media. The latter change was seen in the rats with sustained high blood pressure longer than 6 to 12 months. In this study, marked fall of blood pressure was seen in YSHR – SR though it was seen in all groups. This result shows that BN acts most effectively to the rats in hypertonic state (hypertrophic stage) though it also acts to normotensive rats because BN probably subsides physiologic tonus of vascular smooth muscle. Vasodilatative effect was recognized in YSHR – SR and both YWKY and EWKY while it was not recognized in ESHR – SR. This result suggests that vasculartonus and reactivity are higher not only in YSHR – SR but also in normotensive WKY than in ESHR – SR which are in the state of arteriolar sclerosis or necrotic stage.

To conclude, these results suggested that bunazosin hydrochloride, a selective blockade of postsynaptic alpha – adrenoreceptor is of anti – hypertensive effect for the hypertensives in hypertonic stage but of no effect for the hypertensives with arteriolar smooth muscle destruction caused by prolonged hypertension.

References

Igarashi, T., Nakajima, Y. and Ohtake, S. (1982) : Antihypertensive effect of combined treatment with alpha – and beta – adrenergic blockers in the spontaneously hypertensive rat. Jpn. J. Pharmacol. 31, 361 – 368.

Irinoda, K., Matsuyama, S. and Takahashi, S. (1970) : The narrowing of retinal arterioles in systemic hypertension. A clinical and experimental study revealing functional and organic narrowing in man as well as rats. Excerpta Medica International Congress Series No. 222, Ophthalmology, 912 – 920.

Kawasaki, T., Uezono, K. et al. (1981) : Antihypertensive effect of E – 643, a new alpha – adrenargic blocking agent. Eur. J. Clin. Pharmacol. 20, 399 – 405.

Okamoto, K. and Aoki, K. (1963) : Development of a strain of spontaneously hypertensive rats. Jpn. Circ. J. 27, 282 – 293.

Shoji, T. (1981) : Comparison of pre – and postsynaptic alpha – adrenoreceptor blocking effect of E – 643 in isolated vas deferens of the rat. Jpn. J. Pharmacol. 31, 361 – 368.

Yoshimoto, H. and Takahashi, S. (1977) : Retinal arterioles in the spontaneously hypertensive rats and other experimental hypertensive rats. Jpn. J. Ophthalmol. 21, 157 – 175.

Enhanced emotional responses with aging in stroke-prone spontaneously hypertensive rats (SHRSP)

Hiroshi Ogawa, Tomoyo Tanaka, Sukenari Sasagawa, Sawako Akai *, Tetsuo Akai *, Masaya Takahashi * and Motonori Yamaguchi *

*Department of Hygiene, Kinki University School of Medicine, 377-2 Ohno-Higashi, Osaka-Sayama city, Osaka 589 * Research Department, Institute of Pharma Research, Development and Medical Science, Nihon Schering KK, 2-6-64, Nishimiyahara, Yodogawa-Ku, Osaka 532, Japan*

INTRODUCTION

It is well known that SHRSP shows the increased locomotor activity compared to the age-matched Kyo:Wistar rats (WKY). It is also reported that SHRSP shows a marked hyperactivity associated with induction of stroke. However, behavioral changes with aging and involvement of central nervous systems in those behavioral changes in SHRSP are poorly understood. In the present study, in order to characterize behavioral changes with aging in SHRSP, emotional responses as well as locomotor activity were compared with those of WKY. Next, to clarify functional correlations of the SHRSP brain to the behavioral changes, behavioral effects of central acting drugs and autoradiographical binding patterns of $[^3H]$-neuroreceptor ligands with brain slices were examined. Moreover, magnetic resonance imaging (MRI) was performed to follow up in situ changes in the brain of individual animal.

MATERIALS AND METHODS

Male animals of SHRSP and the age-matched male WKY were housed singly in cages and maintained on SP diet (Funabashi, Japan). In the behavioral study, the emotional responses such as startle response, struggle response, attack response and vocalization were scored by the method of Shibata et al., (1982) with slight modification (Kobayashi et al., 1991). The spontaneous locomotion was evaluated by measuring ambulation and rearing in the open field. Blood pressure was measured by the tail-pulse pick-up method without anesthesia. In the binding study, at 4 and 5 weeks of age when the locomotor activity and the startle response significantly elevated, respectively, six animals per each group were sacrificed by decapitation. The brains were immediately removed and frozen with dry ice for autoradiographical binding studies as reported previously (Akai et al., 1991). The bindings of specific $[^3H]$-ligands to 5-HT$_{1A}$, 5-HT$_2$, α_1, α_2, β, D_1, D_2 and mACh receptors were quantified by an image analysis system (RAS 3000, Amersham Japan). In the MRI study, animals at the age of 8 weeks were given the SP diet and 1% NaCl solution as a drinking water to accelerate generation of stroke. The T1- and T2-weighted MR images were collected on a 4.7 T MRI system (GE Instruments, U.S.A.) in anesthetized rats as reported previously (Takahashi et al., 1991). After the MRI, animals were killed to examine the histological changes.

RESULTS

SHRSP showed an increased ambulatory and rearing behaviors on and after 3 weeks of age compared to the age-matched WKY. Both SHRSP and WKY showed no marked emotional response until 4 weeks of age. However, the emotional responses, especially startle response, were markedly enhanced in SHRSP on and after 5 weeks of age as shown in **Fig. 1**. On the other hand, the blood pressure of SHRSP gradually increased after 5 weeks of age, and reached to 220-240 mmHg after 12 weeks of age. At the age of 16-24 weeks, further increases of the locomotor activity and the emotional responses (attack and startle responses) in SHRSP occurred for 1-2 days. One day after the occurrence of these behavioral changes, the T2-weighted MR images indicated hyperintense areas in the occipital cortex. Judging from the pathological examination, these hyperintense areas corresponded to neurodegenerative areas of edema, softening in the brain regions. The T1-weighted MR images after injection of the contrast media Gd-DTPA also showed smaller hyperintense areas in the occipital cortex. In the case of SHRSP showing no further behavioral changes and WKY, neither abnormal MRI signal nor histological change was detected.

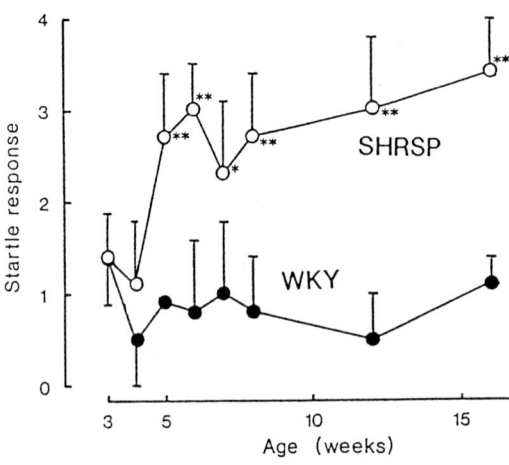

Fig. 1. Enhancement of startle response in SHRSP (O) with aging. The vertical bars indicate the standard deviation of the mean (N=8-16).
*; $p<0.05$, **; $p<0.01$ vs. WKY (●).

Table 1. Changes in densities of neuroreceptors in SHRSP at 4 and 5 weeks of age

Receptor		Brain region	Increase (Av. %, vs. WKY)	
			4 week-old	5 week-old
Serotonin	$5-HT_2$	COR, STR, ACB	55, 43, 37	NS
	$5-HT_{1A}$	HIP	NS	14
Adrenalin	α_1	SEP, OT	NS	31, 22
	α_2	–	NS	NS
	β	–	NS	NS
Dopamine	D_1	FC	NS	57
		STR	15	18
	D_2	–	NS	NS
Acetylcholine	mACh	CER	23	26

NS; Not significant.
ACB; Accumbens nucleus, CER; Cerebellum, COR; Cortex, FC; Frontal cortex, HIP; Hippocampus, OT; Olfactory tubercle, SEP; Septum, STR; Striatum.

The $5-HT_{1A}$ agonist 8-OH-DPAT suppressed the enhanced startle response in SHRSP, while the $5-HT_2$ agonist DOI and the D_1 agonist SKF38393 suppressed the increased locomotor activity. The α_2 agonist clonidine suppressed the increased blood pressure in SHRSP. Densities of $5-HT_2$ receptors in cortex, accumbens nucleus and striatum of SHRSP were 37-55 % higher than those of WKY at 4 weeks of age, and these densities of SHRSP decreased at 5 weeks of age (**Table 1**). Subsequently, no significant difference in those densities was observed between SHRSP and WKY at 5 weeks of age. Densities of $5\text{-}HT_{1A}$ receptors in hippocampus of SHRSP were around 14 % higher than those of WKY at both 4 and 5 weeks of age, but it was statistically significant at 5 weeks of age. Densities of α_1 receptors in septum and olfactory tubercle and those of D_1 receptors in frontal cortex of SHRSP were 22-57 % higher than those of WKY at 5 weeks of age. At both 4 and 5 weeks of age, densities of D_1 receptors in striatum and those of mACh receptors in cerebellum of SHRSP were 15-26 % higher than those of WKY. There was no difference in the densities of α_2, β and D_2 receptors between SHRSP and WKY.

DISCUSSION

Emotional response (startle response) of SHRSP was markedly enhanced on and after 5 weeks of age. The on-set time of the enhancement of startle response was different from that of the increases in locomotor activity and blood pressure. In addition, drug-sensitivity on the former was also different from that on the latter. These results suggest involvement with different mechanism for those induction in SHRSP. Further increases of the locomotor activity and the attack and startle responses in SHRSP were found to occur for 1-2 days at the age of 16-24 weeks upon an appearance of cerebral damage caused by stroke.

SHRSP was also found to show marked changes in densities of $5\text{-}HT_2$ receptors as well as D_1 and α_1 receptors in the specific brain regions of SHRSP between 4 and 5 weeks of age, while densities of D_1 and mACh receptors in the other specific brain regions of SHRSP increased at both 4 and 5 weeks of age. These findings suggest that functional changes in central serotonergic as well as dopaminergic and noradrenergic systems of SHRSP may be involved in the enhanced startle response. Furthermore, the enhanced locomotor activity of SHRSP may be related to the functional change in dopaminergic and cholinergic systems.

CONCLUSION

We suggest that functional change in serotonergic and dopaminergic systems of brain may be mainly involved in the enhanced emotional responses and the enhanced locomotor activity, respectively, while specific neuronal damage after stroke may result in the excess behavioral hyperactivity in SHRSP.

REFERENCES

Akai, T., Yamaguchi, M., Tanaka, T., Ogawa, H. and Sasagawa, S. (1991): Involvement of central serotonergic systems in enhanced startle response in SHRSP. Jpn. Heart J., (in press).

Kobayashi, S., Tanaka, T., Akai, T., Yamaguchi, M., Ogawa, H. and Sasagawa, S. (1991): Enhanced emotional response in stroke-prone spontaneously hypertensive rats. Jpn. Heart J., (in press).

Takahashi, M., Fritz-Zieroth, B., Yamaguchi, M., Ogawa, H., Tanaka, T. and Sasagawa, S. (1991): Magnetic resonance imaging on cerebral disorders with stroke in stroke-prone spontaneously hypertensive rats. Jpn Heart J., (in press).

Shibata, S., Yamamoto, T. and Ueki, S. (1982): Differential effects of medial, central and basolateral amygdaloid lesions on four models of experimentally induced aggression. Physiol. Behav. 28: 289-294.

Exaggerated renal vascular responses to different stresses in spontaneously hypertensive rats

Hiroshi Kawamura, Masahiro Maki, Kazutoshi Komatsu, Keiji Hara, Kenkin Suzuki, Satoru Ito, Wataru Usui, Tadao Yasugi and Michinobu Hatano

2nd Department of Internal Medicine, Nihon University School of Medicine, 30-1 Oyaguchi Kamimachi, Itabashi-Ku, Tokyo 173, Japan

INTRODUCTION
The spontaneously hypertensive rats (SHR) exhibits exaggerated cardiovascular responses to various environmental stimuli, compared to the control rats (Yamori, 1969). Although renal arteries respond greatly to environmental stimuli, the increments in arterial pressure (AP) and heart rate (HR) do not differ between the two strains during stimuli. There would be some hemodynamic adjustment to buffer the pressor response to environmental stimuli and renal responses would differ to the quality of stress rather than to the quantity of stress. Therefore, the purpose of the present study was to test the hypotheses that renal arteries respond differently with different environmental stimuli.

METHODS
Mature male SHR (averaging 20 week old) and age-sex matched Wistar-Kyoto rats (WKY) from the colony of the Nihon University Animal Center were used in the study. Animals were housed individually on a regular light/dark cycles and had free access to laboratory chow and tap water. On the day of flow probes instrumentation, the rats were anesthetized with the inhalation of a gas mixture of 75 % nitrous oxide, 0.5 % halothane and 24.5 % oxygen. Then they were implanted with a Doppler flow probe (diameter 0.2 mm) on the left renal artery. After the chest was opened through a midsternal incision, another Doppler flow probe (diameter 2 mm) was implanted around the ascending aorta to monitor cardiac output (CO). Then, they were allowed to recover from the operation. One week later, the left femoral artery was cannulated for recording mean arterial pressure (MAP). MAP was directly monitored in conscious rats using a pressure transducer. Total peripheral resistance (TPR) was obtained by dividing MAP by CO, and renal vascular resistance (RVR) by dividing MAP by renal blood flow (RBF). Then animal were placed in the plexiglass test chamber. The hemodynamic parameters were simultaneously recorded on a multichannel polygraph. Control MAP, heart rate (HR) and RBF were taken for each animal while it was quiet resting. Other hemodynamic

parameters were also taken while it was on stress. Air blow stress (AB) was given to rats for 10 sec and shaking stress (SS) was also given for 10 sec (100 cycles/min).
The results are presented as the mean ± one standard error of the mean. The F-test was used for the analysis of variance. Student's t-tests of paired and unpaired variates of the analysis of significance. Probability levels of less than 0.05 were considered significant.

RESULTS

The control MAP was higher in SHR than in WKY (145 ± 4 vs. 92 ± mmHg, $P < 0.01$). The control HR was higher in SHR than in WKY (423 ± 63 vs. 392 ± 51, $P < 0.01$). The control CO did not differ between SHR and WKY (6.6 ± 0.6 vs. 7.7 ± 0.5 KHz, n.s.). The control TPR was higher in SHR than in WKY (22.3 ± 2.28 vs. 14.7 1.0 KHz, $P < 0.01$). The control RBF did not differ between SHR and WKY (8.0 ± 1.2 vs. 6.3 ± 1.0 KHz, n.s.).
During AB, MAP and HR increased in both strains (MAP, SHR: 181 ± 5, WKY: 104 ± 9 mmHg; HR, SHR: 440 ± 58, WKY 399 ± 51 beats/min, all $P < 0.01$, respectively). However, RBF decreased in both the two strains during AB (SHR, 3.9 ± 0.6 KHz; WKY, 4.6 ± 0.8 KHz, all $P < 0.01$, respectively). This reduction of RBF is greater in SHR than in WKY ($P < 0.05$). The increment in % RVR was greater in SHR than in WKY (153 ± 16 vs. 135 ± 6 %, $P < 0.01$). During SS, MAP, HR and TPR increased in SHR and WKY. The reduction of RBF occurred but was not different between SHR and WKY. The % RVR increased in SHR and WKY, and this % RVR was greater during SS than AB (SHR, 149 ± 12 %; WKY, 123 ± 2 %, all $P < 0.01$, respectively). During AB, the increment % RVR in SHR and WKY were not so much greater as that during SS.

DISCUSSION

SHR is reported to be hyperactive in renal arteries to AB, compared to carotid and mesenteric arteries (Ito, 1991). However, another report indicates mesenteric arteries is more hyperactive than renal arteries which has been done using electrical foot shock (Kirby, 1984). Therefore, the quality of stress is important to assess the hemodynamic effect by stress. Our present results also support Ito's data. Furthermore, renal arteries are demonstrated to be hyperactive during mental stress in SHR and this responses in renal arteries were characteristic to the defense reaction for both SHR and WKY (Folkow 1982). The increased resting SHR HR in present study indicates increased sympathetic nerve activity which increased during environmental stress. This observation is also in agreement with previous report (Lundin, 1980). SS increased MAP and HR in SHR, which are also agreement with another report (Hallback, 1974). However, reduction in RBF during SS was similar to those in WKY. RVR changes also occurred in SHR to AB but not so pronounced as to SS. The most pronounced difference in RBF occurred during SS but not AB. The possible explanation of this different renal responses between AB and SS may depend upon the quality of stress. The increase in % RVR during AB is considerably augmented in SHR compared to WKY, suggesting that SHR appeared to have reduced threshold in the responses to AB. The results of the present study indicate that renal hemodynamic response of the SHR and WKY to stress are different even though pressor responses is equivalent during the two kind of stress. Different exaggerated sympathetic drive to renal arteries would lead to different level of increased vasoconstriction in the renal arteries.

SUMMARY

The result of the present study demonstrates that renal arterial vasoconstriction in SHR is more exaggerated than WKY to air blow stress and that renal vasoconstriction is greater in shaking stress than in air blow stress. This renal vasoconstrictive response may be stress-specific and may depend on the quality of stress.

REFERENCES

Folkow, B. (1982): Physiological aspects of primary hyper tension. Physiol. Rev. 62: 347-504

Hallback, M., and Folkow B. (1974): Cardiovascular responses to acute mental "stress" in spontaneously hypertensive rats. Acta Physiol. Scand. 90: 684-698

Ito, S., Kawamura, H., et al (1991): Regional vascular responses to two acute stressor in spontaneously hypertensive rats. Nichidai Igakuzasshi (in Japanese).

Lundin, S.A., and Hallback, M. (1980): Background of hyperkinetic circulatory state in young spontaneously hypertensive rats. Cardiovascular. Res. 14: 561-56

Kirby, K.F., Callahon, M.F., et al (1984): Regional vascular responses to an acute stressor in spontaneously hypertensive and Wistar-Kyoto rats. J. Autonomic Nerv. Syst. 20: 185-188

Yamori, Y., Matsumoto, M. et al (1969): Augumentation of spontaneous hypertension of chronic stress in rats. Jpn. Circ. J. 33: 399-409

Role of renin in the cardiovascular response to acute stress in conscious Sprague Dawley and spontaneously hypertensive rats

H.G. Spanos, R. Di Nicolantonio and S.L. Skinner

Department of Physiology, Melbourne University, Parkville, Victoria 3052, Australia

Summary
We examined the role of the renin angiotensin system (RAS) on the pressor response to acute air jet stress in Sprague Dawley (SD) and Spontaneously Hypertensive Rats (SHR). Despite a higher absolute pressor response in SHR's, the relative maximum response was similar in both strains. The SD's displayed a transient bradycardia while SHR's responded with tachycardia suggesting a reduced baroreceptor control of heart rate (HR) compared to the SD. The pressor response in SD but not the SHR was accompanied by an elevated plasma renin activity (PRA) indicating a refractory role of the RAS in the SHR response to stress.

Introduction
The interaction of environmental and genetic factors is important in hypertension development. In the rat environmental stress (nasal stimulation by air jet) produces a pressor response together with an increased renal sympathetic nerve activity (RSNA) and anti-natriuresis which, unlike the pressor response, are abolished by adrenoceptor antagonists (Koepke et al 1986). We suspect that angiotensin may also be involved in the pressor response to air jet. Increased RSNA is known to increase renin release which can cause hypertension (Laragh 1987). Elevated PRA accompanies developing hypertension in crowded CBA mice (Vander et al 1978) and in acutely stressed SD rats (Porter 1989, Vander et al 1977). Conversely Harrap et al (1984) found no evidence of sustained hypertension in crowded SD rats despite an elevated PRA. The prevailing view is that the SHR is more responsive to stress than its normotensive relation the Wistar Kyoto (WKY; Lundin et al 1984), thus highlighting the genetic component of hypertension. Here we examine the possible role of angiotensin release in the pressor responses to air jet stimulation in SHR and an unrelated genetic normotensive strain (SD).

Materials and Methods
Conscious (10-12 weeks) male SD and SHR rats had their BP and HR recorded continuously on a polygraph from an indwelling carotid artery cannula connected to a Statham pressure transducer (P23Db). At least 36 hrs after surgery 2 SD and 2 SHRs were placed in separate holders side by side and while one of each pair of rats served as control (group C) the other (group E) was stimulated for 10 min with an air jet delivered at 15 psi and 20 l/min from 4mm tubing placed 5 cm from the rat's nose. Systolic (S), Mean (M) and Diastolic (D) BP and HR data was analysed during the 1st, 5th and 10th min of the air jet stimulus and at 3x10 min intervals before (control) and after (recovery). Heart rate per min was determined by counting the beats in the first 6 s of each time period. After the 30 min recovery period the experiment was repeated so that group C received the air jet stimulus and group E served as control. Blood samples (0.3ml) for plasma PRA were taken directly into 3U heparin from the carotid cannula 5 min before, during the first 3 min and at 30 min after the air jet. PRA was measured by RIA of angiotensin I generated during

incubation of plasma at pH 7.4 for 120 min at 37ºC in the presence of EDTA, NEM (N-ethylmaleimide) and benzamidine (6,8, & 30 mmol/l). Other than incubation, the assay was carried out on ice. The amount of angiotensin I formed ranged from 50 to 500 fmol and resulted from the hydrolysis of less than 1% of the endogenous angiotensinogen substrate. Data were pooled for groups C and E and analysed by ANOVA and paired t-test.

Results

Table 1 shows the pressor and HR responses of E and C groups of rats to air jet stimulation. There were no significant differences between groups before the air jet. In both strains a maximum pressor response ($P<0.01$) occurred during the first 6 s of the air jet. Controls showed an attenuated response at this time ($P>0.15$). For the remainder of the stimulation period the pressor response in both strains diminished but was still significantly elevated in the SHR ($P<0.05$). Although the magnitude of the maximum pressor response was higher in the SHR, the percentage increase from control levels was not different between these strains viz: 41% vs 42% for SBP, 25% vs 18% for MBP, and 32% vs 34% for DBP (SHR vs SD). The SD responded with an immediate bradycardia of 13% upon air jet stimulation, opposite to the SHR tachycardia

TABLE 1 Effect of Air Jet Stimulation on BP (mmHg) and HR (bpm) of SD and SHR Showing Means ± sem for Experimental (E) and Control (C) Groups

		BEFORE[#]	DURING AIR JET			AFTER[#]
			0.1min	5min	10min	
SYSTOLIC BP						
SHR:	E	183 ±3.8	258 ±8.3*	210 ±7.6*	211 ±5.0*	185 ±7.2
	C	206 9.0	225 10.3	192 6.3	191 9.4	187 6.6
SD:	E	126 6.8	179 8.0*	132 7.7	130 7.7	126 8.6
	C	129 6.2	146 10.3	128 8.8	128 9.5	124 8.3
MEAN BP						
SHR:	E	163 4.0	204 7.4*	179 4.7*	179 2.9*	162 4.9
	C	169 5.8	183 4.0	166 4.7	167 7.8	166 5.0
SD:	E	115 6.3	136 9.7	119 7.6	119 7.9	114 8.7
	C	119 5.3	123 6.8	115 8.0	117 8.4	112 7.8
DIASTOLIC BP						
SHR:	E	137 3.9	181 8.1*	152 6.0*	154 4.9*	141 4.7
	C	145 5.3	163 5.6	145 2.8	146 4.8	140 4.0
SD:	E	104 7.2	139 6.8*	110 8.7	112 8.3	106 9.0
	C	110 5.0	118 7.2	111 8.1	106 8.5	104 8.9
HEART RATE						
SHR:	E	401 11.6	429 14.2	472 11.5*	469 13.3*	385 11.2
	C	394 13.6	413 14.7	431 26.0	448 21.4*	370 7.7
SD:	E	396 10.8	346 29.7*	420 23.0	439 13.5*	402 14.3
	C	399 12.4	412 12.2	412 19.4	438 16.2	402 13.0

[#] Average of 3x10 min control readings before or after nasal air jet stimulation.
* $P<0.05$, compared to values before air jet stimulation.

TABLE 2 Effect of Air Jet Stimulation on PRA (nmol/l/hr) of SD and SHR Showing Means ± sem Before (5 min), During (3 min) and After (30 min) Air Jet

		BEFORE	DURING	AFTER
SHR:	E	0.97 ±0.38	1.15 ±0.24	1.51 ±0.76
	C	1.41 0.94	1.74 0.71	1.97 0.82
SD:	E	0.19 0.11	3.92 1.89*	2.28 1.35
	C	0.94 0.46	0.64 0.35	2.14 1.05

* $P<0.05$, compared to values before air jet stimulation.

of 7%. However with continued stimulation HR increased in both strains but more so in the SHR, thus at 5 and 10 min of air jet the respective increase in HR was 6% & 11% ($P<0.05$) in the SD and 18% ($P<0.001$) & 17% ($P<0.001$) in the SHR. Both HR and BP returned to resting values within 10 min after the air jet ceased. The pressor response to air jet stimulation was paralleled by an increase in PRA that was significant ($P<0.05$) for the SD only (Table 2). Control PRA's were not different in either strain.

Discussion

The direct pressor measurements confirmed our previous findings (Spanos et al 1990) that air jet stimulation results in an immediate transient pressor response that is proportionally similar in SD and SHR. The smaller responses in the C group support the observations of Fisher & Tucker (1991) that air jet noise alone can produce a significant pressor response in borderline hypertensive rats suggesting that the air jet stimulus has an auditory and a tactile component. The brevity of the pressor response in the C group suggests that the auditory component represents only a small part of the total response. The immediate pressor response in both C and E groups is consistent with one that is predominantly sympathetically mediated, whereas the sustained, albeit diminished response seen only in E groups could be due to an hormonal response supplementing the neural one. This appears to be the case with the SD where PRA rose significantly during the air stress. Similar pressor and PRA responses in SD rats to air jet stimulation were reported by Porter (1989). Conversely, the absence of an elevated PRA in the SHR suggests a minor role for the RAS in their response to air stress which supports the view that sympathetic hyperactivity (Lundin et al 1984) alone accounts for the pressor response in the SHR. This view is further supported by the immediate elevation in HR during air stress, indicating a reduced baroreceptor control of HR in SHR compared to the SD. A similar difference in HR response to air stress exists between the SHR and WKY (Lundin et al 1984). Whether the sympathetic hyperactivity is strictly a neural response or is wholly or in part due to an increase in plasma catecholamines remains to be determined.

References

Fisher, L.D. & Tucker, D.C. (1991): Air jet noise exposure rapidly increases blood pressure in young borderline hypertensive rats. *J. Hypertension* 9, 275-282.

Harrap, S.S., Louis, W.J. & Doyle A.E. (1984): Failure of psychosocial stress to induce chronic hypertension in the rat. *J. Hypertension.* 2, 653-662.

Koepke, J.P., Jones, S & DiBona, G.F. (1986): Hypothalamic B-adrenoceptor control of renal nerve sympathetic nerve activity and urinary sodium excretion in conscious spontaneously hypertensive rats. *Cir. Res.* 58, 241-248.

Laragh, J.H. (1987) Role of the Renin-Angiotensin-Aldosterone axis in human hypertensive disorders. In *The Kidney in Hypertension.* ed. N.M. Kaplan, B.M. Brenner, & J.H. Laragh, pp 35-51, New York: Raven Press.

Lundin, S., Ricksten, S.E. & Thoren, P. (1984): Interaction between "mental stress" and baroreceptor reflexes concerning effects on heart rate, mean arterial pressure and renal sympathetic activity in conscious spontaneously hypertensive rats. *Acta Physiol. Scand.* 120, 273-284.

Porter, J.A. (1989): Stress can enhance the renin response to reduced renal perfusion pressure. *Am. J. Physiol.* 256, R554-R559.

Spanos, H.G., Di Nicolantonio, R. & Morgan, T.O. (1990): Comparison of SHR and SD responses to air jet stimulation. *High Blood Pressure Res. Council Aust.* Abstr. p70.

Vander, A.J., Henry, J.P., Stephens, P.M., Kay, L.L. & Mouw, D.R. (1978): Plasma renin activity in psychosocial hypertension of CBA mice. *Cir. Res.* 42, 496-502.

Vander, A.J., Kay, L.L., Dugan, M.E. & Mouw, D.R. (1977): Effects of noise on plasma renin activity in rats. *Proc. Soc. Exp. Biol. Med.* 156, 24-26.

Acknowledgements

This study was supported by the National Heart Foundation of Australia. We thank Miss B. Rees for conducting the PRA assays.

Spectral analysis of short-term oscillations in blood pressure and heart rate in hypertensive rats of the Lyon strain

Jocelyne Blanc, Marie-Laure Grichois, Madeleine Vincent *, Jean Sassard * and Jean-Luc Elghozi

*Laboratoire de Pharmacologie, CNRS I 6167, Faculté de Médecine Necker-Enfants Malades, 156, rue de Vaugirard, 75015 Paris and * Département de Physiologie et Pharmacologie clinique, CNRS URA 606, Faculté de Pharmacie, 8, avenue Rockefeller, 69373 Lyon Cedex 08, France*

INTRODUCTION

We recently developed a spectral analysis technique for instantaneous BP in rats, in order to test fluctuations in BP and heart rate (HR) in the frequency domain (Japundzic et al. 1990). We have shown that clonidine markedly reduced the amplitude of BP and HR oscillations in one frequency region (195-605 mHz) that depends on the activity of the autonomic nervous system (Grichois et al. 1990). We recently characterized the spectral BP and HR profiles in response to an air jet stimulation administered to normotensive Wistar rats (Blanc et al. 1991). Julien et al. (1988) have shown that an increased lability of blood pressure (BP), as reflected by the enhancement of its spontaneous variability and a stronger response to an environmental stressor, develops with hypertension in LH rats. In the present work, both the spontaneous variability of BP and HR and the BP and HR responses to emotional stress were studied in LL, LN and LH rats. In addition, we tested whether clonidine was able to affect the autonomic component of the reaction to stress.

METHODS

Groups of 8 LL, LN and LH male rats belonging to the 40th and 41st generation of these strains were used (Vincent et al. 1984). Experiments were performed in conscious unrestrained animals between 15 and 16 weeks of age. Experiments were started 1 h after the rats had been connected to the pressure transducer and injection syringe. Each rat was recorded 4 times with a 5 min recording period. The first two recordings ie resting period and stress session were initiated 15 min after a saline injection (200 µL/kg). The second recording started 5 min after the onset of a stress elicited by means of a jet of air blown into the cage at a constant 100 kPa pressure. Air jet was switched off at the end of this recording period. After a recovery period lasting 20 to 30 min, allowing the values of BP and HR to return to their resting levels, a third recording was performed 15 min after a clonidine injection (10 µg/kg, 200 µL/kg). At the end of this recording, a jet of air was blown again into the cage, and a fourth recording was performed after 5 min. BP signal processing and spectrum analysis have been detailed elsewhere (Japundzic et al. 1990). Comparisons within each group of animals were made using a two-way analysis of variance followed by an othogonal partitioning. Comparisons between the 3 groups of rats were made using a one-way analysis of variance.

RESULTS

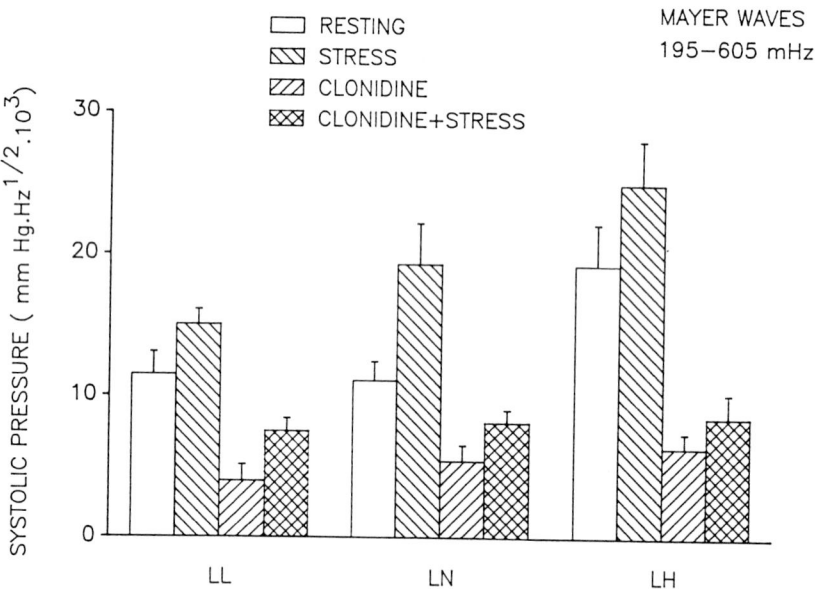

Fig. 1. Area of the 195-605 mHz component (Mayer waves) of the systolic BP spectra in the three groups of rats. Columns represent mean results (n = 8) and the vertical line the s.e.m. Statistical differences are included within the results section.

Fig.1 shows the integrated systolic BP spectra of the 195-605 mHz region corresponding to Mayer waves in the 3 groups of rats. In the resting state LH rats exhibited significantly higher areas than LL and LN rats ($P < 0.01$). Stress amplified Mayer waves ($P < 0.01$ for LN animals). Clonidine markedly reduced Mayer waves in the 3 groups ($P < 0.01$ for LL, $P < 0.05$ for LN and $P < 0.001$ for LH, for the comparison with resting levels). The second stress amplified Mayer waves in those clonidine-treated rats but the levels were still below the resting values. We also compared the response to the first stress (2nd recording - 1st recording values) to the response to stress administered in clonidine-treated rats (4th recording - 3rd recording values) using a paired t test. The responses to stress in these two conditions (without or with clonidine) were quantitatively similar in each group of rats.

DISCUSSION

This study showed that hypertensive LH rats exhibited at rest a high variability of systolic BP, as reflected by the area of the 195-605 mHz spectral region. Julien et al. (1988), using the standard deviations of the BP time series, already reported an increased variability of BP in LH rats, compared to low BP (LL) and normotensive (LN) rats. Our study indicates that the mechanism of this increased variability in LH rats could depend upon a sympathetic activation, which controls the amplitude of the Mayer waves (Japundzic et al. 1990). The 3 groups of rats developed pressor and tachycardic responses to an aversive air jet stimulation, together with an increased amplitude of the Mayer waves. We did not observe in our conditions quantitative differences in the response to stress between the 3 groups, in contrast to Julien et al. (1988) who reported an increased susceptibility to stress in LH rats. Clonidine markedly reduced the oscillations in the 195-605 mHz region in the 3 groups, as previously described in Wistar rats (Grichois et al. 1990, Blanc et al. 1991). Interestingly, another stress was still able to amplify the Mayer waves. The responses to the stressor administered after clonidine were similar to those observed without clonidine. This demonstrates that the opposite effects of clonidine and stress on Mayer waves were additive. In conclusion the present results suggest an increased BP variability in LH rats related to an activation of the sympathetic nervous system. Clonidine markedly reduced Mayer waves in the 3 groups of animals. A mild stress amplified the BP oscillations in the 195-605 mHz region. This effect was still observed after clonidine, which is an indication that the drug does not prevent the response to stress.

REFERENCES

Blanc, J., Grichois, M.L. and Elghozi, J.L. (1991): Effects of clonidine on blood pressure and heart rate responses to an emotional stress in the rat: a spectral study. Clin. Exp. Pharmacol. Physiol. 18: 000-000.

Grichois, M.L., Japundzic, N., Head, G.A. and Elghozi, J.L. (1990): Clonidine reduces blood pressure and heart rate oscillations in the conscious rat. J. Cardiovasc. Pharmacol. 16:449-454.

Japundzic, N., Grichois, M.L., Zitoun, P., Laude, D. and Elghozi, J.L. (1990): Spectral analysis of blood pressure and heart rate in conscious rats : effects of autonomic blockers. J. Auton. Nerv. System 30: 91-100.

Julien, C., Cerutti, C., Kandza, P., Barrès, C., Su, D., Vincent, M. and Sassard, J. (1988): Cardiovascular response to emotional stress and spontaneous blood pressure variability in genetically hypertensive rats of the Lyon strain. Clin Exp. Pharmacol. Physiol. 15: 533-538.

Vincent, M., Sacquet, J. and Sassard, J. (1984): The Lyon strains of hypertensive, normotensive and low-blood-pressure rats. In Handbook of Hypertension. Vol. 4: Experimental and Genetic Models of Hypertension, ed W. de Jong, pp. 314-327. Amsterdam: Elsevier.

Effects of sympathectomy on overall blood pressure variability and its spectral components in unanesthetized unrestrained rats

Anna Daffonchio, Cristina Franzelli, Marco DiRienzo, Paolo Castiglioni, Agustin J. Ramirez, Giuseppe Mancia and Alberto U. Ferrari

Semeiotica Medica and Clinica Medica Generale, Centro Fisiologia Clinica e Ipertensione and CNR, Ospedale Maggiore, Unviersità di Milano, Milano, Italy

The sympathetic nervous system is believed to have multifold influences on blood pressure variability: first, the sympathoexcitation associated with behavioral events such as exercise or emotion is known to favor marked blood pressure alterations, i.e. to enhance blood pressure variability (Mancia et al 1983 a; Littler et al., 1978; Mancia et al., 1983 b), although it is not known whether similar effects on blood pressure variability are exerted under conditions of spontaneous behavior in the absence of any excitatory stimuli. Second, evidence from human and animal experiments suggests that rhythmic cardiovascular variations in the mid- to low-frequency range are related to sympathetic activity (Akselrod et al., 1981; Pagani et al., 1986), although a definitive proof that this is the case is still lacking and the specificity of this relationship, i.e. whether oscillations in certain spectral regions are entirely accounted for by sympathetic influences, is far from being established. In order to get insight into the above mentioned unsettled issues we examined the effects of sympathectomy on overall blood pressure variability and on its spectral components in unanesthetized unrestrained normotensive rats.

METHODS

<u>Animal preparation, surgery and protocol</u>. Normotensive 10- to 12-week-old Wistar-Kyoto rats (n=10) were used. Chemical sympathectomy was produced by i.p. injections of of 6-hydroxydopamine (150 mg/kg every 2-3 days for one week), while an equal number of control animals received vehicle. Under ketamine anesthesia, each animal was chronically instrumented with an arterial and a venous catheter, which were periodically flushed by a 0.5% heparin solution. The rat was placed in a wide individual cage in which it could move, explore, eat and drink ad libitum. Care was taken to minimize environmental disturbances to the animal. Following a 24 hour recovery time, the arterial catheter was connected to a Statham P23Dc transducer to measure arterial blood pressure and heart rate, the latter being obtained by tachographic conversion of the pulsatile pressure signal. Both variables were continuously

displayed on an ink-writing Grass 7D polygraph (Quincy, MA, USA). Before the experiment proper began, the effectiveness of sympathectomy was assessed from the pressor and tachycardic response to an iv bolus injection of tyramine, 100 ug/kg. After a 30 min interval the blood pressure signal was recorded continuously for 90 min and stored on a tape recorder (Racal Store 4, Southampton, UK) for subsequent computer analysis.

Data analysis. The recorded blood pressure trace was scanned beat-to-beat by a computer, sampled at 250 Hz, digitized on 12 bits and edited from inadequate portions of the signal. The computer was programmed to provide the following: 1) systolic blood pressure mean and variance, the latter being taken as the measure of overall blood pressure variability, and 2) spectral powers, obtained by the fast Fourier transform technique, of the systolic blood pressure oscillations in the high- (3.0-0.8 Hz), mid- (0.6-0.1 Hz) and low- (0.1-0.025 Hz) frequency bands calculated over consecutive 100-sec periods after removal of non stationary blocks. Average values were calculated in both groups for the above parameters. Statistical comparisons between sympathectomized and control rats was performed by the Wilcoxon non-parametric rank test; a $p<0.05$ was taken as the level of statistical significance.

RESULTS

Sympathectomy was associated with a mild reduction in systolic blood pressure (117 ± 4 mmHg in the sympathectomized vs $138\pm$ mmHg in the control rats, means+SEM, $p<0.05$) with no significant change in pulse interval. In response to tyramine injection, the rises in blood pressure and heart rate observed in the sympathectomized rats were respectively 85.0% and a 90.4% smaller than those observed in the control rats (both $p<0.01$). Overall blood pressure variability was significantly greater in the sympathectomized than in the control rats, the respective variances amounting to 80.5 ± 7.5 and 52.2 ± 6.0 mmHg2 ($p<0.05$). On the other hand, the effects of sympathectomy on systolic blood pressure power spectra were different in the different frequency bands, the sympathectomized rats exhibiting no change in high-frequency power (3.5 ± 0.6 vs 4.2 ± 0.6 mmHg2, p=ns), a reduction in mid-frequency power (2.5 ± 0.3 vs 6.9 ± 1.4 mmHg2, $p<0.05$) and an increase in LF power (14.1 ± 1.9 vs 9.5 ± 1.7 mmHg2, $p<0.05$) as compared to the control rats.

DISCUSSION

Our study provides evidence on two major new points. First, the influence on blood pressure variability exerted by the sympathetic nervous system critically depends on its degree of activation: whereas a hyperactive sympathetic system may favor an enhanced blood pressure variability, the opposite phenomenon, i.e. a buffering of the blood pressure variations, occurs when tonic sympathetic activity is low such as during a spontaneous undisturbed behavior. Second, the relationship between sympathetic activity and blood pressure power spectral components is complex: sympathectomy had as expected no effect on high-frequency blood pressure waves which rather depend on vagal and ventilatory influences (Akselrod et al., 1981; Koepchen, 1984). On the other hand, our data indicate that the mid-frequency oscillations are indeed related to sympathetic activity, as previously suggested (Pagani et al., 1986; Parati et al., 1990); however, persistence of more than 35% of the mid-frequency power after sympathectomy also suggests that these oscillations are not specifically related to sympathetic factors and rather depend to a sizeable extent also on non-sympathetic factors. Finally, the power of the low-frequency blood pressure oscillations was about 50% greater in sympathectomized as compared to intact rats: in lack of any direct evidence helping to interpret this intriguing phenomenon, one may view it as to unmask the existence of a low-frequency blood pressure oscillator which in the intact animal, however, would be prevented from expressing its effects on the spectral profile by overriding sympathetic influences able to shift part of the power towards the mid-frequency portion of the spectrum. An alternative explanation may be that the enhancement in low-frequency blood pressure oscillations is non-specifically associated with interventions that disrupt normal cardiovascular regulatory mechanisms: this possibility is suggested by our recent finding in cats of a marked increase in low-frequency blood pressure power following sino-aortic denervation (DiRienzo et al., 1990).

REFERENCES

Akselrod S, Gordon D, Ubel FA, Shannon DC, Barger AC, Cohen RJ (1981). Power spectrum analysis of heart rate fluctuation: a quantitative probe of beat to beat cardiovascular control. Science 213:220-223.

DiRienzo M, Castiglioni P, Omboni S, Ferrari AU, Ramirez AJ, Bertinieri G, Parati G, Pedotti A, Mancia G (1990). Sino-aortic denervation and power spectra of systolic blood pressure and pulse interval in conscious cats. J Hypertension 8(Suppl. 3):s58 (Abstract).

Koepchen HP (1984). History of studies and concepts of blood pressure waves. In: Miyakava K, et al (eds) Mechanisms of blood pressure waves. Tokyo, Japan Sci Soc Press/Berlin Springer-Verlay, 3-23.

Littler W, West MJ, Honour AJ, Sleight P (1978). The variability of arterial pressure. Am Heart J 95:180-186.

Mancia G, Ferrari A, Gregorini L, Parati G, Pomidossi G, Bertinieri G, Grassi G, Di Riezo M, Pedotti A and Zanchetti A (1983a). Blood pressure and heart rate variabilities in normotensive and hypertensive human beings. Circ Res 53:96-104.

Mancia G, Bertinieri G, Grassi G, Parati G, Pomidossi G, Ferrari A, Gregorini L, Zanchetti A (1983b). Effect of blood pressure measurement by the doctor on patients' blood pressure and heart rate. Lancet 2:695-698.

Pagani M, Lombardi F, et al (1986). Power spectral analysis of heart rate and arterial pressure variabilities as a marker of sympatho-vagal interaction in man and conscious dog. Circ Res 59:178-193.

Parati G, Castiglioni P, DiRienzo M, Omboni S, Pedotti A, Mancia G. Sequential spectral analysis of 24-hour blood pressure and heart interval in humans (1990). Hypertension 16:414-421.

A new method to assess statistical dependence : application to the relationships between systolic blood pressure and heart rate

Michel Ducher, Catherine Cerutti, Marie-Paule Gustin and Christian Z. Paultre

URA CNRS 606, Faculté de Pharmacie, 8, avenue Rockefeller, 69008 Lyon, France

INTRODUCTION

Continuous recordings of systolic blood pressure (SBP) and heart rate (HR) over long periods (up to 24 hours) exhibit an important spontaneous variability over time. As far as both parameters are involved in various cardiovascular regulations, SBP and HR values may not vary independently. Relationships between SBP and HR had already been described in cats (Bertinieri et al., 1988) or in dogs (Anderson et al., 1979) using classical linear methods. In this work, a probabilistic approach was used to quantify the dependence between the values of two parameters continuously recorded. This method was then applied to the study of the relationships between SBP and HR values obtained in rats during spontaneous activity.

MATERIAL AND METHODS

Animals
Fifteen rats were dispatched in 3 groups : 1) 5 male adult Wistar Kyoto (WKY) rats used as controls ; 2) 5 chronic sinoaortic denervated (SAD) male adult rats (Krieger et al., 1964) ; 3) 5 male adult rats with an early chronic destruction of the peripheral sympathetic nerves by guanethidine (SNX) (Julien et al., 1990).

Systolic blood pressure and heart rate recordings
SBP and HR were continuously recorded beat to beat using a computer data acquisition system (Gustin et al., 1990). This experiment was carried out during 24 hours in control WKY rats, including resting and activity periods, and 30 minutes in the other rats (SAD, SNX).

The Z coefficient

A dependence coefficient (Z) was defined from the properties of the conditional probability. Considering two probabilistic events A and B, the probability to observe B when A is observed is P(B/A) = P(A,B)/P(A) with P(A) the probability to observe A and P(A,B) the probability to observe A and B. The statistical independence between A and B is defined by P(B/A) = P(B), the complete dependence between A and B by P(B/A) = 1, and the complete exclusion of B by A by P(B/A) = 0. For intermediate values, P(B/A) expresses the partial dependency (P(B) < P(B/A) < 1) of B on A and the partial exclusion (0 < P(B/A) < P(B)) of B by A. Z used the difference P(B) - P(B/A) normalized so as to obtain values between -1 (complete exclusion) and 1 (complete dependency). This analysis may be applied to two parameters, the numerical values of which are expressed as ordinal modalities ; a probabilistic event is therefore one modality of one parameter. When considering SBP and HR values, the modalities chosen were amplitude intervals of 10 mmHg for SBP and 30 bpm for HR. The results were presented with a 3 dimensional representation of Z as a function of SBP and HR modalities.

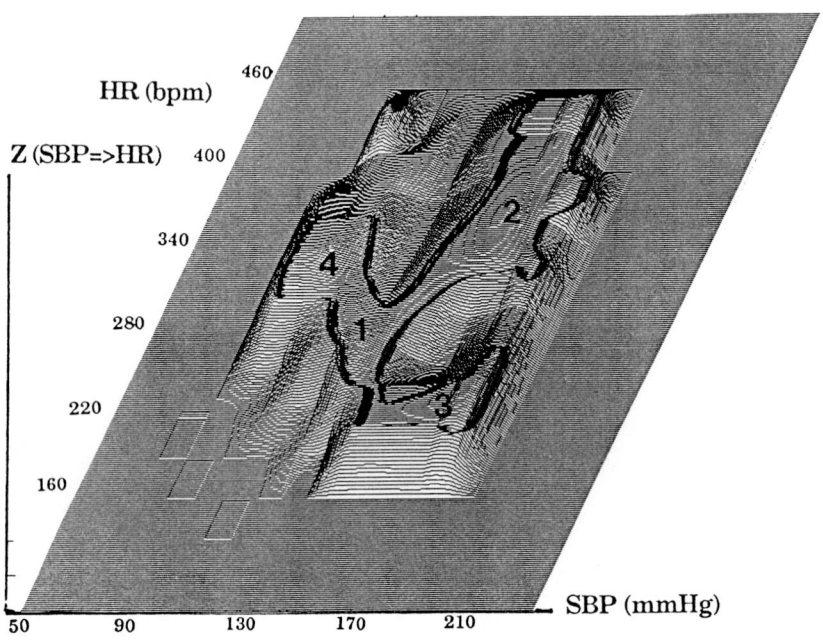

Figure 1.
Three dimensional representation of Z as a function of SBP and HR recorded during 24 hours in one control WKY rat. The Z = 0 level is underlined with dark and delimits zones where Z > 0.

RESULTS

In control rats, five zones of dependence between SBP and HR were obtained in a highly reproducible way. As shown in figure 1, zone 1 containing the set point (mean values of SBP and HR) represents 25 ± 10 % (mean ± sd) of the recorded beats and such a zone was found in rats from all the groups ; zone 2 represents 20 ± 1 % (mean ± sd) of the recorded beats, was enhanced during physical activity, decreased during resting and vanished in SNX rats and therefore could be related to sympathetic nervous activity ; zones 3 and 4, represent 6 ± 2 % (mean ± sd) of the 24 hour recorded beats, were enhanced during resting, vanished in SAD rats and so could be related to the cardiac baroreflex activity. In addition zone 4 disappeared in SNX rats.

DISCUSSION

The use of a coefficient, to quantify the dependence between two parameters, based on the conditional probability characteristics is not common in statistics. Most of the classical methods are based on variance and covariance (Anderson et al., 1979). They allow to study relationships using small samples but they need an a priori model to describe the relationships. In our experiments, a large amount (about 500,000 per 24 h) of data is obtained and so the probabilistic approach is well suited ; in addition, this method is heuristic. Concerning the results, it appears that only 50 to 60 % of the cardiac beats recorded during 24 hours are found into a zone of dependence. This indicates that this method is able to exhibit a dependence relationship between rare events. As far as zone 2 did not exist in SNX rats and was enhanced during physical activity which is associated with an increase in sympathetic nervous activity, it could be related to the sympathetic tone. Zones 3 and 4 represent only a small amount of cardiac beats but the causality between SBP and HR in these zones is high. The disappearance of zone 4 in SNX and SAD rats suggests that zone 4 is related to the sympathetic component of the baroreflex. In SNX rats, the sympathetic component is destroyed whereas the vagal one is still functional. Zone 3 vanished in SAD but not in SNX rats which suggests that zone 3 is related to the vagal component of the cardiac baroreflex. In conclusion, we have developed a software using a new method of dependence analysis between two parameters. The use of these programs for the studies of SBP and HR relationships in freely moving conscious rats allowed to describe the different components of the SBP and HR control, and especially the sympathetic and vagal components of the spontaneous cardiac baroreflex. Therefore this method may represent a powerful new tool to examine the relationships between cardiovascular parameters.

We acknowledge the Institut National de la Santé et de la Recherche Médicale for its financial support (CRE 89-5001/11).

REFERENCES

Anderson, D.E., Yingling, J.E. and Sagawa, K. (1979) : Minute to minute covariations in cardiovascular activity of conscious dogs. *Am. J. Physiol.* 236, H434 - H439.

Bertinieri, G., Di Rienzo, M., Cavallazzi, A., Ferrari, A.U. and Mancia, G. (1988) : Baroreceptor reflex by blood pressure monitoring in unanesthetized cats. *Am. J. Physiol.* 254, H377-H383.

Gustin, M.P., Cerutti, C. and Paultre, C.Z. (1990) : Heterogeneous computer network for real time hemodynamic signal processing. *Comput. Biol. Med.* 20, 205 -215.

Julien, C., Kandza, P., Barrès, C., Lo, M., Cerutti, C. and Sassard, J.(1990) : Effects of sympathectomy on blood pressure and its variability in conscious rats. *Am. J. Physiol.* 259, H1337 - H1342.

Krieger, E.M. (1964) : Neurogenic hypertension in the rat. *Circ. Res.* 15, 511 - 521.

Growth factors

Facteurs de croissance

Effects of hypertension on cellular growth of arterial tissue

Aram V. Chobanian

Boston University School of Medicine, Whitaker Cardiovascular Institute, 80 East Concord Street, Boston, MA 02118, USA

Abstract

This paper reviews data from our own and other laboratories regarding the effects of hypertension and antihypertensive therapy on growth changes in arterial tissue and the relationship of such changes to arterial injury. Recent studies have shown that a large number of agents including known growth factors are capable of stimulating growth of cultured arterial smooth muscle cells (SMC) and endothelial cells. Several of these growth promoters and inhibitors have been shown to be expressed in arterial cells, suggesting that autocrine or paracrine effects may participate in regulating cellular growth. In addition, several vasoconstrictive agents have been shown to stimulate cellular growth while vasodilators may be growth inhibitory, suggesting a close relationship between cell growth, vascular structure, and vascular tone. We have shown that hypertension causes an accumulation of SMC and macrophages in the arterial intima in association with increase in expression of transforming growth factor beta (TGF-ß1) and the beta receptor for platelet-derived growth factor (PDGF). Similar changes were observed as a result of increasing age in spontaneously hypertensive (SHR) and Wistar-Kyoto (WKY) rats. In contrast, myocardial expression of PDGF-beta receptor was unaffected while that of TGF-ß1 was decreased with both age and hypertension, suggesting different modes of regulation of these genes in aorta and heart. Antihypertensive drugs may have vasculoprotective effects against arterial disease induced by balloon-catheter injury, hypercholesterolemia, and aging as well as hypertension. Calcium channel blockers and angiotensin converting enzyme (ACE) inhibitors have been shown to reduce intimal plaque formation after balloon injury. Beta blockers, calcium channel blockers, and the ACE inhibitors may also reduce atherosclerotic plaque formation caused by hypercholesterolemia. The mechanisms for the vasculoprotective actions are unknown although effects on cell growth may play an important role, particularly following balloon injury.

Hypertension has a potent effect on the growth of arterial cells, but the mechanism for the effect and the relationship of the growth changes to the development of vascular abnormalities induced by hypertension have not been well-defined. This paper reviews the current data on the action of growth factors on arterial cells and the effects of experimental hypertension and of vasoactive agents on growth factor expression in vascular tissue. Where data are available, comparisons are made between the changes observed in the spontaneously hypertensive rat and other hypertensive models. In addition, the effects of age as well of hypertension are examined.

Influence of Growth Factors on Smooth Muscle Cells (SMC)

Cell culture studies have indicated that a wide variety of agents may act to stimulate smooth muscle cell (SMC) growth (Schwartz et al., 1990; Owens, 1989). These include traditional growth factors such as platelet-derived growth factor (PDGF), acidic and basic fibroblast growth factors (FGF), insulin growth factor-I and II (IGF-I and II), epidermal growth factor (EGF), and transforming growth factor beta (TGF-ß). In addition, several vasoconstrictive agents appear to be growth promoters including angiotensin II, norepinephrine, epinephrine, serotonin, vasopressin, and endothelin.

Smooth Muscle Cell Growth Factors

Platelet-derived growth factors	Angiotensin II
Interleukin I	Arginine vasopressin
Fibroblast growth factors	Endothelin
Epidermal growth factor	Serotonin
Transforming growth factor beta	Nicotine
Insulin growth factor-1	Neurokinin A
Low density lipoproteins	Substance K
Fibronectin	Substance P
Fibrin	Thrombospondin
Catecholamines	

Adapted from Schwartz et al. (1990) Physiol. Rev. 70:1177.

Addition of angiotensin II to cultured SMC stimulates the expression of protooncogenes and of the A-chain of PDGF (Taubman et al., 1989; Naftilan et al., 1989). In vivo infusion of the alpha-adrenergic agonists phenylephrine and norepinephrine also increases PDGF A-chain and protooncogene expression (Majesky et al., 1990). Furthermore, growth promoters as PDGF may cause vasoconstriction (Berk et al., 1986). These common effects are most likely mediated through rise in intracellular calcium, which stimulates growth as well as contraction.

At least two classes of antihypertensive drugs, ACE inhibitors and calcium channel blockers, have been reported to inhibit SMC growth. Evidence is also accumulating that other vasodilator agents as nitric oxide (Garg & Hassid, 1989) and atrial natriuretic factor (Johnson et al., 1988) also are growth inhibitors. These relationships between cellular growth and vascular tone may be important in the vascular remodeling which occurs as a result of the increase in blood pressure or of other stimuli injurious to the arterial wall. A list of SMC growth inhibitors is shown in Table 2.

<u>Smooth Muscle Cell Growth Inhibitors</u>

Transforming growth factor beta
Tumor necrosis factor
Heparin
Nitric oxide
Atrial natriuretic factor
Angiotensin converting enzyme inhibitors
Calcium channel blockers
Colchicine
Growth factor antibodies
Somatostatin analogues
Steroids

<u>Growth Factors and Endothelial Cells</u>

Several growth promoters and inhibitors for endothelial cells also have been identified (Schwartz et al., 1990). These include acidic and basic fibroblast growth factors, TGF-ß, and gamma-interferon.

Fibroblast growth factors and TGF-ß may have angiogenic as well as growth regulatory effects (Schwartz et al., 1990).

<u>Effects of Hypertension on Cellular Growth and Growth Factor Expression</u>

Hypertension has been shown to increase ^{3}H-thymidine labeling of both endothelial and SMC in the SHR (Schwartz et al., 1986; Schwartz & Benditt, 1977). In aortic explants taken from rats with DOC-salt hypertension or in the SHR, the rate of proliferation of SMC is greater than that observed in normotensive controls (Haudenschild et al., 1985; Grunwald et al., 1987). In rat models of hypertension, blood pressure elevation may stimulate either hypertrophy or hyperplasia of arterial SMC. With most forms of chronic hypertension, including that seen in the SHR, SMC hypertrophy, which often is associated with nuclear polyploidy, appears to be the characteristic response (Owens, 1989; Owens & Schwartz, 1982; Owens & Schwartz, 1983; Lichtenstein et al., 1986). On the other hand, acute elevation of blood pressure caused by aortic constriction has been shown to induce SMC hyperplasia in rabbit and rat arteries (Bevan et al., 1976; Owens & Reidy, 1985). In addition, SMC hyperplasia rather than hypertrophy appears to be the typical response to hypertension in mesenteric resistance vessels of the SHR (Mulvany et al., 1985).

Angiotensin II and arginine vasopressin have been shown to induce hypertrophy of cultured SMC maintained in serum-free medium (Geisterfer et al., 1988; Geisterfer & Owens, 1989), although SMC hyperplasia has been observed when the cells are grown in serum-rich medium (Campbell-Boswell & Robertson, 1981). Such findings have suggested that these vasoactive hormones are only partial growth factors that can initiate cell growth and increase cell size but that require the presence of other growth factors in order to cause cell division (Owens, 1989).

The mechanisms involved in the increased growth of arterial cells caused by hypertension are unknown. We have reported that DOC-salt hypertension increases steady-state mRNA levels of TGF-ß, but without affecting levels of both chains of PDGF, EGF, acidic and basic FGF, or IGF I and II. Of interest is the observation that TGF-ß may act as either a growth promoter or inhibitor and may cause hypertrophy and polyploidy of cultured arterial SMC (Owens et al., 1988).

Increased expression of TGF-ß also was observed in the SHR as compared to WKY controls from 5 to 40 weeks of age (Figure 1)(Sarzani et al., 1991b).

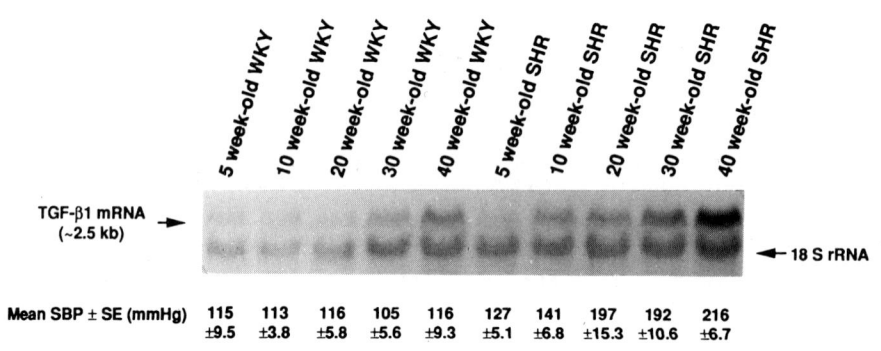

FIG. 1. Northern blot analyses of steady-state mRNA levels of transforming growth factor ß1 (TGF-ß1) in aorta of WKY and SHR rats of 5, 10, 20, 30, and 40 weeks of age. Each lane contains 20 µg of total RNA. The mean ± S.E. of systolic blood pressure in each group is shown at the bottom of each lane. Note the increases in steady-state mRNA levels at all ages with the SHR and the increases at 30 and 40 weeks in the WKY. The levels in the SHR are greater than those in age-matched WKY except at 5 weeks. A second band at the level of 18S RNA was detected when the SmaI-SmaI TGF-ß1 cDNA fragment was used.

[Reproduced with permission from Sarzani et al., 1991[b].

In these normotensive controls as well as in the SHR, there was an age-related increase in TGF-ß1 expression. In contrast, in cardiac tissue, steady-state mRNA appeared unaltered by hypertension and decreased progressively with age.

Although PDGF A- and B-chain expression appeared unaffected by hypertension, changes were observed in aortic steady-state mRNA levels for the PDGF-ß receptor which binds the PDGF B-chain. DOC-salt hypertension was associated with a three-fold rise in expression of aortic PDGF-ß receptor (Sarzani et al., 1991b). No similar rise was observed with the PDGF-α receptor expression. Aortic PDGF-ß receptor expression was also increased considerably in SHR as compared with WKY rats (Sarzani et al., 1991a), and, as with TGF-ß1 expression, an age-related rise in expression was present in SHR and WKY rats (Figure 2).

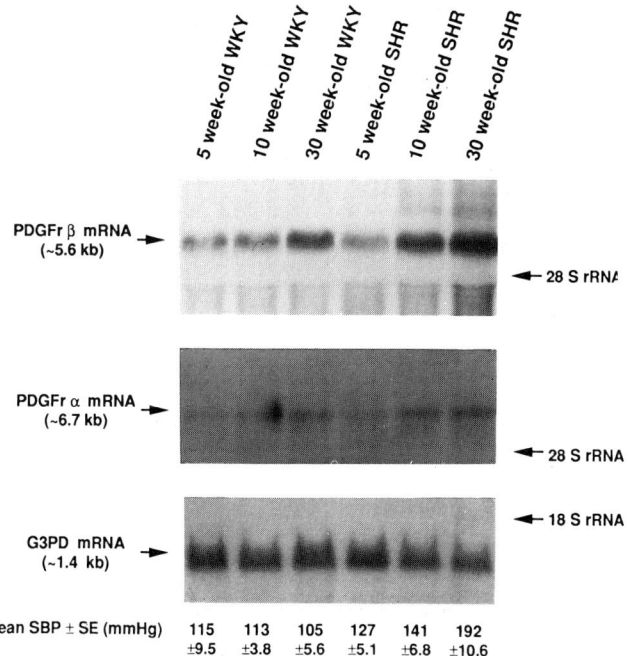

FIG. 2. Northern blot analyses of aortic RNA from WKY and SHR rats of 5, 10, and 30 weeks of age. Each lane contains 20 μg of total aortic RNA. The RNA for each sample was pooled from three aortas. The mean ± S.E. of systolic blood pressure in each group is shown at the bottom of each lane. Shown are the effects of age on aortic PDGF-receptor-ß (PDGF r ß, upper panel), PDGF-receptor-α (PDGF r α, middle panel) and glyceraldehyde-3-phosphate dehydrogenase (G3PD, lower panel) steady-state mRNA.

[Reproduced with permission from Sarzani et al., 1991[b].

Cardiac PDGF-ß receptor mRNA was unaffected by hypertension in the DOC-salt treated rats and appeared reduced in the SHR as compared to WKY rats (Sarzani et al., 1991b). Thus, aortic and cardiac expression of both TGF-ß1 and PDGF-ß receptors appears regulated differently in response to hypertension even though both organs respond to the blood pressure elevation with cellular hypertrophy.

It should be remembered that our studies have not investigated actual quantity of these growth factors and receptors but rather only the steady-state mRNA levels. Thus, the biological significance of the changes remains to be demonstrated. However, recent reports have suggested that changes in levels of the PDGF receptors may be important in mediating PDGF effects which include stimulation of SMC hypertrophy or hyperplasia, chemotaxis, and mitogenesis (Owens, 1989; Ross et al., 1986).

In addition, the cells responsible for the changes in expression of both TGF-ß1 and PDGF-ß receptor with hypertension have not been determined as yet.

Hypertension appears to promote entry of monocytes and other leucocytes into the arterial intima and any of these cell types as well as vascular endothelial cells and SMC could be responsible for the observed changes.

Hypertension and Connective Tissue Matrix

The changes in growth of vascular cells caused by hypertension might be related in part to its effects on the extracellular matrix. Recent studies have indicated that interactions between extracellular proteins and integrin cell receptors may alter phenotypic characteristics and growth of vascular cells, perhaps by causing change in the shape of these cells (Ingber, 1990). Of particular interest in this regard is fibronectin, a large extracellular matrix protein which has been reported to induce functional changes in endothelial cells (Madri et al., 1989) and to modify the phenotype of SMC from contractile to synthetic state (Hedin et al., 1988). We have recently been examining the influence of experimental hypertension on fibronectin expression, synthesis, and accumulation in the aorta. Steady-state mRNA levels of fibronectin were elevated markedly in DOC-salt hypertension and following angiotensin II-infusion (Takasaki et al., 1990). The changes were rapid, occurring within 3 days of angiotensin II administration. In addition, total amount and synthesis of fibronectin were increased in aortic rings taken from each of these 3 hypertensive models (Saouaf et al., 1991).

Blood pressure and age-related increases in aortic fibronectin expression, synthesis, and content also were observed in SHR and WKY rats. The changes in gene expression are illustrated below.

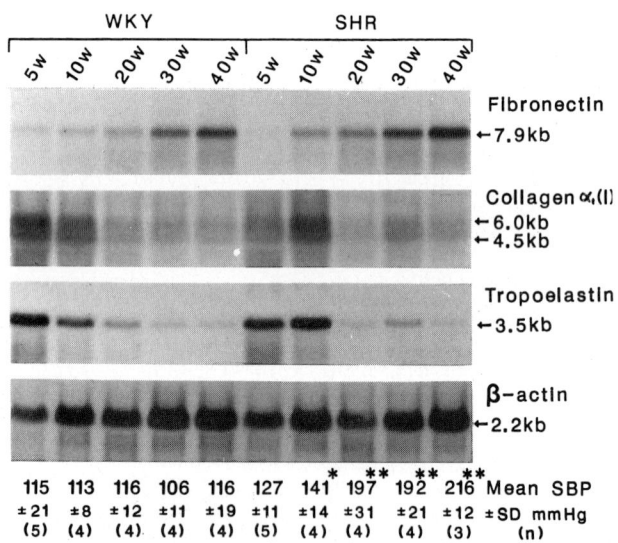

FIG. 3. The effect of age and hypertension on the steady-state mRNA level for fibronectin in rat aorta. Total aortic RNA from SHR and WKY rats of different ages (5 to 40 weeks) were used for Northern blot analysis of fibronectin, collagen $\alpha_1(I)$, tropoelastin, and ß-actin. The same nylon membrane was rehybridized for the four different probes.

[Reproduced with permission from Takasaki et al., 1990.]

Further studies are warranted to determine whether the early responses of fibronectin to hypertension play a role in mediating the effects of hypertension on cellular growth or whether they merely reflect a secondary effect of hypertension on connective tissue synthesis by SMC.

Effects of Antihypertensive Drugs on Vascular Cell Growth and Disease

Several recent studies have suggested that certain antihypertensive drugs may inhibit the development of vascular disease caused by balloon injury of an artery, hypercholesterolemia, aging or blood pressure elevation. Some of these vasculoprotective effects may be related to inhibitory effects of the drugs on cellular growth.

Balloon Injury -- The model of balloon injury provides an in vivo system for examining the growth-inhibiting properties of antihypertensive drugs. The lesion which develops appears highly proliferative in nature, and it has been reported recently that intravenous administration of antibodies to platelet-derived growth factor reduces the size of the plaque developing in rat carotid artery following balloon injury (Ferns et al., 1991). Both calcium channel blocking drugs and ACE inhibitors also may affect this process. Isradipine, a dihydropyridine derivative, reduced plaque size caused by balloon-injury of the rat carotid artery (Handley et al., 1986). A reduction in intracellular calcium caused by the drug might be responsible for this action since such reduction could inhibit cellular migration and proliferation, processes considered important in the pathogenesis of the plaque.

The ACE inhibitors cilazapril and captopril both have been reported to inhibit plaque formation in the rat carotid artery model (Powell et al., 1989). ACE inhibitors reduce angiotensin II levels and thereby influence cellular growth. In addition, the bradykinin elevation resulting from ACE inhibition also could play a role in reducing proliferative activity. Some recent data suggest that the reduction in plaque size caused by ACE inhibition may not occur in all species or under differing experimental conditions. Although a beneficial action of ACE inhibition following balloon injury has been apparent in the rat and guinea pig, no effect of cilazapril on intimal hyperplasia was demonstrable in the baboon (Hanson et al., 1991). The clinical implications are as yet unknown but studies are currently in progress to determine the effects of ACE inhibition in patients who have undergone balloon angioplasty of their coronary arteries.

Atherosclerosis -- Beta adrenergic blockers, calcium channel blockers, and ACE inhibitors appear capable of reducing the development of atherosclerosis in hypercholesterolemic, normotensive animals. The obvious feature common to all of these drugs is their ability to lower blood pressure, which could have a protective effect on the vasculature, even in normotensive animals, by altering hemodynamic stresses on the arterial wall. Another common property is their potential to reduce cellular growth either by reducing sympathetic activity (beta blockers and ACE inhibitors), angiotensin II levels (beta blockers and ACE inhibitors), or cellular calcium content (calcium channel blockers). The reader is referred to a recent review of the topic for a further discussion of the potential mechanisms (Chobanian, 1990).

With beta adrenergic and calcium channel blockers, anti-atherosclerotic effects were observed in cholesterol-fed animals (Chobanian et al., 1985; Kaplan et al., 1987; Henry & Bentley, 1981; Havel, 1983), but no inhibition was apparent in the Watanabe heritable hyperlipidemic rabbit with a deficit in the cellular receptor for low density lipoproteins (Lichtenstein et al., 1989; VanNiekerk et al., 1984). However, ACE inhibition may reduce atherosclerosis in the WHHL (Chobanian et al.,

1990) as well as in the cholesterol-fed cynomolgus monkey (Aberg & Ferrer, 1990). Our studies have demonstrated that captopril therapy causes a decrease in cellularity of aortic atherosclerotic lesions in the WHHL (Chobanian et al., 1990), although it is unknown whether this action is related directly to a growth-inhibitory effect.

Hypertension -- Some antihypertensive drugs may correct some of the arterial cellular abnormalities induced by hypertension. We have observed that propranolol inhibits the development of nuclear polyploidy in aortic SMC of DOC-salt hypertensive rats (Leitschuh & Chobanian, 1987). Captopril also has been reported to decrease the extent of polyploidy in the SHR (Owens, 1987). We also have observed decrease in intimal cell accumulation by blood pressure lowering in DOC-salt hypertensive rats and in the SHR (Haudenschild et al., 1981). On the other hand, the extracellular abnormalities such as the accumulation of collagen and elastin are much more difficult to reverse (Brecher et al., 1978; Haudenschild et al., 1980). Growth factor abnormalities induced by hypertension also may be reversed by therapy. Reduction of blood pressure to control levels in the DOC-salt hypertensive rat by dietary sodium restriction and chlorothiazide administration caused decreases in steady-state mRNA levels of TGF-ß1 (Sarzani et al., 1989) and the PDGF-beta receptor (Sarzani et al., 1991b). Fibronectin mRNA levels and total quantity of aortic fibronectin also were essentially normalized by reversal of hypertension (Takasaki et al., 1990; Saouaf et al., 1991).

Aging -- Aging is associated with vascular changes that are similar to those observed with hypertension (Chobanian, 1989). As noted above, abnormalities in arterial cellular growth and in growth factor expression appear similar with both conditions. In addition, we have demonstrated that prolonged blood pressure lowering in the normotensive WKY rat as well as in the SHR may prevent age-related changes in the arterial wall. A combination of reserpine, hydralazine, and chlorothiazide caused reduction in intimal thickness and in accumulation of cellular components (Haudenschild & Chobanian, 1984).

In conclusion, a close relationship appears to exist between the growth of vascular cells and the development of arterial disease in response to hypertension and other potentially injurious stimuli. Certain antihypertensive drugs may influence the growth properties of arterial cells and could have a vasculoprotective action independent of blood pressure lowering.

REFERENCES

Aberg, G., and Ferrer, P. (1990): Effects of captopril on atherosclerosis in cynomolgus monkeys. J. Cardiovasc. Pharmacol. 15, S-65-S-72.
Berk, B.C., Alexander, R.W., Brock, T.A., Gimbrone, M.A. Jr., and Webb, R.C. (1986): Vasoconstriction: A new biological activity of platelet-derived growth factor. Science 232, 87-90.
Bevan, R., Marthens, E., and Bevan, J. (1976): Hyperplasia of vascular smooth muscle in experimental hypertension in the rabbit. Circ. Res. 38, II-58-II-62.
Brecher, P., Chan, C.T., Franzblau, C., Faris, B., and Chobanian, A.V. (1978): Effects of hypertension and its reversal on aortic metabolism in the rat. Circ. Res. 43, 561-569.
Campbell-Boswell, M., and Robertson, A. (1981): Effects of angiotensin II and vasopressin on human smooth muscle cells in vitro. Exp. Molec. Path. 35, 265-276.
Chobanian, A.V. (1989): Arterial wall characteristics in hypertension and aging. In Handbook of Hypertension. Vol. 12: Hypertension in the Elderly, ed. A.

Amery & J. Staessen, pp. 8-23. Amsterdam: Elsevier Science Publishers BV.

Chobanian, A.V. (1990): The effects of ACE inhibitors and other antihypertensive drugs on cardiovascular risk factors and atherogenesis. Clin. Cardiol 13, 43-48.

Chobanian, A.V., Brecher, P., and Chan, C. (1985): Effects of propranolol on atherogenesis in the cholesterol-fed rabbit. Circ. Res. 56, 755-762.

Chobanian, A.V., Haudenschild, C.C., Nickerson, C., and Drago, R. (1990): Antiatherogenic effect of captopril in the Watanabe heritable hyperlipidemic rabbit. Hypertension 15, 327-331.

Ferns, G.A.., Raines, E.W., Sprugel, K.W., Motani, A.S., Reidy, M.A., and Ross, R. (1991): Inhibition of neointimal smooth muscle accumulation after angioplasty by an antibody to PDGF. Science 253, 1129-1132.

Garg, U.C., and Hassid, A. (1989): Nitric oxide-generating vasodilators and 8-bromo-cyclic guanosine monophosphate inhibit mitogenesis and proliferation of cultured rat vascular smooth muscle cells. J. Clin. Invest. 83, 1774-1777.

Geisterfer, A., Peach, M.J., and Owens, G.K. (1988): Angiotensin II induces hypertrophy, not hyperplasia, of cultured rat aortic smooth muscle cells. Circ. Res. 62, 749-756.

Geisterfer, A.A., and Owens, G.K (1989): Arginine vasopressin induced hypertrophy of cultured rat aortic smooth muscle cells. Hypertension 14, 413-420.

Grunwald, J., Chobanian, A.V., and Haudenschild, C.C. (1987): Smooth muscle cell migration and proliferation: Atherogenic mechanisms in hypertension. Atherosclerosis 67, 215-222.

Handley, D.A., VanValen, R.G., Melden, M.K., and Saunders, R.N. (1986): Suppression of rat carotid lesion development by the calcium channel bocker PN 200-100. Am. J. Path. 124, 88-93.

Hanson, S.R., Powell, J.S., Dodson, T., Lumsden, A., Kelly, A.B., Anderson, J.S., Clowes, A.W., and Harker, L.A.: Effects of angiotensin converting enzyme inhibition with cilazapril on intimal hyperplasia in injured arteries and vascular grafs in the baboon. Hypertension (in press).

Haudenschild, C.C., and Chobanian, A.V. (1984): Blood pressure lowering diminishes age-related changes in the rat aortic intima. Hypertension 6, I-62-I-68.

Haudenschild, C.C., Grunwald, J., and Chobanian, A.V. (1985): Effects of hypertension on migration and proliferation of smooth muscle in culture. Hypertension 7, I-101-I-104.

Haudenschild, C.C., Prescott, M.F., and Chobanian, A.V. (1980): Effects of hypertension and its reversal on aortic intimal lesions of the rat. Hypertension 2, 33-44.

Haudenschild, C.C., Prescott, M.F., and Chobanian, A.V. (1981): Aortic endothelial and subendothelial cells in experimental hypertension and aging. Hypertension 3, I-148-I-153.

Hedin, U., Bottger, B.A., Forsberg, E., Johansson, S., and Thyberg, J. (1988): Diverse effects of fibronectin and laminin on phenotypic properties of cultured arterial smooth muscle cells. J. Cell Biol. 107, 307-319.

Henry, P.D., and Bentley, K.I. (1981): Suppression of atherosclerosis in cholesterol-fed rabbits treated with nifedipine. J. Clin. Invest. 68, 1366-1369.

Ingber, D.E. (1990): Fibronectin controls capillary endothelial cell growth by modulating cell shape. Proc. Natl. Acad. Sci. 87, 3579-3583.

Johnson, A., Lermioglu, F., Garg, U.C., Morgan-Boyd, R., and Hassid, A. (1988): A novel biological effect of atrial natriuretic hormone: Inhibition of mesangial cell mitogenesis. Biochim. Biophys. Res. Commun. 152, 893-897.

Kaplan, J.R., Manuck, S.B., Adams, M.R., Weingand, K.W., and Clarkson, T.B. (1987): Inhibition of coronary atherosclerosis by propranolol in behaviorally predisposed monkeys fed on atherogenic diet. Circulation 76, 1364-1372.

Leitschuh, M., and Chobanian, A.V. (1987): Inhibition of nuclear polyploidy by propranolol in aortic smooth muscle cells of hypertensive rats. Hypertension 9, III-106-III-109.

Lichtenstein, A.H., Brecher, P., and Chobanian, A.V. (1986): Effects of deoxycorticosterone-salt hypertension on cell ploidy in the rat aorta. Hypertension 8, II-50-II-54.

Lichtenstein, A.H., Drago, R., Nickerson, C., Prescott, M.F., Lee, S.Q., and Chobanian, A.V. (1989): The effect of propranolol on atherogenesis in the Watanabe heritable hyperlipidemic rabbit. J. Vasc. Med. Biol. 1, 248-254.

Madri, J.A., Pratt, B.M., and Tucker, A.M. (1989): Endothelial cell behavior after denudation injury is modulated by transforming growth factor-ß1 and fibronectin. Lab. Invest. 60, 755-765.

Majesky, M.M., Daemen, M.J.A.P., and Schwartz, S.M. (1990): α_1-Adrenergic stimulation of platelet-derived growth factor A-chain gene expression in rat aorta. J. Biol. Chem. 265, 1082-1088.

Mulvany, M., Baandrup, U., and Gundersen, H. (1985): Evidence for hyperplasia in mesenteric resistance vessels of spontaneously hypertensive rats using a three-dimensinal dissector. Circ. Res. 57, 794-800.

Naftilan, A., Pratt, R., and Dzau, V. (1989): Induction of c-fos, c-myc and PDGF A-chain gene expressions by angiotensin II in cultured vascular smooth muscle cells. J. Clin. Invest. 83, 1419-1424.

Owens, G.K. (1987): Influence of blood pressure on development of aortic medial smooth muscle cell hypertrophy in spontaneously hypertensive rats. Hypertension 9, 178-187.

Owens, G.K. (1989): Control of hypertrophic versus hyperplastic growth of vascular smooth muscle cells. Am. J. Physiol. 26, H1755-H1765.

Owens, G.A., Geisterfer, A., Yang, Y., and Komoriya, A. (1988): Transforming growth factor beta induced growth inhibition and cellular hypertrophy in cultured vascular smooth muscle cells. J. Cell Biol. 107, 771-780.

Owens, G., and Reidy, M. (1985): Hyperplastic growth response of vascular smooth muscle cells following induction of acute hypertension in rats by aortic coarctation. Circ. Res. 57, 695-705.

Owens, G.K., and Schwartz, S.M. (1982): Alterations in vascular smooth muscle mass in the spontaneous hypertensive rat. Role in cellular hypertrophy, hyperploidy and hyperplasia. Circ. Res. 51, 280-289.

Owens, G.K., and Schwartz, S.M. (1983): Vascular smooth muscle cell hypertrophy and hyperploidy in the Goldblatt hypertensive rat. Circ. Res. 53, 491-501.

Powell, J.S., Clozel, J.-P., Muller, R.K.M., Kuhn, H., Hefti, F., Hosang, M., and Baumgartner, H.R. (1989): Inhibitors of angiotensin-converting enzyme prevent myointimal proliferation after vascular injury. Science 245, 186-188.

Ross, R., Ranes, E.W., and Bowen-Pope, D.F. (1986): The biology of platelet-derived growth factor. Cell 46, 155-169.

Rouleau, J.-L., Parmley, W.W., Stevens, J., Wilkman-Cofflet, J.W., Mahley, R.W., and Havel, R.J. (1983): Verapamil suppresses atherosclerosis in cholesterol-fed rabbits. J. Am. Coll. Cardiol. 1, 1453-1460.

Saouaf, R., Takasaki, I., Eastman, E., Chobanian, A.V., and Brecher, P. (1991): Fibronectin synthesis in the rat aorta in vitro. Changes due to experimental hypertension. J. Clin. Invest. 88, October, 1991 (in press).

Sarzani, R., Arnaldi, G., and Chobanian, A.V. (1991[a]): Hypertension-induced changes of platelet-derived growth factor receptor expression in rat aorta and heart. Hypertension 17, 888-895.

Sarzani, R., Arnaldi, G., Takasaki, I., Brecher, P., and Chobanian, A.V. (1991[b]): Effects of hypertension and aging on PDGF and PDGF receptor expression in rat aorta and heart. Hypertension 18, Suppl. III (in press).

Sarzani, R., Brecher, P., and Chobanian, A.V. (1989): Growth factor expression in aorta of normotensive and hypertensive rats. J. Clin. Invest. 83, 1404-1408.

Schwartz, S.M., Benditt, E.P. (1977): Aortic endothelial cell replication. I. Effects of age and hypertension in the rat. Circ. Res. 41, 248-255.

Schwartz, S.M., Campbell, G.R., and Campbell, J.H. (1986): Replication of smooth muscle cells in vascular disease. Circ. Res. 41, 248-255.

Schwartz, S.M., Heimark R.L., and Majesky, M.W. (1990): Developmental mechanisms underlying pathology of arteries. Physiol. Rev. 70, 1177-1209.

Takasaki, I., Chobanian, A.V., Sarzani, R., and Brecher, P. (1990): Effect of hypertension on fibronectin expression in the rat aorta. J. Biol. Chem. 265, 21935-21939.

Taubman, M.B., Berk, B.C., Izumo, S., Tsuda, T., Alexander, R.W., Nadal-Ginard, B. (1989): Angiotensin II induces c-fos mRNA in aortic smooth. Role of Ca^{2+} mobilization and protein kinase C activation. J. Biol. Chem. 264, 526-530.

Van Niekerk, J.L.M., Hendriks, Th., DeBoer, H.H.M., and Van't Laar, A. (1984): Does nifedipine suppress atherogensis in WHHL rabbits? Atherosclerosis 53, 91-98.

Résumé

Cet article résume les résultats obtenus par nous-mêmes et par d'autres laboratoires concernant les effets de l'hypertension et des traitements antihypertenseurs sur la croissance du tissu artériel et ses relations avec les lésions artérielles. Des travaux récents ont montré qu'un grand nombre de substances, incluant les facteurs de croissance connus, peuvent stimuler la croissance des cellules musculaires lisses de la paroi artérielle (CML) ainsi que celle des cellules endothéliales. Plusieurs de ces promoteurs ou inhibiteurs de croissance se sont révélés être exprimés dans les cellules artérielles suggérant ainsi que des actions autocrine ou paracrine puissent participer à la régulation de la croissance cellulaire. En outre, de nombreux agents vasoconstricteurs ont été démontrés capables de stimuler la croissance cellulaire alors que les vasodilatateurs sembleraient l'inhiber, ce qui suggère une relation étroite entre la croissance cellulaire, la structure vasculaire et le tonus des vaisseaux. Nous avons montré que l'hypertension provoque une accumulation de ces CML et de macrophages dans l'intima artérielle, ceci en association avec une expression accrue du Transforming Growth Factor ß (TGF-ß1) et du récepteur ß pour le Platelet-Derived Growth Factor (PDGF). Des résultats similaires ont été observés comme conséquence de l'âge chez les rats spontanément hypertendus (SHR) et chez des rats Wistar Kyoto (WKY). A l'inverse, l'expression myocardique du récepteur ß du PDGF n'était pas modifiée, alors que celle du TGF-ß1 était diminuée à la fois par l'âge et par l'hypertension, ce qui suggère que la régulation des gènes correspondants dans l'aorte et le coeur est soumise à des modalités de régulation différentes. Les antihypertenseurs pourraient exercer des effets vasculo-protecteurs contre les lésions artérielles provoquées par un cathéter à ballonnet, une hypercholestérolémie, l'âge, de même que par l'hypertension. Les antagonistes calciques et les inhibiteurs de l'enzyme de conversion de l'angiotensine ont prouvé leur capacité à réduire la formation de la plaque intimale après une lésion par ballonnet. Les ß-bloqueurs, les bloqueurs des canaux calciques et les inhibiteurs de l'enzyme de conversion de l'angiotensine pourraient aussi réduire la formation de la plaque athéroscléreuse provoquée par l'hypercholestérolémie. Le mécanisme de cette action vasculo-protectrice reste inconnu, encore que les effets sur la croissance cellulaire puissent y participer de façon importante et ce tout spécialement lorsqu'il s'agit des lésions par ballonnet. L'hypertension a des effets marqués sur la croissance des cellules artérielles, toutefois son mécanisme d'action ainsi que les relations entre les changements de croissance et le développement des lésions vasculaires induites par l'hypertension, restent à caractériser. Cette revue résume les données disponibles sur l'action des facteurs de croissance sur les cellules artérielles, les effets de l'hypertension expérimentale ainsi que des molécules vaso-actives sur l'expression des facteurs de croissance dans le tissu vasculaire. Chaque fois que possible des comparaisons sont faites entre les modifications observées chez le rat spontanément hypertendu et dans d'autres modèles d'hypertension. Enfin les effets de l'âge comme ceux de l'hypertension sont résumés.

Vasculotropin/VEGF hypersecretion by vascular smooth muscle cells from spontaneously hypertensive rats : a paracrine loop ?

Jean Plouët, Hafida Moukadiri, Laurence Gouzi, Bernard Malavaud and Marie-Madeleine Ruchoux

Centre de Recherche de Biochimie et Génétique Cellulaires, 118, route de Narbonne, 31062, Toulouse, France

Several laboratories have shown that smooth muscle cells (VSMC) cultured from aorta of spontaneously hypertensive rats (SHR) grew faster than their normotensive littermates Wistar-Kyoto (WKY) and were hypersensitive to the mitogenic effects of fetal calf serum (Yamori, 1981; Haudenschild, 1985) and other growth factors such as Epidermal Growth Factor, EGF, (Hadrava, 1989) and Platelet Derived Growth Factor A, PDGF-AA, (Resink, 1990). The factors enhancing the proliferation of VSMC from SHR as compared to their normotensive counterparts might therefore constitute important signals leading to the process of maladaptative structural remodelling.

We purified recently a new growth factor (Plouët et al, 1989), which is in vivo a strong inducer of the neovascularization (Favard et al, 1991). Since its mitogenic activity seemed to be restricted to vascular endothelial cells, we called it Vasculotropin (VAS). In the same time other groups purified a similar angiogenic factor, the Vascular Endothelial Growth Factor, or Vascular Permreability Factor. The cloning of the cDNA showed that VAS sequence shares 18-16% homology with that of PDGF A and B chains and therefore belongs to the sis oncogene family.

Since whether a cultured cell expresses VAS or VAS receptors, never both (Moukadiri et al 1991), it seems that VAS acts through a paracrine mechanism. We therefore looked onto the physiological relevance of a paracrine action of VAS inside the vascular wall.

Vasculotropin expression in SHR and WKY VSMC.

The conditioned medium of VSMC was chromatographied on heparin affinity columns and eluted by a stepwise gradient and the fractions assayed for VAS content. It appeared that VAS is secreted constitutively by VSMC, as shown in Fig 1A, at a level (0.1 ng/ml) Parallel experments showed that VAS is not synthesized by aortic endothelial cells. The constitutive secretion of SHR-VSMC was 10 times higher than that of WKY-VSMC (Fif 1B). However the secretion of VAS was stimulated in a parallel extent by phorbol myristate acetate. VAS had no mitogenic or haptotaxic effect on these cells.

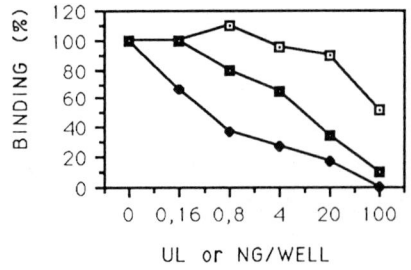 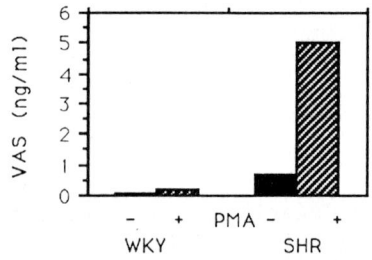

Fig.1. VAS secretion by bovine (A) and rat VSMC (B). (A)Inhibition of the binding of radiolabeled VAS was to fetal aortic endothelial cells by purified VAS (   ), or conditioned medium of VSMC untreated (   ), or treated 48 hours with 5 ng/ml of bFGF. (B) VAS radioreceptor assay of the conditioned medium of VSMC cultured from WKY or SHR stimulated or not by PMA.

Vasculotropin stimulates Endothelin-1 secretion by endothelial cells.

To assess a role to the hypersecretion of VAS by SHR-VSMC, it was tempting to determine whether VAS might take part to the endothelial-driven control of the vascular tone. Endothelins are known as the more potent vasoconstrictors synthesized by the endothelial cells; we therefore examined the ability of the endothelial cells to regulate their Endothelin-1 secretion through a VAS-dependant mechanism.
Confluent bovine aortic endothelial cells were incubated in serum free conditions in the presence of several putative modulators, and the Endothelin-1 concentration in the conditioned medium was assessed in a sensitive radioreceptor-assay (L.G. et al, in preparation). It appeared that VAS enhanced the ET secretion in a time and dose dependant fashion. This response was not related to the mitogenic effect of VAS since several growth factors mitogenic for these cells, such as FGF, Interferon g, or Interleukine 1, failed to enhance the Endothelin-1 secretion, whereas other angiogenic factors such as transforming growth factor b or Interleukine 4 induced a potent release of Endothelin-1. This effect occured in a smaller extent in arteries than in vein derived endothelial cells.

Vasculotropin-Endothelin-1 : a paracrine loop?

Should the constitutive hypersecretion of vasculotropin by vascular smooth muscle cells cultured from spontaneously hypertensive rats play a role in the physiopathology of arterial hypertension, it would require the existence of a paracrine loop since this growth factor does not bind to these cells.

The SHR-VSMC exhibit an increased growth rate and an enhanced reactivity to growth factors. These properties might result from growth factors synthesis and growth factors receptors expression abnormalities. Both PDGF-AA and TGFb transcripts are induced in SHR-VSMC as well as in their normal counterparts by the potent vasoconstrictors angiotensin II and Endothelin-1 (Hahn et al, 1991). However a dissociation between transcripts induction and growth factor secretion occured and thus the actual contribution of these growth factors to the hyperproliferation remained unknown.

Vasculotropin might sustain the hyperproliferation, despite its lack of mitogenicity for VSMC. Therefore it should act through the activation of other mitogens synthesized outside the VSMC. Endothelin-1 was one candidate since it is released from the endothelial cells and promotes the contraction and the proliferation of the smooth muscle cells. These data provide a new clue as to the paracrine control of the muscle cell proliferation. It remains to investigate the effects of vasculotropin on the secretion of Endothelin-1 by aortic endothelial cells cultured from WKY or SHR rats. In addition to its endothelial actions, vasculotropin is mitogenic for human IL2 dependant lymphocytes (Praloran et al, 1991) and therefore it might be involved, through lymphocytes-endothelium interactions, in the inflammatory reaction leading to atherosclerosis.

REFERENCES

Hadrava, V., Tremblay, J., & Hamet, P. (1989): Abnormalities in growth characteristics of aortic smooth muscle cells in spontaneously hypertensive rats. *Hypertension* 13, 589-597.

Hahn, A.W.A., Resink, T.J., Bernhardt, J., Ferracin, F. & Bühler, F.R. (1991): Stimulation of autocrine Platelet Derived Growth Factor AA-homodimer and Transforming Growth Factor b in vascular smooth muscle cells. *Biochem. Bioph. Res. Commun.* 178, 1451-1458.

Haudenschild, C.C., Grundwald, J. & Chobanian, A.V. (1985): Effects of hypertension on migration and proliferation of smooth muscle in culture. *Hypertension* 7(suppl.1), 101-104.

Moukadiri, H., Favard, C., Bikfalvi, A. & Plouët, J. (1991): Biosynthesis of vasculotropin and expression of vasculotropin receptors by cultured cells. *Biothech. Growth Factors;* Paoletti F., Mantovani, G. Eds, Karger, (in press).

Plouët, J. & Shilling, J. & Gospodarowicz, D. (1989): Isolation and characterization of a newly identified endothelial cell mitogen produced by At-T20 cells. *Embo. J.* 9, 3801-3806.

Praloran, V., Mirshahi, S.S., Favard, C., Moukadiri, H. & Plouët, J. (1991): Vasculotropin is mitogenic for normal human lymphocytes. *C.R.A.S.* 313, III, 21-26.

Yamori, Y. & Igawa, T., Kanbe, T., Kihara, M., Nara, Y. & Horie, R. (1981): Mechanism of structural vascular changes in genetic hypertension: analysis on cultured vascular smooth muscle cell from spontaneously hypertensive rats. *Clin. Sci.* 61, 121s-123s.

Differential autocrine responses of SHR- and WKY-VSMC to stimulation with vasoactive peptides

Alfred W.A. Hahn, Stefan Regenass, Therese J. Resink, Fabrizia Ferracin and Fritz R. Bühler

Department of Research, University Hospital Basel, Hebelstrasse 20, CH 4031 Basel, Switzerland

SUMMARY: Responses of quiescent vascular smooth muscle cells from spontaneously hypertensive and Wistar-Kyoto rats to stimulation with a selected number of growth factors- and vasoconstrictor peptides were established for autocrine platelet- derived growth factor AA (PDGF -AA) and transforming growth factor ß (TGF ß).The interrelationship between PDGF, TGF ß and vasoconstrictors was investigated in experiments using the pure peptides individually for stimulation of PDGF -AA and TGF ß peptide secretion. Both growth factors enhanced their own and one anothers transcript expression.
The results demonstrated that in spontaneously hypertensive rats, an established animal model of hypertension, the steady state balance of this set of growth factors may be disturbed. Defects involved may be attributable to alterations in the secretory machinery and/or amount of autocrine growth factor produced.

INTRODUCTION AND RESULTS: Aberrant regulation of cell proliferation plays a crucial role in the pathogenesis of many diseases including hypertension. The morphologic smooth muscle lesion associated with hypertension has been suggested to represent a maladaption of "autoregulatory" mechanisms responsible for local control of blood flow (Cowley, 1990) involving factor(s) which can stimulate active vasoconstriction and DNA synthesis/cell replication (Schwartz et al.,1990; Naftilan et al., 1989; Hahn et al., 1990) like angiotensin II and endothelin-1. In some tissues there is evidence for a local production of Ang II (Campbell, 1987), while for ET-1 autocrine production in VSMC has been demonstrated (Hahn et al., 1990). Within blood vessels a limited local production of ET-1 and/or Ang II therefore may play an important regulative role in the modulation of VSMC function including contraction, extracellular matrix- and autocrine growth factor production. PDGF -AA is one of the peptide factors that may maintain and/or provoke modulation of the VSMC state of differentiation (Corjay et al., 1989). In addition there is evidence that TGF ß can counteract cellular responses to PDGF (Anzano et al., 1986) and therefore exert growth inhibiting effects on VSMC (for review see Moses et al., 1990). De- regulation of either the production or balance of these peptides or their modulation of VSMC function may well contribute to those vessel wall changes (e.g. myointimal thickening) typical of hypertension.

<u>Secretion of PDGF-AA homodimer by VSMC.</u> Secretion of metabolically labelled PDGF-AA into culture medium was determined by immunoprecipitation and electrophoresis (Fig. 1). Relative amounts of $[^{35}S]$- PDGF-AA secreted (30-31 KD peptide dimer) were assessed by densitometric analysis of autoradiograms. For growth arrested, non- stimulated VSMC incubated in the presence of $[^{35}S]$- methionine, minute amounts of radiolabelled PDGF-AA could be detected only in the medium from SHR-derived cells (arbitrary OD units of 0.6). However inclusion of either Ang II, ET-1 or TGFß during the 16 hr metabollic labelling period resulted in secretion of $[^{35}S]$- PDGF-AA from both SHR- and WKY- VSMC (Fig. 3A) (respective arbitrary OD units were 4.0 and 3.8 in response to Ang II and 3.0 and 3.0 in response to TGFß). The secretion response of SHR-VSMC (arbitrary OD units 14.8) to ET-1 was, however, ~3 fold greater than that of WKY-VSMC (arbitrary OD units 5.5). Additionally, only SHR-VSMC secreted $[^{35}S]$- PDGF-AA (arbitrary OD units 1.5) in response to this homodimer (Fig.1A). PDGF-BB stimulated secretion of labelled peptides from SHR-VSMC (arbitrary OD units 2.2) and to a minor extent in WKY-VSMC (arbitrary OD units 0.5)(Fig.1A).

The kinetics of PDGF-AA secretion in response to Ang II were studied in pulse-chase experiments. Quiescent VSMC from SHR- and WKY (at equivalent cell numbers of 1.5×10^7) were exposed to 1 nM Ang II for 5 hrs, then incubated in methionine- free medium for 1 hr before pulse- (30 min. with [^{35}S]- methionine) chase. Secreted immunoreactive [^{35}S]- peptide was readily detectable in media from SHR- and WKY-VSMC after 30 mins of chase (Fig.1B). For WKY- VSMC maximal peptide secretion occurred within 1 hr of chase and thereafter declined to undetectable levels within 2.5 hrs of chase. In contrast, maximal secretion of [^{35}S]- PDGF-AA from SHR- VSMC occurred between 1.5-2 hrs of chase and thereafter decreased to undetectable levels after 3 hrs of chase (Fig 1B).

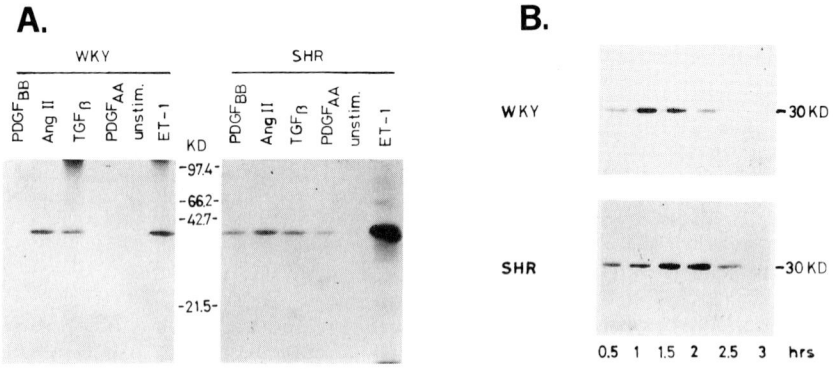

Figure 1: <u>Immunoprecipiation of PDGF-AA secreted by rat VSMC</u> stimulated with different vasoconstrictor peptides (Ang II, ET-1; 1nM each) and growth factors (PDGF-AA, PDGF-BB; 2ng/ml each and TGFβ ; 2.5 ng/ml) (Panel A). Panel B: Pulse- chase analysis of autocrine PDGF-AA homodimer in response to Ang II (10^{-8}M) stimulation.

<u>Stimulation of TGFβ production in SHR- and WKY- VSMC.</u> The secretion of TGFβ from VSMC was examined by Western blot analysis of concentrated and desalted media from stimulated cells. Both SHR- and WKY-VSMC secreted TGFβ following 16 hrs exposure to either Ang II (1nM), ET-1 (1nM) or TGFβ (2.5ng/ml) (Fig. 2). The data in Fig. 2B for TGFβ secreted from TGFβ stimulated VSMC have been corrected for that immunoreactivity due to exogeneously added TGFβ. The amount of TGFβ secreted in response to ET-1, TGFβ and Ang II was greater (p at least < 0.05) for SHR- VSMC than WKY- VSMC (Fig 2B). However, the most interesting observations were that PDGF-BB induced TGFβ secretion from WKY- VSMC only, and that neither SHR- nor WKY-VSMC secreted detectable levels of TGFβ in response to PDGF-AA (Fig. 2B).

DISCUSSION: In culture, SHR- VSMC exhibit an increased growth rate as well as hyperreactivity in response to various peptide factors when compared to VSMC of normotensive controls. Therefore, differential (auto-) stimulated secretion of autocrine PDGF-AA by SHR- and WKY VSMC may relate to the vascular pathologies observed in SHR and to cell surface expression of different PDGF α and ß receptor complements.

We have demonstrated the absence of PDGF-α receptors on cultured WKY VSMC (Resink et al., 1990). Moreover, the PDGF-AA autocrine responses described here suggest that cellular responses triggered via different PDGF receptor dimers are not equivalent. Additonally, neither SHR- nor WKY secreted TGFβ in response to PDGF-AA stimulation and only WKY- VSMC secreted this peptide in response to PDGF-BB. These results, which demonstrate a dissociation between transcript induction and peptide secretion, suggest an important role for posttranscriptional regulation processes in the control of autocrine growth regulator production. Similar dissociative observations have been made for the expression of thrombospondin transcripts and secretion of the glycoprotein (Majack et al., 1985). In the light of these findings, it is possible to propose that interactions between growth regulators constitute an important mechanism in controlling production of autocrine growth factors. Especially the secretion of PDGF-AA in response to ET-1 in both WKY- and, more pronounced in SHR- VSMC may not only add to the long lasting vasoconstrictor effect of ET-1, but also influence expression of PDGF cell surface receptors, since PDGF itself can down- regulate its own receptors (Escobedo et al., 1989).

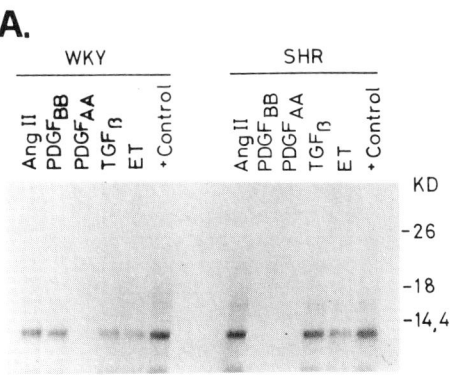
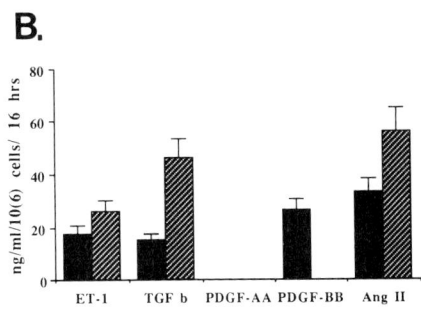

Figure 2: <u>Western blot of immunoreactive TGFβ secreted by rat VSMC</u> after stimulation with different vasoconstrictor peptides (Ang II, ET-1; 1nM each) and growth factors (PDGF-AA, PDGF-BB; 2ng/ml each and TGFβ ; 2.5 ng/ml) using TGF ß antiserum and [^{125}I]- labeled second antibodies (Panel A). Panel B displays the results (mean ± SD, n=3) from densitometric analyses normalized with respect to control (50 ng TGFβ) absorbance values.

ACKNOWLEGEMENT: This study was supported by the Swiss National Fund grant no. 31- 29275.90

REFERENCES

Anzano, M.A. et al. (1986): Anchorage- independent growth of primary rat embryo cells is induced by platelet- derived growth factor. J Cell Physiol 126: 312-18

Campbell, D.J. (1987): Circulating and tissue angiotensin systems. J Clin Invest 79: 1-6

Cowley, A.W. (1980) In: Laragh JH, ed.Topics in hypertension, New York: Yorke Medical Books, pages 184-200

Corjay, M.H. et al. (1989): Differential effect of platelet- derived growth factor- versus serum-induced growth on smooth muscle alpha actin and non-muscle beta actin expression in cultured rat aortic smooth muscle cells. J Biol Chem 264: 10501- 6

Escobedo, J.A. et al. (1988): Platelet- derived growth factor receptors expressed by cDNA transfection couple to diverse groups of cellular responses associated with cell proliferation. J Biol Chem 263: 1482-87

Hahn, A.W.A. et al. (1990): Stimulation of endothelin mRNA and secretion in rat vascular smooth muscle cells: a novel autocrine function. Cell Regulation 1: 649- 659

Majack, R.A. et al. (1985): Platelet-derived growth factor and heparin-like glycosaminoglycans regulate thrombospondin synthesis and deposition in the matrix by smooth muscle cells. J Cell Biol 101: 1059-70

Moses, H.L. et al. (1990): TGFß stimulation and inhibition of cell proliferation: new mechanistic insights. Cell 63: 245-7

Naftilan, A.J. et al. (1989): Induction of platelet-derived growth factor a-chain and c-myc gene expression by angiotensin II in cultured rat vascular smooth muscle cells. J Clin Invest 83:1419- 24

Resink, T.J. et al. (1990): Specific growth stimulation of cultured rat vascular smooth muscle cells by platelet- derived growth factor A-chain homodimer. Cell Regulation 1: 821-31

Schwartz, S.M. et al. (1990) In: Hypertension, Pathophysiology, Diagnosis and Management, Raven Press Ltd., New York

Upregulation of adrenal, renal and vascular growth factors in salt fed hypertensive Dahl rats

Mohinder P. Sambhi, Narayan Swaminathan, Hong Wang and Hong Mei Rong

Hypertension Research Laboratory, Hypertension Section, Department of Medicine, Veterans Administration Medical Center, Sepulveda and UCLA School of Medicine, Los Angeles, CA 91343, USA

ABSTRACT

Participation of peptide growth factors in the vascular proliferative response, as a contributory factor to the development of hypertension is proposed but not established. The mRNA expression of transforming growth factor (TGF-B_1), epidermal growth factor (EGF), EGF receptor (EGFR) and platelet derived growth factor (PDGF-B) was examined in aorta, kidney, heart, and adrenals from Dahl rats of susceptible strain (DS/Jr), given high salt (DS-S) or normal salt diet (DS-N) for 4 wks. Significant upregulation of TGF-B_1 gene in the adrenal and EGFR gene in the kidney occurred, with a marked downregulation of EGF in the adrenal, kidney, and heart in DS-S. The kidney and aorta showed increased EGF binding sites. The results show a tissue specific pattern of *in vivo* expression, and demonstrate that EGFR can be differentially upregulated in the presence of suppressed EGF in the kidney and post transcriptionally upregulated in aorta. Adrenal TGF-B_1 and renal EGFR may have an important role in the genesis of vascular proliferation in salt induced hypertension, and these effects are consistent with and may represent endocrine action of the adrenals.

INTRODUCTION

The underlying mechanisms or the sequence of events leading to sustained hypertension with high salt feeding in Dahl rats remains to be defined (Rapp, 1984; Tobian, 1984). Extensive search for specific mediators has included vasoconstrictor sympathetic neuroeffector mechanisms (Mark, 1991), sodium retaining or hypertensinogenic steroids (Rapp & Dahl, 1971), and undefined natriuretic factors (Taisuke et al., 1991). Potential involvement of peptide growth factors in the progression and chronic maintenance of the hypertensive state, through the genesis of cardiovascular proliferative response has been increasingly appreciated (Schwartz, 1984; Lever, 1986; Chobanian, 1990) but remains to be established. The present studies were undertaken to examine the mRNA expression of growth factors in salt induced hypertension in Dahl rats.

METHODS AND MATERIAL

DS-S rats (7 weeks obtained from HSD, Indiana) were fed for four weeks either high salt (8% NaCl) diet (n=8) or normal salt (n=6) and were allowed to drink water ad libitum. After sacrifice, the heart, kidney, adrenals, liver, and aorta (from the beginning of the aortic arch to the abdominal bifurcation) were removed. Total RNA was extracted from the tissues as described by Chromczynski and Sacchi (1987). Quantification of mRNA was performed by slotblot hybridization using ^{32}P labelled specific riboprobes. The probes were prepared from their respective cDNAs in plasmids obtained from ATCC (EGFR, pE7; EGF, PhEGF-121; TGF-B_1, PhTGF-B_1; PDGF-B, PMS-1). The fragments produced by specific enzymic cleavage were inserted into suitable vectors and subcloned. A 0.7 kb Eco R1-Hind III fragment (representing the tyrosine kinase message at the 3′ end of EGFR mRNA from the EGFR cDNA in plasmid pE7) was cloned into pGEM 4Z. Similarly a 0.54 kb Eco R1 fragment of the PhEGF-121, 2.0kb EcO R1 fragment of PhTGF-B and 2.0 kb Bam H1 fragment of PSM-1 were subcloned into the vector pGEM-3Z. ^{32}P labelled riboprobes were prepared using reagents and protocols from Promega. The slot blots (0.03-0.5 ug total RNA) were hybridized with the probes, washed, cut and counted in a Beckman LS-7000 liquid scintillation counter. Plots of the concentration of total RNA blotted versus cpm were analyzed by linear regression. Plots with regression coefficients, (r<0.9, p<0.05) were compared and the significance of the difference in the slopes determined to estimate the relative abundance of the specific mRNA in the tissues. The binding kinetics of ^{125}I labelled EGF to the membranes isolated from the kidney, heart and aorta were studied as described by Swaminathan and Sambhi (1991).

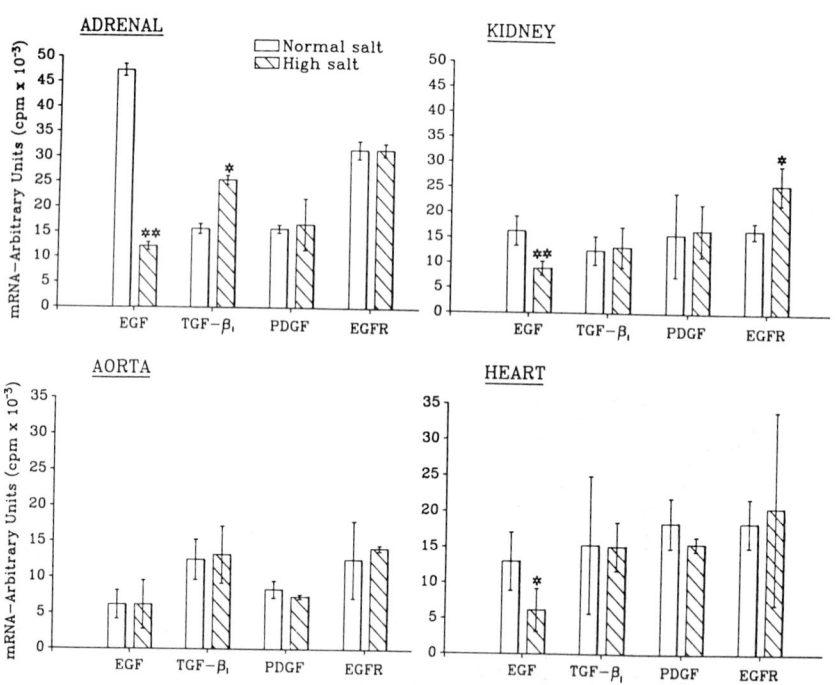

Fig. 1. Growth factor mRNA levels in Dahl rats tissues.

RESULTS

In DS-S a marked elevation in systolic BP (173± 2.9 vs 133± 6.9 mm Hg, p<0.001), occurred as compared with DS-N rats. Mean body weight did not differ (382±9 vs 370±7 g, NS). The quantification of the mRNA transcripts of the four growth factors examined in Dahl rats on normal or high salt diet,is shown in Fig 1.

Three major findings emerging as effects of high salt diet are: (1) The upregulation of TGF-B_1 mRNA in the adrenals, (15.7±1.0 vs 25.4±0.9 arbitrary mRNA units, p<0.05); (2) down regulation of EGF mRNA expression in the adrenals (47.3±1.2 vs 12.2±0.8, p<0.001), kidneys (16.3± 2.9 vs 8.9±1.4, p<0.01) and in the heart (13.0 ± 4.1 vs 6.2±3.0, p<0.05); (3) elevation of EGFR mRNA levels (16.7±1.6 vs 25.8±3.9, p<0.05) in the kidney tissue. PDGF-B mRNA expression levels did not change in any of the tissues examined. The results of EGF binding to tissue membrane preparations indicated a significant increase in EGF binding sites in the aorta and kidney tissues, with heart tissue showing no change. B_{max} of EGF binding in the aorta of DS-S vs DS-N was significantly higher (34.2 ±5.1 vs 10.6 ± 0.28 fmoles /mg protein, p<0.01) with no significant change in Kd (1.25±0.12 vs 1.11±0.10 nM). The findings were similar in the kidney (B_{max}, 1.4±.25 vs

0.81 ± 0.08, $p<0.05$). Tyrosine phosphorylation units (functional activity of EGFR) in aortic membranes without added EGF were similar in the two groups on high and normal salt (812 ± 98 cpm /mg protein vs 995 ± 109), but increased to (4048 ± 329 vs 2420 ± 212, $p\leq0.01$) following the addition of EGF. Phosphorylation units were based on counts (^{32}P) in the precipitated proteins and specifity of tyrosine phosphorylation was shown by its 70% inhibition by a specific inhibitor genestein (Clegg & Sambhi, 1989).

DISCUSSION

High salt in genetically susceptible rats resulted in marked hypertension and an upregulation of TGF-B_1 gene expression singularly in the adrenal. In view of the experimental evidence in vitro (Assoian et al.,1984), the observed effects in other tissues on EGF and EGFR can be considered as secondary to the upregulation of TGF-B_1, which is secreted from tissues as a latent form in plasma (Miyazono et al., 1988), capable of being picked up and activated in other tissues (Wakefield et al., 1990). Thus potential endocrine effects of adrenal TGF-B_1 can be proposed. Salt induced hypertension in Dahl model, does not develop in the absence of the adrenals (Iwai et al., 1969) and can be humorally transmitted to a parabiotic partner (Dahl et al., 1969). In the aortic tissue increased EGF binding with no change in EGFR mRNA expression may be attributed to post translational changes. It is suggested that a primary or dominant factor in the genesis of salt induced hypertension may be the upregulation of adrenal TGF-B_1 leading to transcriptional changes in the EGF-EGFR system in the kidney and post transcriptional changes in EGFR in the aorta.

REFERENCES:

Assoian, R.K., et al. (1984): Transforming growth factor beta controls receptor levels for epidermal growth factor in NRK fibroblasts. Cell. 36,35-41.

Chobanian, A.V. (1990): Corcoran lecture: adaptive and maladaptive responses of the arterial wall to hypertension. Hypertension. 15, 666-674.

Clegg,K., & Sambhi, M.P. (1989): Inhibition of epidermal growth factor mediated DNA synthesis by a specific tyrosine kinase inhibitor in VSM cells of the SHR J. Hypertension 7 (supple 6): S144-145.

Cromczynski, P. & Sacchi, N. (1987): Single step method of RNA isolation by acid guanidinium thiocyanate-phenol-chloroform extraction. Anal. Biochem. 12, 156-159.

Dahl, L.K. et al. (1969): Humoral transmission of hypertension: evidence from parabiosis. Circ. Research. Vols. XXIV and XXV. I, 121-133.

Iwai, J. et al. (1969): Effect of adrenalectomy on blood pressure in salt fed, hypertension prone rats, failure of hypertension to develop in absence of evidence of adrenal cortical tissue. J. Exp. Med. 129, 663-678.

Lever, A.F. (1986): Slow pressor mechanisms in hypertension: a role for hypertrophy of resistance vessels. J. of Hypertension. 4, 515-524.

Mark, A.L. (1991): Sympathetic neural contribution to salt-induced hypertension in Dahl rats. Hypertension. 17, I-86-I-90.

Miyazono, K. et al. (1988): Latent high molecular weight complex of transforming growth factor B_1. J. Biol. Chem. 263, 6407-6415.

Rapp, J. (1984): Characteristics of Dahl salt-susceptible and salt-resistant In Handbook of Hypertension, Vol. 4, Experimental and Genetic Models of Hypertension, ed. W. de Jong, pp. 286-295. Elsevier Science Publishers B.V.

Rapp, J.P., & Dahl, L.K. (1971): Adrenal steroidogenesis in rat bred for susceptibility and resistance to the hypertensive effect of salt. Endocrinology. 88, 52.

Schwartz, S.M. (1984): Smooth muscle proliferation in hypertension. Hypertension. 6, I-56-I61.

Swaminathan, N. & Sambhi, M.P. (1991): Increased epidermal growth factor receptor levels in the adult SHR kidney. Fed. Am. Soc. Exp. Biol. Vol 5 (4), A662 (Abstr.)

Taisuke, I. et al. (1991): Renal sodium handling and sodium transport inhibitor in salt-sensitive essential hypertension. J. of Hypertension. 9, 49-54.

Tobian, L. (1984): Renal sodium handling and vascular responsiveness in experimental hypertension with special reference to Dahl rats. In Handbook of Hypertension, Vol. 4: Experimental and Genetic Models of Hypertension, ed. W. de Jong, pp. 135-146. Elsevier Science Publishers B.V.

Wakefield, L.M. et al. (1990): Recombinant latent transforming growth factor B_1, has a longer plasma-half life in rats than active transforming growth factor B_1, and a different tissue distribution. J. of Clin. Invest. 86, 1976-1984.

Flowcytometric analysis of cell cycle of cultured vascular smooth muscle cells from SHR and New Zealand GH rat

Masanori Hamada, E.L. Harris [*], J.A. Millar [*], F.O. Simpson [*], Ichiro Nishio and Yoshiaki Masuyama

Division of Cardiology, Department of Medicine, Wakayama Medical College, Wakayama, Japan and [*] Wellcome Medical Research Institute, Otago University, Dunedin, New Zealand

INTRODUCTION: The arterial wall thickening in hypertension has been one of the major interests in pathogenesis of hypertension for the last two decades. Enhanced cell proliferation of cultured vascular smooth muscle cells (CVSMC) from spontaneously hypertensive rats(SHR) compared to Wistar-Kyoto(WKY) rats has been reported(Yamori et.al., 1981). In our previous studies, we demonstrated the possibility that CVSMC from SHR had short G0 phase duration or that there was a smaller proportion of cells in G0 phase(Hamada et. al.,1990). In this study, we used flowcytometry to compare the proportions of DNA-synthesizing S phase cells in different strains of rats. An advantage of this method is that the obtained values are not influenced by cell protein or difference of cell numbers in individual dishes. The method also makes it possible to evaluate the proportion of cells in G0+G1 and G2+M phases. In this study, we investigated whether an other genetically hypertensive rat strain, the New Zealand genetically hypertensive rat(GH), also shows enhanced CVSMC proliferation. If enhanced cell proliferation of vascular smooth muscle cells is observed also in more than one, this would provide further evidence for a role of abnormal cell growth in the pathogenesis of hypertension.

MATERIALS AND METHODS: Aortic vascular smooth muscle cells were prepared by enzyme digestion method from 20 week old SHR, WKY, GH and N (New Zealand normotensive; closed colony) rats. The details of the culture method have been described elsewhere(Hamada et.al.,1990). Systolic blood pressures were as follows; SHR:175 ± 9.6 mmHg, WKY:108.4 ± 20.1, GH:195.1 ± 8.2, N:117.5 ± 18.5 (mean ± SD, n=4, p<0.01 between SHR and WKY, and between GH and N). Cells were incubated in Dulbecco-modified Eagle's medium; (DMEM: Sigma: St.Louis, USA) supplemented with 10% fetal calf serum (FCS:Gibco:New York) under standard conditions (37°C, 95% air and 5% CO_2). CVSMC in this experiment were used after 4th to 7th passages.

<u>Exp.1: Measurement of cell phase proportions in exponential growth.:</u>
CVSMC were seeded at an approximate density of 4.0×10^5 cells per $27\ cm^2$ and cultured under the standard conditions for 72h. The cells in four dishes for each strain were then separated and counted, and this procedure was repeated every 48h. The medium of the other dishes was renewed with the fresh standard medium every 48h.

Exp.2: The effect of FCS-free medium on exponential growth phase cells:
CVSMC were seeded as described above and cultured for 120 h in the standard medium. Then the cells were washed twice with FCS-free DMEM and cultured in FCS-free DMEM for a further 96 h. The cells in four dishes for each strain of rats were separated and counted at 24 h interval after the medium was switched to FCS-free DMEM.

Exp.3: The response of FCS-deprived cells to FCS:
CVSMC were seeded as described above and cultured for 120 h in the standard medium. Then the medium was switched to FCS-free and maintained for 48 h. The medium was then switched back to the standard medium and cells were collected and counted at 12 h intervals after the medium was switched to the standard medium.

The percentage of S phase cells, as well as G0+G1 phase and G2+M phase, in four different strains of rat was measured by flowcytometry(FACScanTM) with propidium iodide staining of double-stranded DNA. Cell proportion in DNA cell-cycle was calculated by Dean's sum of broadened rectangle (SOBR) model (Dean et.al., 1987). The values are shown as mean±SD of percentage. The data were analyzed by two-tailed Student's "t" test, comparing each hypertensive strain with its control strain.

RESULTS:
Exp.1: Measurement of cell phase proportions in exponential growth.:
Doubling time for SHR and WKY CVSMC were 30.4 ± 2.0 h and 42.9 ± 2.2 h (n=4 rats, difference p<0.01). Comparing doubling times for GH and N CVSMCs were 29.9 ± 2.9 and 25.6 ± 3.2 h(n=4 rats, NS). During exponential growth (at seventh day), the percentage of G0+G1 phase cells was significantly smaller in SHR than in WKY CVSMC (SHR: 64±2.0%, WKY: 82.8±1.3%, difference p<0.001) The percentage of S phase cells during logarithmic growth was significantly greater in SHR than in WKY (SHR: 24.7±2.1%, WKY: 8.5±1.3%, p<0.001). There was no difference between GH and N CVSMCs in the proportions of S phase (GH:7.3±1.3%, N: 7.0±1.4%, NS), G2+M phase (GH: 5.3±0.5%, N: 3.5±1.3%, NS), and G0+G1 phase cells (GH: 87.8±1.3%, N: 88.8±1.0%, NS).

Exp.2:The effect of FCS-free medium on exponential growth phase cells:
When switched to FCS-free DMEM, CVSMCs from GH and N stopped proliferating while WKY CVSMC continued to proliferate slowly. In contrast, SHR CVSMC showed considerable continued proliferation. In SHR, the percentage of S phase cell decreased for the first 48 h and then increased again (8.0±1.2% at 48 h, and 17.5±0.6% at 96 h after medium switch). After FCS deprivation, the percentage of S phase cells decreased greatly in GH and N CVSMC (GH: 2.5±0.6%, N: 3.5±0.6%, at 24 h after medium switch NS). There was no significant difference in cell proportion between GH and N CVSMCs.

Exp.3:The response of FCS-deprived cells to FCS:
The proliferative effect was maximum at 24 h after the switch back to the standard medium In SHR, FCS led to a doubling in the proportion of S phase cells in 24 h (14.5±0.6% in FCS-deprived arrested condition, 28.5±1.7% 24 h after FCS application) and there was little further change over the next 24 h. In WKY, the proportion of S phase cells increased 24 h after FCS to about the same level as in SHR but then diminished gradually. In GH and N CVSMC, FCS application led to a large increase in S phase cells, with a maximum effect at 24 h. There was no noteworthy difference in cell phase proportion between GH and N CVSMCs.

DISCUSSION: The shorter doubling time and increased S phase cells during the exponential growth in SHR compared to WKY CVSMCs represents enhanced cell proliferation. In contrast to Japanese strains, there was no significant difference between GH and N CVSMC in doubling time and no major difference in cell cycle phase during exponential growth. When the four strains are compared together, it is WKY that is slow rather than SHR which is fast. Nevertheless, SHR shows a distinctive characteristics as follows; CVSMC from SHR are unable to attain true quiescence in FCS-free DMEM. The results are quite compatible with our previous finding using [^{3}H]-thymidine incorporation method and SHR cells-conditioned medium(Hamada et.al.,1990).and suggest the production of an autocrine growth factor from CVSMC. The FCS-deprived cells could be stimulated to synthesize DNA by FCS stimulation. The maximum enhancement was obtained at 24 hours after switching from the FCS-free medium to the standard medium, and the maximum effects showed no difference between SHR and WKY CVSMCs and between GH and N CVSMCs. However, SHR cells showed prolonged response to FCS compared to WKY cells. The result suggest a possible hyperresponse to growth factor in SHR cells.

The present study revealed major differences in cell-cycle of CVSMC between SHR/WKY and GH/N. These results indicate that the enhanced proliferation of CVSMCs observed in SHR compared to WKY in FCS-supplemented medium, is not an universal feature in all hypertensive strains of rat.

ACKNOWLEDGMENTS: The authors gratefully acknowledge Dr. E.L Phelan (Wellcome Medical Research Institute, Otago Medical School, Dunedin, New Zealand) for breeding the four different strains of rats. The Dunedin authors acknowledge the support of the Hearth Research Council of New Zealand. Aspect of this work have been reported elsewhere(Hamada et.al.,1991).

REFERENCES:

Yamori Y, Igawa T, Kanbe T, Kihara M, Nara Y, Horie R(1981):.Mechanisms of structural vascular changes in genetic hypertension:analyses on cultural vascular smooth muscle cells from spontaneously hypertensive rats. Clin. Sci.61:121s-123s.

Hamada M, Nishio I, Baba A et al(1990): Enhanced DNA synthesis of cultured vascular smooth muscle cells from spontaneously hypertensive rats.Atherosclerosis 81:191-198.

Hamada M, Harris E, Millar JA and Simpson FO(1990):Temporal differences in the cell cycle of cultured vascular smooth muscle cells from spontaneously hypertensive and normotensive Wistar-Kyoto rats. J.Vasc Med Biology 2:136-141.

Dean PH.(1987): Data analysis and cell kinetics research.techniques in cell cycle analysis, Gray JW and Darzynkiewicz Z.(Eds), Humana Press, Clifton, N.J., Chapter 8.

Hamada M, Millar JA, Simpson FO, Harris EJ.(1991):Flowcytometric analysis of cell cycle of cultured aortic smooth muscle cells from two strains of genetically hypertensive rats. J. Cardiovasc. Pharmacol., 16(suppl 7): s9-s11.

Dissociation of hypertension and genetically enhanced cell growth in skin fibroblasts of F2 hybrid SHR/WKY rats

Pascale Guicheney, Karen Soussan, Rossella Rota and Eric Dausse

Clinique Néphrologique, Hôpital Necker, 75015 Paris, France

It is well-known that significant structural cardiovascular changes are adaptative responses to high blood pressure. Nevertheless several investigators have reported cardiac and peripheral vascular hyperplasia and hypertrophy in young spontaneously hypertensive rats (SHR) compared to WKY rats preceding the development of high blood pressure levels (Gray, 1984; Kunes et al, 1987). Some has suggested that a genetic susceptibility to proliferation of the vascular system may be a primary mechanism involved in the development of high blood pressure (Folkow, 1986; Lever, 1986). Increased growth rate and reactivity of vascular smooth muscle cells (VSMC) derived from SHR compared with normotensive WKY in culture has been demonstrated by numerous laboratories (Yamori et al, 1981; Baudouin-Legros et al 1990). We recently observed in skin fibroblasts from newborn SHR a proliferative advantage and an increased reactivity to serum, epidermal growth factor (EGF) and angiotensin II (Guicheney et al, 1991) as it has been described for VSMC (Scott Burden et al, 1989; Baudouin et al, 1990). This suggests the existence of an intrinsic abnormality in vascular and non-vascular cells of mesodermal origin affecting one or several mechanisms which control cell proliferation.. We thus studied growth and reactivity of skin fibroblasts from F1 and F2 hybrid SHR/WKY rats to determine whether the proliferative advantage is a primary genetic cause of high blood pressure in SHR according to the experimental approach detailed by Rapp (1983).

METHODS

SHR and their normotensive control strain Wistar-Kyoto rats (WKY) were obtained from Janvier Breeding Laboratories (France). A F1 hybrid strain was obtained by crossing female SHR with male WKY. Fourteen couples of F1 rats gave birth to 73 male rats forming the F2 hybrid SHR/WKY generation. Blood pressure was measured by tail plethysmography on conscious animals on at least three separate occasions between 14 and 16 weeks of age and the average of the measurements was taken as the blood pressure for the rats. Fibroblasts from adult rats were obtained from a piece of back skin by explant technique and cultured in Modified Eagle's Medium (MEM) supplemented with 10 % fetal calf serum (FCS) as previously described (Guicheney et al, 1990). To determine proliferation rate, the fibroblasts were seeded at the concentration of 30,000 cells/cm2. DNA content/well was determined using bisbenzimid as fluorescent probe and cells were counted using a Coulter counter (Coultronics, France). Cell doubling time was calculated according to the following equation : DT = (t - to) x log2/ (log N - log No) where to and t are day 1 and day 3 after seeding and No and N, the cell number or the well DNA content at to and t. Quiescent cells for 3H-thymidine incorporation were obtained by incubation of confluent cells for 24 h with 0.5% FCS in MEM The reinitiation of DNA synthesis was induced by 10 ng/ml EGF in the presence of 0.5 µCi/ml ^{3}H-thymidine (Amersham) and 0.5 mM unlabeled thymidine. Twenty-four hours later, the nuclear ^{3}H-thymidine incorporation was determined (Guicheney et al, 1991).

RESULTS

F1 hybrid SHR/WKY rats had intermediate mean blood pressure (BP) and relative heart weight between SHR and WKY (Table 1). The BP of the 73 male F2 hybrid rats ranged from 120 to 190 mm Hg. Rats have been divided in 3 groups according to their BP. The "low pressure" group (n=18) represented 24.7 % of the rats, with a BP lower than 140 mmHg. The "median pressure" group (n= 36) is formed by 49.3 % of the rats with a BP between 140 and 155 mm Hg and the "high pressure" group (n= 19) included 26 % of the rats having a BP higher than 155 mm Hg. Mean heart weight and heart weight on body weight ratio were significantly higher in the "high pressure" group compared to the "low pressure" group confirming the role of high blood pressure level on the development of hypertrophy (table 1). Nevertheless, the relative heart weights were not closely related to mean blood pressure in the male F2 population, although a weak significantly positive correlation was obtained ($r=0.319, P=0.006, n=73$).

Table 1
Biological characteristics of male SHR, WKY, F1 and F2 rats.

	Blood pressure	Body weight (g)	Heart weight (mg)	HW/BW (mg/g)	n
WKY	120.6±2.2	445.9 ±14.7	1085 ±55	2.41 ±0.04	8
SHR	173.9 ±3.1	304 8 ±8.5	957 ±29	3.13 ±0.04	8
F1	151.5 ±2.7	383.3 ±6.7	1047 ±15	2.73 ±0.02	15
F2 "LP"	131.8 ±0.9	421.6 ± 9.5	1053 ±23	2.50 ±0.04	18
F2 "HP"	163.2 ±2.0***	429.8 ± 8.6	1143 ±31*	2.66 ±0.05**	19

Skin fibroblasts were cultured from 21 rats belonging to the "low" and the "high pressure" groups. Their growth rates were studied both by cell counting and by cell DNA content determination. A high degree of correlation was observed between the values obtained with these two methods ($r=0.903, P<0.001, n=21$). The distribution of the values in the "low pressure" group did not differ from that in the "high pressure" group, as is the case for the means (Table 2). Since in newborn rat fibroblasts, EGF stimulates DNA synthesis much greater in SHR than in WKY strains (Guicheney et al, 1990), we studied the effects of added EGF upon 3H thymidine incorporation in F2 fibroblasts. The percentages of stimulation were similar between the two groups (F2"LP": 332 ±36 over basal and F2"HP": 267 ±26 %).

Table 2
DNA doubling times of WKY, SHR, F1 and F2 fibroblasts
(* p= 0.002, SHR versus WKY, Student's t test)

	x ± SEM	n
SHR	37.2 ± 2,3 *	8
WKY	53.9 ± 3.6	6
F1	44.4 ± 5.3	9
F2 "LP"	47.5 ± 4.1	11
F2 "HP"	44.6 ± 3.2	10

We also tested whether cell growth correlated with the cardiac hypertrophy within individual rat of the F2 generation. For the whole F2 rats and for the "high pressure" group there was no correlation between DNA doubling times and the relative heart weights. In contrast, for the "low pressure" group, cardiac hypertrophy tends to be associated with shorter doubling times, although the correlation was only of borderline significance ($r= 0.546, p= 0.079, n= 11$).

DISCUSSION

We previously observed that cultured skin fibroblasts from SHR exhibited an enhanced growth rate in presence of 10 % fetal calf serum and an higher sensitivity to EGF compared to WKY rat fibroblasts (Guicheney et al, 1991). Comparable observations have been reported for vascular smooth muscle cells derived from aorta of these rats (Yamori et al 1981, Scott-Burden et al 1989 Baudouin-Legros et al 1990). In addition, cardiac, renal and vascular polyploidy and/or hypertrophy have been reported in various strains of genetically hypertensive rats at birth and even in utero (Gray 1984, Kunes et al 1987, Eccleston-Joyner & Gray 1988). This enhance proliferation capacity may be a genetic trait of these strains responsible for cardiovascular enlargement but its role as causing factor in blood pressure increase has not been clearly demonstrated in SHR.

An enhanced growth and reactivity to serum of adult and newborn SHR fibroblasts compared to WKY ones has been observed. The scope of this study was to determine whether this genetically inherited growth capacity is responsible for differences in blood pressure since genetic differences between SHR and control rats may be due to a genetic drift unrelated to high blood pressure. F2 rats were examined at four months of age. It appears clearly from our results that the enhanced fibroblast growth capacity is not associated with high blood pressure levels. The cell doubling times were identical in fibroblasts derived from the "low" or from the "high blood pressure" group. Similar results were obtained for reactivity to EGF. These results are in agreement with those of Mulvany who has studied media:lumen ratio of resistance vessels from SHR/WKY F2 populations; this author concluded that increased structure per se did not appear to be a major determinant of the blood pressure elevation (1988). In the F2 population, heart weights were not closely related to mean blood pressure as it has been previously noticed (Tanase et al.1982; Grassi de Gende,1988). Indeed it is established that the relative organ weights in hypertensive individuals reflect both the intrinsic organ growth capacity and the growth induced by deleterious effects of increased blood pressure. Relative organe weight in normotensive individuals preferentially reflects intrinsic organ growth capacity. In "low pressure" F2, cardiac hypertrophy tends to be negatively correlated with skin fibroblast doubling times. Similar measurements in newborn F2 rats without hypertension would allow to ascertain whether cardiac development in SHR and growth of skin fibroblasts in culture are controlled by the same genetic factors.

These observations suggest that the increased growth capacity observed in SHR does not play a determinant role in high blood pressure development. Nevertheless, it is possibly involved in the neonatal cardiac and vascular enlargement and, through the induction of irreversible vascular changes, it may play an important role in the maintenance of hypertension.

REFERENCES

Baudouin-Legros, M., Guicheney, P., Meyer, P. (1990): Enhanced cell proliferation in essential hypertension. J. Cardiov. Pharmacol. 16(suppl1): S1-S3.

Eccleston-Joyner, C.A., Gray, S.D. (1988): Arterial hypertrophy in the fetal and neonatal spontaneously hypertensive rat. Hypertension 12: 513-518.

Folkow, B. (1987): The structural cardiovascular factor in primary hypertension - pressure dependence and genetic reinforcement. J. Hypertens. 4 (suppl3): S51-S56.

Grassi de Gende, A.O. (1987): Evaluation of right and left ventricular size in SHR-Wistar hybrids. Am. J. Physiol.255: H587-H591.

Gray, S.D. (1984): Spontaneous hypertension in the neonatal rat. Clin. Exp. Hypertens.[A],6: 755-781.

Guicheney, P., Wauquier, I., Paquet, J.L., Meyer, P. (1991): Enhanced response to growth factors and to growth factors and to angiotensin II of spontaneously hypertensive rat skin fibroblasts in culture. J. Hypertens. 9: 23-27.

Kunes, J., Pang, S.C., Cantin, M., Genest, J., Hamet, P. (1987): Cardiac and renal hyperplasia in newborn spontaneously hypertensive rats. Clin. Sci. 72: 271-275.

Lever, A.F. (1986): Slow pressor mechanisms in hypertension: a role for hypertrophy of resistance vessels. J. Hypertens. 4: 515-524.

Mulvany, M.J. (1988): Resistance vessel structure and function in the etiology of hypertension studied in F2-generation hypertensive-normotensive rats. J. Hypertens. 6: 655-663.

Rapp, J.P. (1983): A paradigm for identification of primary genetic causes of hypertension in rats. Hypertension 5 (suppl 1): I-198-I-203.

Scott Burden, T., Resink, T.J., Baur, U, Bürgin, M., Bühler, F.R. (1989): Epidermal growth factor responsiveness in smooth muscle cells from hypertensive and normotensive rats. Hypertension 13: 295-304.

Tanase, H., Yamori, Y., Hansen, C.T., Lovenberg, W. (1982): Heart size in inbred strains of rats. Part 1. genetic determination of the development of cardiovascular enlargement in rats. Hypertension 4: 864-872.

Yamori, Y., Igawa, T., Kanbe, T., Kihara, M., Nara, Y., Horie, R. (1981): Mechanisms of structural vascular changes in genetic hypertension: analysis on cultured vascular smooth muscle cells from spontaneously hypertensive rats. Clin. Sci. 61: 121s-123s.

Participation of proteolysis and transforming growth factor β_1 activation in growth of cultured vascular smooth muscle cells from spontaneously hypertensive rats

Noboru Fukuda, Johanne Tremblay and Pavel Hamet

Centre de Recherche Hôtel-Dieu de Montréal, Université de Montréal, Pavillon Marie-de-la-Ferre, 3850, rue Saint-Urbain, Montréal H2W 1T8, Québec, Canada

SUMMARY Transforming growth factor-ß1 (TGFß$_1$) is a bifunctional growth factor which we have previously shown to be increasingly expressed in vascular smooth muscle cells (VSMC) from spontaneously hypertensive rats (SHR). The present study demonstrates TGFß$_1$ proteosynthesis in VSMC. TGFß$_1$ activation by plasmin as well as the growth inhibitory effect of proteinase inhibitors support the possibility that in SHR VSMC, TGFß$_1$ is present in an active form. The implication of TGFß$_1$ in enhanced VSMC growth in SHR is confirmed by the inhibitory effect of the antisense oligonucleotide to TGFß$_1$. Increased TGFß$_1$ expression and activation are potentially associated with augmented SHR VSMC proliferation.

INTRODUCTION It has been demonstrated that proliferation of cultured vascular smooth muscle cells (VSMC) from spontaneously hypertensive rats (SHR) is increased in response to growth factors (Hamet et al. 1988, Hadrava et al, 1989). We recently reported that the accumulation of transforming growth factor-ß$_1$ (TGFß$_1$) mRNA in SHR VSMC is higher than in cells from normotensive Wistar Kyoto (WKY) rats, and DNA synthesis is enhanced in response to exogenous TGFß$_1$ in SHR at a high cell density without any effect in WKY rats (Hamet et al. 1991). TGFß is usually secreted in culture in a biologically latent form (Sporn et al. 1987, Miyazono et al. 1988), which can be activated by proteolytic processes (Lyons et al. 1988, Sato et al. 1990). There has been no report of TGFß synthesis in VSMC. The present study was designed to investigate TGFß$_1$ peptide synthesis in VSMC, and to evaluate the role of endogenous TGFß$_1$ in VSMC SHR growth, employing proteinase as TGFß activator, proteinase inhibitors and the antisense oligonucleotide of TGFß$_1$.

METHODS Cultured VSMC were obtained by the explant method from the thoracic aortae of male WKY rats and SHR (Charles River, Canada). The cells were characterized as described previously (Hadrava et al. 1989), and were used between 8-18 passages. The VSMC were made quiescent by incubation in Dulbecco's modified Eagle medium (DMEM) with insulin, transferrin, and selenium for 48-72 hours. Immunoprecipitation of ^{35}S-cysteine labelled TGFß$_1$ in VSMC was performed by incubation with [^{35}S]cysteine in cysteine-free DMEM for 20 hours. The medium and acid-ethanol extract of cells were precipitated with rabbit serum (Gibco Labs., Burlington, Ontario, Canada) and Staphylococcus aureus (Bethesda Research Laboratory, Gaithersburg, MD, USA), after which the samples were incubated with rabbit anti-human TGFß$_1$ (R and D System, Minneapolis, Minn., USA). The immunoreactive TGFß$_1$ was subjected to electrophoresis. DNA synthesis in VSMC was determined by [^{3}H]thymidine incorporation into newly-synthesized DNA of quiescent VSMC. VSMC conditioned medium from WKY rats or SHR with serum-free DMEM was treated with plasmin to activate endogenous TGFß$_1$. The treated, conditioned medium was then added to VSMC from WKY rats and SHR for the bioassay of TGFß$_1$ production. The reaction was stopped by the addition of a proteinase inhibitor, aprotinin. Sense (CCC ATG CCG CCC TCG GGG) and antisense (CCC CGA GGG CGG CAT GGG) oligonucleotides selected from cDNA of rat TGFß$_1$ spanning the initial codon were kindly provided by Dr. Francis Gossard of the Biotechnology Research Institute, Montreal, Canada.

RESULTS The immunoprecipitation of ^{35}S-cysteine labelled VSMC and medium with an antibody to TGFß$_1$ indicated that TGFß$_1$ is synthesized and secreted from aortic smooth muscle cells in culture (data not shown). Plasmin, known to activate the latent form of TGFß, significantly ($p < 0.05$) inhibited DNA synthesis in VSMC at a low cell density (5×10^3 cells/cm^2), and significantly ($p < 0.01$) increased it at a high cell density (10^5 cells/cm^2). The addition of increasing doses of plasmin to VSMC from WKY and SHR produced a biphasic response of [^{3}H]thymidine incorporation (Figure 1A). SHR VSMC grew faster than cells from WKY rats after plasmin stimulation in the presence of 0.2% calf serum at a high cell density (Figure 1A). The fold stimulation of DNA synthesis by plasmin (0.1 U/ml) was, however, significantly ($p < 0.01$) greater in WKY (4.3-fold) than in SHR cells (1.9-fold). The addition of higher concentrations (5 or 10%) of calf serum diminished the difference in plasmin-induced DNA synthesis between both strains. The VSMC-conditioned medium from SHR VSMC significantly ($p < 0.05$) increased DNA synthesis in cells from WKY rats but not from SHR (not shown). The proteinase inhibitors, aprotinin, calpastatin and leupeptin (Figure 1B), significantly inhibited DNA synthesis in VSMC from SHR but not from WKY rats.

Three μM of antisense oligonucleotide to TGFß$_1$ significantly ($p < 0.01$) suppressed DNA synthesis in VSMC from both strains at a high cell density. These decreases in DNA synthesis by the antisense oligonucleotide were greater in SHR than in WKY cells compared to sense oligonucleotide as a control (Table 1).

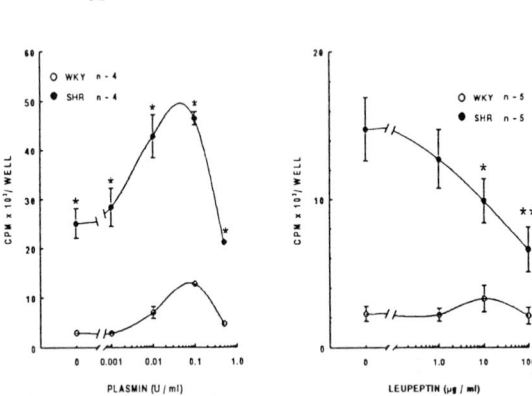

Figure 1. Panel A.
Effects of plasmin on DNA synthesis in VSMC (from WKY and SHR) at a high cell density.
*: $p < 0.01$ vs WKY rats

Figure 1. Panel B.
Effects of leupeptin on DNA synthesis in VSMC (from WKY and SHR) at a high cell density.
*: $p < 0.05$; **: $p < 0.01$ vs values at 0 ng/ml.

Table 1. Effect of antisense oligonucleotide to TGFß$_1$ on DNA synthesis in VSMC from WKY rats and SHR.

		[^{3}H]thymidine incorporation CPM x 10^3 /WELL		
Oligonucleotide	n	WKY rats	n	SHR
Sense	5	5361 ± 269	5	14359 ± 464
Antisense	5	4143 ± 266*	5	8708 ± 1907*

Values are means ± SE. *: $p < 0.01$ vs sense oligonucleotide.

DISCUSSION The role of endogenous TGFß$_1$ in the growth of SHR VSMC has not yet been well determined. The present experiment revealed that TGFß$_1$ is synthesized in VSMC and suggests an autocrine effect on VSMC growth. There is evidence that rapidly growing, transformed cells exhibit high proteolytic activity (Laiho and Keski-Oja, 1989). In this study, the fold stimulation of DNA synthesis by plasmin was greater in WKY rats than in SHR, despite the faster growth of SHR VSMC. Our interpretation of the biphasic curve seen in Figure 1A is that its upward portion is related to the activation of endogenous TGFß$_1$, while at the highest dose, proteolytic activity leads to cell disruption, as confirmed by morphological observations (data not shown). In addition, several proteinase inhibitors suppressed DNA synthesis in VSMC from SHR but not from WKY rats. These findings indicate that VSMC from SHR have higher endogenous proteolytic activity under basal conditions, which may activate TGFß$_1$. On the other hand, the VSMC-conditioned medium from SHR but not from WKY rats increased DNA synthesis, suggesting that SHR VSMC produce a larger amount of TGFß, including latent and mature forms. This observation extends our previous data on elevated mRNA accumulation TGFß$_1$ in VSMC from SHR (Hamet et al. 1991). It can be concluded from our results with antisense oligonucleotide to TGFß$_1$ that the higher proteolytic activity in SHR VSMC may lead to increased TGFß$_1$ activation potentially associated with enhanced SHR VSMC proliferation.

ACKNOWLEDGEMENTS These studies were suppored by a grant from the Medical Research Council of Canada (MA-10803). Noboru Fukuda is a fellow from the Heart and Stroke Foundation of Canada and Johanne Tremblay is a scholar from Fonds de Recherche en Santé du Québec. The authors thank Monique Poirier and Carole Long for their technical assistance throughout these investigations, Louise Chevrefils for preparing and Ovid Da Silva for editing this manuscript.

REFERENCES

Hadrava, V., Tremblay, J., Hamet, P.: Abnormalities in growth characteristics of aortic smooth muscle cells in spontaneously hypertensive rats. Hypertension 1989;13:589-597

Hamet, P., Hadrava, V., Kruppa, U., Tremblay, J.: Vascular smooth muscle cell hyper-responsiveness to growth factors in hypertension. J. Hypertens. 1988;6(suppl. 4):S36-S39

Hamet, P., Hadrava, V., Kruppa, U., Tremblay, J.: Transforming growth factor ß1 expression and effect in aortic smooth muscle cells from spontaneously hypertensive rats. Hypertension 1991;17:896-901

Laiho, M., Keski-Oja, J.: Growth factors in the regulation of pericellular proteolysis: A review. Cancer Res. 1989;49:2533-2553

Lyons, R.M., Keski-Oja, J., Moses, H.L.: Proteolytic activation of latent transforming growth factor-ß from fibroblast-conditioned medium. J. Cell Biol. 1988;106:1659-1665

Miyazono, K., Hellman, U., Wernstedt, C., Heldin, C.: Latent high molecular weight complex of transforming growth factor ß1; Purification from human platelets and structural characterization. J. Biol. Chem. 1988;263:7646-7654

Sato, Y., Lyons, T.R., Moses, H., Rifkin, B.: Characterization of activation of latent TGFß by co-culture of endothelial cells and pericytes or smooth muscle cells. A self-regulating system. J. Cell Biol. 1990;111:757-763

Sporn, M.B., Roberts A.B., Wakefield, L.M., de Crombrugghe, B.: Some recent advances in the chemistry and biology of transforming growth factor-ß. J. Cell Biol. 1987;105:1039-1045

Heart and vessels

Cœur et vaisseaux

Mechanical and contractile properties of *in situ* isolated mesenteric artery in normotensive (WKY) and spontaneously hypertensive rats (SHR)

Hong Y. Qiu, Bruno Valtier, Harry A.J. Struyker-Boudier and Bernard I. Lévy

INSERM U.141, Hôpital Lariboisière, 75010 Paris, France

Summary

Mesenteric artery was studied in situ in 22 twelve-week-old WKY rats and 22 age matched SHRs. A segment of mesenteric artery (external diameter 450-550 µm) was exposed for video-microscopic measurement. The diameter was measured under basal, active (phenylephrine 10^{-6} M) and passive (potassium cyanide 0.1mg/ml) smooth muscle conditions for transmural pressures ranging from 0-200 mmHg. After the experiment, the artery was fixed and the wall cross sectional area was measured in transverse sections (19.1 ± 0.3 10^3 µm^2 and 14.6 ± 0.2 10^3 µm^2 in SHRs and in WKY rats respectively, p<0.001). From diameter, pressure, and wall thickness values, mesenteric compliances (µl/mmHg), distensibilities (mmHg^{-1}), wall tensions (N/m) and wall stresses (kPa) were calculated under basal, active and passive conditions. Active tension and active stress were defined as differences in wall stresses and wall tensions calculated under passive and active conditions. Comparative studies of WKY rats and SHRs when arteries were studied at the respective operating pressures indicate: 1) stiffer mesenteric arteries in SHRs than in WKY rats, 2) similar wall stresses in mesenteric arteries from WKY and SHRs despite larger wall tensions in the hypertensive group, 3) the reactivity to phenylephrine, larger in SHRs than in WKY mesenteric arteries, could be primarily related to the enhanced sensitivity of the SHR's smooth cells and less to the increased smooth muscle mass in the arterial wall from the hypertensive rats.

Introduction

Hypertension is associated with structural and functional abnormalitie of the small arteries. The mechanical properties of these small arteries were studied and the pressure-diameter relation were determined using myograph mounted rings of arteries (Mulvany MJ et al., 1976; 1978) or " in vitro" cannulation segments methods (Halpern W. and Kelly M.,1991). However, the " in vitro" methods have some disadvantages, especially, the longitudinal stress of the studied arteries is not kept at its "in vivo" value, and whatever the skilfulness of the experimentator, the excision procedure of the studied segment of artery cannot be atraumatic. We have developed an experimental model of "in situ" isolated rat mesenteric artery to determine the pressure-diameter relation in more physiological and potentially less traumatic conditions.

Methods

Experimental model:

After anesthesia with intraperitoneal sodium pentobarbital (50mg/kg), a median laparotomy was performed and the last loop of small intestine was exposed on a laboratory-built plastic container

including an optical glass parallelepiped. The preparation was immediately irrigated by a buffered Tyrode's solution (pH = 7.4) maintained at 38°C. The mesenteric arteries and arcades were neither fixed nor stretched. A short segment of mesenteric artery (about 3 mm) of a second generation branch (diameter 450-550 μm) was gently dissected. A video camera was mounted on the binocular lens and allowed to record video images. The final magnification of the system was x100. Every arterial branch located downstream of the observed segment of artery except one was then ligated with silk thread 9/0. A removable micro-clamp was placed on the last branch.
Finally, a polyethylene catheter was introduced into the first generation branch of the mesenteric artery. This catheter was filled with Tyrode's albumin (4%) solution and connected to a manometer with adjustable pressure levels. After removing the clamp from the distal segment of the mesenteric artery, the observed mesenteric artery was filled with the flushing solution.
The segment of isolated artery was submitted to study steady pressures ranging from 0 to 200 mmHg per steps of 25 mmHg. The external diameter of the artery was measured at each pressure step.
The mean arterial pressure was continuously recorded from the right carotid.

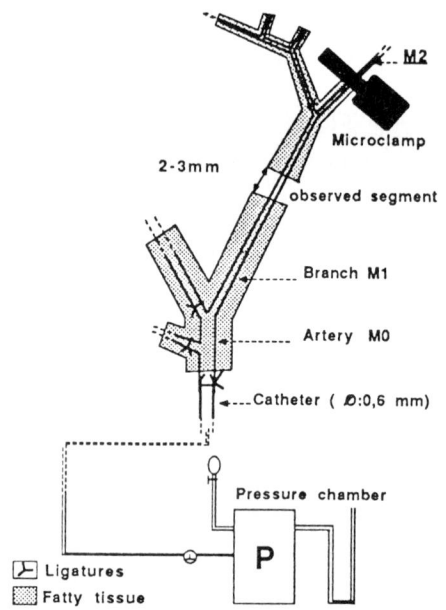

2) <u>Experimental protocol</u>:

Experiments were performed under <u>basal conditions</u>, under <u>active smooth muscle conditions</u> (phenylephrine 10^{-6} M) and under <u>passive smooth muscle conditions</u> (potassium cyanide 0.1mg/ml). At the end of every experiment, the mesenteric artery was fixed with a solution containing glutaraldehyde (2.5%) buffered with sodium cacodylate (0.1M) and paraformaldehyde (2%). The wall vessel cross sectional area was determined in transverse sections.

3) <u>Calculation of mechanical parameters</u>:

Using the measured values of the "in situ" arterial external diameter (D_e, μm) from 0 to 200 mmHg and the wall cross sectional area (CSA, μm^2) measured after the experiment, several parameters were calculated: 1) Wall thickness (h, μm): $h = CSA / \pi \cdot D_e$, 2) internal diameter (Di, μm) $Di = De - 2.h$, 3) vessel volume (Vi, μl): $Vi = \pi \cdot D_i^2 / 4$, 4) compliance per unit length (C, μl/mmHg. mm) of the observed segment of mesenteric artery was defined, for each pressure step, as: $C = \Delta V/\Delta P$, where ΔV is the volume change induced by a transmural pressure variation ΔP (25mmHg) in a segment of 1 mm length of the artery, 5) vessel distensibility (Dist, 10 mmHg^{-1}) was defined, as the Compliance (C) divided by the initial internal volume: $Dist = C / Vi$, 6) tangential wall tension (T, N/m): $T = P \cdot D_i/2$, 7) tangential wall stress (s, kPa): $s = T/h$. The active wall stress was calculated as the difference in wall stress calculated, at a given pressure, under active and passive conditions. Similarly, active wall tension was calculated from active and passive wall tension values.

Results (mean±SEM)	Mean Arterial Pressure (mmHg)	Heart Rate (beats/minute)	Body weight (g)	Cross Sectional Area (μm2)
SHR(n=22)	154+15	394±12	288+12	19033±342
WKY(n=22)	104+11	354±3	320+15	14563±208

Table 1 summarizes the results of mean arterial pressure, heart rate, body weight, and cross sectional area obtained in SHRs and WKY rats.

	WKY (P=100 mm Hg)			SHR (P=150 mm Hg)		
	Basal	Phenylephrine	KCN	Basal	Phenylephrine	KCN
xtern Diameter	490±13	466±21	503±21	571±11	526±23	581±11
ompliance	897±195	531±168	383±87	219±83	529±130	149±66
stensibility	4.75±1.03	3.59±1.33	2.16±0.45	0.85±0.4	2.61±0.76	0.63±0.29
all tension	3.36±0.08	2.97±.14	3.26±.14	5.41±0.11	4.52±0.56	5.63±0.13
all Stress	260±18	303±22	357±28	311±17	431±68	548±38
tive Tension			0.26±0.06			0.55±14
tive Stress			54.4±13.			102±28

Table II summarizes the mesenteric arterial diameters and the mecanical parameters measured and calculated at the mean operating pressure under basal, active and passive conditions. The mean operating pressure is defined as the mean arterial pressure of the animals (roughly 100 mmHg in WKY and 150 mmHg in SHR).

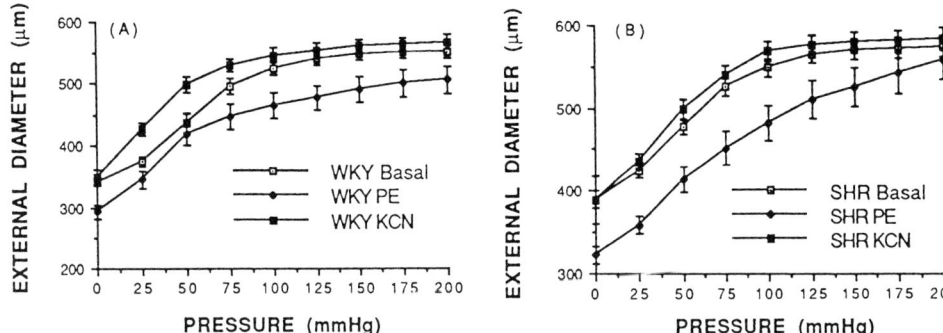

Fig1 shows the diameter-pressure relations in WKY (A) and SHR (B) under basal, active (PE), and passive (KCN) smooth muscle conditions. At low pressure, the vessels exhibited large changes in diameters with each step change in pressure, whereas at high pressure, diameter changes per pressure increase were minor.

Conclusion

In conclusion, the present method for studying the mechanical properties, the reactivity and the sensitivity of the in situ localized mesenteric artery (400-550 μm) offers a new possibility to explore the behavior of small arteries in the intact rat. This "in situ" method provides results markedly different of those obtained from "in vitro" myograph mounted arteries. Comparative studies of normotensive WKY rats and SHRs indicate 1) stiffer arteries in SHRs than in WKY rats when mechanical properties were compared at their respective physiological operating pressure values, 2) an increase in tangential forces measured at physiological operating pressure values in arteries from the hypertensive strain, 3) similar wall stress (forces normalized by the wall thickness) in both normotensive and hypertensive rats despite large differences in operating arterial pressure.

References

Halpern, W., Kelly, M. (1991): In vitro methodology for resistance arteries. Blood Vessels. 28: 245-251.

Mulvany, M.J., Halpern, W., (1976): Mechanical properties of vascular smooth muscle cell in situ. Nature Lond. 260: 617-619.

Mulvany, M.J., Hansen, P.K., Aalkjaer, C. (1978) Direct evidence that the greater contratility of resistance vessels in spontaneously hypertensive rats is associated with a narrowed lumen, a thickened media, and an increased number of smooth muscle cell layers. Cir Res. 43: 845-864.

Sympatho-adrenal system and development of cardiac and vascular amplifier properties in SHR

P.I. Korner, A. Bobik, C. Oddie and P. Friberg

Baker Medical Research Institute and Alfred Hospital, Melbourne, Australia

Medial hypertrophy of the resistance vessels, in conjunction with narrowing of the lumen, play an important role in the 'amplified' resistance responses of the hypertensive circulation (Folkow, 1982). In addition, the concentrically hypertrophied left ventricle (LV) amplifies stroke volume volume and cardiac output (Broughton & Korner, 1986). Together, the cardiovascular amplifiers contribute to the maintenance of the elevated blood pressure (BP) and, in SHR, they may be important in the initiation of hypertension (Adams et al, 1989).

In previous studies of the sympathetic neural ablation in SHR, using antinerve growth factor antibody (ANGFA) plus guanethidine, the hypertension was attenuated but not completely prevented (Lee et al, 1987). The regime destroys sympathetic nerves, but leaves intact the adrenal medullary catecholamines, which could affect the hypersensitive heart and vasculature. Since cardiac hypertrophy was not prevented in the previous study, we added a period of treatment with prazosin to the immuno–chemical sympathectomy regime. In tissue culture catecholamines promote myocardial hypertrophy through α–adrenoceptor stimulation (Simpson, 1985) and we wished to determine whether prazosin prevented both LV and vascular hypertrophy *in vivo*.

METHODS.

Series 1 was performed to test the effects on vascular amplifier properties and LV hypertrophy at 4 weeks of age. There were 3 groups of rats:– 1) Control SHR (n=13) and WKY (n=17), which received no treatment except vehicle injections, at the same times as the other groups. 2) Sympathectomy Only (Sx) SHR (n=6) and WKY (n=6), which were given ANGFA from day 2 of age (d2) to d7 (50–150μl), followed by intraperitoneal (i.p.) injections of guanethidine monosulfate (50 mg/kg/d) from d8 to the end of wk4. 3) Sympathectomy + prazosin (Sxp) SHR (n=6) and WKY (n=6), which received the same regime as Sx rats, plus prazosin HCl (0.25 μg/kg/d, i.p.) from d8 to wk4. At the end of 4 weeks, measurements were made of the animals' body weight (BW), LV/BW ratio and of the resistance properties of the isolated hindquarters (HQ) (Adams et al, 1989). In addition, tissue norepinephrine concentration [NE] was measured in LV, kidney, forelimb muscle and adrenal gland (Adams et al, 1989). In 15 SHR (n=15) treated with Sx, tissue [NE] was determined until the age of 50 weeks. Because the results suggested significant re–innervation (Bobik, Korner & Oddie, unpublished data), we modified the ANGFA + guanethidine regime in Series 2.

Series 2 consisted of:– 1) Untreated control SHR and WKY rats [SHR$_c$ (n=20) and WKY$_c$ (n=20)]; 2) Sympathectomized + prazosin treated SHR and WKY [SHR$_{sxp}$ n=16) and WKY$_{sxp}$ (n=2), that had received ANGFA from d2–d7, followed by guanethidine (50 mg/kg/d, i.p.), from d8 to wk8 and by prazosin (0.125 μg/kd/d, i.p) from wk3–wk6. In these animals BW and tail cuff systolic BP were measured every week, starting from 4 wk. At 21 and 35 wk, we determined LV/BW ratio and HQ resistance properties.

The methodology, including that for measuring [NE], was similar to that of Adams et al (1989). For HQ perfusion we used 1.5% dextran T-70 (Pharmacia, Sweden) in Tyrodes solution (123 mM NaCl, 4.3 mM KCl, 0.83 mM $MgCl_2.6H_2O$, 0.5 mM $NaH_2PO_4.2H_2O$, 25 mM $NaHCO_3$, 5.55 mM d–glucose, 2.5 mM $CaCl_2.2H_2O$) aerated with 95% O_2 + 5% CO_2. In series 1, we determined the perfusion pressure (PP) at full dilatation at flows of 5, 10 and 15 ml/min/100 g HQ weight. Following this we determined PP at maximum constriction (PP_{max}), using injections of methoxamine, plus boluses of angiotensin II (AngII) and vasopressin. In series 2, full sigmoidal log dose methoxamine - resistance responses curves were obtained during constant flow perfusion at 10 ml/min/100 g HQ; from these we determined PP (i.e. vascular resistance) at full dilatation (PP_{min}), PP_{max}, average slope and ED_{50} (Adams et al, 1989).

RESULTS

Series 1.
At 4 wk, the BW of untreated rats (75.4 ± 2.1 g) was greater than in Sx rats (60.2 ± 3.1 g) and in Sxp rats (48 ± 2.6 g) (P for diff < 0.0001). In each group, BW of SHR and WKY rats were similar. Denervation was satisfactory in both Sx and Sxp groups, with [NE] in LV, kidney ranging from 1–10% of values in untreated controls. The important finding was that in Sx and Sxp rats, adrenal [NE] was greatly raised, with concentrations, respectively, 48% and 98% above corresponding controls.

In young rats, from 40–200 g, LV/BW ratio falls steeply as BW increases. For any given BW, LV/BW ratio is higher in SHR than in WKY, with the regression lines parallel in the two strains. In each strain, the observed LV/BW ratio was compared with the expected ratio from regression functions calculated from the LV/BW–BW relationship, obtained from an earlier series. Expressing observed LV/BW ratio as a percentage of expected (=100%) and determining SEM by 1–way ANOVA, LV/BW ratios were:– 1) *Control rats*: SHR 101 ± 2.5%, WKY 100 ± 2.5%; 2) *Sx rats*: SHR 104 ± 2.5%, WKY 99 ± 2.5%; 3) *Sxp rats*:– SHR 93 ± 2.5% , WKY 109 ± 2.5%. In SHR_{sxp} animals, LV/BW ratio was thus smaller than expected (P ≤ 0.05), suggesting that the addition of prazosin had prevented development of LV hypertrophy in SHR. Moreover, comparison with the Sx group suggests that following sympathetic denervation, the increase in adrenal catecholamines maintains LV hypertrophy in SHR.

During full dilatation of the HQ vessels there is a linear relationship between PP and flow, with the regression lines parallel in SHR and WKY (Adams et al, 1989). For a given flow, PP was significantly higher in SHR than in WKY, with the intercept differences at flow of 10 ml/min/100g averaging:– 4.9 ± 0.9 mmHg (*control rats*), 7.9 ± 1.7 mmHg (*Sx rats*) and 2.5 ± 1.1 mmHg (*Sxp rats*). Thus, in Sxp rats the between–strain difference in PP was reduced compared with control rats (P= 0.05). However, in Sx rats, where adrenal catecholamines were increased, the between–strain difference was somewhat greater than in controls.

PP_{max} was higher (P < 0.01) in SHR than in WKY in all 3 groups. the values in the 3 groups were (in mmHg):– *Controls*— SHR 204, WKY 174; *Sx rats*:– SHR 220, WKY 196; *Sxp rats*— SHR 189, WKY 167. Thus, the between strain difference was not affected by any of the treatments. However in Sxp rats, PP_{max} was lower in both strains compared with corresponding values in the other two groups.

Series 2.
In the control group, the BW at a given age was less in SHR_c than in WKY_c, with the difference in plateaus of the growth curve, averaging ≃ 12%. In young SHR_{sxp}, BW was lower than in SHR_c, though the difference was less than in series 1, probably due to the lower dose of prazosin. By 12 wk of age, the growth rates of SHR_{sxp} and SHR_c was identical.

In control rats (SHR_c and WKY_c), BP increased progressively from 4 to 35 weeks, as did the difference between strains:— *4 weeks:*— SHR$_c$ 127, WKY$_c$ 109, Δ=4.9 ± 2.2 mmHg; *21 weeks:*— SHR$_c$ 188, WKY$_c$ 123, Δ= 45.4 ± 4.6 mmHg; *35 weeks:*— SHR$_c$ 196, WKY$_c$ 138, Δ = 58 ± 5.2 mmHg. Thus, in the SHR$_{sxp}$ group, hypertension was completely prevented. Indeed, before age 21 wk, their BP was below that of WKY$_c$ rats, with values at age 4, 21 and 35 wk averaging 109, 128 and 138 mmHg. In WKY$_{sxp}$ rats, BP stayed close to values of WKY$_c$ rats over the period at which observations were made, from 4–21 wk.

The Sxp regime prevented development of LV hypertrophy in SHR. The average LV/BW ratios at 21 and 35 weeks in controls were:— SHR$_c$ 3.1 ± 0.06, WKY$_c$ 2.3. In SHR$_{sxp}$ and WKY$_{sxp}$ the ratios were 2.3 ± 0.04 and 2.3. In the control groups, resistance properties showed the usual between–strain differences, with SHR$_c$ having greater PP$_{min}$, PP$_{max}$ and average slope than WKY$_c$. In SHR$_{sxp}$ the between–strain difference compared to WKY$_c$ and WKY$_{sxp}$ was reduced rather than abolished.

Sxp treatment produced marked and prolonged depletion of tissue [NE], with values at 21 and 35 weeks ranging from 4–8% of controls in LV, kidney and skeletal muscle. In SHR$_{sxp}$, adrenal [NE] was approximately 100% above controls at 21 wk, similar to the 4 wk findings. However, at 35 wk it had returned to control level (SHR$_c$).

DISCUSSION.

Immuno–chemical sympathectomy plus α–adrenergic blockade with prazosin, completely prevented the development of hypertension, in contrast to previous studies where the effects of the adrenal catecholamines could influence cardiovascular function (Lee et al, 1987). The earlier studies had shown that Sx prevented the development of structural changes in the mesenteric resistance vasculature, but that cardiac hypertrophy was unaffected. It follows that the prevention of LV hypertrophy in the present study by a relatively brief period of prazosin treatment, must have been an important factor in the complete suppression of hypertension in the SHR$_{sxp}$ group. The present findings suggest that trophic effects of catecholamines mediated through α–adrenoceptors have a specific action in the development of LV hypertrophy in SHR. This is the first *in vivo* demonstration of such an effect, though this has previously been demonstrated in tissue culture (Simpson,1987). The between strain difference in PP$_{min}$ was reduced by Sxp treatment, but somewhat enhanced in the presence of elevated adrenal [NE] in the Sx group. This suggests that α–adrenoceptor–mediated sympathetic effects may also affect vascular changes. The present findings support the hypothesis that both LV hypertrophy and vascular hypertrophy are necessary for the development of hypertension in SHR.

References.

Adams, M., Bobik, A. and Korner, P.I. (1989): Differential development of vascular and cardiac hypertrophy in genetic hypertension. Hypertension 14: 191–202.
Broughton, A. and Korner, P.I. (1986): Left ventricular pump function in renal hypertensive dogs with cardiac hypertrophy. Am.J.Physiol. 251: H1260–H1266.
Folkow, B. (1982): Physiological aspects of primary hypertension. Physiol.Rev. 62: 347–504.
Lee, R.M.K.W., Triggle, C.R., Cheung, D.W.T. and Coughlin M.D. (1987): Structural and functional consequences of neonatal sympathectomy on blood vessels of spontaneously hypertensive rats. Hypertension 10: 328–338.
Simpson, P. (1985): Stimulation of hypertrophy of cultured neonatal rat heart cells through an $α_1$–adrenergic receptor and induction of beating through an $α_1$– and $β_1$– adrenergic receptor interaction. Circ.Res. 56: 884–894.

Acknowledgements.

The study was supported through grants from the National Heart Foundation of Australia, the National Health & Medical Research Council and the Alfred Hospital Research Fund. We are grateful to Peter Kanellakis for excellent technical assistance.

Sympathetic hyperinnervation of the coronary artery in the stroke-prone spontaneously hypertensive rat

Ryo Tabei, Mari Kondo, Tatsuhiko Miyazaki, Takashi Fujiwara *,
Miho Terada and Yukihiko Watanabe

Department of Pathology and Laboratory Animal Center *, Ehime University School of Medicine, Ehime 791-02, Japan

SUMMARY

The distribution of fluorescent adrenergic nerve fibers in coronary arteries was examined in stroke-prone spontaneously hypertensive rats (SHRSP) aged 10, 30, 60, 90 and 180 days, by the glyoxylic acid method. The results were compared with those in age-matched normotensive Wistar Kyoto (WKY) rats. The distribution pattern of fluorescent nerve fibers in the coronary arteries of both strain showed a constant meshwork pattern throughout the entire examination period. The distribution density of adrenergic nerve fibers in coronary arteries of SHRSP was significantly higher ($p<0.01$ and 0.05) than that of WKY rats at all ages studied. The difference in nerve fiber density between SHRSP and WKY rats reached a peak at 60 days of age and gradually decreased with age. The present study suggests that sympathetic hyperinnervation is an important factor in the development and maintenance of hypertension in SHRSP.

INTRODUCTION

Protein and catecholamine synthetic activities in the superior cervical and stellate sympathetic ganglia of the SHR have been shown to be greater than those in the WKY rat by light microscopic autoradiography (Kondo, 1986; 1987). However, there have been no data on the distribution density of sympathetic adrenergic fibers in the coronary arteries, the fibers of which are mainly derived from the stellate ganglion. In the present study, we aimed to confirm our previous results by examining the adrenergic innervation density in the coronary artery of SHRSP from the prehypertensive to the established hypertensive stages.

MATERIALS AND METHODS

The animals used in this study were 10, 30, 60, 90 and 180-day-old male SHRSP and age-matched WKY rats. Six animals of each age from both strains were anesthetized, perfused with 120 ml PBS followed by 150 ml of 2 per cent glyoxylic acid (Furness and Costa, 1975). After removing of coronary arteries, they were immersed in the same glyoxylic acid solution for 40 min at room temperature, stretched on nonfluorescent glass slides as whole mounts, and dried at room temperature for 20 min. These preparations were incubated at 100°C for 7 min and mounted with paraffin oil. Catecholamine fluorescent nerve fibers of the arteries were photographed at a magnification of x250 with a Zeiss photomicroscope. The distribution density of adrenergic nerve fibers of each coronary artery was measured by quantitative image analysis using VIDAS (Karl-Zeiss). Density of the fluorescent nerve fibers was expressed as the percentage of the area of a blood vessel occupied by fluorescent nerve fibers.

RESULTS

Perivascular nerve fibers exhibited a green fluorescence characteristic of noradrenaline (Kawai and Ohhashi,1986). Varicose adrenergic nerve fibers showed a constant meshwork pattern at all ages examined of both strains (Fig.1). The distribution density of adrenergic nerve fibers in SHRSP increased markedly until 60 days of age and decreased gradually thereafter. On the other hand, the nerve density in WKY rats continuously increased with age.

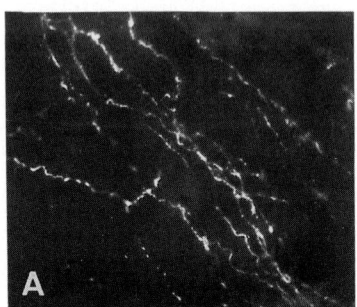 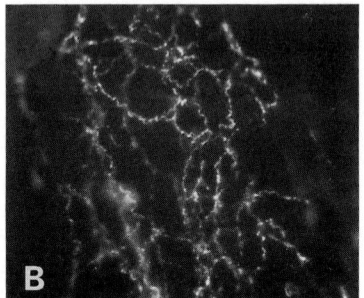

Fig. 1. Photomicrographs showing noradrenergic nerve fibers of the coronary arteries in 60-day-old WKY (**A**) rats and SHRSP (**B**).

Table 1. Distribution density of adrenergic nerve fibers in coronary arteries of SHRSP and WKY at various ages

Days after birth	SHRSP	WKY	1) difference
10	11.7±2.5*	8.4±1.1	X1.4
30	12.3±1.5**	7.5±1.4	X1.6
60	19.8±3.1**	11.5±1.7	X1.7
90	18.0±2.0**	13.2±1.0	X1.4
180	17.0 2.2*	13.7 1.7	X1.2

Values are means±SEM
 * $P<0.05$ compared with WKY
 ** $P<0.01$ compared with WKY
 1) These ratios obtained by dividing the values in SHRSP by those in WKY rats

The nerve fiber density of the coronary artery was significantly higher in SHRSP than age-matched WKY rats ($p<0.01$ and 0.05) at all ages examined (Table 1). The difference in the nerve density between SHRSP and WKY rats increased from 10 to 60 days after birth, reached a peak (x1.7) and then decreased.

DISCUSSION

The distribution density of perivascular sympathetic nerve fibers in SHR has been investigated in various peripheral arteries such as the mesenteric, jejunal, and caudal arteries at the prehypertensive, developing and established stages of hypertension by fluorescence and electron microscopy. In the present study, the density of adrenergic nerve fibers of the coronary arteries in SHRSP increased rapidly from 30 days to 60 days of age and decreased gradually thereafter, although those in WKY rats increased gradually with age as reported in normal rats (Amenta, 1988). Increased sympathetic innervation in the coronary arteries of SHRSP may reasonably be assumed to be caused by hyperfunction of the stellate ganglia (Kondo, 1986;1987). Sympathetic nerves are known to alter vascular smooth muscle cells, both through direct, rapid action and long-term regulatory and trophic effects (Bevan, 1984). Hyperinnervation by sympathetic nerves on the blood vessels in SHRSP during the prehypertensive stage, via a trophic effect, may cause a hypertrophy and/or hyperplasia of smooth muscle cells in the media. Our results suggest that vascular adrenergic sympathetic hyperinnervation is a primary factor in the development of hypertension and may also be involved in the maintenance of hypertension in SHRSP (Kawamura et al. 1989).

REFERENCES

Amenta, F., and Mione, M.C. (1988): Age-related changes in the noradrenergic innervation of the coronary arteries in old rats: a fluorescent histochemical study. J. Auton. Nerv. Syst. 22: 247-251.

Bevan, R.D. (1984): Trophic effects of peripheral adrenergic nerves on vascular structure. Hypertension (Suppl 3) 6: 19-26.

Furness, J.B., and Costa M. (1975): The use of glyoxylic acid for the fluorescence histochemical demonstration of peripheral stores of noradrenaline and 5-hydroxytryptamine in whole mounts. Histochemistry 41: 335-352.

Kawai, Y., and Ohhashi, T. (1986): Histochemical studies of the adrenergic innervation of canine cerebral arteries. J. Auton. Nerv. Syst. 15: 103-108.

Kawamura, K., Ando, K., and Takebayashi, S. (1989): Perivascular innervation of the mesenteric artery in spontaneously hypertensive rats. Hypertension 14: 660-665.

Kondo, M. (1986): Autoradiographic study of ^{3}H-lysine uptake by superior cervical and stellate ganglia in prehypertensive spontaneously hypertensive rats. Virchows Arch. B 52: 299-304.

Kondo, M. (1987): Autoradiographic study of ^{3}H-DOPA uptake by superior cervical and stellate ganglia of spontaneously hypertensive rats during the prehypertensive stage. Virchows Arch. B 54: 190-193.

Autoradiographic localization and quantitation of cardiac β-adrenoceptor subtypes in SHR

Roger J. Summers, Seigo Fujimoto, Helen Pak, Daen Soukseun and Peter Molenaar

Department of Pharmacology, University of Melbourne, Parkville, Victoria 3052, Australia

Development of hypertension with age in spontaneously hypertensive rats (SHR) is associated with increased sympathetic activity, cardiac hypertrophy and impaired responsiveness to β-adrenoceptor stimulation. Evidence for changes in cardiac β-adrenoceptors is controversial. In SHR with cardiac hypertrophy and heart failure (Yamada et al., 1984) or in 14 to 18 week old SHR (Bohm et al., 1988) a decrease in the number of myocardial β-adrenoceptors has been reported. However there are also reports of no change in β-adrenoceptors (Bhalla et al., 1980).

Many studies have shown (see Standen, 1978) that the sympathetic innervation to the rat heart is sparse at birth and develops rapidly over the first 4 to 5 weeks of the postnatal period. However the development of the nerves does not parallel that of the receptors which appear prior to the establishment of the innervation (Pappano, 1976). Thus, driven left atria from rats < 2 weeks of age show supersensitive inotropic responses to noradrenaline (Standen, 1978). Here we have utilized quantitative autoradiography to localize and delineate the β-adrenoceptor subtypes in a variety of cardiac regions in age matched WKY and SHR and determine how the receptors alter during development of hypertension.

Hearts were dissected from age matched WKY and SHR (24 days and 11 weeks old) so that the sections contained AV node (AVN), bundle of His (BH), left (LBB) and right bundle branch (RBB) as well as atrial (IAS) and ventricular myocardium (IVS) (Molenaar et al., 1990). The sectioning, mounting, pre-incubation, and labelling of the β-adrenoceptor subtypes with $(-)[^{125}I]$ CYP (50 pM) and CGP 20712A (100 nM; β_1-adrenoceptor selective or ICI 118551 (70 nM; β_2-adrenoceptor selective) were as described previously (Molenaar et al., 1990). After 14 days exposure film images were quantitated using the MCID system using ^{125}I standards in heart paste. Every 10th slide was stained with haematoxylin and eosin for histology. The density of β_1- and β_2-adrenoceptors was determined by the inhibition of $(-)[^{125}I]$ CYP binding by CGP 20712A (100 nM) and the calculations for determining the proportions of the β-adrenoceptor sybtypes (Molenaar et al., 1990).

Results are expressed as mean ± SEM. Statistical differences between groups was determined using Student's t-test.

Drugs used were (−)-CYP (Sandoz Basel, Switzerland); CGP 20712A (2-hydroxy-5[2-((2-hydroxy-3-(4-((1-methyl-4-trifluoromethyl] 1H-imidazole-2-yl)-phenoxy)propyl) amino)ethoxy)-benzamide monomethane sulphonate) (Ciba-Geigy AG, Basel, Switzerland); Sodium ^{125}I (Amersham Int, Bucks, UK); ICI 118551 [erythro-DL-1(7-methylindan-4-yl-oxy)-3-isopropylamino-butan-2-ol] (ICI, Wilmslow, Cheshire, UK); Guanosine triphosphate, Boehringer, Australia)

RESULTS

The density of β-adrenoceptors in the pacemaker and conducting tissues was higher than in myocardium in both WKY and SHR. The ratios in AVN, BH, LBB and RBB to those in IVS and IAS were 1.36-2.14 (IVS, 24d) and 1.73-2.78 (IVS, 11w) and 1.45-2.28 (IAS, 24d) and 1.52-2.55 (IAS, 11w). β-Adrenoceptor density decreased with age in all areas between 24 days and 11 weeks by 16.0-41.0% in WKY and by 25.3-41.3% in SHR (Table 1). At 24 days there was no significant difference in the β-adrenoceptor density in any of the areas studied although there was a tendency for the levels to be higher in WKY than SHR and in the pacemaker and conducting regions for there to be somewhat larger amounts of β_2-adrenoceptors in SHR which in LBB were significantly higher than in WKY (P<0.05). At 11 weeks of age the β-adrenoceptor density although lower in all areas still showed no significant differences between SHR and WKY except for BH where total β-adrenoceptor levels were higher in WKY. When the receptors were delineated into β_1- and β_2-adrenoceptor subtypes there was a tendency for an increase in β_2-adrenoceptors particularly in the pace-maker and conducting regions of SHR. Only in RBB were these significantly different (P<0.05). However, when the proportions of β-adrenoceptor subtypes are expressed as a percentage of the total β-adrenoceptor population, the 24 day old animals showed a mean β_2-adrenoceptor proportion which was higher in most areas of the pacemaker and conducting region and this was significant (P<0.05) for RBB (Figure 1). However no such differences were apparent for the myocardial areas (IVS, IAS). However by 11 weeks of age in all of the areas measured in the pace-maker and conducting regions the proportions of β_2-adrenoceptors were significantly higher whereas in the myocardial regions the differences were not significant (Figure 1).

	24 days			
	β_1-ar (a mole/mm^2)		β_2-ar (a mole/mm^2)	
	WKY	SHR	WKY	SHR
AV	86.7± 9.0	60.5±12.3	23.6± 3.5	23.8± 2.3
BH	50.2±11.7	51.1±14.9	23.9± 4.5	29.5± 2.0
LBB	42.5± 2.8	36.0±13.3	18.8± 3.2	37.0± 5.4*
RBB	54.2± 9.7	29.1± 7.9	27.6± 5.2	39.8± 2.3
IVS	32.3± 4.1	31.6± 4.4	9.7± 1.0	8.7± 1.1
IAS	33.5± 4.7	39.2± 4.8	8.9± 0.9	9.7± 0.7

	11 weeks			
	β_1-ar (a mole/mm^2)		β_2-ar (a mole/mm^2)	
	WKY	SHR	WKY	SHR
AV	46.0± 7.2	36.5± 4.9	22.2± 2.0	26.5± 3.1
BH	51.4± 8.8	21.2± 3.5*	21.6± 1.5	26.2± 2.1
LBB	34.4± 3.0	28.3±11.1	12.6± 3.6	25.0± 4.7
RBB	34.7± 2.8	32.3± 8.2	19.1± 1.7	29.7± 1.4*
IVS	20.9± 1.6	17.1± 1.9	6.4± 0.4	6.2± 0.6
IAS	22.2± 3.2	23.4± 2.4	6.2± 0.6	8.1± 1.1

Table 1. Comparison of β-adrenoceptor subtype concentrations in cardiac regions of WKY and SHR at 24 days and 11 weeks of age (n=3-6). AV=AV node; BH=bundle of His; LBB & RBB=bundle branches; IVS & IAS=interventricular and interatrial septum. * significant P<0.05.

DISCUSSION

The present study uses quantitative autoradiographic techniques to examine the distribution and density of cardiac β-adrenoceptor subtypes in the SHR and WKY. The method utilizes a single concentration of ligand to measure binding and assumes that changes in binding result from differences in density of receptors rather than changes in affinity. Between SHR and WKY and with age binding affinity has been shown to remain constant (Masuyama & Fukuda, 1989). At 24 days,

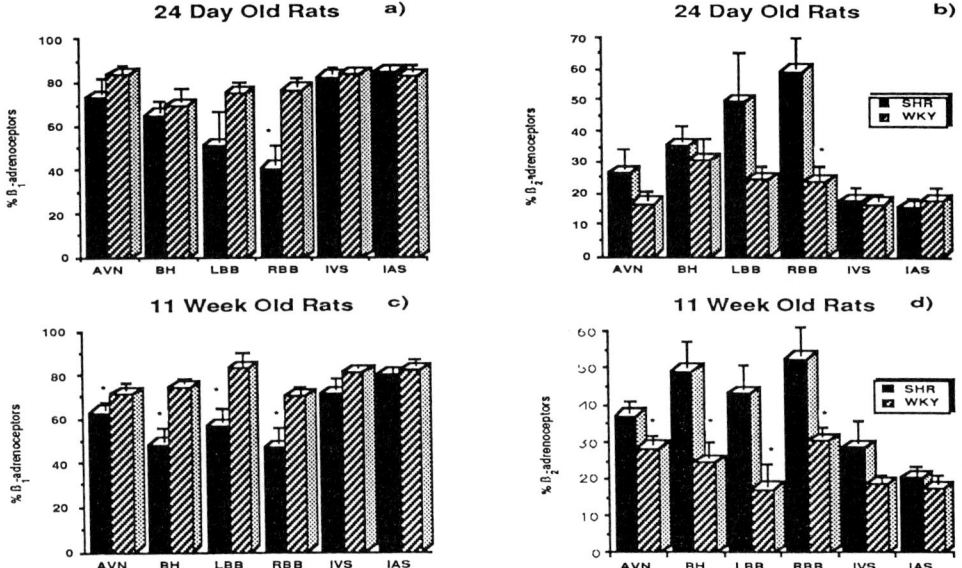

Figure 1. Proportions of β-adrenoceptor subtypes in WKY and SHR heart regions

and before development of hypertension, β-adrenoceptor density in pacemaker and conducting regions of both SHR and WKY was higher than in myocardial areas. There were no significant differences in receptor concentrations between SHR and WKY although mean receptor concentrations in WKY appeared to be higher in most areas. Increased densities of β_2-adrenoceptors were only significant in LBB. However the proportion of β_2-adrenoceptors showed signs of increasing in SHR. A higher concentration of β-adrenoceptors in young rats confirms earlier reports (Masuyama & Fukuda, 1989; Woodcock et al., 1978) and is probably associated with the low level of adrenergic innervation at this age (see Standen, 1978). At 11 weeks, β-adrenoceptor concentrations were still similar between SHR and WKY but the proportion of β_2-adrenoceptors was now clearly higher in SHR in pacemaker and conducting regions although not in myocardium. The major finding of this study was that rather than changes in the overall β-adrenoceptor population between SHR and WKY the development of hypertension was most clearly associated with an increase in the proportion of β_2-adrenoceptors in the pacemaker and conducting regions of the heart in SHR.

REFERENCES

Bhalla, R.C., Sharma, R.V. and Ramanthan, S. (1980): Ontogenetic development of isoproterinol subsensitivity on myocardial adenylate cyclase and β-adrenergic receptors in spontaneously hypertensive rats. *Biochim. Biophys. Acta.* 632, 497–506.
Bohm, M., Beuckelmann, D., Diet, F., Feiler, G., Lohse, M.J. and Erdmann, E. (1988): Properties of cardiac alpha– and beta–adrenoceptors in spontaneously hypertensive rats. *Naunyn–Schmiedeberg's Arch. Pharmacol.* 338, 383–391.
Masuyama, Y. and Fukuda, K. (1989): Adrenoceptors in experimental hypertension. *Clin. Exp. Hypertens. Theory and Practice* A11 (Supp 1) 31–42.
Molenaar, P., Smolich, J.J., Russell, F.D., McMartin, L.R. and Summers, R.J. (1990): Differential regulation of β_1– and β_2–adrenoceptors in guinea–pig atrial ventricular conducting system after chronic (–)-isoprenaline infusion. *J. Pharmacol. Exp. Ther.* 255, 393–400.
Standen, N.B. (1978): The postnatal development of adrenoceptor responses to agonists and electrical stimulation in rat isolated atria. *Br. J. Pharmacol.* 64, 83–90.
Woodcock, E.A., Funder, J.W. and Johnston, C.I. (1978): Decreased cardiac β–adrenoceptors in hypertensive rats. *Clin. Exp. Pharmac. Physiol.* 5, 545–550.
Yamada, S., Ishima, T., Tomita, T., Hayashi, M., Okada, T. and Hayashi, E. (1984): Alterations in cardiac alpha and beta adrenoceptors during the development of spontaneous hypertension. *J. Pharmacol. Exp. Ther.* 228, 454–460.

Echocardiographic evaluation of left ventricular function and left ventricular hypertrophy in SHR

Hikaru Nishimura, Masakuni Ueyama, Tamiko Oka, Jiro Kubota, Hisashi Hanada, Michihiro Suwa and Keishiro Kawamura

The 3rd Department of Internal Medicine, Osaka Medical College, 2-7 Daigakumachi, Takatsuki, Osaka 569, Japan

INTRODUCTION

Ultrasonic echocardiography (UCG) has widely been used in evaluation of hemodynamics and left ventricular mass (LVM) in humans. However, UCG has not yet been utilized in determining cardiac function and LVM in small animals such as rats. The purpose of this study was to determine the usefulness of UCG in the evaluation of LV function and LVM in SHR and Wistar rats. We compared cardiac output (CO) and LVM measured by UCG with those obtained by invasive method.

MATERIALS AND METHOD

Fifteen-week-old SHR (n=13) and Wistar rats (n=12) were used. Conscious blood pressure and pulse rate were measured by the tail-cuff method. Under pentobarbital anesthesia (50mg/kg body weight, i.p.), a venous catheter (PE50) was inserted to the right atrium through the right jugular vein to be used for injection. A thermistor-tipped catheter was introduced via the right carotid artery to the ascending aorta to determine CO with the thermodilution method (Cardiotherm 500^R, Columbus Instruments, USA). After shaving the anterior chest, rats were placed prone on a board with a 3cm-window. A 7.5 MHz transducer (HP Sonos 100^R, Hewlett-Packard, USA) was directed upward on the anterior chest through a latex pack filled with diluted ultrasound gel. Short-axis images were obtained at several levels of the left ventricle by moving rats until the short-axis image of the LV cavity was circular, indicating essentially perpendicular intersection of the left ventricle by the ultrasonic beam. Under the guidance of this two-dimensional echocardiogram, LV end-diastolic external diameter (ED), internal diameter (Dd) and end-systolic internal diameter (Ds) were measured on M-mode recording. Simultaneous measurement of CO with the thermodilution method (Richardson et al., 1962) was performed by injecting 0.1 ml of normal saline. Heart rate was obtained by electrocardiogram. At the completion of hemodynamic study, diastolic arrest was induced by intravenous injection of 2% procaine. After a careful removal of the atria and right ventricle, LV weight was determined. Echocardiographic parameters were calculated as follows: LV end-diastolic volume (EDV) = Dd^3, end-systolic volume (ESV) = Ds^3, stroke volume (SV) = EDV-ESV, CO = SV x heart rate. LVM = 1.05 x $4\pi/3$ x 1.5 x (ED^3-Dd^3), where 1.05 is specific gravity of the myocardium and 1.5 is derived from the assumption that the long axis of the left ventricle is 1.5 times the short axis.

RESULTS

Conscious systolic blood pressure and pulse rate were significantly higher in SHR than in Wistar rats (216±16 vs 128±14 mmHg, P<0.001; 486±39 vs 427±26 beats/min, P<0.05, respectively). Body weight of SHR was smaller than in their counterparts (316±18 vs 436±12 g, P<0.01). In SHR, CO simultaneously obtained by UCG and the thermodilution was 76.0±16.8 and 89.1±9.3 ml/min, r=0.71, P<0.05). In Wistar rats, CO determined by UCG (123±26 ml/min) was well correlated with that obtained by the thermodilution (114±14 ml/min)(r=0.82, P<0.05). Echo-derived LVM in SHR (0.77±0.08 g) was correlated with anatomic LVM (0.83±0.04 g) (r=0.69, P<0.05). LVM in Wistar rats was 0.92±0.17 g with UCG and 1.02±0.78 g at autopsy; there was a significant correlation between these values (r=0.79, P<0.05).

DISCUSSION

Several formulae have been proposed to estimate LVM by M-mode UCG in humans, indicating a significant correlation between echocardiographic and necropsy LV mass (Devereux, 1987). We determined UCG-derived LVM based on the assumption that the left ventricle is ellipsoidal (Devereux et al., 1977):LVM was calculated as total LV volume minus cavity volume times coefficent. There was a good correlation between echocardiographic and anatomical LVM both in the hypertensive and normotensive rats, although the correlation was better in Wistar rats. The poorer correlation in SHR may be due to limitations of M-mode echocardiography in abnormally shaped left ventricle, as LV hypertrophy is already present in 15-week-old SHR (Kawamura, et al., 1976). Clinically, the validation of LV volume determination by UCG is well established (Fortuin, et al., 1971). In this study, we calculated echo-derived CO by determining LV volume, demonstrating a close correlation between echo-derived CO and CO obtained by the thermodilution. These results indicate that UCG is a useful noninvasive method in evaluating cardiac function and LVM in both hypertensive and normotensive rats. However, further studies are required in establishing echocardiographic method in SHR because of severe LV hypertrophy.

REFERENCES

Devereux, R.B. & Reichek, N. (1977): Echocardiographic determination of ventricular mass in man: anatomic validation of the method. Circulation 55,613-618.
Devereux, R.B. (1987): Detection of left ventricular hypertrophy by M-mode echocardiography. Anatomic validation, standardization, and comparison to other methods. Hypertension 9 (suppl II), II-19-II-26.
Fortuin, N.J. Hood, W.P. Jr. Sherman, M.E. and Craige, E. (1971):Determination of left ventricular volumes by ultrasound. Circulation 44,575-584.

Kawamura, K. Kashii, C, and Imamura, K. (1976): Ultrastructural changes in hypertrophied myocardium of spontaneously hypertensive rats. Jpn. Circ. J. 40,1119-1145.

Richardson, A.W. Cooper, T. and Pinakatt, T. (1962): Thermodilution method for measuring cardiac output of rats by using a transistor bridge. Science 135,317-318.

Inhibition of cardiac ACE does not reduce left ventricular mass in salt-loaded spontaneously hypertensive rats

Vincent Mooser, Alexandra Katopothis, Stephen B. Harrap and Colin I. Johnston

University of Melbourne, Department of Medicine, Austin Hospital, Heidelberg 3084, Victoria, Australia

INTRODUCTION

The beneficial effect of ACE inhibitors on the development of left ventricular hypertrophy (LVH) in spontaneously hypertensive rats (SHR) (Sen et al, 1980; Michel et al, 1984; Clozel & Hefti, 1988) might be due not only to the reduction of ventricular afterload, but also to the reduced generation of angiotensin II (ANG II) at the tissue level, this hypothesis being reinforced by the fact that ANG II has been shown to have growth factor properties on the myocardium (Khairallah & Kanabus, 1983).

To differentiate between these 2 factors, the effect of enalapril on cardiac ACE, the circulating components of the renin angiotensin system (RAS), blood pressure (BP) and left ventricular mass (LVM) was evaluated in SHR, with modulation of the antihypertensive properties of enalapril by salt loading.

METHODS

Twenty seven male 9 to 10 week old SHR of the strain Okamoto were allocated into 3 experimental groups : 8 control rats were given distilled water to drink; another group of 8 rats received enalapril 2 mg/kg/day in distilled water as a drinking solution, and 11 rats received enalapril at the same dose, but in saline 1 %. Systolic BP was measured weekly by using the tail cuff method in conscious animals. After 8 weeks, animals were killed, and trunk blood collected for biochemical assays. Plasma enalaprilat was measured by radio-inhibitory binding assay (Jackson et al, 1987). Plasma renin activity, blood angiotensin I (ANG I), plasma ANG II were determined by radioimmunoassay (Johnston et al, 1980), ANG II being measured directly on plasma, without prior extraction. The heart of 2 animals in each group, and one kidney of each animal were used for quantitative in vitro autoradiography, performed as described by Chai et al (1987). Data are expressed as mean +/- SEM.

RESULTS

Plasma levels of the drug, as well as the degree of ACE inhibition achieved by enalapril at the tissue and plasma levels were comparable in both treatment groups, as evidenced by quantitative autoradiography and by the ratio ANG I/ANG II (table 1).

Table 1. Tissue and plasma ACE inhibition in 2 groups of SHR treated for 8 weeks by enalapril either given in water or saline 1 % as a drinking solution, as compared to a control group given water only.

	Control	Enalapril in water	Enalapril in saline
Plasma enalaprilat (ng/ml)	0	14 +/- 5	25 +/- 7
Tissue ACE inhibition (percent dpm)			
heart	0	17	9
kidney	0	33	37
Plasma RAS			
ANG II (ng/ml)	89 +/- 27	85 +/- 17	40 +/- 15**##
ANG I/ANG II	16 +/- 3	28 +/- 5*	38 +/- 4*

* $p < 0.05$; ** $p < 0.01$ vs control
$p < 0.01$ vs enalapril in water

However, the effect of ACE inhibition on BP and LVM was markedly attenuated in salt loaded animals (table 2).

Table 2. Effect of enalapril 2 mg/kg/day for 8 weeks on BP and LVM

	Control	Enalapril in water	Enalapril in saline
Initial BP (mm Hg)	161 +/- 6	177 +/- 2*#	160 +/- 2
Final BP (mm Hg)	218 +/- 2	172 +/- 2**##	201 +/- 5**
LVM (mg/g)	3.11 +/- 0.03	2.74 +/- 0.03 **##	3.14 +/- 0.04

* $p < 0.05$; ** $p < 0.01$ vs control
\# $p < 0.05$; ## $p < 0.01$ vs enalapril in water

DISCUSSION

The present study was designed to differentiate the effect of the reduced ventricular afterload induced by enalapril from ACE inhibition per se in the development of LVH in SHR.

Despite a comparable level of enalaprilat in plasma and a similar degree of ACE inhibition in tissue and plasma, salt loading profoundly attenuated the antihypertensive effect of enalapril, but also completely abolished the preventive effect of the drug on the development of LVH. Furthermore, saline itself appeared to inhibit the release of renin and was associated with a lower level of ANG II in plasma.

Our data therefore strongly suggest that the preventive effect of ACE inhibitors on the development of LVH in SHR is mainly due to the decreased ventricular load and not directly to ACE inhibition per se, and raise the question of the importance of ANG II as an independant growth factor in LVH.

REFERENCES

Chai, S.Y., Mendelsohn F.A.O., Paxinos, G. (1987) : Angiotensin converting enzyme in rat brain visualized by quantitative in vitro autoradiography. Neuroscience 20, 615-627.

Clozel, J.P. & Hefti, F. (1988) : Cilazapril prevents the development of cardiac hypertrophy and the decrease of coronary vascular reserve in spontaneously hypertensive rats. J. Cardiovasc. Pharmacol. 11, 568-572.

Jackson, B., Cubela, R., Johnston, C.I. (1987) : Measurement of angiotensin-converting enzyme inhbititors in serum by radioinhibitor binding displacement assay. Biochem. Pharmacol. 36, 1357-1360.

Johnston, C.I., Millar, J.A., Casley, J.D., McGrath, B.P., Matthews, P.G. (1980) : Hormonal responses to angiotensin blockade : comparison between receptor antagonism and converting enzyme inhibition. Circ. Res. 46 (Suppl 1), I128-I134.

Khairallah, P.A. & Kanabus, J (1983) : Angiotensin and myocardial protein synthesis. In Perspectives in cardiovascular research, ed Tarazi, R.C. & Dunbar, J.B. New York : Raven Press.

Michel, J.B., Salzmann, J.L., de Lourdes Cerol, M., Dussaule, J.C., Azizi, M., Croman, B., Camilleri, J.P., Corvol, P.(1984) : Myocardial effect of converting enzyme inhibition in hypertensive and normotensive rats. Am. J. Med. 84 (Suppl 3A), 12-21.

Sen, S., Tarazi, R.C., Bumpus, F.M. (1980) : Effect of converting enzyme inhibitor (SQ 14,225) on myocardial hypertrophy in spontaneously hypertensive rats. Hypertension 2, 169-176.

Myocardial vulnerability in cardiac hypertrophy : comparison of hypertensive and normotensive rat drug-induced myocardial changes

Hiroyuki Ito, Mikinori Torii and Tsuneyuki Suzuki

Department of Pathology, Kinki University School of Medicine, Osaka 589, Japan

SUMMARY

In order to ascertain myocardial cell vulnerability of hypertrophied heart, myocardial changes following isoproterenol administration were compared between SHRSP and WKY. Incidence of abnormal ECG and level of serum α-HBD after isoproterenol injection were markedly higher in SHRSP than in WKY, indicating myocardial vulnerability of SHRSP heart. Na/K-ATPase activity, a plasma membrane marker enzyme, was lower in treated SHRSP than in control and also treated WKY. Similar results were obtained for ICDH, a mitochondria marker enzyme, but not for lysosomal enzymes. These findings indicate the membrane abnormality in SHRSP hypertrophied myocardium. This may be a important causative factor for myocardial vulnerability.

INTRODUCTION

Due to elevation in blood pressure, SHR or SHRSP exhibit such myocardial changes as degeneration, necrosis and/or interstitial fibrosis as well as hypertrophy. Since Wexler (1979) had reported the myocardial changes in SHR heart after isoproterenol administration, several reports are now available on SHR myocardial changes after certain drug administration (Herman et al. 1985, Herrmann et al. 1987, Tisne-Versailles et al. 1985). These findings collectively suggest myocardial cell vulnerability of SHR hypertrophied heart. In the present experiment, in order to ascertain hypertrophied heart myocardial vulnerability, we used SHRSP, a rat strain evidencing severe hypertension and cardiac hypertrophy, to examine myocardial changes following administration of high doses of isoproterenol in comparison with those in normotensive WKY.

MATERIALS AND METHODS

1. Animals

Six- and 16-week-old male SHRSP and 16-week-old WKY were used in this experiment. They were maintained in our laboratory in an air-conditioned room at 23°C., fed a stock chow diet (Funabashi SP, Chiba, Japan) and given tap water ad lib. Blood pressures were taken once a week using the tail pulse pick-up method. Myocardial necrosis was produced by a single subcutaneous injection of isoproterenol (150 mg/kg). Control rats were injected with physiologic saline.

2. Methods

Electrocardiograms were taken on rat chest without anesthesia as previously reported (Chichibu et al. 1982). ECG abnormality was graded primarily from Grade 0 to Grade 3 by measuring the elevation or depression of the ST segment at a section 3-4 msec from the Q wave.

Serum α-HBD activity was measured spectrophotometrically using an RABA Super spectrograph (Chugai Co Ltd., Tokyo).

For the histological examination, the heart was fixed in a 10% buffered formalin solution and stained with either Hematoxyline-Eosin or Mallory-Azan stain. Lactic dehydrogenase (LDH) was histochemically examined and electronmicroscopical observations were carried out under standard conditions.

In order to biochemically analyze the myocardial changes, 4-month-old rats were decapitated under light ether anesthesia 24 hours after isoproterenol injection. The left ventricles and septa were isolated and homogenized in 0.25 M sucrose-10 mM Tris buffer (pH 7.4). By the standard centrifugation method, mitochondrial and microsomal fractions were obtained. Isocitrate dehydrogenase (ICDH), N-acetyl b-glucosaminidase (NAGA) and acid phosphatase (AcP) activities were measured using mitochondrial fraction , and 5'-nucleotidase and Na/K-ATPase activities were assayed in microsomal fraction. All enzyme assay were carried out spectrophotometrical method.

RESULTS

1. ECG changes

After injection of isoproterenol, the ECG show typical infarction curves on the first and second days following injection, but beyond the third day, ST elevations gradually decreased and ST depressions became prominent. Such ST changes were found mainly in left-side lead, indicating that acute myocardial damage had occurred in a wide area of the anterior-lateral portion of the left ventricle and apex. Histologicaly, the Mallory-Azan stain are more homogeneous and dense in the injured muscles than they are in the uninjured muscles and for lesions such as these LDH staining is weak and uneven, indicating diffuse LDH leakage from the injured muscle. At 24 hours after injection of isoproterenol, electronmicroscope revealed marked degeneration and destruction of the myocardium.

For the incidence rates for ST changes during the first 3 days following injection of isoproterenol, almost all of the mature SHRSP showed marked ST changes (93.2 %), with about half of the total SHRSP population showing high (Grade 3) degrees of change. However the incidence of ST changes was lower for young SHRSP (54.6 %). And, when these changes did occur, they were graded as being less severe (Grade 1 or 2) than those of the mature SHRSP. In WKY, on the other hand, about half of the rats did not evidence any ECG changes; the incidence rate for ST change being only 25.6%.

2. Alteration of serum α-HBD

In comparison with pre-injection values, serum α-HBD had increased significantly in all of the strains examined within 24 hours of injection of isoproterenol. Remarkable differences were also found within the strains, i.e., mature SHRSP showed the highest levels while young SHRSP, like WKY, evidenced the lowest. Beyond 24 hours, however, α-HBD levels decreased rapidly and no significant differences were seen between the strains by just the 3rd day following injection. These results suggest that mature SHRSP are more susceptible to severe myocardial isoproterenol-induced damage than are either young SHR or WKY.

3. Enzyme changes in myocardium

SHRSP ICDH activity, mitochondria marker enzyme, was lower than that of WKY ($p<0.01$). In addition, for both strains, ICDH activity was lower in the treated groups than in the control groups. Similar results were obtained for Na^+/K^+-ATPase, plasma membrane marker enzyme; SHRSP activity being lower than that of WKY and, for both strains, treated group activity being lower than that of the control. No significant difference was found for 5'-nucleotidase, another plasma membrane marker enzyme, between WKY and SHRSP non-treated groups. No statistically significant differences were found for ACP or NAGA activities, lysosomal enzymes, not only between non-treated WKY and non-treated SHRSP but also between the experimental and control groups for both strains.

DISCUSSION

In this study, myocardial changes after isoproterenol injection were examined and compared between severe hypertensive and normotensive rats using two different methods: electrocardiograms and measurement of serum α-HBD activity. By these two different examination, it was clearly shown that myocardial changes were more severe in SHRSP myocardium than those in WKY; this means myocardial cell vulnerability in SHRSP hypertrophied heart.

In the present study, five different enzymes were examined following injection of isoproterenol. No significant differences were found for 5'-nucleotidase, ACP or NAGA, whereas significant differences were seen for Na^+/K^+-ATPase and ICDH activities. Since Na^+/K^+-ATPase, one of the plasma membrane marker enzymes, is related to Na-K exchange through the plasma membrane as well as because ICDH is a typical marker mitochondria enzyme, the lowering of these enzyme activities in SHRSP in comparison to WKY, as well as in isoproterenol-treated rats in comparison to their respective controls, suggests alterations in sodium and potassium metabolism in the myocardium as well as disturbances in mitochondrial energy production. On the other hand, the lysosome marker enzymes NAGA and ACP, did not differ, neither between SHRSP and WKY nor between the treated and control groups. This means that lysosome fluctuation may not be a major cause for early isoproterenol injection-induced changes in the myocardium. We have also examined several enzyme changes in SHR myocardium in relation to myocardial cell vulnerability and reported that membrane-related enzymes such as 5'-nucleotidase and Na/K-ATPase were lower in 16-week-old SHR than in age-matched WKY (Torii et al. 1990). Therefore, plasma-membrane abnormality is likely to common characteristics of SHR and/or SHRSP hypertrophied heart and this may be a important causative factor for myocardial cell vulnerability.

REFERENCES

Chichibu, S., Kitagawa, C., Ito, H., and Okamoto, K. (1982): ECG patterns and the potential field profile on the thoracic surface of the rat. Acta Med. Kinki Univ. 7:13-27.
Herman, E.H., El-Hage, A.N., Ferrans, V.J. and Ardalan, B. (1985): Comparison of the severity of the chronic cardiotoxicity produced by doxorubicin in normotensive and hypertensive rats. Toxicol. Appl. Pharmacol. 78: 202-214.
Herrmann, H.J., Massow, S., Moritz, V., Norden, C. and Kuhre, C. (1987): Peculiarities of adriamycin cardiotoxicity in spontaneously hypertensive rats (SHR). Biomed. Biochim. Acta 46: s593-s596.
Tisne-Versailles, J., Constantin, M., Lamar J.C. and Pourries, B. (1985): Cardiotoxicity of high doses of isoproterenol on cardiac heamodynamics and metabolism in SHR and WKY rats. Arch. Int. Pharmacodyn. 273: 142-154.
Torii M., Ito, H. and Suzuki, T. (1990): Some enzyme characteristics of spontaneously hypertensive rats myocardium. Jpn. Circ. J. 54: 688-694.
Wexler, B.C. (1979): Isoprenaline-induced myocardial infarction in spontaneously hypertensive rats. Cardiovasc. Res. 13:450-458.

Cardioprotective effect of indapamide on experimental ischemia and reperfusion in rats

François Boucher, Sylvie Pucheu, Christian Schatz *, David Guez *
and Joël de Leiris

*Laboratoire de Physiologie Cellulaire Cardiaque, Université Joseph Fourier, B.P. 53X, 38041 Grenoble and
* Institut de Recherches Internationales Servier, 6, place des Pléïades, 92415 Courbevoie, France*

Indapamide is a non-thiazide chlorosulfamoyl diuretic, which is used in clinical practice for its antihypertensive properties. Recent studies using in vitro models of artificial membranes, biomembranes and cell cultures, have demonstrated an antioxidant effect of indapamide, comparable to that of alpha-tocopherol (Tamura et al., 1990; Uehara et al., 1990). Indapamide therefore has the potential to eliminate oxygen derived free radicals (ODFR).

It has been suggested that during post-ischemic myocardial reperfusion, short life oxygen radicals are produced (Das & Engelman, 1990). In a previous study, we have shown that pretreatment with indapamide in rats was capable of inducing the disappearance of an electron spin resonance (ESR) signal in post-ischemic coronary effluents of hearts in the presence of the spin trap DMPO (Boucher et al., 1991). This result suggested the possibility of an interaction between ODFR and indapamide in the pathophysiological situation of ischemia/reperfusion.

In the present study, we evaluated the effect of indapamide treatment on the function of an isolated rat heart model, submitted to experimental conditions of ischemia and reperfusion. Since ODFR are known to cause some detrimental effects on cellular ultrastructure by initiating membrane-lipid peroxidation, we also studied following post-ischemic reperfusion, the effect of indapamide on post-ischemic alterations in the mitochondrial membranes, evaluated by electron microscopy.

Materials and methods :

Thirty male adult Wistar rats (240-270 g body weight) were used for all the studies and separated into two homogenous groups. Indapamide, suspended in an aqueous solution of gum arabic (20 g/l) was administered orally at 3 mg/kg b.w./day for 7 days to 15 animals. The control animals (n=15) received a similar pretreatment using the vehicle only (gum arabic at 2%). At the end of the treatment, the heart was excised and rapidly perfused according to Neely et al. (1967) at 37°C (working heart perfusion) with a Krebs-Henseleit buffer containing glucose (11 mM) and DMSO (0.1% for indapamide solubility). The perfusion fluid for indapamide-treated rat hearts contained 10^{-4}M indapamide.

After a 20 min perfusion under control normoxic conditions, the hearts were submitted to a global and total ischemia at 37°C for 15 minutes, followed by 15 minutes of reperfusion under pre-ischemic conditions at the end of which lactate dehydrogenase (LDH) activity was measured in 0.5 ml of coronary effluent (Wroblewski & LaDue, 1955).

Indices of cardiac function were measured or calculated during the pre-ischemic perfusion and at the end of reperfusion : aortic output in ml/min (AO), heart rate in bts/min (HR) and aortic peak systolic pressure in mmHg (APSP). The product HRxAPSP was taken as an index of oxygen consumption.

Following reperfusion, the 10 hearts of both groups were used for the determination of i) organic hydroperoxides (HPO) content (Heath & Tappel, 1976), and ii) the activities of glutathione peroxidase (GPx) (Flohe & Günzler, 1984) and of superoxide dismutase (SOD) (Marklund, 1976). Five other hearts of both groups were perfused with a 2.5% glutaraldehyde solution (25°C) for electron microscopy.
Biopsies were taken from the medial part of the left ventricular free wall of each heart excluding the epicardium and the endocardium. 16 longitudinal 500Å-thick sections were cut and examined with an electron microscope (Zeiss). Six micrographs (magnification x 4400) were taken of each myocardial ultrathin section. The mitochondria were then classified in four different categories (A : normal mitochondria ; B : swollen mitochondria ; C : mitochondria exhibiting some membrane disruption ; D : mitochondria exhibiting severe membrane disruption) according to the degree of morphological alterations.
Results were expressed as mean ± standard error of the mean (sem) and compared using the Student t-test. Qualitative measurements of mitochondrial impairments were compared using a chi^2-test corrected for continuity by the Yates method. In all studies, $p<0.05$ was considered significant.

Results :

As shown in Table 1, treatment with indapamide led to an improvement in the post-ischemic cardiac function recovery which was accompanied by a highly significant increase in the oxygen consumption index (HRxAPSP).

Table 1 : Effect of indapamide on functional parameters evaluated 15 minutes after post-ischemic reperfusion of isolated rat hearts. Abreviations are given in the text. **$p<0.01$; ***$p<0.001$ indapamide vs control.

Group	Nb of hearts recovering a measurable function	AO (ml/min)	HR (bts/min)	APSP (mmHg)	HRxAPSP (x10-3)
Control	2/10	6.5±4.7	195±16	195±16	2.3±1.5
Indapamide	7/10	*** 17.2±4.5	** 270±18	** 270±18	** 6.5±1.6

LDH release appeared significantly lower in the indapamide-treated group after 15 min of post-ischemic reperfusion (Table 2).
Myocardial HPO content decreased significantly in the treated group, whereas SOD and GPx activities remained unchanged (Table 2).

Table 2 : Effect of indapamide on biochemical parameters evaluated 15 minutes after post-ischemic reperfusion of isolated rat hearts. abreviations are given in the text. *$p<0.05$ indapamide vs control.

Group	LDH release (U/min/g)	SOD (U/mg prot)	GPx (U/g prot)	HPO (µmol/g prot)
Control (n=10)	18.2±1.8	15.6±3.7	940±281	23.5±3.1
Indapamide (n=10)	* 10.8±0.3	16.9±2.1	893±130	* 20.5±2.2

Finally, in the treated group, the percentage of D type mitochondria (severe membrane disruption) appeared to be less whereas the number of normal mitochondria (A type) was significantly higher (Fig. 1).

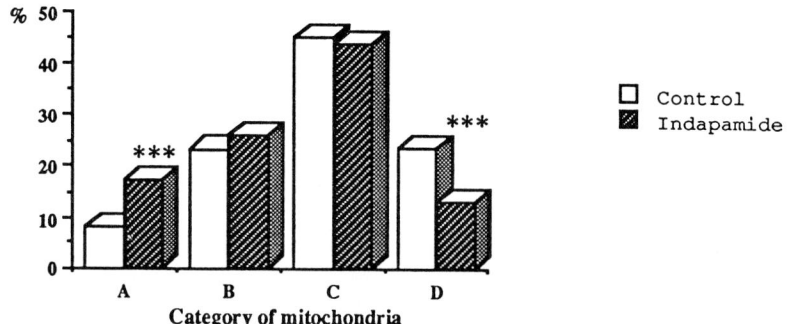

Fig. 1 : Effect of indapamide on mitochondrial ultrastructure in isolated rat hearts submitted to ischemia and reperfusion. For explanations of the different types of mitochondria, see the text. ***p<0.001. number of mitochondria observed : i) control group : 1424 ; ii) treated group : 1511.

Discussion :

The present data indicate that indapamide may significantly improve the post-ischemic recovery of cardiac function in an isolated rat heart model submitted to a short period of total and global ischemia and then reperfused. This functional improvement is accompanied by i) a significant decrease of post-ischemic lactate dehydrogenase release, an effect which is generally considered as indicative of a decrease in ischemia-induced cell membrane damage, ii) a significant decrease in organic hydroperoxide accumulation in the myocardial tissue, which can be considered as indicative of a reduction in the ischemia-induced lipid peroxidation process, and iii) a better preservation of mitochondrial membrane integrity. The latter could partially explain the beneficial effect of indapamide treatment reported in the present work. Indeed, indapamide which has been shown to possess antioxidant properties, could act as a free radical scavenger, and thereby reduce the degree of oxygen radical-induced reperfusion injury to the ischemic isolated rat heart.

References :

Tamura, A., Sato, T., and Fujii, T. (1990) : Antioxidant activity of indapamide and its metabolites. Chem. Pharm. Bull. 38: 255-257.
Uehara, Y., Shirahase, H., Nagata, T., Ishimitsu, T., Morishita, S., Osumi, S., Matsuoka, H., and Sugimoto, T. (1990) : Radical scavenging effects of indapamide on prostacyclin generation in vascular smooth muscle cells in rats. Amer. J. Hypertension 15: 216-224.
Das, D.K., and Engelman, R.M. (1990) : Mechanism of free radical generation during reperfusion of ischemic myocardium. In Oxygen radicals : Systemic Events and Disease Process, eds D.K. Das and W.B. Essman, pp. 97-121. Karger.
Boucher, F.R., Schatz, C.J., Guez, D.M., and de Leiris, J.G. (1991) : Beneficial effect of indapamide in experimental myocardial ischemia. Amer. J. Hypertension. (in press).
Neely, J.R., Liebermeister, H., Battersby, E.J., and Morgan, H.E. (1967) : Effect of pressure developpment on oxygen consumption by isolated rat heart. Amer. J. Physiol. 212: 804-814.
Heath, R.L., and Tappel, A.L. (1976) : A new sensitive assay for the measurement of hydroperoxides. Anal. Biochem. 76: 184-191.
Flohe, L., and Günzler, W.A. (1984) : Assays of glutathione peroxidase. Meth. Enzymol. 105: 114-121.
Marklund, S.L. (1976) : Spectrophotometric study of spontaneous disproportionation of superoxide anion radical and sensitive direct assay for superoxide dismutase. J. Biol. Chem. 251: 7504-7507.
Wroblewski, F., and La Due, J.S. (1955) : Lactic dehydrogenase activity in blood. Proc. Soc. Exptl. Biol. Med. 90: 210-213.

Cardiac and aortic sarcolemmal Na^+/Ca^{2+} exchange and Ca^{2+}-ATPase activities in SHR and WKY

Isabelle Drubaix, Isabelle Berrebi-Bertrand, Nadim Kassis, Yves Leclercq and Lionel G. Lelièvre

Laboratoire de Pharmacologie des Transports Ioniques Membranaires, Université Paris 7, 2, place Jussieu, 75251 Paris Cedex 05, France

It is yet unknown whether transarcolemmal Ca^{2+} movements involved in muscle relaxation are similar in aortas and hearts of SHR and/or WKY rats. The sarcolemma-bound Ca^{2+} transports involved are the Na^+/Ca^{2+} exchange and the Ca^{2+}-ATPase. The goal of this study was i) to determine the *in vitro* activities of these two systems and ii) to characterize putative differences according to tissues and WKY or SHR.

In heart, the low resting cytoplasmic Ca^{2+} level is maintained by the transarcolemmal Ca^{2+} efflux via sarcolemmal Na^+/Ca^{2+} exchange (Reeves 1985) and Ca^{2+}-ATPase (Rega and Garrahan 1986) and by the ATP-dependent Ca^{2+} uptake into the sarcoplasmic reticulum (Carafoli 1987). In rat, the contribution in the total Ca^{2+} transport capacity of the Na^+/Ca^{2+} exchange averaged 20% (Bers et al 1990) whereas sarcolemmal Ca^{2+}-ATPase contributed for less than 5% (Caroni et al 1982). A previous study (Pernollet et al 1981) showed that Na^+/Ca^{2+} exchange and Ca^{2+}-ATPase activities were higher in SHR than in WKY. However, in WKY and SHR aortas, the activities of these two functions have not yet been established.

The heart to body weight ratio (mg/g) was 2.74 in WKY whereas it averaged 3.55 in SHR, *i.e* a mean degree of cardiac hypertrophy of 30% in SHR. We have not observed any morphological or weight changes in aortas from either WKY or SHR animals.
Sarcolemmal vesicles from WKY and SHR rat hearts and aortas were isolated by the same procedure (Drubaix et al 1991) and consisted of a homogeneous population of sealed inside-out vesicles. No sealed right-side-out vesicles could be detected.

The specific activities of the cardiac Na^+/Ca^{2+} exchange and Ca^{2+}-ATPase are listed in Table I.

Table I. Na^+/Ca^{2+} exchange and Ca^{2+}-ATPase activities in cardiac and aortic vesicles from WKY and SHR rats.

	Na^+/Ca^{2+} exchange (a,c)	Ca^{2+}-ATPase (b,d)
WKY heart	1.37 ± 0.52 (n = 27)	8.22 ± 3.82 (n = 13)
SHR heart	1.02 ± 0.41 ** (n = 27)	9.16 ± 4.60 NS (n = 16)
WKY aorta	2.29 ± 0.53 (n = 27)	9.10 ± 1.30 (n = 12)
SHR aorta	2.18 ± 0.43 NS (n = 27)	7.00 ± 2.21 NS (n = 12)

(a) : The Na^+/Ca^{2+} exchange activity was measured (Hanf et al 1988) by the Na^+- dependent $^{45}Ca^{2+}$ influx at a potential of -85 mV i.e. the resting membrane potential in vivo .
(b) : The Ca^{2+}-ATPase activity was assayed as the ATP-dependent $^{45}Ca^{2+}$ accumulated in 18 minutes. The reaction initiated by addition of sarcolemmal vesicles was carried out at 37°C in 160mM KCl, 100μM $^{45}CaCl_2$, 20mM Imidazole/HCl pH 7.4 plus 4mM of either Mg-ATP or $MgCl_2$ for total and basal activities, respectively.
(c) : nmoles Ca^{2+}/mg prot. 2 sec, (d) : nmoles Ca^{2+}/mg prot. 18 min.
** : $p < 0.005$, NS : Not Significant, as compared to WKY.

The Ca^{2+}-ATPase did not seem to be altered in heart preparations from both WKY and SHR whereas Na^+/Ca^{2+} exchange activity was 25% decreased in SHR heart. This decrease could be due to the 30% hypertrophy of heart muscle in SHR. Indeed, a similar decrease (30%) in Na^+/Ca^{2+} exchange activity was also observed in Wistar rat heart hypertrophied by pressure overload (Hanf et al 1988).
Na^+/Ca^{2+} exchange and Ca^{2+}-ATPase activities were similar in WKY and SHR aortic preparations (Table I).

As a conclusion : in the SHR cardiovascular system, only the cardiac Na^+/Ca^{2+} exchange seems to be affected. Indeed, in hearts and aortas from both WKY and SHR, we found similar specific activities of Ca^{2+}-ATPase.

Thus, of particular interest is the tissue (- specific ?) distribution of the Na^+/Ca^{2+} exchanger. In aorta, the Na^+/Ca^{2+} exchange activity was up to 100% increased as compared to the cardiac one. The molecular basis of this difference occurring in both WKY and SHR rats could be quantitative (increased number of functional exchangers and/or higher turnover rates) and/or qualitative (altered Ca^{2+} and/or Na^+ sensitivities). Moreover, inasmuch as at least three isoforms of the cardiac Na^+/Ca^{2+} exchanger exist (Drubaix et al 1991) a new question arises : does an aortic isoform of the Na^+/Ca^{2+} exchanger exist?

REFERENCES.

Bers, D.M. Lederer, W.J., and Berlin, J.R. (1990). Intracellular Ca transients in rat cardiac myocytes: role of Na^+/Ca^{2+} exchange in excitation contraction coupling. Am.J.Physiol. 258 : C944-C954.

Carafoli, E. (1987). Intracellular Ca homeostasis. Ann. Rev. Biochem. 56 : 395-433.

Caroni, P. Zurini, M., and Clark, A. (1982). The calcium-pumping ATPase of heart sarcolemma. in "Transport ATPases" Ann. N.Y. Acad.Sci. 402 : 402-421. Ed. E. Carafoli. et A. Scapa.

Drubaix, I., Kassis, N., and Lelièvre, L.G. (1991). At least three functional isoforms of the cardiac Na^+/Ca^{2+} exchange exist. Ann. N.Y. Acad. Sci. (in press).

Hanf, R. Drubaix, I. Marotte, F. and Lelièvre, L.G. (1988). Rat cardiac hypertrophy. Altered sodium-calcium exchange activity in sarcolemmal vesicles. FEBS.Letters. 236 : 145-149.

Pernollet, M.G. Devynck, M.A, and Meyer, P. (1981). Abnormal calcium handling by isolated cardiac plasma membrane from spontaneously hypertensive rats. Clinical.Science. 61 : 45S-48S.

Reeves, J.P. (1985) The sarcolemmal sodium-calcium exchange system. Curr.Top.Memb.Transp. 25 : 77-127.

Rega, A.F., and Garrahan, P.J. (1986). The Ca^{2+} pump of plasma membranes. in CRC press Inc. Boca Raton, Florida.1-162.

Intracellular sodium ion content in vascular smooth muscle cells from normotensive and spontaneously hypertensive rats

Klaus Kisters, *Ernst-Rudolf Krefting, Claus Spieker, *Ute Scholz, Martin Tepel, Karl-Heinz Rahn and Walter Zidek

Medizinische Poliklinik der Universität, * Medizinische Physik der Universität, Albert-Schweitzer-Strasse 33, W-4400 Münster, Germany

Summary

Whereas numerous studies on Na^+ transport of blood cells in hypertension have been performed, little is known on Na^+ handling in vascular smooth muscle cells in primary hypertension. Therefore we measured Na^+ content in smooth muscle cells from aortas of normotensive (n=13, systolic pressure 120,1 ± 8,9 mm Hg) and spontaneously hypertensive rats (n=13, systolic pressure 195,4 ± 11,8 mm Hg) aged 3 months using energy-dispersive electronprobe X-ray microanalysis. With this method electrons are shot on carbon-coated cryosections of a thickness of 3 µm, frozen in liquid propane at -190 °C. Thereby electrons are displaced from their atomic shell and with the rearrangement of electrons by refilling the inner shells an X-ray emission specific for each element is measured with a scanning electron microscope fitted with an energy-dispersive X-ray analyzer. Cross sections of the abdominal aorta were examined. The sites of measurements were proved to be intracellular optically and by measuring phosphate content. Measurements of intracellular Na^+ content were done at 7 sites in each cryosection. In normotensive animals Na^+ content in aortic smooth muscle cells was 0,71 ± 0,08 g/100 g of dry weight (mean values ± SD), whereas Na^+ content in hypertensive smooth muscle cells was 1,25 ± 0,20 g/100 g of dry mass (p<0,01).
The study shows that by energy-dispersive electronprobe microanalysis Na^+ content of vascular smooth muscle can be evaluated. Furthermore, the pronounced increase in Na^+ content of hypertensive aortic smooth muscle cells suggests that changes in Na^+ transport of vascular smooth muscle play a role in the pathogenesis of spontaneous hypertension.

Key words: Na^+, vascular smooth muscle, spontaneously hypertensive rats, hypertension, electronprobe X-ray microanalysis

Introduction

Numerous disturbances of cellular electrolyte metabolism have been described in primary hypertension (D'Amico, 1958; Losse et al., 1960).

In most studies, blood cells of essential hypertensive patients were used. Comparatively few data are available to test possible analogies between electrolyte metabolism in any type of blood and in arterial smooth muscle cells. Therefore electronprobe microanalysis was performed in aortic smooth muscle cells from normotensive and spontaneously hypertensive rats to test cellular Na^+ handling in essential hypertension.

Methods

Aortae from 13 spontaneously hypertensive rats (SHR, systolic pressure 195,4 $\pm$ 11,8 mm Hg) and from 13 normotensive rats (WKY, 120,1 $\pm$ 8,9 mm Hg) aged 3 months were used. The aortae were frozen in liquid propane cooled with liquid nitrogen at a temperature of about -190 °C. Then cryosections of 3 μm were lyophilized. For the electronprobe microanalysis, an electron microscope with an X-ray detector was used. When the electrons of the incoming beam strike an atom in the specimen, energy characteristic for each element becomes free. For quantification, the continuum method developed by Hall was used (Goldstein et al., 1981). Intracellular sites of measurements were identified by the morphology and by simultaneous measurements of sulfur and phosphorus being markedly elevated in the intracellular space as compared to extracellular concentrations. In each aorta, mean values of 5 intracellular measurements at different sites were calculated. Na^+ content was expressed in g/kg dry weight of the tissue. For statistical analysis unpaired Student's t test was used.

Results

In SHR intracellular Na^+ content was 12,5 $\pm$ 2,0 g/kg dry weight as compared to 7,1 $\pm$ 0,8 g/kg dry weight in WKY (mean values $\pm$ SD, p<0,01, Fig. 1.).

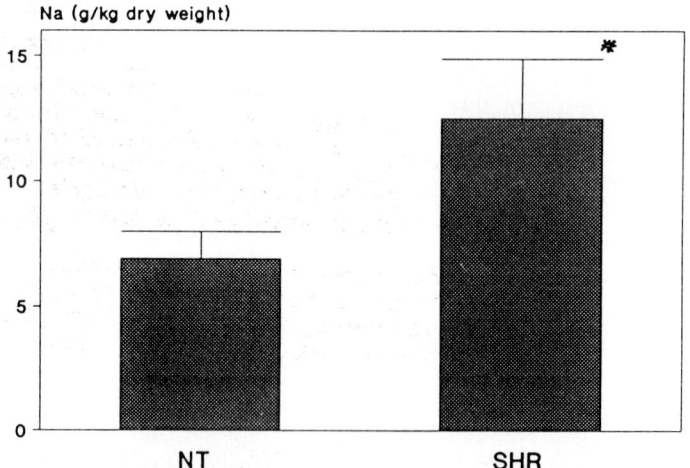

Fig. 1. Intracellular Na^+ content in aortic smooth muscle cells from normotensive (NT) and spontaneously hypertensive rats (SHR)(mean values $\pm$ SD, * =p<0,01).

Discussion

There are only few data on intracellular Na^+ content in arterial smooth muscle cells from hypertensive animals. Elevated intracellular Na^+ concentrations in arterial smooth muscle cells in one kidney, one clip hypertensive rats were described by Tobian & Binion (1952), whereas Massingham and Shevde (1973) found principally unchanged total Na^+ content in aortae from genetically hypertensive rats without distinguishing between intra- and extracellular Na^+ content. The inhibition of Na^+, K^+-ATPase has been postulated to cause hypertension as a consequence of elevated intracellular Na^+ concentrations (De Wardener & Clarkson, 1985). Increased intracellular Na^+ concentrations have been claimed to cause vasoconstriction by increasing Na^+-Ca^{++} exchange (Blaustein, 1977), by increasing the sensitivity of arterial smooth muscle to noradrenaline (Aronson, 1984), or by decreasing the lumen:wall ratio of resistance vessels (Folkow, 1978). The reasons for elevated intracellular Na^+ concentrations of vascular smooth muscle cells in essential hypertension may be disturbances in Na^+, K^+-cotransport (Garay et al., 1980), Na^+ - H^+ exchange (Livne et al., 1987), Na^+ - K^+-countertransport (Poston, 1987) and open-channel block of Na^+ channels by intracellular Mg^{++} (Pusch, 1990). Although the present results cannot evaluate the relative roles of these possible mechanisms, the findings demonstrate that there are analogies in Na^+ handling in aortic smooth muscle cells of SHR to those detected in blood cells from hypertensive animals or human subjects.

References

Aronson, J.K. (1984): The role of the Na^+, K^+ - ATPase in the regulation of vascular smooth-muscle contractility and its relationship to essential hypertension. In Biochem. Soc. Trans. 12: 943-945.
Blaustein, M.P. (1977): Sodium ions, calcium ions, blood pressure regulation and hypertension: a reassessment and a hypothesis. In Am. J. Physiol. 232: C165-C173.
D'Amico, G. (1958): Red cell sodium and potassium in congestive heart failure, essential hypertension and myocardial infarction. In Am. J. Med. Sci. 236: 156-161.
De Wardener, H.E., Clarkson, E.M. (1985): Concept of natriuretic hormone. In Physiol. Rev. 65: 658-759.
Folkow, B. (1978): Cardiovascular structural adaption: its role in the initiation and maintenance of primary hypertension. The Fourth Volhard Lecture. In Clin. Sci. Mol. Med. 55: 3-22.
Garay, R.P., Dagher, G., Pernollet, M.G., Devynck, M.A., Meyer, P. (1980): Inherited defect in a Na^+, K^+, co-transport system in erythrocytes from essential hypertensive patients. In Nature 284: 281-283.
Goldstein, J.T., Newbury, D.E., Echlin, P., Joy, D.C., Fiori, C., Lifshin, E. (1981): Scanning electron microscopy and X-ray microanalysis. In New York: Plenum Press.
Livne, A., Balfe, J.W., Veitch, R., Marquez-Julio, A., Grinstein, S., Rothstein, A. (1987): Increased platelet Na^+ - H^+ exchange rates in essential hypertension: application of a novel test. In Lancet I: 533-536.
Losse, H., Wehmeyer, H., Wessels, F. (1960): Der Wasser- und Elektrolytgehalt von Erythrozyten bei arterieller Hypertonie. In Klin. Wschr. 38: 393-395.
Massingham, R., Shevde, S. (1973): The ionic composition of aortic smooth muscle from A. S. - hypertensive rats. In Br. J. Pharmacol. 47: 422-424.
Pusch, M. (1990): Open-channel block of Na^+ channels by intracellular Mg^{++}. In Eur Biophys J 18: 317-326.
Poston, L. (1987): Endogenous sodium pump inhibitors: a role in essential hypertension? In Clin. Sci. 72: 647-655.
Tobian, L. Jr., Binion, J.T. (1952): Tissue cations and water in arterial hypertension. In Circulation 5: 754-758.

Arterial mechanical properties in Dahl sensitive rats

Hervé Bouaziz, Athanase Benetos, Bernard I. Levy and Michel Safar

INSERM U.337, Hôpital Broussais, 96, rue Didot, 75674 Paris Cedex 14, France

INTRODUCTION

Alterations of the elastic properties of the large arteries are common phenomenon in hypertension (1). These alterations reduce the buffering function of the elastic arteries and participate to increase left ventricular afterload (2). On the other hand such changes of the large arteries can play a role in the development of atherosclerotic lesions.

In animal models a decrease in the elastic properties is often observed in hypertensive animals (3,4). It is not very clear whether these changes are only due to high pressure levels or preceed the development of hypertension. The aim of this study was to assess in rats prone to hypertension, large arteries alterations were present even before the development of hypertension. For that we studied the mechanical properties of the carotid artery in Dahl sensitive rats with or without chronic salt loading and in SHR and WKY rats.

MATERIAL AND METHODS

Thirty nine male Dahl sensitive rats were used in these experiments (Mollergaard Breeding Center, Skensved, Denmark). The rats were delivered to our animal house at 7 weeks of age. Therefore they were divided in 4 groups : Dahl sensitive rats under standard low salt diet (DSL, .4% NaCl n = 9) ; Dahl sensitive rats under high salt diet (DSH, 7% NaCl n = 10) ; WKY (n = 9) and SHR (n = 12) under normal salt diet. On the day of the experiment, the rats were anesthetized with intraperitoneal pentobarbital (60 mg/kg). The right femoral artery and the left carotid artery were cannulated for direct arterial pressure recording and arterial compliance measurments. The carotid compliance was evaluated in situ using a previously described method (3). In brief the left carotid artery is isolated and connected with a manometer pressurized at adjustable pressure values. This preparation allows us to exclude in situ 14-20 mm carotid to be studied.

To start the measurements, the segment of the isolated artery is submitted to a pressure of 25 mmHg for 5 minutes, and the position of the meniscus is noted. The artery is then submitted to 50 mmHg pressure steps. The movement of the meniscus is noted at 30 seconds, then every 1 minute for 3 minutes for each step. The increase in the arterial volume is recorded from 25 to 175 mmHg. The static compliance of the isolated segment of the artery is calculated for each level of pressure as the ratio of the volume increase for a given change of pressure ($\Delta V/\Delta P$). For statistical comparisons the values of compliance were normalized by the length of the isolated arterial segment.

STATISTICS

All results were expressed as mean ± SEM blood pressure and compliance values of the different groups were compared by one way ANOVA. A $p < .05$ was considered significant.

RESULTS

Duration of hypertension and MBP levels were similar in the 2 groups of hypertensive rats (DSH : 185 ± 7 mmHg, SHR : 180 ± 6 mmHg) (mean ± SEM). MBP was significantly lower in the 2 other groups ($p < .001$) (DSL : 140 ± 6 mmHg ; WKY 121 ± 4 mmHg). In DS groups and SHR pressure/volume curves were similar and significantly lower than in WKY rats. ($p < .001$) (Fig).

Fig. shows compliance values in the different groups of rats

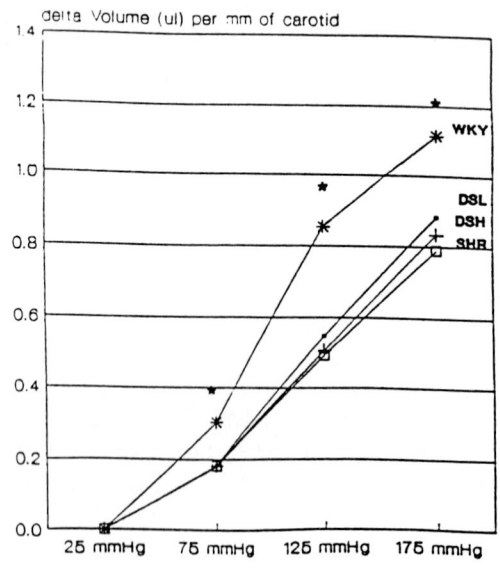

DISCUSSION

In this study we evaluated the values of carotid artery compliance in Dahl sensitive rats under different NaCl diets and in SHR and WKY rats of the same age. Dahl sensitive rats are known to develop hypertension when fed a high salt diet (5,6). Moreover previous studies showed that these rats frequently develop arterial and arteriolar lesions (7,8).

For that we used a method able to measure the arterial compliance in vivo, in situ with respect of the anatomy, vascularisation and innervation of the carotid artery. This method has already been validated in different studies (3). In the present study using this model we observed that compliance values in Dahl sensitive rats were not modified after salt loading. As compared to the other studied groups, DS rats present compliance values close with those observed in SHR and significantly lower of the values we recorded in normotensive rats (WKY) (fig). These results show that DS rats present low compliance values even before the development of salt dependant hypertension. This suggest that in this rat strain, prone to develop hypertension genetical factor seem to be involved in large arteries alterations.

REFERENCES

1 - Safar, M. & London G. (1987): Arterial and venous compliance in sustained essential hypertension. Hypertension 10, 133-139.

2 - Merillon, J.P., Motte, G. et al (1982): Inter-relation entre les propriétés physiques du système artériel et la performance ventriculaire gauche lors du vieillissement et dans l'hypertension artérielle. In: Brutsaert DL., Ed. L'hypertension ventriculaire gauche. Paris, Masson, 95-104.

3 - Levy, B.I., Michel, J.B. et al (1988): Effects of chronic inhibition of converting enzyme on mechanical and structural properties of arteries in rats renovascular hypertension. Circulation Research 63, 227-237.

4 - Cox, RH (1979): Comparison of arterial wall mechanics in normotensive and spontaneously hypertensive rats. Am J Physiol 237, H159-H167.

5 - Dahl, L.K., Heine, M. et al (1962): Role of genetic factors in susceptibility to experimental hypertension due to chronic excess salt ingestion. Nature 194: 480.

6 - Rapp, J.P. (1982): Dahl salt-susceptible and salt-resistant rats. Hypertension 4,753-763.

7 - Boegehold, M. & Kotchen, T (1990): Effect of dietary salt on the skeletal muscle microvasculature in Dahl rats. Hypertension 15, 420-426.

8 - Lee, RMKW &Triggle, C. (1986): Morphometric study of mesenteric arteries from genetically hypertensive Dahl strain rats. Blood Vessels 23,: 199-224.

Effect of angiotensin II on the number of smooth muscle cells in the SHR aorta

M.J. Black, J.F. Bertram [1] and J.H. Campbell [2]

Baker Medical Research Institute, Commercial Road, Prahran 3181, Victoria, Australia, [1] Department of Anatomy, University of Melbourne, Parkville 3052, Victoria, Australia and [2] Department of Anatomy, University of Queensland, St Lucia 4072, Australia

INTRODUCTION

Hypertension is characterised by hypertrophy of the arterial tree. This hypertrophy is linked to decreased compliance of the large elastic arteries and increased peripheral resistance due to encroachment of the wall on the lumen of small resistance vessels. Both hypertensive animals and humans have an enlarged medial layer compared to normotensives, hence it is of particular interest to determine the factors that control vascular smooth muscle cell growth within the artery wall. Several lines of evidence suggest that angiotensin II (AII) can play a major role in initiating vascular smooth muscle growth. In culture, vascular smooth muscle cells undergo a marked induction of hypertrophy in the presence of AII, accompanied by the enhanced mRNA expression of the proto-oncogenes c-fos and c-myc (Campbell et al, 1991). A role for AII contributing to vascular hypertrophy in primary hypertension has been largely based on the ability of ACE inhibitors to markedly attenuate the development of vascular hypertrophy in the spontaneously hypertensive rat (SHR) (Christensen et al, 1989). However, ACE inhibitors also elevate bradykinin (Erdös, 1975) and this could, at least in theory, contribute to the prevention of vascular hypertrophy.

The aim of this study is to more directly ascertain the contribution of angiotensin II in the induction of aortic hypertrophy during the developmental phase of the SHR, with special emphasis on its effects on vascular smooth muscle cell growth and proliferation. These responses of AII are determined using optical disectors (Gundersen et al, 1988) to estimate the total number of smooth muscle cells in the descending thoracic aortae of rats. The optical disector is one of the new generation of unbiased stereological counting methods. Unlike traditional stereological methods for counting cell nuclei, and thereby cells, these new unbiased methods do not require assumptions with respect to nuclear shape, size distribution or orientation.

MATERIALS AND METHODS

Animals

Male SHR were obtained from a colony maintained at the Baker Medical Research Institute, Melbourne, Australia since 1986 and derived originally from the breeding stock of Dr Yukio Yamori (Izumo, Japan). All animals were housed individually and food and water administered ad libitum. From 4 weeks of age systolic blood pressure was determined at twice weekly intervals in conscious rats maintained at an ambient temperature of 28°C using a photoelectric tail-cuff pulse detection system (IITC Inc., Woodland Hills, California, USA).

Drug Treatment and Surgical Procedures
Perindopril (S9490-3) an ACE inhibitor was administered in the drinking water at a dosage of 1mg/kg/day to two experimental groups of rats from 7 to 15 weeks of age. In the first group SHR were treated with perindopril. The second group was, in addition, infused with AII (20ng/min). The untreated SHR were used as controls.

At age 7 weeks the rats were anaesthetised (Ketalar 50mg/kg, Rompun 6mg/kg) and Alzet osmotic minipumps (Model 2ML4) placed subcutaneously on the animals back with the outflow catheters leading subcutaneously to the right jugular vein. Saline was infused via minipumps in rats not receiving AII. Following 4 weeks infusion the rats were lightly anaesthetized (Ketalar 40mg/kg, Rompun 7mg/kg) and the minipumps replaced through a small cutaneous incision. All rats were sacrificed at 15 weeks of age.

Estimation of the total number of smooth muscle cells in the descending thoracic aorta
The aortae were perfusion fixed at maximum dilatation using 5% glutaraldehyde in 0.1M phosphate buffer (pH 7.3). The descending thoracic aortae (from the subclavian branch point to the diaphragm) were excised, cleaned of excess fat and connective tissue, placed in agar, and sliced into 2mm rings using a razor blade fractionator (Gundersen *et al*, 1988). Every second ring (the first was chosen at random) was processed for embedding in glycolmethacrylate, and exhaustively sectioned at approximately 20μm. Every 10th section was sampled (with the first section chosen at random) and stained with haematoxylin and eosin. The numerical density of smooth muscle cells in the combined volume of media and intima ($Nv_{smc,mi}$) was estimated with optical disectors which were selected using a systematic uniform random scheme. Smooth muscle cells were counted at a final magnification of approximately 2,250x (Gundersen *et al.*, 1988). The combined volume of the media and intima in aorta, V_{mi}, was estimated using the Cavalieri principle (see Gundersen *et al*, 1988). The sampled sections were projected at a final magnification of 95x onto an orthogonal grid. The number of points counted per vessel in order to estimate volume using the Cavalieri principle ranged from 170 to 330. An unbiased estimate of the total number of smooth muscle cells in an aorta, $N_{smc,mi}$ was obtained by multiplying the volume of media and intima, (V_{mi}, obtained with the Cavalieri principle) by smooth muscle cell numerical density ($Nv_{smc,mi}$, obtained using optical disectors):

$$N_{smc,mi} = V_{mi} \times Nv_{smc,mi}$$

Statistics
The statistical significance of drug treatment and AII infusion on medial cross-sectional area and the number of cells/descending thoracic aorta was determined by a one way analysis of variance and its effect on systolic blood pressure by a two way analysis of variance. Values are expressed as means ± standard error of the mean.

RESULTS

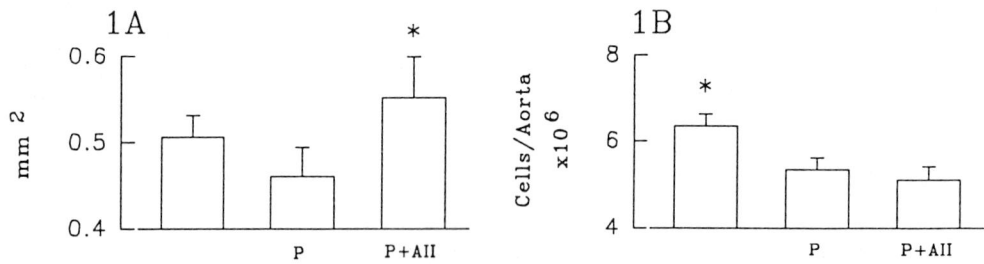

Fig. 1A. Aortic medial cross-sectional area (a measurement of aortic hypertrophy) in untreated, perindopril treated and perindopril treated plus AII infused SHR.
Fig. 1B. Estimation of the number of smooth muscle cells in the descending thoracic aorta as determined by an optical disector/cavalieri combination in the untreated, perindopril treated and perindopril treated plus AII infused SHR. (*p <0.05 from P treatment)

Perindopril inhibited the development of hypertension such that systolic blood pressure remained at normotensive levels (<150mmHg). Simultaneous infusion of AII raised blood pressure in the perindopril treated group to hypertensive levels. After one week infusion mean systolic blood pressure (SBP) = 175 ± 8mmHg and after 8 weeks infusion mean SBP = 201 ± 9mmHg, which in the corresponding SHR SBP averaged 146 ± 7mmHg and 175 ± 5mmHg respectively.

Perindopril treatment tended to reduce medial cross-sectional area (mean = 0.460 ± 0.075mm² in perindopril treated compared to mean = 0.506 ± 0.025mm² in the untreated SHR) however this difference did not reach significance (Fig. 1A). Concomitant infusion of AII markedly increased ($p<0.01$) the cross-sectional area of the aorta in perindopril treated rats (mean = 0.552 ± 0.046mm²), Fig. 1A.

AII infusion did not significantly affect the number of smooth muscle cells within the aortic wall. In contrast, perindopril treatment significantly reduced ($p<0.02$) the number of smooth muscle cells within the descending thoracic aortic media (Fig. 1B); this effect was not attenuated by infusion of AII. (mean = 5.35×10^6 ± 0.26 cells/descending thoracic aorta, and mean = 5.02×10^6 ± 0.30 cells respectively).

DISCUSSION

The major finding of this study is that the number of smooth muscle cells in the SHR aorta does not appear to be influenced by AII infusion. However the AII mediated increase in medial cross-sectional area suggests that it can influence blood vessel growth. At present one can only speculate as to whether this effect is indirect, a consequence of raising blood pressure, or a direct effect on blood vessel growth. The recent finding by Prewitt *et al*, 1990 that ACE inhibition in one kidney one clip rats reduced vascular hypertrophy but not the hypertension, suggests that it may be at least partially be a direct effect. Noradrenaline infusion in perindopril treated SHR, which also elevates blood pressure, has no effect on medial cross-sectional area (unpublished observations, M.J Black).

It is conceivable that perindopril treatment in SHR may inhibit vascular smooth muscle proliferation either by a direct effect of the drug on the smooth muscle or indirectly through its potentiation of bradykinin formation (Erdös *et al*, 1975). Bradykinin could potentially influence vessel growth possibly acting through the endothelium, and the medial smooth muscle cells may be inhibited in such a way that they are unresponsive to stimuli such as AII or increased blood pressure.

ACKNOWLEDGEMENTS: Supported in part by Servier Institute for International Research and the Australian National Heart Foundation.

REFERENCES

Campbell, J.H., Tachas, G., Black, M.J., Cockerill, G., & Campbell, G.R. (1991): Molecular biology of vascular hypertrophy. In *Pharmacology of cardiac and vascular remodeling*, ed. J.F.M. Smits. et al., pp 3–11. Steinkopff Verlag Darmstadt.

Christensen, K.L., Jespersen, L.T., & Mulvany, M.J. (1989): Development of blood pressure in spontaneously hypertensive rats after withdrawal of long-term treatment related to vascular structure. *J. Hypertens.* 7, 83–90.

Erdös, E.G. (1975): Angiotensin I converting enzyme. *Circ. Res.* 36, 247–255.

Gundersen, H.J.G., Bagger, P., Bendtsen, T.F., Evans, S.M., Korbo, L., Marcussen, N., Moller, A., Nielsen, K., Nyengaard, J.R., Pakkenberg, B., Sorensen, F.B., Vesterby, A., & West, M.J. (1988): The new stereological tools: disector, fractionator, nucleator and point sampled intercepts, and their use in pathological research and diagnosis. *APMIS* 96, 857–881.

Prewitt, R.L., Wang, D.H. (1990): Captopril reduces aortic and microvascular growth in hypertensive and normotensive rats. *Hypertension* 15, 68–77.

Arterial wall distensibility in hypertensive rats

Daniel Hayoz, Michel Niederberger, Blaise Rutschmann, Hans R. Brunner and Bernard Waeber

Division d'Hypertension, Centre Hospitalier Universitaire Vaudois, Lausanne, Switzerland

Introduction

The purpose of our study was to determine whether vascular alterations induced by chronic hypertension modify mechanical properties of the arteries. Vascular smooth muscle cell hypertrophy and extracellular matrix modifications in the media are responsible for arterial wall thickening (1-4). It is today possible to measure continuously in the anesthetized rat the internal diameter of the carotid artery simultaneously with intra-arterial pressure using a new non-invasive device (5). In the present study we measured the mechanical behavior of the common carotid artery of 16-week-old spontaneously hypertensive rats (SHR) treated for 6 weeks with either the ACE inhibitor captopril or the arteriolar dilator hydralazine. Treated and untreated rats were compared to normotensive controls (WKY rats).

Methods

Ten 16-week old normotensive male rats (WKY) and 30 age- and sex-matched spontaneously hypertensive rats (SHR) were used. The SHR were allocated to 6 week treatments with either captopril (n = 10), hydralazine (n = 9) or vehicle (tap water; n = 10). The drugs were administered in drinking water (captopril, 25 mg/30 ml of water, hydralazine, 5 mg/30 ml of water).
Anesthesia was induced with ether and then maintained with fluothane (1.5%). The right external carotid artery was cannulated with a catheter (PE 50) filled with a heparinized 0.9% NaCl solution. Intra-arterial pressure and heart rate were monitored using a computerized data acquisition system (6). The internal diameter of the left external carotid artery was measured at the same time using an A-Mode ultrasonic echo-tracking device (5). Ten successive diameter-pressure recordings were obtained for each animal in a five minute period. The apparatus allows measurements of the internal carotid artery diameter variations with a precision close to one micron. This degree of resolution is made possible by oversampling (5000 arterial diameter measurements per second) and averaging 16 consecutive values. For the recordings, a 10-MHz probe is positioned perpendicularly over the artery without direct contact with the skin. The Doppler technique is used for guidance of the probe and an ultrasonic gel is employed for signal transduction.
The simultaneous and continuous acquisitions of internal arterial diameter and blood pressure are processed on line to compute a diameter (or cross-section) -pressure relationship. The latter is

subsequently converted into a distensibility-pressure curve. This curve fits best with an arctangent function first described by Langwouters (7).
Arterial cross-sectional distensibility (D) is the inverse of the Peterson elastic modulus, and represents the arterial compliance normalized for the cross-section (s). [$D = (1/s) * \partial$ cross-section/∂ pressure] Data are reported as means ± SEM. A one way analysis of variance was used to compare the baseline characteristics of the experimental groups. Differences were considered significant for p values < 0.05. Statistical analysis of compliance-pressure and distensibility-pressure curves were done using a multivariate analysis based on Hotelling T2 considering compliance values at three arbitrarily defined blood pressures in the range of measured values.

Results

Under halothane anesthesia, captopril- and hydralazine-treated hypertensive rats and WKY normotensive controls displayed overlapping blood pressures (Figure 1), allowing statistical comparisons between the distensibility-pressure curves. Vehicle-treated SHR exhibited clearly higher blood pressure values. There was no significant difference in heart rate between the 4 groups of animals (SHR: Vehicle = 324 ± 11, captopril = 348 ± 22 and hydralazine = 318 ± 12 b/min; WKY = 316 ± 21 b/min). Left ventricular mass adjusted to total body weight was significantly (p<0.01) reduced in treated-SHR in comparison to untreated SHR (3.19 ± 0.11 g/kg) (Table 1).

Table 1

Hemodynamic parameters and left ventricular mass of the different groups of rats under anesthesia

	WKY	SHR		
	Vehicle	Vehicle	Captopril	Hydralazine
Systolic BP (mm Hg)	169±2***	218±2	170±5***	182±3***
Diastolic BP (mm Hg)	135±2***	176±3	137±5***	151±2***
Heart rate (bpm)	316±21	324±11	348±22	318±12
Left ventricular mass per kg (g/kg)	2.41±0.03**	3.19±0.11	2.51±0.05**	2.68±0.06**

Mean ± SEM *p<0.05 **p<0.01 ***p<0.001 versus SHR vehicle

Figure 1. shows the cross-sectional distensibility as a function of intra-arterial blood pressure recorded synchronously in the controlateral carotid artery. There was no statistically significant difference in the distensibility-pressure curves between the treated SHR and the normotensive controls, although distensibility tended to be enhanced by the two antihypertensive agents. Because of the absence of overlapping blood pressures between untreated SHR and WKY animals, the distensibility-pressure curves cannot be subjected to statistical analysis. These curves appear however to represent the direct continuation of one another.

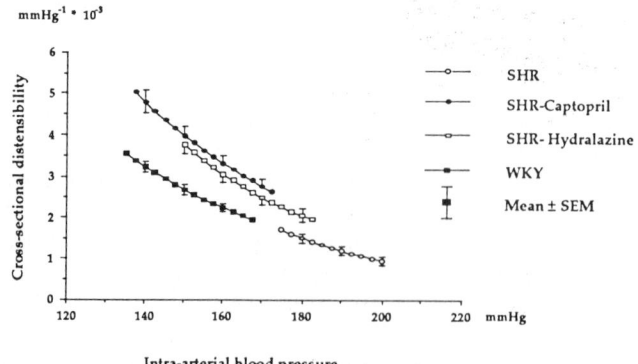

Legend Figure 1

Relationships between cross-sectional distensibility of the carotid artery and intra-arterial pressure established in spontaneously hypertensive rats (SHR) and normotensive controls (WKY). The 16-week old animals were studied after a 6 week treatment with either captopril or hydralazine administered in drinking water. Untreated animals received only water.

Discussion

This study performed in intact young spontaneously hypertensive rats shows the impact of drug-induced blood pressure reductions on distensibility-pressure curves using a new ultrasound A-Mode echotracking device. The two drugs, the ACE inhibitor captopril and the arterial dilator hydralazine, were equally effective in lowering blood pressure but, as anticipated, ACE inhibition with captopril led to a more pronounced regression of cardiac hypertrophy (8,9).

The major advantage of our technique is derived from the fact that the arterial diameter and the intra-arterial pressure are recorded continuously over the entire pulse pressure range. The arterial distensibility can therefore be related to each pressure actually measured in these animals. The determinations were performed at the carotid artery, a typical elastic artery. By this approach no significant difference was found between captopril- or hydralazine-treated hypertensive rats and their normotensive untreated WKY counterparts, although a trend towards an increased distensibility was apparent after treatment. Moreover, the distensibility-pressure curves established in untreated hypertensive animals appeared to be the direct extension of the corresponding curves determined in WKY rats. These data may seem rather surprising since there is general agreement that arterial wall thickening, already present in young SHR, is associated with increased stiffness (10). They are however in agreement with previous observations made using the same echotracking system in patients with essential hypertension and in normotensive subjects (11). In this clinical setting also, the hypertensive disorder did not result a decrease in arterial distensibility, at least as assessed at the level of the radial artery, a medium-size muscular artery.

The experiments reported here were carried-out in rather young rats treated for only a few weeks. Further studies involving older hypertensive animals are needed first to ensure whether long-term blood pressure control changes the mechanical properties of the arterial wall and secondly to relate mechanical behavior with morphometric analysis.

References

1. Warshaw DM, Mulvany MS et al., (1979): Mechanical and morphological properties of arterial resistance vessels in young and old spontaneous hypertensive rats. Circ Res; 45: 250-259.
2. Chobanian AV, Prescott MF et al., (1984): The effects of hypertension on the arterial walls. Exp Mol Pathol; 41: 153-169.
3. Folkow B. (1982) : Physiological aspects of primary hypertension. Physiol Rev; 62: 347-504.
4. Hart MN, Heistad DD et al., (1980): Effect of chronic hypertension and sympathetic denervation on wall/lumen ratio of cerebral vessels. Hypertension; 2: 419-423.
5. Tardy Y, Meister JJ et al., (1991): Non-invasive estimate of the mechanical properties of peripheral arteries from ultrasonic and photoplethysmographic measurements. Clin Phys Physiol Meas; 12: 39-54.
6. Flückiger JP, Gremaud G et al., (1989): Measurement of sympathetic nerve activity in the unanesthetized rat. J Appl Physiol; 67: 250-255.
7. Langwouters GJ, Wesseling KH et al., (1984): The static elastic properties of 45 human thoracic and 20 abdominal aortas in vitro and the parameters of a new model. J Biomechanics; 17: 425-435.
8. Sen S, Tarazi RC et al., (1980): Effect of converting enzyme inhibitor (SQ 14,225) on myocardial hypertrophy in spontaneously hypertensive rats. Hypertension; 2: 169-176.
9. Freslon JL, Giudicelli JF. (1983): Compared myocardial and vascular effects of captopril and dihydralazine during hypertension development in spontaneously hypertensive rats. Br J Pharmac; 80: 533-543
10. Michel JB, Salzmann JL et al., (1990): Effect of hypertension and vasodilator treatment on arterial wall structure. In: Atkinson J., Capdeville C. Zannad F., eds: Coronary and cerebrovascular effects of antihypertensive drugs. Cambridge, Transmedica; 205-218.
11. Perret F, Hayoz D et al., (1990): Arterial compliance : is it necessarily decreased in hypertensive patients. 13th Scientific Meeting of the International Society of Hypertension Montréal, Canada.; Abst: S82 P3.17.

Effects of indapamide on the mechanical properties of the mesenteric artery in spontaneously hypertensive rats (SHR)

Hong Y. Qiu, Bruno Valtier, Christian Schatz *, David Guez * and Bernard I. Lévy

INSERM U.141, Hôpital Lariboisière, 75010 Paris, and * Institut de Recherches Internationales Servier, 92415 Courbevoie, France

Summary

The effects of chronic treatment with indapamide (3mg/kg/day) on the structure and function of the mesenteric artery were studied in SHRs using an experimental model of "in situ" localized mesenteric artery. Indapamide (n=12) or placebo (n=12) were given to 8-week-old rats for 4 weeks. After anesthesia and laparotomy, a segment of mesenteric artery was exposed for video- microscopic measurements. The diameter-pressure relationships were established under active conditions (phenylephrine 10^{-6} M), and passive conditions (potassium cyanide) for transmural pressure ranging from 0-200 mmHg. This studied segments were then fixed and the wall cross sectional area (CSA) were measured in transverse sections. Active wall stress and tension were defined as the differences in wall stresses and wall tensions calculated for active and passive conditions. Systolic arterial pressure and mesenteric CSA were decreased in treated rats (197 ± 15 mmHg vs 211 ± 12 mmHg, $p<0.05$, 16230 ± 1048 μm^2 vs 19033 ± 1082 μm^2, $p<0.05$). In both groups, mesenteric diameters were smaller under active than under passive condition without significant changes in treated vs untreated group. The active wall tension was lower in treated (0.4 ± 0.19 N/m) than in untreated rats (1.19 ± 0.62 N/m, $p<0.05$). However, there were no differences in active wall stress in both groups (103 ± 47 kPa and 134 ± 30 kPa). These results suggest that chronic treatment with indapamide induced a reduction of the mesenteric arterial smooth muscle mass associated with a marked decrease in its maximal contractile tone. The latter was related to the smooth muscle mass reduction and not to alteration of the vascular muscle contratility.

Introduction

Indapamide is an antihypertensive agent with diuretic activity and specific vascular effects in man (Royer RJ, 1976) and in animal (Kyncl J, et al., 1975). The specific vascular effects of indapamide is to reduce total peripheral resistance (Canicave JCl, et al., 1977) and to decrease vascular reactivity (Finch L, 1977). The aim of this study was to test the effects of chronic treatment of indapamide on the mesenteric arterial structure and function in spontaneously hypertensive rats (SHR).

Methods

1) Preparation of animals

Twenty-four 8 week-old SHRs were separated into treated (n=12) and untreated (n=12) groups. Treated SHRs received 3mg/kg indapamide by gavage in 1ml arabic gum daily during 28 days. At the same time, untreated SHRs received 1ml arabic gum by gavage. Standard rat diet and water was provided ad libitum. Systolic blood pressure (tail-cuff method), heart rate and body weight were measured before and after treatment. At the end of the treatment (28 days latter), all rats were used for study of the mechanical properties of the mesenteric artery.

2) Experimental model

After anesthesia with sodium pentobarbital (50mg/kg ip), a median laparotomy was performed and the last loop of small intestine was exposed on a laboratory-built plastic container including an optical glass piece. The preparation was immediately irrigated by a buffered Tyrode's solution (pH = 7.4) maintained at 38°C. The mesenteric arteries and arcades were neither fixed nor stretched. A short segment of mesenteric artery (about 3 mm) of a second generation branch (diameter 300-400 µm) was gently dissected A video camera was mounted on the binocular lens and allowed to record video images (magnification x100). Every arterial branch located downstream of the observed segment of artery except one was then ligated. A removable micro-clamp was placed on the last branch. Finally, a polyethylene catheter was introduced into the first generation branch of the mesenteric artery. This catheter was filled with Tyrode's albumin (4%) solution and connected to a manometer with adjustable pressure levels. After removing the clamp from the distal segment of the mesenteric artery, the observed mesenteric artery was filled with the flushing solution. The segment of isolated artery was submitted to pressure ranging from 0 to 200 mmHg per steps of 25 mmHg. The external diameter of the artery was measured at each pressure step.

Experiments were performed under active smooth muscle conditions (phenylephrine 10^{-6} M) and under passive smooth muscle conditions (potassium cyanide 0.1mg/ml for 30 minutes). At the end of the experiment, the mesenteric artery was fixed with a glutaraldehyde (2.5%) and paraformaldehyde (2%) buffered solution. The wall vessel cross sectional area was determined in transverse sections.

3) Calculation of mechanical parameters

Using the measured values of the "in situ" arterial external diameter (D_e, µm) and the wall cross sectional area (CSA, µm^2), several parameters were calculated at each pressure: 1) Wall thickness (h, µm): h = CSA/ $\pi \cdot D_e$, 2) internal diameter (D_i, µm) : D_i= D_e - 2·h, 3) tangential wall tension (T, N/m) T = P · D_i /2, 4) tangential wall stress (s, kPa) s = T/h. The active wall stress was calculated as the difference in wall stress, at a given pressure, under active and passive conditions. Similarly, active wall tension was calculated from active and passive wall tension values.

Results (mean ±SEM)

		Treated SHRs		Untreated SHRs
Systolic Pressure	Day 1	192 ± 4		193±6
	Day 28	197 ± 4	--★--	211±4
Heart rate	Day 1	368 ±12		358±8
	Day 28	424 ±16		394±12
Body weight	Day 1	200 ± 5		200±4
	Day 28	270 ± 4		288±2
Wall cross sectional area	Day 28	16229 ± 1048	--★--	19032±1082

Table1 summarizes the results of systolic arterial pressure (mmHg), heart rate (beats/min), body weight (g), and wall cross sectional area (µm^2) obtained in treated and untreated SHRs. Systolic arterial pressure and mesenteric CSA were decreased in treated rats (·p<0.05).

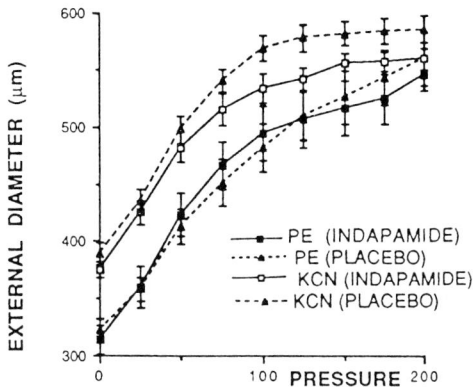

FIG1: Variation of external diameter response with transmural pressure for treated group (INDAPAMIDE) and untreated group (PLACEBO) under active vascular smooth muscle (PE) and passive vascular smooth muscle condition (KCN).

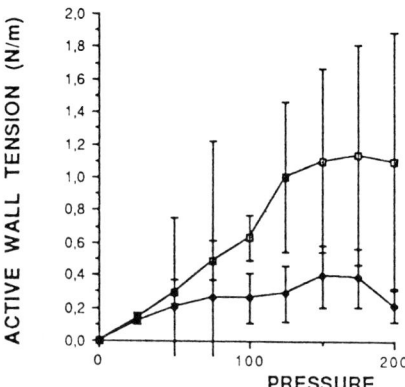

FIG 2 (A): Variation of active wall tension response with transmural pressure in two groups (open symbols = untreated group, closed symbols = treated group)

Fig 1 shows that the mesenteric external diameters in treated and untreated groups were smaller under active than under passive conditions for all transmural pressures. No difference was found in diameters measured in treated and untreated SHRs.

Fig 2: Active wall tension (A) and active wall stress (B) vs transmural pressures in treated and untreated groups. The active wall tension was lower in treated ($p<0.05$) than in untreated rats. However, there were no differences in active wall stress in both groups.

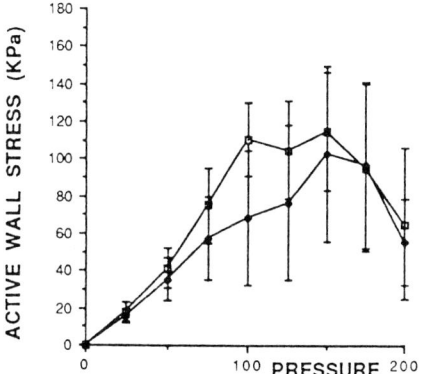

FIG 2(B): Variation of active wall stress with transmural pressure in two groups (open symbols = untrated group, closed symbols = treated group)

Conclusion

Chronic treatment with indapamide slightly decreases the arterial pressure in SHRs. However there was a significant decrease in mesenteric arterial cross sectional area in the treated rats. The significant reduced reactivity to phenylephrine in mesenteric arteries from SHRs treated with indapamide was related to the treatment-induced reduction of the arterial mass. The unchanged active wall stress in treated SHRs suggests that the sensitivity to phenylephrine of smooth muscle cells was not affected by indapamide.

References

Canicave, J.C.I., Lesber, F.X. (1977): Measurement of peripheral resistance by carotid pulse wave recording: Study of a vasopressor and an antihypertensive agents. Curr Med Res Opin. 5: suppl; 1: 79-82.

Finch, L., Hicks, P.E., Moore, R.A. (1977): The effects of indapamide on vascular reactivity in experimental hypertension. Curr Med Res Opin. 5: 44-54.

Kyncl, J., Oheim, K., Seki, T., Solles, A. (1975): Antihypertensive effect of indapamide in various experimental models. Arzneimittel Forsch. 25: 1491-1495.

Royer, R. (1976): Progress in the treatment of arterial hypertension: Clinical approach arising from a french multicentre study. Sem Hôp Paris 52: 365-368.

The effects of a K+ channel opener, BRL 38227, on blood pressure and vascular thromboxane A_2 generation in Dahl salt-sensitive rats

Nobuhito Hirawa, Satoshi Umemura, Yasuo Tokita, Yoshiyuki Toya, Koichi Sugimoto, Nobuyoshi Takagi, Yoshio Kato, Toshio Ikeda and Masao Ishii

Second Department of Internal Medicine, Yokohama City University, 3-9, Fukuura, Kanazawa-ku, Yokohama 236, and Division of Nephrology, Kantoh Teishin Hospital, 5-9-22, Higashigotanda, Shinagawa-Ku, Tokyo, 141, Japan

Introduction A newly synthesized K+ channel opener, BRL 38227, has been shown to dilate artery through hyperpolarisation and inhibiting calcium channels of smooth muscle cells in rats (Hof, 1988; Coldwell, 1987; Kajioka, 1991). However, the effect of this agent was not known in Dahl salt-sensitive rats. Recent studies showed the anti-hypertensive drugs modify the eicosanoid system of vasculature and the kidney (Hirawa, 1991; Uehara, 1991; Numabe, 1989). Thus, this study examined the effect of BRL 38227 on blood pressure, thromboxane A2 (TXA2) generation from aorta, atrial natriuretic peptide (ANP)- cyclic GMP (cGMP) system and renin-angiotensin-aldosterone system in Dahl salt-sensitive rats.

Materials and methods After a 5-week high salt period (4% NaCl diet), blood pressure and heart rate were measured under a conscious condition using the tail cuff method in sixteen 9-week-old Dahl salt sensitive rats. They were given 500 ug/kg of BRL 38227 (n=9) or vehicle (n=7) using the stomach tube once a day for 2 weeks. On the following day of the last administration of the BRL 38227 or vehicle, blood samples were obtained, then the aortas were removed. Aortic strips were incubated with a phosphate buffer solution (PBS) at 37°C for 30 mins. The generated thromboxane A2 was measured as thromboxane B2 (TXB2), stable metabolite of TXA2 using sensitive radioimmunoassay (RIA) (Uehara, 1987). To investigate the direct effect of BRL 38227 on TX generation from the aortas of Dahl salt sensitive rats, aortic strips were incubated with PBS containing BRL 38227 (10^{-10} to 10^{-6}M) and the generated TXA2 was measured with RIA. Plasma renin activity (PRA), plasma concentration of aldosterone (PAC), ANP and cGMP were measured by RIA. Serum electrolytes were measured using flame-photometer.

Results After administration of the agent on the last day of the treating period, blood pressure decreased significantly at 2 hours (159 ± 7 vs. 247 ± 7 mmHg, p<0.01; BRL 38227 vs. vehicle), 5 hours (161 ± 4 vs. 244 ± 6 mmHg, p<0.01) and 24 hours (215 ± 6 vs. 248 ± 6, p<0.01). The body weights of the two groups did not differ significantly (353 ± 4 vs. 346 ± 6 g, BRL 38227 vs. vehicle). Serum electrolyte (Na+: 150 ± 1 vs. 150 ± 1 mEq/l, K+: 4.9 ± 0.1 vs. 4.9 ± 0.2 mEq/l), PRA (1.9 ± 0.6 vs. 1.4 ± 1.1 ngA1/ml/hr) and PAC (71 ± 12 vs. 73 ± 11 pg/ml), ANP (71 ±14 vs. 79 ± 16 pg/ml) and cGMP (94 ± 13 vs 69 ± 5 pmol/ml) did not differ significantly between the

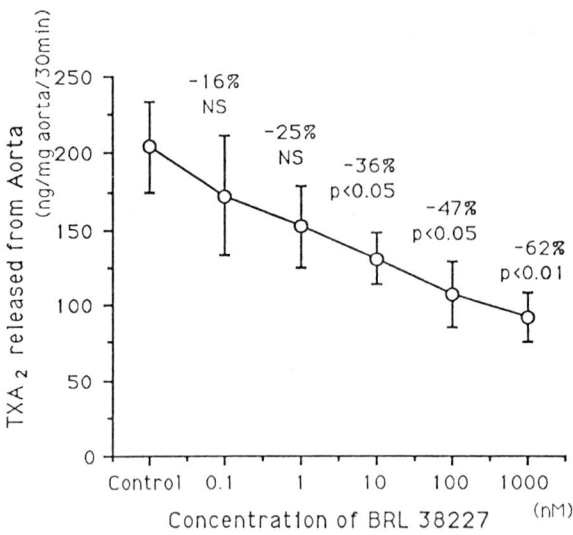

Figure 1. Direct effect of BRL38227 on the production of thromboxane A2 from aortic strips of Dahl salt-sensitive rats. (n=8)

two groups. However, the vascular TXA2 generation decreased significantly with BRL38227 treatment (0.38 ± 0.06 vs. 0.61 ± 0.05 ug/mg dry tissue weight/30 mins, p<0.01). Furthermore, BRL 38227 reduced the TXA2 generation dose-dependently in the incubation media with the concentration of BRL 38227 at 10^{-8} to 10^{-6}M (Figure 1).

Discussion In this study, we demonstrated that chronic BRL 38227 treatment attenuated the elevation of blood pressure in Dahl salt sensitive rats fed on a 4% NaCl diet. Blood pressure reduction was already observed at 2 hours after administration of BRL 38227 and was continued for 24 hours and this antihypertensive effects were sustained for the whole period of treatment (2 weeks). The mechanisms of antihypertensive effect of BRL 38227 treatment in salt-induced hypertension are not clear. However, like other rats, hyperpolarisation of smooth muscle cells by opening K^+ channel and inhibiting Ca^{++} channel may be the main mechanisms, because PRA, PAC, ANP and cGMP did not change with this treatment. In addition to these antihypertensive mechanisms, attenuation of TXA2 formation seems to be another mechanism of antihypertensive effect of this agent as discussed below. In the preparation of aortic strips, thromboxane formation was directly inhibited with BRL 38227 treatment and in viva system this effect of inhibiting thromboxane formation was also demonstrated by in subchronic treatment of oral administration for 2 weeks. Since thromboxane A2 is known to be a potent vasopressor substance, the inhibition of its generation may induce vasodilation and contribute to the antihypertensive effect of BRL 38227 shown in the present study. Furthermore, recent study showed that thromboxane itself stimulate the vascular smooth muscle cell growth and proliferation (Ishimitsu, 1988). Thus, the attenuation of the thromboxane generation, as shown in the BRL-treated Dahl salt sensitive rat, seems to be a favorable effect in respect of vascular hypertrophy. In summary, present study suggests that BRL 38227 has an antihypertensive effect in Dahl salt sensitive rats and that this effect may be partly due to a decrease in vascular TXA2 generation by this agent.

Acknowledgements The authors acknowledge Dr. Yoshio Uehara for a gift of antibody of thromboxane B2. We greatfully thank Smithkline-Beecham Co., Ltd, Tokyo, Japan for a gift of BRL 38227 (Lemakalim) . We also thank Ono Pharmaceutical Co., Ltd, Osaka, Japan for a gift of eicosanoids for radioimmunoassay.

References

Coldwell, M.V. and Howlett, D.R. (1987): Specificity of action of the novel antihypertensive agent, BRL 34915, as a potassium channel activator. Biochem. Pharmacol. 36: 3663-3669.

Hirawa, N., Uehara, Y., Numabe, A., Ikeda, T., Yagi, S., Sugimoto, T. and Ishii, M. (1991): Inhibitory effects of beta adrenoceptor antagonist, atenolol, on the thromboxane system in the kidney of spontaneously hypertensive rats. Prostaglandins Leukot. Essent. Fatty Acids 43: 93-98.

Hof., R.P., Quast, U., Cook, N.S. and Blarer, S. (1988): Mechanism of action and systemic and regional hemodynamics of the potassium channel activator BRL34915 and its enantiomers. Circ. Res. 62: 679-686.

Ishimitsu, T., Uehara, Y., Ishii, M., Ikeda T., Matsuoka, H. and Sugimoto. T. (1988): Thromboxane and vascular smooth musc cell growth in genetically hypertensive rats. Hypertension 12: 46-51.

Kajioka, S., Nakashima, M., Kitamura, K. and Kuriyama, H. (1991): Mechanisms of vasodilatation induced by potassium-channel activators. Clin. Sci. 81: 129-139.

Numabe, A., Uehara, Y., Hirawa, N., Takada, S. and Yagi, S. (1989): Effect of thiazide diuretics on vascular eicosanoid system of spontaneously hypertensive rats. J.Hypertens. 7: 493-499.

Uehara, Y., Tobian, L., Iwai, J. and Sugimoto, T. (1987): Alterations of vascular prostacyclin and thromboxane A2 in Dahl genetical strain susceptible to salt-induced hypertension. Prostaglandins. 33: 727-738.

Uehara, Y., Numabe, A., Hirawa, N., Kawabata, Y., Iwai, J., Ono, H., Matsuoka, H., Takabatake, Y., Yagi, S. and Sugimoto T. (1991): Antihypertensive effects of cicletanine and renal protection in Dahl salt-sensitive rats. J. Hypertens. 9: 719-728.

Genetics

Génétique

… Genetic Hypertension. Ed J. Sassard. Colloque INSERM/John Libbey Eurotext Ltd. © 1992, Vol. 218, pp. 295-296

Polymerase chain reaction-based DNA fingerprinting in the spontaneously hypertensive rat : a new method of genetic analysis

Robert Di Nicolantonio, Takashi Imai [3], Katsumi Ikeda [2], Yasuo Nara [2], Akiyoshi Fukamizu [1], Yukio Yamori [2], Eiichi Soeda [3] and Kazuo Murakami [1]

Department of Physiology, University of Melbourne, Parkville, Victoria 3052, Australia, [1] Gene Experiment Centre, University of Tsukuba, Tsukuba, Ibaraki 305, Japan, [2] Department of Pathology, Shimane Medical University, Izumo 693, Japan and [3] Tsukuba Life Science Centre, Riken, Tsukuba, Ibaraki 305, Japan

Despite extensive pathophysiological investigation the mechanism of the elevated blood pressure (BP) of the spontaneously hypertensive rat (SHR) of the Okamoto strain remains unknown. Very early studies showed that the elevated BP of the SHR had a genetic component and that relatively few genes were involved (Tanase et al., 1970). However it is only recently that newer, more powerful molecular biological techniques have been used to re-examine the genetic basis for the elevated BP of the SHR (Samani et al., 1989; Yagisawa et al., 1990) and other genetically hypertensive rat strains (Samani et al., 1990). The development of the polymerase chain reaction (PCR; Mullis & Faloona, 1987) has allowed the rapid amplification of specific DNA sequences against a complex mixture of genomic sequences. Using this technique we have established a genetic "fingerprinting" technique which utilises repetitive DNA sequences found at irregular intervals throughout the rat and human genome (Witney & Furano, 1984; Nelson et al., 1989). Using PCR primers homologous to such repetitive elements we have been able to synthesise DNA spanning such units and visualise them as a ladder of discrete bands upon gel electrophoresis. This allows ready comparisons of fingerprint patterns between normal individuals and those with congenital diseases. Major gene insertions or deletions will result in altered lengths between repetitive units and therefore band shifts on the PCR-fingerprint. Here we report the first use of this method in comparing the SHR, Wistar Kyoto (WKY) and Sprague Dawley (SD) genome.

Genomic DNA was extracted, using standard phenol/chloroform protocols, from four different rat strains; original progenitor SHR and WKY, SD and a commercially available WKY. PCR buffers, polymerase and deoxynucleotides were obtained from a commercial source (GeneAmp PCR Reagent Kit, Perkin Elmer Cetus). Each PCR incubation contained 1 μl PCR buffer (Tris/KCl/MgCl$_2$/Gelatin), 0.4 μl dNTP mixture(2.5 mM each), 0.05 μl Taq polymerase (0.01 U Amplitaq), 1 μl DNA (35 ng), 0.4 μl primer (25 μM) and 2.15 μl water making a total volume of 5 μl. 20 μl of light mineral oil (Sigma) was placed over the mixture in 0.5 ml reaction vessels (GeneAmp Reaction Tubes, Perkin Elmer Cetus) and placed into the wells of a Perkin Elmer Cetus Thermocycler (N801-0101). The following conditions were found to provide optimal amplification of DNA sequences:

STEP		
1	94°C,	1 min
2	60°C,	1 min
3	74°C,	1 min

The reaction was run for 20 cycles with a 15 second extension of step 3 per cycle. The primer used had the following sequence; AGAAAGAAGAGGTCAAGGCC (5'-3'; Alonso et al., 1983). Following incubation the mixture was electrophoresed on a vertical 5% acrylamide gel for 3 hours at 110 V (constant voltage). Lamda/Hind III and Phi X174/Hinc II digests were co-run as size markers. Following electrophoresis the gel was stained in ethidium bromide and photographed over an UV lamp.

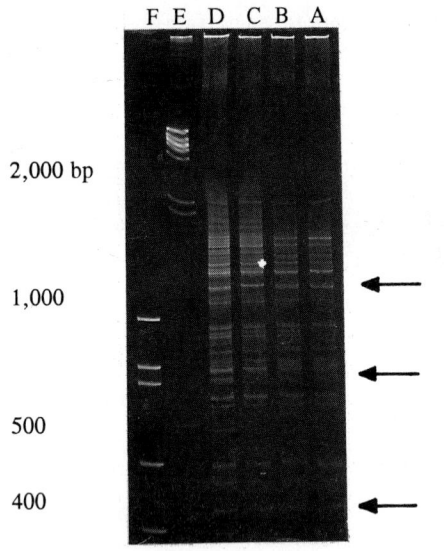

Fig.1. PCR fingerprints of progenitor SHR (lane A), WKY (B), commercially available WKY (C), and SD (D). Lanes E and F represent Lamda/Hind III and Phi X174/Hinc II digest size markers. The upper arrow indicates a band duplication found only in the commercially available WKY and SD. The middle arrow indicates a band shift in the commercially available WKY and the lowest arrow shows a band duplication in the WKY and triplication in the SHR.

As can be seen from Fig.1 there is a large degree of homology between the PCR fingerprints of the rats from the four different colonies. However some clear differences exist in the form of band shifts or deletions, band duplications and band triplications. Clearly though some of the band differences are not associated with high blood pressure. For example the band shift identified in the commercially available WKY (Fig.1, middle arrow) is not found in the SHR, WKY or SD. Thus some differences in fragment profiles could occur in noncoding regions of the genome or relate to RFLPs in genes unrelated to hypertension. Breeding studies, as proposed by Rapp (1983), would be required before candidate fragments were chosen for further characterisation.

Thus, unlike traditional fingerprinting, PCR-fingerprinting selectively amplifies a series of discrete DNA bands more easily excised and characterised. Of equal importance, PCR-fingerprinting increases the possibility of detecting polymorphic genes not previously known, or not thought of as contributing to hypertension and may also provide probes for screening of a cDNA library.

Alonso, A., Kuhn, B., and Fischer, J. (1983): An unusual accumulation of repetitive sequences in the rat genome. *Gene*, 26, 303-306.
Morris, B.J. (1991): Molecular genetics links renin to hypertension. *Mol. Cell. Endocr.*, 75, C13-C18.
Mullis, K.B. and Faloona, F.A. (1987): Specific synthesis of DNA *in vitro* via a polymerase-catalyzed chain reaction. *Methods Enzymol.*, 155, 335-350.
Nelson, D.L., Ledbetter, S.A., Corbo, L., Victoria, M.F., Ramirez-Solis, R., Webster, T.D., Ledbetter, D.H. and Caskey, C.T. (1989): Alu polymerase chain reaction: a method for rapid isolation of human specific sequences from complex DNA sources. *Proc. Natl. Acad. Sci.*, 86, 6686-6690.
Rapp, J.P. (1983): A paradigm for identification of primary genetic causes of hypertension in rats. *Hypertension*, 5(suppl 1), 1-198-1-203.
Samani, N.J., Brammar, W.J. and Swales, J.D. (1989): A major structural abnormality in the renin gene of the spontaneously hypertensive rat. *J. Hypertension*, 7, 249-254.
Samani, N.J., Vincent, M., Sassard, J., Henderson, I.W., Kaiser, M.A., Brammar, W.J. and Swales, J.D. (1990): Analysis of the renin gene intron A tandem repeat region of Milan and Lyon hypertensive rat strains. *J. Hypertension*, 8, 805-809.
Tanase, H., Suzuki, Y., Ooshima, A., Yamori, Y. and Okamoto, K. (1970): Genetic analysis of blood pressure in spontaneously hypertensive rats. *Jap. Circ. J.*, 34, 1197-1212.
Witney, F.R. and Furano, A.V. (1984): Highly repeated DNA families in the rat. *J. Biol. Chem.*, 259, 10481-10492.
Yagisawa, H., Emori, Y. and Nojima, H. (1991): Phospholipase C genes display restriction fragment length polymorphisms between the genomes of normotensive and hypertensive rats. *J. Hypertension*, 9, 303-307.

Genetic analysis of the spontaneously hypertensive rat (SHR), Wistar-Kyoto rat (WKY) and their F_2 generation using 26 human variable number of tandem repeats (VNTR) markers

T. Nabika, Y. Nara *, K. Ikeda *, M. Sawamura *, J. Endo and Y. Yamori *

*Departments of Laboratory Medicine and Pathology *, Shimane Medical University, Izumo 693, Japan*

SUMMARY

1) F2 rats obtained from crossmating between stroke-prone spontaneously hypertensive rats (SHRSP) and Wistar Kyoto rats (WKY) were genetically analyzed by the DNA fingerprinting using 26 human variable number of tandem repeats (VNTR) probes.
2) Seventeen of 26 VNTR probes exhibited polymorphic bands between SHRSP and WKY when they were hybridized with the genomic DNA digested by Hae III or Rsa I.
3) Thirty-seven informative bands given by 8 VNTR probes were studied in 35 F_2 rats. The result indicated that 37 bands represented 26 different genetic loci and they were divided into 22 groups that did not have close linkages with one another.
4) The segregation study indicated that a polymorphic band detected by MCT96.1 might segregate with high blood pressure in F_2 rats.
5) These results suggested that the DNA fingerprinting analysis using VNTR probes is useful both in the construction of a linkage map and in the segregation study of high blood pressure in F_2 rats.

INTRODUCTION

Spontaneously hypertensive rats (SHR) have been the most widely studied model animals for essential hypertension. SHR are thought to have more than two "hypertensive" genes of which interaction causes hypertension (Tanase, H. et al., 1970). To elucidate these "hypertensive" genes in SHR, it is essential to get a genomic map made up of the marker loci that distinguish polymorphisms between SHR and normotensive control rats such as Wistar-Kyoto rats (WKY). However, the genomic map of the rat is far from completion. In the present study, we thus studied genomic polymorphisms between SHR and WKY by the DNA fingerprinting analysis using human VNTR probes to get a linkage map of SHR.

METHODS

F_2 generation rats were obtained through interbred of F_1 hybrids that were made by crossbreeding between SHRSPA$_3$/Izm and WKY/Izm. Blood pressures were measured once every 2-3 weeks and the end of the 12 months' observation period, F_2 rats were sacrificed and genomic DNA was extracted from the livers. The DNA was digested with restriction endonucleases, Hae III or Rsa I. The digested DNA was then fractionated by electrophoresis on 1% agarose gel and capillary transferred onto nylon membrane.

Prehybridization and hybridization were performed at 60°C in 6x SSC, 0.5% SDS with and without 5x Denhardt solution, respectively. Twenty-six human VNTR probes were generously provided by Dr. Y. Nakamura, Cancer Institute, Tokyo, Japan (Nakamura, Y. et al. 1987). These probes were labeled by the random primer method. After hybridization was completed, the memrane was washed under a low stringency condition (3 times in 2x SSC, 0.1% SDS at room temperature for 60 min) to get fingerprinting patterns. Autoradiogram was taken at -80°C for 2 to 7 days.

RESULTS AND DISCUSSION

Seventeen of 26 VNTR probes were found to distinguish polymorphic bands between SHRSPA$_3$/Izm and WKY/Izm. We performed the linkage analysis of 37 polymorphic bands detected by 8 VNTR probes (Table 1) in 35 F_2 rats. When DNA fingerprints represented by different probes were compared with each other, we found that 4 bands were detected by multiple probes. Further, LOD scores of 636 pairs of the bands revealed that 7 of 37 bands made up 3 linkage groups (Table 2). Other bands showed no close linkages with one another. As a result, we obtained 37 polymorphic bands which represented 26 different genetic loci that were divided into 22 groups having no close linkages with one another. This result indicated that a single VNTR probe detected 2.8 independent genetic loci on average. This figure is substantially lower than the value in the mouse, in which a single VNTR probe detected 14.9 polymorphisms (Julier, C. et al., 1990). The condition of hybridization and/or washing may be critical to get large number of polymorphic bands.

In addition, we performed the segregation study of the 37 polymorphic bands with high blood pressure in F_2 rats. Thirty-three F_2 rats that had blood pressures either above 189 mmHg (HBP group, 16 rats) or below 160 mmHg (LBP group, 17 rats) were selected from 75 F_2 rats, and we examined whether the distributions of the polymorphic bands were distorted between the two groups of F_2 rats. The results of χ^2 test indicated that a band detected by MCT96.1, one of VNTR probes, exhibited weak distortion in the distribution of the bands ($p<0.05$) between HBP and LBP groups. This distorted distribution may be false positive because the p value (0.05) is not stringent enough (Rise, M.L. et al., 1991), however, this strategy allows rapid screening of many polymorphic bands in the segregation study of high blood pressure.

Table 1 Numbers of polymorphic bands detected between SHRSP and WKY by 8 VNTR probes

	YNZ2	MCT96.1	YNM3	KKA12	YNZ132	MCK2	EFD64.1	JCZ30
Hae III	6	6	4	6	3	3	4	1
Rsa I	4	n.d.	n.d.	n.d.	n.d.	n.d.	n.d.	n.d.

n.d.: not determined

Table 2 Three linkage groups detected by VNTR probes

Group	Linked Bands			Θ	Zmax
1	#5/KKA12	-	#3/MCT96.1	0.01	4.24
2	#2/YNZ2	-	#1/JCZ30	0.05	8.02
3	#5/YNZ2	-	#4/EFD64.1	0.05	3.23
	#4/EFD64.1	-	#1/MCT96.1	0.05	3.23
	#1/MCT96.1	-	#5/YNZ2	0.05	6.45

LOD scores of each pair of bands were calculated against multiple recombinant fractions, θ ($0<\theta<0.5$). Maximal LOD scores (Zmax) and recombinant fractions at which Zmax were obtained (Θ) were represented with pairs of polymorphic bands tested. Pairs of the bands with Zmax over 3 were assumed to have positive linkages.

REFERENCES

Julier, C., De Gouyon, B., Georges, M., Guenet, J-L., Nakamura, Y., Avner, P., Lathrop, G.M. (1990): Minisatellite linkage maps in the mouse by cross-hybridization with human probes containing tandem repeats. *Proc. Natl. Acad. Sci. USA* 87:4585-4589.

Nakamura, Y., Leppert, M., O'Connell, P., Wolff, R., Holm, T., Culver, M., Martin, C., Fujimoto, E., Hoff, M., Kumlin, E., White, R. (1987): Variable number of tandem repeat (VNTR) markers for human gene mapping. *Science* 235:1616-1622

Rise, M.L., Frankel, W.N., Coffin, J.M., Seyfried, T.N. (1991): Genes for epilepsy mapped in the mouse. *Nature* 253: 669-673.

Tanase, H., Suzuki, Y., Ooshima, A., Yamori, Y., Okamoto, K. (1970): Genetic analysis of blood pressure in SHR. *Jpn. Circ. J.*. 34: 1194-1212.

Identification of a hypertensinogenic gene in spontaneously hypertensive rats

Naoharu Iwai, Shigeyuki Chaki and Tadashi Inagami

Department of Biochemistry, Vanderbilt University School of Medicine, Nashville, TN 37232, USA

We have recently isolated a gene (1), designated as Sa, which is ten times more abundantly expressed in the kidneys of spontaneously hypertensive rats (SHR) than in those of Wistar-Kyoto rats(WKY). To test the hypothesis that the Sa gene is one of the genes responsible for the high blood pressure in SHR, we examined whether the SHR genotype of the Sa gene was associated with higher blood pressure than the WKY genotype of the Sa gene in the F2 rats.

Male SHR and female WKY used to produce F1 rats were derived from rats originally derived from those obtained from Taconic Farm. Since heterogeneities in WKY(2) and in SHR(3) have been reported, the genotypes of the Sa gene and the renin gene were checked in all parental rats. The parental rats were then crossed to produce F1 rats that were then inter-crossed to produce 67 male F2 rats. At 24-26 weeks of age, the blood pressure was carefully measured by the tail cuff microphonic manometer method. Fourteen rats of low blood pressure phenotype(<128 mmHg) and fifteen rats of high blood pressure phenotype(>145 mmHg) were selected, and the genotypes of the Sa and renin gene of these rats were analysed by the Southern blotting method. The genotype analysis of the renin gene was included in view of the previous report that the renin gene genotypic difference was not associated with the high blood pressure(4).

The restriction fragment length polymorphism(RFLP) in the Sa gene was observed by the restriction enzyme Stu I, and the RFLP of the renin gene was observed by HindIII (Fig. 1). As shown in the Table 1, the frequency of the SHR genotype of the Sa gene in the high blood pressure group was significantly different ($p<0.025$ by Fisher's exact probability test) from that in the low blood pressure group. On the other hand, no statistical difference was observed in the frequency of the SHR or WKY genotype of the renin gene between the two groups.

Taking into consideration that the Sa gene is differentially expressed between the kidneys of SHR and WKY from the 4th week of age, it is highly likely that that the Sa gene is one of the genes responsible for the high blood pressure in SHR.

The expression of the Sa gene was reassessed in other tissues by using the competitive polymerase chain reaction method(5). The Xba I(97)-Msc I(961) fragment of the Sa cDNA (1) was subcloned into pBluescript II KS(+) (Stratagene), designated as pSA. pSA was digested by with Nsi I and Nco I, was blunt-ended by the Klenow treatment, and was self ligated. The resultant plasmid contained the cDNA fragment which lacked the region between the Nsi I(177) and Nco I(287) sites. This plasmid was linealized with XhoI and the sense strand deletion-mutated RNA was synthesized by T7 RNA polymerase. Total RNA from various tissues and the deletion-mutated RNA of various amount were mixed, and were reverse-transcribed. The resultant cDNA mixture was amplified by the polymerase chain reaction method using the following two oligonucleotides as primers: 5'-(GAAGAGCTCAAGATCACTGACTTGTGAGCT)-3'(101-130), and 5'-(CAGGGAACAGGCTTCTGTGAGTATGTTGGC)-3'(621-592). The amplification of the Sa mRNA and the deletion-mutated RNA by these two primers should give 521 and 411bp fragments, respectively. With this method, the expression levels of the Sa gene in the central nervous system of WKY were found to be more than ten times higher than those of SHR. As shown in the Fig. 2, the expression level of the Sa gene in the brain of F2 rat was well correlate to the genotype of the Sa gene of each rat.

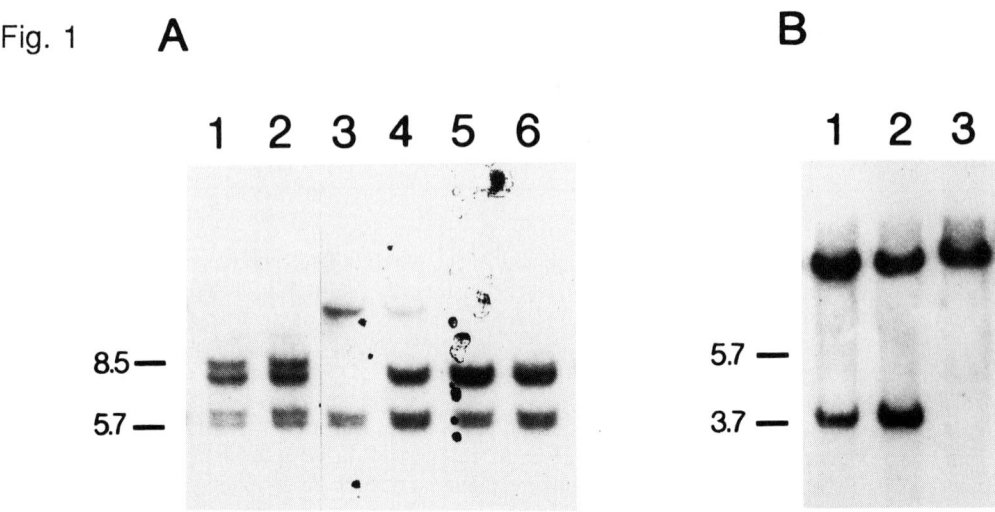

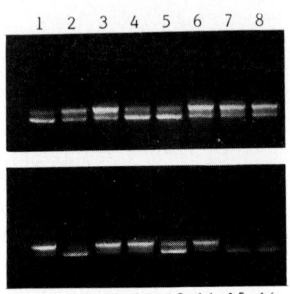

Fig.2

Fig.1A Southern blot of Sa gene
  1. Brown-Norway 2. Fisher 3. SHR
  4. F-1 5. WKY 6. Lewis
Fig.1B Southern blot of renin gene
  1. F-1 2. WKY 3. SHR

Fig.2 Expression levels in the brains of F2
  Twenty micrograms of the total brain RNA was combined with two picograms of the deletion mutated RNA. The genotype of each rat was as follows:
    SHR. 1,4,5,10,13,15,16
    WKY. 2,6,7,9,11
    F-1. 3,8,12,14

Heterogeneities among WKY(2) and SHR(3) have been reported. It is reasonable to think that those observed genetic drifts may occur at loci not involved in the blood pressure regulation, and the important loci may be homogeneous among various SHR and among WKY. However,as pointed out by Rapp et al.(6), the genetic back ground is important in the expression of the blood pressure effects of a given locus. Therefore, it is possible that a given genotype,which is hypertensinogenicin a F2 population derived from one source, may not be hypertensinogenic in F2 populations derived from other sources. A discrepancy between the two results(4,7) may be interpreted by this mechanism. In this sense, our current results may be applicable only to the F2 rats generated in the present study. However, it is concluded that the Sa gene is one of the genes regulating blood pressure, and the Sa gene can be one of the genes responsible for the genetic form of spontaneous hypertension. Whether the SHR genotype of the Sa gene can be hypertensinogenic in other genetic backgrounds than WKY can be tested by the use of RFLPs observed in other normotensive inbred strains of Lewis rat, Brown-Norway rat, and Fisher rat(Fig. 1), in which the expression levels of the Sa gene in the kidney are all comparable to that in WKY(Data not shown).

TABLE 1. Genotypes of the F2 rats

Genotype	HIGH 15 rats — number of rats with given genotypes in Sa gene and (renin gene)	LOW 14 rats — number of rats with given genotypes in Sa gene and (renin gene)
SHR	8 (5)	1 (2)
F1	6 (7)	3 (6)
WKY	1 (3)	10 (6)

To apply Fisher's exact probability test, the rats whose genotypes were F1 and WKY were categorized in one group.

REFERENCE

1. Iwai N and Inagami T   Hypertension 17, 161-169, (1991)
2. Kurtz TW, Montano M, Chan L, and Kabra P   Hypertension 13, 188-192, (1990)
3. Nabica T, Nara Y, Ikeda K, Endo J, and Yamori Y   Hypertension 18, 12-16, (1991)
4. Lindpainter K, Takahashi S, and Ganten D   J.Hypertens. 8, 763-773, (1990)
5. Iwai N, Yamano Y, Chaki S, et al.   Biochem.Biophys.Res.Commun. 177, 299-304, (1991)
6. Rapp JP, Wang SM, and Dene H   Am.J.Hypertens. 3, 391-396, (1990)
7. Kurtz TW, Simonet L, Kabra PM, Wolfe S, Chan L, and Hjelle BL   J.Clin.Invest. 85, 1328-1332, (1990)

Abnormal structure and expression of *hsp70* genes in hypertension

Pavel Hamet, Dewen Kong, Toshihiko Hashimoto, Yu-Lin Sun, Gilles Corbeil, Michal Pravenec [1], Jaroslav Kunes [1], Pavel Klir [1], Vladimir Kren [2] and Johanne Tremblay

Centre de Recherche Hôtel-Dieu de Montréal, Université de Montréal, 3850, rue Saint-Urbain, Pavillon Marie-de-la-Ferre, Montréal, Québec, Canada H2W 1T8, [1] Institute of Physiology, Czechoslovak Academy of Sciences, Prague and [2] Institute of Biology, Faculty of Medicine, Charles University, Prague, Czechoslovakia

SUMMARY The major stress gene *hsp70* is abnormally expressed *in vivo* as well as in cultured vascular smooth muscle cells, due to a higher transcription rate in genetically hypertensive rats and mice. Using human *hsp70* probe for hybridizing Southern blots of genomic DNA digested with Bam HI enzyme, a restriction fragment length polymorphism (RFLP) was revealed between spontaneously hypertensive rats (SHR) and various normotensive strains. This polymorphism in SHR was associated with 15 mmHg of blood pressure and maps into the RT1 complex in the rat. A RFLP was also observed with XbaI restriction enzyme in spontaneously hypertensive mice using the murine *hsp68* probe. These structural modifications of *hsp70* gene may be functionally relevant to abnormalities in thermosensitivity in hypertension.

INTRODUCTION Stressful environments modify the expression of hypertension. The working hypothesis of our group is that the response to stress is genetically determined. Among stressful environmental agents known to have an impact on blood pressure, we selected heat as a stimulus. Our past results have demonstrated that thermosensitivity correlates with hypertension and is determined by a distinct *locus* (*Tms*) in spontaneously hypertensive mice (SHM). Since thermosensitivity persists at the level of vascular smooth muscle cells (VSMC) as well as in neonatal cardiomyocytes from spontaneously hypertensive rats (SHR), we undertook to analyze candidate genes of cellular thermosensitivity. The heat stress genes HSP70 are expressed by a variety of environmental stimuli in all cells. Anomalies in the transcription of the heat stress gene HSP70, accompanied by abnormal mRNA accumulation and a transient increase in HSP70 protein, have been reported by our group (Hamet et al., 1990). We, therefore, studied anomalies of HSP70 gene expression in more details and searched for a restriction fragment length polymorphism (RFLP) in genetically hypertensive rats and mice.

METHODS Cultured VSMC were obtained by the explant method from thoracic aortae of male Wistar-Kyoto rats (WKY) and SHR supplied by Charles River Canada, St. Constant, Quebec, Canada. The cells were characterized as described previously (Hadrava et al., 1989) and used between the 5th and 19th passages. VSMC quiescence was induced by incubation in Dulbecco's Modified Eagle Medium (DMEM) containing insulin, transferrin and selenium (ITS) for 72 hrs. Total RNA was extracted by the acid guanidium thiocyanate method, electrophoresed, blotted and hybridized with human ^{32}P-*hsp70* probe obtained from Dr. R.I. Morimoto (Northwestern University, Evanston, IL, USA). Genomic DNA was extracted, digested by restriction enzymes and hybridized with human ^{32}P-labelled *hsp70* by standard methods. Inbred strains, SHR and BN.lx (progenitors of HxB/BxH recombinant inbred strains), and RT1 congenic rats, SHR.1N and BN.lx.1K were obtained from the Czechoslovak Academy of Sciences and the Department of Biology, Faculty of Medicine, Charles University, Prague.

RESULTS Heat shock-induced accumulation of *hsp70* mRNA was greater *in vivo* as well as *in vitro* in spontaneously hypertensive rodents as compared to their normotensive controls. An example of this exaggerated accumulation in cultured VSMC is illustrated in Figure 1. In these experiments, cells were submitted to heat stress at 43 °C for 0, 10, and 20 min. The upper part of the figure illustrates a typical Northern blot experiment and the lower part represents mean of 6 separate experiments expressed as a ratio of *HSP70* to ß-actin. It is now well recognized that heat-induced *hsp70* transcription is regulated at the level of heat stress element (HSE), a cognate sequence in the promoter region of *HSP*. Transcription is triggered by binding of a trimeric heat stress transacting factor (HSTF) to the HSE of *HSP70*. This protein complex is a cytosolic factor that binds *HSP70* which acts as a negative regulator.

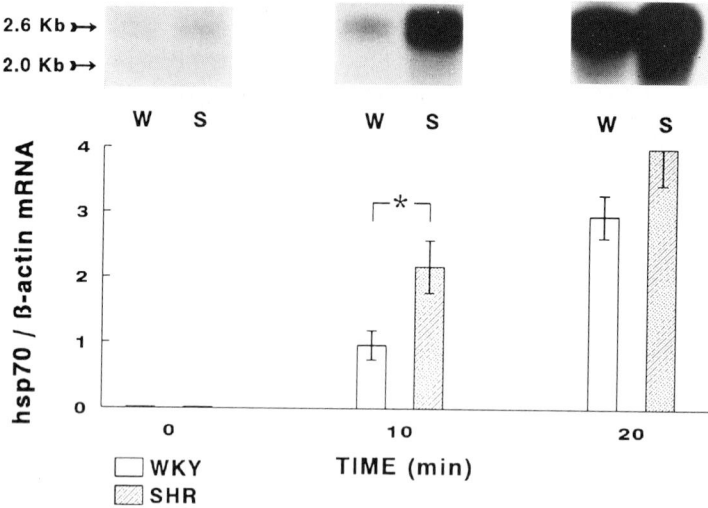

Figure 1. Time-dependent expression of HSP70 in cultured aortic smooth muscle cells from WKY and SHR. Cells were heat stressed at 43 °C for the times indicated. The upper panel indicates a typical Northern blot experiment of HSP70 mRNA accumulation. W, WKY; S, SHR. The lower panel illustrates the mean of 6 different experiments of HSP70/ß-actin mRNA. p < 0.05.

A gel retardation assay, using a ^{32}P-labelled double-stranded oligonucleotides spanning the HSE sequence as a probe, revealed that HSTF activation is more rapid and complete in cells from SHR than normotensive WKY rats (Hashimoto et al., 1991). However, since *HSP70* mRNA accumulation is only transient, it is also possible that insufficient levels of HSP70 protein or an anomaly in the protein product may in turn lead to a defect in *HSP70* transcription. This possibility is supported by the fact that although transiently enhanced, there is in fact lower *de novo* cellular ^{35}S-methionine-labelled HSP70 synthesis in the cytosol of hypertensive cells at later times (Hamet et al., 1990). Since the abnormality may occur at the gene level, we undertook to search for a polymorphism of *HSP70* (Hamet et al., 1991). Our data are summarized in Table 1.

TABLE 1. RFLP OF *HSP70* IN SEVERAL INBRED AND CONGENIC RAT STRAINS

Rat strain (human *HSP70* probe, Bam HI)	Polymorphic fragments	
	3.0	4.4
WKY	+	+
SHR (Prague)	+	-
SHR (Charles River)	+	-
SHR (Taconic)	+	-
BN	-	+
BN.1K	+	-
SHR.1N	-	+

It is clear from this Table that SHR of various origins carry only one polymorphic allele of 3.0 kb after digestion with Bam HI restriction enzyme and hybridization with human *hsp70* or murine *hsp68* probe. BN rats have only a 4.4 kb fragment whereas both fragments are found in the WKY strain. At present, we cannot exclude the possibility that the two bands in WKY are due to heterozygocy. The congenic strains (BN.1K and SHR.1N) enabled us to map this polymorphism into the RT1 complex of the rat. Additional studies in recombinant inbred (RI) strains demonstrated that those with the RT1 *k* haplotype carry the 3.0 fragment while those with the RT1 *n* haplotype have the 4.4 kb fragment. Thus, structural modifications apparently exist in *HSP70* and only further investigations will establish the link between these abnormalities and the expression and/or protein stability. A partial restriction map of *HSP70* from normotensive BN and WKY as well as SHR is

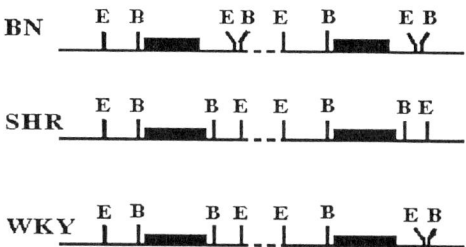

Figure 2. Comparison of the HSP70 restriction map between BN, SHR and WKY rats. E, Eco R1, B, Bam HI restriction enzymes.

illustrated in Fig. 2. In this Figure, we suggest that there are at least two copies of *hsp70* in the RT1 complex and that the difference between BN and SHR progenitors is in the length of the Bam HI fragment while the Eco RI fragment is of identical length. In contrast, in WKY, one of the regions corresponds to that observed in SHR while the other is similar to that in the BN strain. Noticeably, a similar restriction map, as seen in BN, is demonstrated in the Sprague-Dawley strain.

DISCUSSION Our studies revealed that thermosensitivity, which is evident in several genetically hypertensive animals models, is accompanied by abnormalities in the expression of a major heat stress gene, *HSP70*. A transient increase in mRNA accumulation may lead to a higher turnover of *HSP70*, and lower steady state levels of the protein with time may be responsible for the diminished defence mechanisms of hypertensives. Lower protein synthesis has been reported by Klimanskaya et al. (1991) in embryo fibroblasts from SHR. These abnormalities tend to support our contention of an abnormal negative feedback in the regulation of transcription. Diminished *HSP70* binding to HSTF would lead to an exaggerated transcription rate. We report here a RFLP of *HSP70* in SHR that maps into the RT1 major histocompatibility complex, which has been previously demonstrated (Pravenec et al., 1989) to correlate with hypertension in RI strains. In addition, our studies show that all RI strains with the *k* haplotype have a 3.0 kb allele of *HSP70*. The blood pressure difference between all strains with the 3.0 kb fragment including RI strains with BN and SHR progenitors vs those with the 4.4 kb fragment, is 15 mmHg. Furthermore, using the same probe under high stringency conditions, which allowed us to visualize only RT1-linked *HSP70* genes by Southern blot, we observed abnormal *HSP70* mRNA accumulation from an *HSP70* gene most probably located in the RT1 complex. This represents evidence that the abnormal *HSP70* expression is associated with 15 mmHg of blood pressure. Therefore, genes in the major histocompatibility *locus* potentially closely related with *HSP70* are responsible for a major difference in blood pressure, thus contributing to the pathogenesis of hypertension.

REFERENCES

Hadrava V, Tremblay J, Hamet P: Abnormalities in growth characteristics of aortic smooth muscle cells in spontaneously hypertensive rats. Hypertension 13: 589-597, 1989

Hamet P, Tremblay J, Malo D, Kunes J, Hashimoto T: Genetic hypertension is characterized by the abnormal expression of a gene localized in major histocompatibility complex, HSP70. Transplantation Proc 22:2566-2567, 1990

Hamet P, Kong D, Pravenec M, Kunes J, Kren V, Klir P, Sun YL, Tremblay J: RFLP of *hsp70* gene, localized in the RT1 complex, is associated with hypertension in SHR. Hypertension, submitted 1991

Hashimoto T, Mosser RD, Tremblay J, Hamet P: Increased accumulation of *hsp70* mRNA due to enhanced activation of heat shock transcription factor in spontaneously hypertensive rats. J Hypertens, submitted 1991

Klimanskaya IV, Lukashev ME, Postnov YuV. Heat shock protein (HSP) synthesis in normotensive and spontaneously hypertensive rat embryo fibroblasts (REF). Abstracts of the Fifth European Meeting on Hypertension, Milan, Italy, June 7-10, 1991 (No. 337)

Pravenec M, Klir P, Kren V, Zicha J, Kunes J. An analysis of spontaneous hypertension in spontaneously hypertensive rats by means of new recombinant inbred strains. J Hypertens 7: 217-222, 1989

Correct expression of the transgene in the brain of hypertensive transgenic mice carrying the rat angiotensinogen gene

Bernd Bunnemann, Shoji Kimura, John J. Mullins, Frank Zimmermann, Detlev Ganten and Michael Kaling

German Institute for High Blood Pressure Research and Department of Pharmacology, University of Heidelberg, Im Neuenheimer Feld 366, D-6900 Heidelberg, Germany

In recent years, the transgenic animal methodology has found entry into cardiovascular research and several transgenic animals have been generated, having physiological and/or pathophysiological alterations due to transgene expression (Mockrin et al., 1991). The first successfully generated transgenic rats harbouring the mouse ren-2 gene showed severe hypertension despite low circulating renin and angiotensin II (ANG II) concentrations (Mullins et al., 1990). This suggested a probable involvement of local tissue renin-angiotensin systems (RAS) in cardiovascular homeostasis independently of the circulating RAS.

Angiotensinogen (AOGEN), expressed from a single gene in a variety of different tissues, is cleaved by the subsequent actions of renin and converting enzyme to the vasoactive hormone ANG II. Therefore overexpression of AOGEN in vivo is likely to result in increased ANG II levels which in turn might lead to cardiovascular effects. Based on this hypothesis and on the fact that mouse renin is capable of cleaving rat AOGEN, we generated transgenic mice, TGM(rAOGEN), carrying the rat AOGEN gene including 1.6Kb of 5'flanking sequences (Tanaka et al., 1984). Two independent transgenic mouse lines, TGM(rAOGEN)123 and TGM(rAOGEN)92 with different phenotypes respectively, hypertensive and normotensive, were established (TABLE 1). Since liver is a main source of circulating AOGEN, overproduction of AOGEN in the liver resulted in elevated plasma AOGEN and ANG II concentrations in hypertensive TGM(rAOGEN)123. In contrast, normotensive TGM(rAOGEN)92 expressed the transgene very low in the liver, and plasma AOGEN concentrations were not altered. However, it seems unlikely that overexpression of AOGEN in the liver accompanied by an enhancement of circulating RAS activity is the sole mechanism responsible for the development of hypertension in TGM(rAOGEN)123. Ohkubo et al. (1990) reported the generation of similar transgenic mice which expressed the rat AOGEN from a heterologous promoter predominantly active in the liver.

TABLE 1. Mean Arterial Blood Pressure of Control and Transgenic Mice

	Control	Normotensive TGM(rAOGEN)92	Hypertensive TGM(rAOGEN)123
Mean Arterial Blood Pressure (mmHg)	107.3±2.8	103.8±4.4	159.2±7.9*

Values are mean ± SEM obtained from age-matched 6 or more male mice. *P<0.01 vs control. Data from Kimura et al., 1992.

TABLE 2. Comparison of Rat Angiotensinogen Gene Expression in Different Brain Areas of the Rat, Normotensive and Hypertensive Transgenic Mice

Brain Area	Rat	Normotensive TGM(rAOGEN)92	Hypertensive TGM(rAOGEN)123
Telencephalon			
Hypocampus	low	—	moderate
Medial amygdaloid nucleus	moderate	—	moderate
Septum	moderate	—	moderate
Diencephalon			
Thalamus			
Paraventricular nucleus	high	—	high
Subthalamic nucleus	moderate	—	high
Epithalamus			
Habenula	moderate	low	high
Preoptic area			
Median preoptic nucleus	high	—	high
Medial preoptic nucleus	moderate		high
Hypothalamus			
Supraoptic nucleus	high	—	high
Suprachiasmatic nucleus	high	low	high
Periventricular nucleus	high	—	high
Arcuate nucleus	high	—	high
Paraventricular nucleus	high	—	high
Mammilary nucleus	moderate	low	moderate
Mesencephalon			
Substantia nigra	moderate	low	high
Central gray	moderate	low	high
Superior colliculi	high	low	high
Interpeduncular nucleus	moderate	low	high
Pons			
Locus coeruleus	high	moderate	high
Central gray	high	moderate	high
Medulla Oblongata			
Nucleus of the solitary tract	high	high	high
Nucleus of the hypoglossal nerve	high	moderate	low
Inferior olivary nucleus	high	high	high
Spinal trigeminal nucleus	low	high	high
Cerebellum			
Purkinje cell layer	high	high	high
Circumventricular Organs and others			
Subfornical organ	high	—	low
Area postrema	moderate	—	—
OVLT	—	—	—
Choroid plexus	—	—	moderate

Minus means not detected. OVLT: Organum vasculosum of the lamina terminalis

Plasma concentrations of the transgene product were similar to the values found in the present hypertensive TGM(rAOGEN)123. However, their mice did not develop hypertension.

High expression of the transgene was found in the brain of both transgenic mouse lines. All conponents of the RAS have been identified within the brain, thus an overexpression of AOGEN in the brain is likely to result in increased central ANG II concentrations. Since previous studies on rat brain (Bunnemann et al., 1990) have localized AOGEN mRNA primarily to areas and nuclei known to participate in ANG II mediated regulations of hormone releases, salt appetite, drinking behaviour and blood pressure (see reveiw; Ganten et al.,1984, Phillips, 1987), we investigated the rat AOGEN mRNA distribution in the brain of both transgenic mouse lines by *in situ* hybridization. We used a species specific radiorabelled cRNA probe to discriminate between the endogenous mouse and the transgene rat AOGEN mRNA. TABLE 2 summerizes the data obtained with both transgenic mouse lines in comparison to the expression pattern of the endogenous AOGEN gene in the rat brain. In the hypertensive TGM(rAOGEN)123, distribution of the rat AOGEN mRNA was very similar to that observed in rats. Highest expression was seen within the nuclei of the thalamus, hypothalamus and medulla oblongata. On the other hand, in normotensive TGM(rAOGEN)92, the expression pattern was aberrant. The transgene mRNA was expressed similaly to TGM(rAOGEN)123 only in the medulla oblongata, but was abscent or expressed differently in other brain areas including the thalamus, hypothalamus and preoptic area. The ANG II of these areas is thought to influence water intake, release of vasopressin and adrenocorticotropin from the pituitary gland, and also to modulate sympathetic nerve activity. These data indicate that correct expression of the AOGEN gene is a prerequisite for the hypertensive phenotype in transgenic mice. Only TGM(rAOGEN)123, which express the transgene in a correct manner, are hypertensive.

In conclusion, we established the hypertensive and normotensive transgenic mice carrying the rat AOGEN gene. They illustrate the concept that an overproduction of AOGEN can cause hypertension and might become useful experimental models especially for study of the brain RAS.

REFERENCES

Bunnemann, B., Fuxe, K., Bjelke, B., and Ganten, D. (1990): The brain renin-angiotensin-system and its possible involvment in volume transmission. In Advances in Neuroscience vol.1, eds K.Fuxe and L.F.Annati, pp. 131-158. New York: Raven Press.

Ganten, D., Lang, R.E., Lehmann, E. and Unger, T. (1984): Brain angiotensin: on the way to becoming a well-studied neuropeptide system. Biochem.Pharmacol. 33: 3523-3528.

Tanaka,T., Ohkubo, H. and Nakanishi, S. (1984): Common structural organization of the rat angiotensinogen and the alpha1-antitrypsin genes. J.Biol.Chem. 259: 8063-8065.

Kimura, S., Mullins, J., Bunnemann, B., Metzger, R., Hilgenfeldt, U., Zimmermann, F., Jacob, H., Fuxe, K., Ganten,D. and Kaling, M.(1992): Elevated blood Pressure in transgenic mice carrying the rat angiotensinogen gene. EMBO.J. (in press).

Mockrin, S.C., Dzau, V.J., Gross, K.W. and Horam, M.J. (1991): Transgenic animals. Hypertens. 17: 394-399.

Mullins, J.J., Peters, J. and Ganten, D. (1990): Fulminant hypertension in transgenic rats harbouring the mouse ren-2 gene. Nature 344: 541-544.

Ohkubo, H., Kawakami, H., Kakehi, Y., Takumi, T., Arai, H., Iwai, M., Tanabe, Y., Masu, M., Hata, J., Iwao, H., Okamoto, H., Yokoyama, M., Nomura, T., Kasuki, M. and Nakanishi, S. (1990): Generation of transgenic mice with elevated blood pressure by introduction of the rat renin and angiotensinogen genes. Proc.Natl.Acad.Sci.USA 87: 5153-5157.

Phillips, M.I. (1987): Functions of angiotensin in the central nervous system. Ann.Rev.Physiol. 49: 413-435.

Genetic Hypertension. Ed J. Sassard. Colloque INSERM/John Libbey Eurotext Ltd. © 1992, Vol. 218, pp. 313-315

Chromosomal mapping of genetic loci associated with hereditary hypertension in the rat

Klaus Lindpaintner [1][2], Pascale Hilbert [3], Detlev Ganten [2][4], Michel Georges [5] and Mark Lathrop [3]

[1] *Department of Cardiology, Brigham and Women's Hospital, Harvard Medical School, Boston, USA;* [2] *Department of Pharmacology and Institute for High Blood Pressure Research, University of Heidelberg, Germany;* [3] *Centre d'Études du Polymorphisme Humain, Paris, France;* [4] *Centre for Molecular Medicine, Berlin, Germany;* [5] *Genmark, Salt Lake City, USA*

Summary

Primary hypertension in humans is recognized as a polygenic, quantitative trait. We have used the stroke prone, spontaneously hypertensive rat (SHRSP) as a model to elucidate genetic loci associated with blood pressure regulation in hypertension. By performing a cosegregation analysis of phenotype and a large array of genetic markers randomly distributed over the genome, we were able to identify two loci, BP-SP1 and BP-SP2 which show highly significant linkage to blood pressure. These loci were subsequently mapped to chromosome 10 and the X-chromosome, respectively. BP-SP1 lies within a linkage group which, by synteny, corresponds to a region on human chromosome 17q which contains the locus for angiotensin converting enzyme (ACE), a key enzyme of the renin-angiotensin pathway. A subsequently developed polymorphic marker for rat ACE mapped within the BP-SP1 linkage group on rat chromosome 10. Our study demonstrates the feasibility and power of genome screening using random markers over the traditional approach of investigating candidate genes. It charts the way for similar analyses in other hypertensive animal models and, eventually, for the study of human hypertension.

Primary hypertension, due to its high prevalence in the population and its deleterious long-term complications, is a clinical entity of major impact both in terms of individual suffering and of health economics. While family and twin studies have provided convincing evidence for a genetic basis of the disease, its heterogeneous and multifactorial nature have so far resisted investigative efforts to elucidate any of the genes involved. The fact that the disease represents a quantitative trait described by a continuous variable further complicates any analysis. Inbred animal models of heritable hypertension offer the advantage of genetic homogeneity; the ability to produce large cross-bred cohorts combined with newly available methodologies allowing the generation of large numbers of polymorphic markers with (ideally) random distribution across the genome now yield the statistical power to analyze complex genetic traits.

The spontaneously hypertensive rat and its close relative, the SHRSP, represent the most widely investigated model for human hypertension; like the human disease, hypertension in these strains is regarded as a polygenic trait with a limited number (2-4) of major causative genes involved (Tanase *et al.* 1970). Studies examining the relationship between blood pressure and a number of physiological and biochemical phenotypes (Harrap, 1986; Yamori, & Okamoto, 1970) as well as polymorphisms of candidate genes (Lindpaintner *et al.* 1990; Kurtz *et al.* 1990) have so far failed to provide any conclusive evidence as to the etiology of hypertension in this strain. We have used a F_2 population bred from SHRSP and their normotensive control strain, the Wistar Kyoto rat, to screen a large number of randomly distributed genetic markers for their association with blood pressure phenotype.

Two groups of F_1-progeny were produced by breeding a male WKY rat with female SHRSP rats (cross 1), and, conversely, a male SHRSP with female WKY rats (cross 2). Subsequent brother-sister mating within each group of F_1-animals provided the study cohort of 115 F_2-progeny. At 14 to 16 weeks of age (when the until then progressive development of hypertension of the SHRSP enters an asymptotic phase) animals underwent hemodynamic studies by femoral artery catheterization, both before and after oral sodium loading (an important environmental factor influencing blood pressure). Systolic and diastolic blood pressure and heart rate were determined under strictly standardized conditions. At sacrifice, tissue was collected, and a number of additional phenotype characteristics, such as body weight and organ weights, were measured.

Genotype analysis was carried out on genomic DNA prepared from either tail-preps or hepatic tissue. Two different sets of genetic markers were developed and examined: DNA fingerprinting was performed by Southern blot analysis of restriction endonuclease-digested DNA hybridized against a panel of human VNTR (very numerous tandem repeats)-probes, and microsatellite typing was performed based on published rat sequence data. VNTR screening identifies multiple bands for any given restriction enzyme-VNTR probe combination; since the presence of multiple bands precludes the identification of corresponding alleles in the two strains, they are scored as dominant markers, i.e. as either present (representing ++ homozygotes and +- heterozygotes) or absent (--). In contrast, microsatellite screening, which is performed by PCR-amplification of polymorphic regions of CA-repeats using specific primers taken from flanking sequences, allows scoring for co-dominant bands, i.e. ++, +-, or --. Using digests with three different restriction enzymes, and a total of 11 different VNTR probes, we found 139 informative polymorphic markers; in addition, a total of 50 polymorphic microsatellite markers were characterized. Microsatellite markers were subsequently anchored to individual chromosomes using a rat-hamster somatic cell hybrid panel, and, where possible, mini-and microsatellite markers were ordered according to linkage groups. A total of 20 chromosome-mapped linkage groups were thus defined, covering all chromosomes except chromosome 15. In addition, 8 linkage groups and 51 singleton markers were defined which could not be assigned a chromosomal localization.

For the detection of linkage, both analysis of variance (corrected for sex and cross) and segregation and linkage analysis were employed. A p-value of <0.0001 was chosen as the critical limit for the detection of linkage to reduce type-1 error. Thus, two chromosomal regions were identified which showed significant linkage to blood pressure data: One linkage group, associated with the rat growth hormone promotor locus (GHP), is located on chromosome 10; the other, represented by a VNTR-band (**PER-Ha-2**), defines a linkage group on the X-chromosome. These two markers have been termed *BP/SP-1* and *BP/SP-2*, respectively.

The GHP locus was found to be tightly linked to sodium-loaded systolic and diastolic blood pressure, with Lod scores of 5.2 and 5.1, respectively. This locus accounts for about 20% of the blood pressure variance. A microsatellite marker at the nerve growth factor receptor locus (NGFRR), located within the same linkage group at a distance of about 12 cM from GHP, was found to be linked, with a Lod score of 4.2, to baseline diastolic blood pressure values, again accounting for approximately 20% of the variance of this variable. Across-species comparison revealed that the region on rat chromosome 10 identified by the GHP linkage group corresponds, by synteny, to a conserved linkage group on mouse chromosome 11 and human chromosome 17q. This association was of particular interest because the gene for angiotensin converting enzyme (ACE) had previously been mapped to this region on chromosome 17q (Mattei *et al.*1989). After developing a polymorphic microsatellite for rat ACE we confirmed the localization of this gene within the same linkage group on chromosome 10, at a 0.02 recombination frequency from GHP. As expected, Lod scores for linkage of the ACE marker with systolic and diastolic blood pressure values were similar to those seen with the GHP marker. The effect of the GHP locus, as well as of the ACE and NGFRR loci, was found to be consistent with a dominant influence on blood pressure of the gene(s) at by these loci.

The finding that sodium-stimulated, but not baseline blood pressure cosegregated with the SHRSP allele of chromosome 10 may, at first glance, be interpreted as indicating that one (or more) gene(s) at this locus may be involved in sodium-sensitivity. While not characterized, such genes are well known to exist, as exemplified by the breeding of the *Dahl* rat strains in which hypertension (in the S-substrain) only develops after exposure to sodium chloride (Dahl et al.1962). In this model, hypertension (i.e. sodium sensitivity) has been demonstrated to cosegregate with a restriction fragment length polymorphism of the first intron of the renin gene (Rapp et al.1989). Similarly, SHRSP (as well as SHR), while primarily studied as a non-sodium-dependent model of hypertension, show significant further elevations in blood pressure in response to dietary sodium loading (Aoki et al.1972). In contrast, blood pressure in WKY has generally been found to respond modestly, or not at all to dietary sodium loading. Studies in human hypertension have also identified sodium-sensitive subgroups which show a strong pattern of familial aggregation and heritability and are characterized by such phenotype markers as haptoglobin (Weinberger et al.1987). Alternatively, when blood pressure is measured in animals receiving a standardized, high sodium diet, the effect of this environmental variable is not only better controlled than on regular chow, but may also be at its saturation point, thus resulting in a higher quality data set with lower variance, yielding the statistical power to identify cosegregating loci.

The locus identified on the X-chromosome is linked to baseline systolic blood pressure with a Lod score of about 3.0. The effect of this locus was calculated to account for more than 60% of the variance of this variable in female animals. In contrast to the chromosome 10 locus, this locus appears to have a co-dominant effect on blood pressure. Of interest, the WKY allele at this locus is associated with higher blood pressures, whereas the SHRSP allele conveys a hypotensive effect. It is of interest that WKY rats are usually found to have somewhat higher blood pressures than other non-hypertensive strains; the effect of this locus may account for this. Also, it is conceivable that the presence of a hypotensive allele at this locus may act as a counterbalancing or permissive factor in the SHRSP ensuring survival at least until the animal has reached reproductive age.

Our study represents the first successful example of how genome-screening approaches, rather than candidate-gene experimentation, may lead to the identification of hypertension- or blood-pressure related genes in mammals. The data presented herein represent, of course, only the first step towards the solution of the riddle of genetic hypertension. Identification and typing of additional polymorphic markers will allow a more comprehensive genome analysis in which chromosomal regions not represented so far will be examined, and additional markers in regions already represented will enable more accurate typing and localization of genes of interest. The long-term goal, of course, will be, eventually, the identification and characterization of specific genes by molecular genetic approaches, and confirmation of their physiological and pathological relevance by whole animal experimentation, using either transgenic techniques or conventional breeding approaches to generate congenic substrains.

References

Aoki, K., Yamori, Y., Ooshima, A., & Okamoto, K. (1972): Effects of high or low sodium intake in spontaneously hypertensive rats. Jap. Circ. J. 36, 539-545.
Dahl, L.K., Heine, M., & Tassinari, L. (1962): Role of genetic factors in susceptibility to experimental hypertension due to chronic excess salt ingestion. Nature 194, 480-482.
Harrap, S.B. (1986): Genetic analysis of blood pressure and sodium balance in spontaneously hypertensive rats. Hypertension 8, 572-582.
Kurtz, T.W., Simonet, L., Kabra, P.M., Wolfe, S., , & Hjelle, B.L. (1990): Cosegregation of the renin allele in the spontaneously hypertensive rat with an increase in blood pressure. J. Clin. Invest. 85, 1328-1332.
Lindpaintner, K., Takahashi, S., & Ganten, D. (1990): Structural alterations of the renin gene in stroke-prone spontaneously hypertensive rats: Examination of genotype-phenotype correlations. J. Hypertension. 8, 763-773.
Mattei, M.G., Hubert, C., Alhenc-Gelas, F., Roeckel, N., Corvol, P., & Soubrier, F. (1989): Angiotensin converting enzyme maps on chromosome 17. Cytogenet. Cell. Gen. 51, 1041.
Rapp, J.P., Wang, S.M., & Dene, H. (1989): A genetic polymorphism in the renin gene of Dahl rat cosegregates with blood pressure. Science 243, 542-544.
Tanase, H., Suzuki, Y., Ooshima, A., Yamori, Y., & Okamoto, K. (1970): Genetic analysis of blood pressure in the spontaneously hypertensive rat. Jpn. Circ. J. 34, 1197-1212.
Weinberger, M.H., Miller, J.Z., Fineberg, N.S., Luft, F.C., Grim, C.E., & Christian, J.C. (1987): Association of haptoglobin with sodium sensitivity and resistance of blood pressure. Hypertension 10, 443-446.
Yamori, Y., & Okamoto, K. (1970): Zymogram analyses of various organs from spontaneously hypertensive rats. A gentico-biochemical study. Lab. Invest. 22, 206-211.

Red cell ion transport in genetic hypertension : recombinant inbred strain study

Hassan K. Bin Talib, Vladimír Křen *, Jaroslav Kuneš, Michal Pravenec and Josef Zicha

*Institute of Physiology, Czechoslovak Academy of Sciences, Vídeňská, CS-142 20 Prague 4, and * Institute of Biology, First Medical Faculty, Charles University, Albertov 4, CS-120 00 Prague 2, Czechoslovakia*

ABSTRACT

Blood pressure of recombinant inbred strains (SHR x BN.lx) cosegregates with inward Na^+ leak but not with $Na^+ - K^+$ cotransport activity or red cell Na^+ content.

Multiple abnormalities revealed by a simple comparison of SHR and WKY rats were proposed to be involved in the pathogenesis of genetic hypertension. They include alterations of ouabain-resistant (OR) ion transport especially augmented cation leak due to an increased passive membrane permeability in SHR erythrocytes (Postnov et al. 1976, Friedman et al. 1977, Wiley et al. 1980, Duhm et al. 1983, Harris et al. 1984, Feig et al. 1985). Consequently a mild elevation of red cell Na^+ content was occasionally observed in SHR (Berglund et al. 1981, Feig et al. 1985, Wauquier et al. 1988). On the other hand, the activity of $Na^+ - K^+$ cotransport system in SHR is still unclear since this system can operate in either direction depending on the transmembrane gradient of respective ions. Due to substantial methodical variations (e.g. Na^+ presence in incubation media) the cotransport in SHR erythrocytes was found to be enhanced (Duhm et al. 1983, Feig et al. 1985, Saitta et al. 1987), unchanged (Wiley et al. 1980, Wolowyk and Slosberg 1983) or reduced (De Mendonca et al. 1985, Rosati et al. 1988). The relationship between particular quantitative traits can be demonstrated using F_2 hybrids or recombinant inbred (RI) strains (Rapp 1987). As far as genetic hypertension in the rat is concerned, the only available set of RI strains is based upon F_2 hybrids of SHR with normotensive BN.lx rats (Pravenec et al. 1989). Our aim was to examine particular components of red cell OR Na^+ and $K^+(Rb^+)$ transport in progenitor strains and their cosegregation with blood pressure (BP) in 20 RI strains.

METHODS

Blood was withdrawn from abdominal aorta of male rats aged 3–4 months. Plasma and buffy coat were removed and samples for red cell Na^+ content (Na^+_i) determination were taken. One half of remaining cells was washed three times with Na^+ medium (137 mM NaCl, 10 mM choline chloride) whereas the rest with Mg^{2+}-sucrose medium (75 mM $MgCl_2$, 85 mM sucrose); both media contained 5 mM glucose, 2.5 mM phosphoric acid, 10 mM MOPS (pH 7.4 with TRIS, 310 mosm/kg H_2O). The incubation (60 min, 37 °C; 40 μl of packed cells in 1.75 ml media) was carried out in either Na^+ or Mg^{2+}-sucrose media supplemented with 3.5 mM RbCl and 5 mM ouabain that was combined in 50% samples with 1 mM furosemide. After the incubation red cells were rapidly washed with ice-cold isotonic choline chloride and hemolysed with 6%

n-butanol. Na^+, Rb^+ and hemoglobin concentrations were determined in hemolysates. Mean values of BP, Na^+_i as well as of furosemide-sensitive (FS) and -resistant (FR) ion fluxes in respective RI strains were used for correlations (cosegregation analysis).

RESULTS

Ouabain-resistant Na^+ net uptake was greater in SHR than in BN.lx red cells incubated in Na^+ media (especially due to augmented FS Na^+ uptake). In contrast with the elevated Na^+ influx red cell Na^+ contents (Na^+_i) were slightly lower in SHR compared to BN.lx rats. OR Na^+ net uptake and its FR component (Na^+ leak) cosegregated with BP of RI strains but this was not true for Na^+_i or any Na^+ flux determined in erythrocytes incubated in Mg^{2+}-sucrose medium. FR Rb^+ uptake (Rb^+ leak) but not FS Rb^+ uptake was enhanced in SHR erythrocytes but BP in RI strains had no relationship to any parameter of Rb^+ transport (irrespective of incubation medium used).

	Na^+ movement			Na^+_i	Rb^+ uptake		
	OR	FS	FR		OR	FS	FR
	Na^+ medium						
SHR	4336±172	1736±113	2600±76	3.09±0.07	855±50	451±36	403±14
BN.lx	3634±195*	1220±194*	2414±76	3.39±0.09*	790±45	452±33	339±13*
r coeff.	0.456*	-0.085	0.435*	0.055	-0.067	-0.096	0.153
	Mg^{2+}-sucrose medium						
SHR	-607±81	-450±46	-158±59	–	791±21	161±16	630±15
BN.lx	-496±76	-426±40	-71±37	–	645±14*	167±33	478±29*
r coeff.	0.299	0.122	0.040	–	-0.140	-0.115	-0.103

Data (means±SEM, n=6) are expressed per 5.2 mmol hemoglobin/l cells; fluxes in μmol . (l cells . h)$^{-1}$, Na^+_i in mmol/l cells; * significant differences (p<0.05) BN.lx versus SHR; r coefficient characterize the relationship of BP in RI strains (n=20) with the respective parameter (* p<0.05)

DISCUSSION

Our data indicate a cosegregation of OR Na^+ uptake and FR Na^+ leak with BP of RI strains whereas there was no relationship of BP to either FS Na^+ net uptake or red cell Na^+ content. The increased passive membrane permeability for sodium may thus be related to the pathogenesis of genetic hypertension in the rat. A contrast between higher rates of OR Na^+ influx in strains with elevated BP and their normal red cell Na^+ contents suggests that ouabain-sensitive Na^+ extrusion is accelerated in these hypertensive strains. This was also true for SHR in which OR Na^+ uptake was high but Na^+_i lower than in normotensive BN.lx rats. Indeed Orlov et al. (1991) demonstrated higher Na^+,K^+-ATPase activity in SHR than in BN.lx erythrocytes. It would be interesting to know whether this difference is due to a greater number of pump sites and/or higher pump Na^+ turnover and whether these parameters would also cosegregate with BP in RI strains. The absence of any significant cosegregation of Rb^+ leak with blood pressure of RI strains is rather surprising because the difference between both progenitor strains was considerable (Orlov et al. 1991). The lack of correlation between Na^+ and Rb^+ leaks in RI strains does not support the idea that in SHR the passive membrane permeability is uniformly elevated for all monovalent cations. Our data do not also confirm the earlier reports on the cosegregation of outward Na^+-K^+ cotransport with BP of SHR x WKY or MHS x MNS F_2 hybrids (Bianchi et al. 1985, Kotelevtsev et al. 1989). The absence of a significant difference in FS Na^+ efflux between SHR and BN.lx erythrocytes (incubated in Mg^{2+}-sucrose media) might be one of the possible explanations.

ACKNOWLEDGEMENT

The authors are grateful to Alexander von Humboldt Foundation (Bad Godesberg, FRG) for a generous bequest of some measuring equipment and PC for data processing. A part of our research was supported by the research grant No 7112 of the Czechoslovak Academy of Sciences, Prague.

REFERENCES

Berglund G., Sigström L., Lundin S., Karlberg B.E. & Herlitz H. (1981): Intraerythrocyte sodium and (Na^+,K^+-activated)-ATPase concentration and urinary aldosterone excretion in spontaneously hypertensive rats. *Clin. Sci.* 60, 229–232.

Bianchi G., Ferrari P., Trizio D., Ferrandi M., Torielli L., Barber B.R. & Polli E. (1985): Red blood cell abnormalities and spontaneous hypertension in the rat. A genetically determined link. *Hypertension* 7, 319–325.

De Mendonca M., Knorr A., Grichois M.-L., Brossard M., Garay R.P., Ben-Ishay D. & Meyer P. (1985): Erythrocyte Na^+ transport systems in three strains of genetically hypertensive rats. *Klin. Wochenschr.* 63 (Suppl. III), 66–69.

Duhm J., Göbel B.O. & Beck F.-X. (1983): Sodium and potassium ion transport accelerations in erythrocytes of DOC, DOC-salt, two-kidney, one clip, and spontaneously hypertensive rats. Role of hypokalemia and cell volume. *Hypertension* 5, 642–652.

Feig P.U., Mitchell P.P. & Boylan J.W. (1985): Erythrocyte membrane transport in hypertensive humans and rats. Effect of sodium depletion and excess. *Hypertension* 7, 423–429.

Friedman S.M., Nakashima M. & McIndoe R.A. (1977): Glass electrode measurement of net Na^+ and K^+ fluxes in erythrocytes of spontaneously hypertensive rat. *Can. J. Physiol. Pharmacol.* 55, 1302–1310.

Harris A.L., Guthe C.C., van't Veer F. & Bohr D.F. (1984): Temperature dependence and bidirectional cation fluxes in red blood cells from spontaneously hypertensive rats. *Hypertension* 6, 42–48.

Kotelevtsev Y.V., Spitkovski D.D., Orlov S.N. & Postnov Y.V. (1989): Interstrain restriction fragment length polymorphism in the c-src correlates with Na,K cotransport and calcium content in hybrid rat erythrocytes. *J. Hypertens.* 7 (Suppl. 6), S112–S113.

Orlov S.N., Petrunyaka V.V., Pokudin N.I., Kotelevtsev Y.V., Postnov Y.V., Kuneš J. & Zicha J. (1991): Cation transport and ATPase activity in rat erythrocytes: a comparison of spontaneously hypertensive rats with normotensive Brown-Norway strain. *J. Hypertens.* 9, No 10 (in press).

Postnov Y. V., Orlov S., Gulak P. & Shevchenko A. (1976): Altered permeability of the erythrocyte membrane for sodium and potassium ions in spontaneously hypertensive rats. *Pflügers Arch.* 365, 257–263.

Pravenec M., Klír P., Křen V., Zicha J. & Kuneš J. (1989): An analysis of spontaneous hypertension in spontaneously hypertensive rats by means of new recombinant inbred strains. *J. Hypertens.* 7, 217–222.

Rapp J.P. (1987): Use and misuse of control strains for genetically hypertensive rats. *Hypertension* 10, 7–10.

Rosati C., Meyer P. & Garay R. (1988): Sodium transport kinetics in erythrocytes from spontaneously hypertensive rats. *Hypertension* 11, 41–48.

Saitta M.N., Hannaert P.A., Rosati C. Meyer P. & Garay R.P. (1987): A kinetic analysis of inward Na^+,K^+ cotransport in erythrocytes from spontaneously hypertensive rats. *J. Hypertens.* 5 (Suppl. 5), S285–S286.

Wauquier I., Pernollet M.-G., Grichois M.-L., Lacour B., Meyer P., & Devynck M.-A. (1988): Endogenous digitalis like circulating substances in spontaneously hypertensive rats. *Hypertension* 12, 108–116.

Wiley J.S., Hutchinson J.S., Mendelsohn F.A.O. & Doyle A.E. (1980): Increased sodium permeability of erythrocytes in spontaneously hypertensive rats. *Clin. Exp. Pharmacol. Physiol.* 7, 527–530.

Wolowyk M.W. & Slosberg B.N. (1983): Hypertension: cation transport and the physical properties of erythrocytes. *Can. J. Physiol. Pharmacol.* 61, 1003–1009.

Pattern of inheritance of the startle-induced heart rate response in the spontaneously hypertensive rat

Morton P. Printz, Rod Casto, M. Anne Spence * and Rita Cantor *

*Department of Pharmacology 0636, University of California San Diego, La Jolla, CA 92093 and * Departments of Psychiatry and Biomathematics, University of California Los Angeles, Los Angeles, CA 90024, USA*

INTRODUCTION

It has generally been assumed that stress will, in the susceptible subject, contribute to or facilitate the development of hypertension. To test this assumption, studies were undertaken to define the differences in cardiovascular responses to a mild stress stimulus between inbred normotensive Wistar-Kyoto (WKY) rats and inbred hypertensive Spontaneously Hypertensive rats (SHR) derived from the Okamoto SHR (Casto et al., 1989; Casto & Printz, 1990). The stress paradigm employed was a repeated airpuff startle stimulus repeated every 45 - 60 seconds over 30 Trials. As reported previously we found that this mild stimulus elicits in both WKY and SHR a transient pressor response which was of greatest magnitude on Trial 1, was maintained over the 30 trials with only slight attenuation and was of greater magnitude in the SHR. In addition, we found that both strains exhibited a tachycardia in a trial-dependent manner; SHR exhibiting tachycardia from Trial 1 on while WKY exhibited bradycardia on Trial 1 which was rapidly attenuated and replaced by tachycardia between Trials 5 - 10.

The distinct phenotypic difference in heart rate response between SHR and WKY permitted a direct test of the relationship between inheritance of the cardiovascular responses to the stressor and the inheritance of hypertension (Casto & Printz, 1998). The first and essential goal was to determine the pattern of inheritance of the heart rate response in the WKY and SHR. The classical Mendelian intercross between two inbred strains was used which tests for independent segregation of the alleles for the different traits under test.

METHODS

The airpuff startle procedures have been described in detail elsewhere (Casto et al., 1989; Casto & Printz, 1990) and will be summarized only briefly. Rats were chronically instrumented with arterial catheters and tests conducted in a special chamber modified for cardiovascular measurements. The stimulus, a 100 msec duration 12.5 psi puff of air was delivered approximately 2 cm above the dorsal thorax. All rats were naive to the startle test. Following cardiovascular stabilization, stimuli were delivered at 30 - 45 second intervals which permitted cardiovascular parameters to return to baseline. Data were obtained by a digital acquisition system (Gould, Cleveland, Ohio) and analyzed using SYSTAT (Evanston, IL). Comparisons among groups were made by one-way analysis of variance (ANOVA). Repeated comparisons within the animals and comparisons between groups were made using a two-way ANOVA for repeated measures. Each ANOVA was followed by a posteriori Tukeys tests when criterion for significance was met. A probability of less than 0.05 was considered significant.

The parental rat strains used for the intercross were bred in La Jolla from breeding stock obtained in 1980 from Charles Rivers Laboratories (Wilmington, MA) and inbred further through successive brother-sister matings. Since we have obtained evidence that these rats may differ from present commercial animals, we will denote them by the subscripts for their lineage. For generation of the intercross progeny, male $SHR_{CR/LJ}$ were crossed with female $WKY_{CR/LJ}$ to produce an F1 generation. The F1 generation was both randomly intercrossed to produce an F2 generation and females back-crossed to parental $SHR_{CR/LJ}$ to generate a back-cross (BC) generation. Male F2 and BC rats were then tested for blood pressure and startle response profile.

RESULTS AND DISCUSSION

The F1 generation was derived from a cross between ten male $SHR_{CR/LJ}$ and ten female $WKY_{CR/LJ}$ which yielded 60 F1 offspring (29 males and 31 females). Brother-sister matings of the F1 yielded 102 F2 from which 38 males were randomly selected for testing. For the backcross (BC) progeny, twelve F1 females were mated to their male $SHR_{CR/LJ}$ parents yielding 70 males and 56 females. From the 70 BC males 64 were selected for startle testing. The inheritance pattern of all components of the cardiovascular response to airpuff stimuli were analyzed and will be reported in detail elsewhere.

TABLE 1. FREQUENCY OF TRIAL 1 BRADYCARDIA TO AIRPUFF STARTLE

Progeny	N*	# Brady.	# Predicted	Deviation From Model
$WKY_{CR/LJ}$	15	15	15	NS
$SHR_{CR/LJ}$	16	0	0	---
F1	19	19	19	NS
F2	38	29	28.5	NS
BC	64	36	32	NS

The pattern of inheritance of the bradycardia response was determined in the progeny and Chi-Square Goodness of Fit tested against a model with bradycardia as a simple autosomal dominant trait (Table 1).

The bradycardia response is inherited in the $WKY_{CR/LJ}$ rat consistent with a single autosomal dominant allele. Likewise, the absence of bradycardia is inherited as a simple recessive trait. When histogram analysis was conducted on the distribution of mean arterial pressures (MAP), evidence for cosegregation of the absence of bradycardia with hypertension became obvious. The MAP of the parental strains differed by 44.2 mmHg (104.5 vs 148.7 mmHg) while the F1 progeny were slightly higher then $WKY_{CR/LJ}$ mothers (116.2 mmHg) as expected (Kurtz et al., 1990). While there was drift of the MAP upwards from the F1 generation for animals exhibiting bradycardia, those which failed to exhibit bradycardia had group mean arterial pressures which were not significantly different from parental SHR (e.g., 145.2 mmHg vs 148.7 mmHg).

The apparent cosegregation of high blood pressure with tachycardia was investigated using the LOD score linkage analysis (Morton, 1955) with the computer program LIPED (Ott, 1974). The results, to be reported in detail elsewhere, indicated that when the F2 and BC populations were analyzed LOD scores greater then 3.0 were obtained for the traits indicating a high probability of genetic linkage of the alleles. The finding that the animals without bradycardia had MAP not significantly different from parental SHR would argue that the linked locus for hypertension is a major contributor to the blood pressure elevation.

It must be recognized that these results may be most applicable to the $WKY_{CR/LJ}$ rats bred in La Jolla since 1980 and denoted by the subscripts. In fact, recent studies (manuscript in preparation) indicate that commercial inbred WKY rats do not show bradycardia to the airpuff stimulus when tested within two to three weeks after arrival. However, these animals will, under the appropriate pharmacological manipulation, demonstrate strong bradycardia responses. The difference between commercial animals and those bred in La Jolla may reside in other genetic factors which compensate for and prevent expression of this phenotypic trait. Further studies comparing the various substrains of WKY and validating the observations reported here are underway.

REFERENCES

Casto, R. and Printz, M.P. (1988): Genetic transmission of hyperresponsivity in crosses between spontaneously hypertensive and Wistar-Kyoto rats. J Hypertension 6(Suppl 4):S52-S54.

Casto, R., Nguyen T., and Printz, M.P. (1989): Characterization of cardiovascular and behavioral responses to alerting stimuli in rats. Am J Physiol 256:R1121-R1126.

Casto, R. and Printz, M.P. (1990): Exaggerated response to alerting stimuli in spontaneously hypertensive rats. Hypertension 16:290-300.

Kurtz, T.W., Casto, R., Simonet, L., and Printz, M.P. (1990): Biometrical genetic analysis of blood pressure in the spontaneously hypertensive rat. Hypertension 16:718-724.

Morton N.E. (1955): Sequential tests for detection of linkage. Am. J Hum Genet 7:277-318.

Ott, J. (1974): Estimation of the recombinant fraction in human pedigrees: Efficient computation of the likelihood for human linkage studies. Am. J Hum Genet 26:588-597.

Characterization of WKY, SHR and SHRSP substrains with fingerprint patterns

Yasuo Nara *, Toru Nabika **, Katsumi Ikeda ***, Makoto Sawamura *, Yukio Yamori *

on behalf of International Study Group on the Genetic Background of SHR and WKY

*Departments of Pathology * and Laboratory Medicine **, Shimane Medical University, Shimane Institute of Health Science ***, Izumo 693, Japan*

SUMMARY

We compared fingerprint patterns with several restriction enzymes and probes among WKY, SHR and SHRSP from several breeders. Since WKY were initially distributed in the world from closed colony maintained at Kyoto University, great number of polymorphisms in fingerprint patterns were observed among breeders. The polymorphisms among SHR were decreased in number and the similar pattern was obtained among SHRSP which were shared after establishment of the inbred strain. These results indicate that each strain can be identified by this method with several restriction enzymes and probes.

INTRODUCTION

Spontaneously hypertensive rats (SHR) selectively bred from Wistar Kyoto rats (WKY) are widely distributed in the world and regard as the most popular animal models for essential hypertension. Many biochemical and physiological markers were compared SHR and WKY, however there have been inconsistent results obtained differnt in SHR and WKY from breeders. These discrepancies might be not only due to different experimental conditions but also to genetical heterogeneities among strains even though they have the same nomenclature, because some SHR were donated from the original corony at Kyoto University before the establishment of the inbred strain, and WKY were donated after 2-3 generations of the sibmating. Each strain is kept inbred in each breeder at present. To understand the discrepant results among the strains, we examined the DNA fingerprint patterns of the representative strains of WKY, SHR and SHRSP available in the world in cooperation with their breeders.

MATERIALS AND METHOD

Male WKY and SHR from Charles River Laboratories (WKY/NCrj, SHR/NCrj) were purchased from Charles River Laboratoris, Atsugi, Japan. WKY, SHR and SHRSP from the NIH strain (WKY/N, SHR/N and SHRSP/N) were sent from the National Institute of Health, Bethesda, Md., in 1987 and have been maintained at our laboratory as inbred colonies. WKY/Ta and SHR/Ta were donated from Takeda Pharmaceutical Company. WKY/G, SHR/G and SHRSP/G were also donated from German Institute for High Blood Pressure Research. WKY/Izm, SHR/Izm and SHRSP/Izm in Shimane Institute of Health Science, Izumo Japan are all direct descendents of the original Kyoto strains. Minisatellite DNA probe myo and ins geneously provided from Professor Ryo Kominami, University of Niigata, Niigata, Japan and YNZ 2 was also generously provided from Dr. Yusuke Nakamura, Cancer Institute, Japanese Foundation for Cancer Research, Tokyo Japan. Genomic DNA of the rats was extracted from the liver by phenol/chloroform extraction. Ten microgams of DNA was digested with 30 units of Hae III, Hin f I and Rsa I for 3-4 hours under the conditions recommended by the manufacturer (Boehlinger-Mannheim, Mannheim, FRG). Digested DNA was electrophoresed, transfered and hybridized with a minisalellite DNA probe according to the reported method (Nabika et al., 1991).

RESULTS AND DISCUSSION

Fig. 1 shows fingerprint patterns of WKY, SHRSP and SHR from different breeders. The highest polymorphisms among several WKY strains were observed by the combination of Hae III and YNZ 2 probe as far as we examined. At lest 6 tipical bands were detected in WKY/Izm compared to WKY/Ta or WKY/G. WKY/Ta expressed rather near patterns to those of WKY/G than that of WKY/Izm. Matsumoto et al., (1991) reported that WKY/izm had the same RT-1 haplotype as SHR but not WKY/N and futher they observed that WKY/Ta did not have the same RT-1 haplotype as SHR. The haplotype of WKY/Ta was the same as WKY/N. These results might exprain the difference in the fingerprint pattern between WKY/Izm and WKY/Ta. WKY/Ta and WKY/G were separated from the colony of WKY maintained at Kyoto University between 1974 and 1975.

In SHR, there wrere two patterns, that is SHR/Izm pattern and SHR/Ta pattern. SHR/Ta and SHR/N were separated from the original SHR strain of Kyoto University at the 7 the generation and the 13 the generation, respectively. SHRSP showed similar fingerprint patterns among the strains maintained at different breeders, because they were separated each breeders from the original SHRSP strains after the 20 the generation. Since WKY/NCrj and SHR/NCrj were derived from NIH strains, there was no typical difference in fingerprint patterns between WKY/N and WKY/NCrj or between SHR/N and SHR/NCrj as far as we examined. Suitable combination of restriction enzymes and probes enables us specify each strain among SHR and WKY. Because of obvious differences in fingerprint patterns detected among various SHR and WKY strains from different breeder's, each SHR and WKY strain should be named with their breeder's name to avoid further confusion due to interstrain variabilities among SHR or WKY.

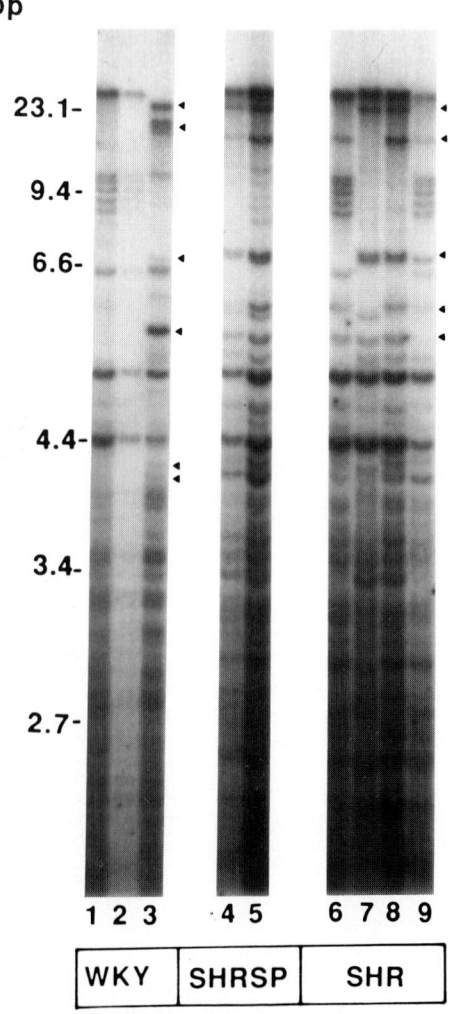

Figure 1 Comparison of DNA fingerprint patterns of WKY, SHR and SHRSP.

Restriction enzyme and probe were used Hae III and YNZ 2, respectively.
Arrow heads show tipical bands of WKY/Izm.

1. WKY/Ta 2. WKY/G
3. WKY/Izm 4. SHRSP/G
5. SHRSP/Izm
6. SHR/Ta 7. SHR/G
8. SHR/Izm 9 SHR/N

REFERENCES

Matsumoto, K., Yamada, T., Natori, T., Ikeda, K., Yamada, J., Yamori Y. (1991): Genetic variability in SHR (SHRSR), SHRSP and WKY strains. *Clin. Exp. Hypertens.* 13: (in press).
Nabika, T., Nara, Y., Ikeda, K., Endo, J., Yamori, Y.(1991): genetic Heterogeneity of the spontaneously hypertensive rat. *Hypertension* 18:12-16.

Genetic analysis for major histocompatibility complex in spontaneously hypertensive rat and its control strain

Kozo Matsumoto, Tohru Sakai, Takahisa Yamada, Takashi Agui, Yasuo Nara *, Yukio Yamori * and Takashi Natori **

*Institute for Animal Experimentation, University of Tokushima Schoool of Medicine, Tokushima 770, Japan; * Shimane Medical University and Japan Stroke Prevention Center, Izumo 693, Japan and ** Otsuka Pharmaceutical Co., Ltd., Tokushima Research Institute, Tokushima 771, Japan*

SUMMARY: SHR, SHRSP, WKY and W lines were screened for RT1 class I and class II antigens by dextran-hemagglutination method and flow cytometry using polyclonal and monoclonal alloantibodies, respectively. The result showed that every SHR and SHRSP strains had $RT1^k$ haplotype in both class I and class II antigens. On the other hand, WKY lines were classified into two major groups having $RT1^k$ and $RT1^l$ haplotypes. Several Japanese WKY strains such as WKY/Izm showed $RT1^k$ haplotype, while most WKY rats derived origin from NIH showed $RT1^l$ haplotype.

Spontaneously hypertensive rat (SHR) and its related strains such as SHRSP and WKY rats are widely used as a model of human hypertensive disease. Since genetic studies on the pathogenesis of hypertension in SHR are in current topics (Hilbert et al., 1991), the exact genetic definition of many sublines of SHR, SHRSP or WKY rats becomes more important. Genetic variability among SHR and its related strains have previously been demonstrated using biochemical genetic markers. Namely, the allele differences were observed at 1 to 3 loci among 25 biochemical genetic loci tested in SHR lines, and at 1 to 2 loci in SHRSP lines, while WKY lines showed large genetic variability (Matsumoto et al., 1991). Furthermore, the data showed that SHR strains and the Wistar rats, which were derived from University of Tokyo supplied from Wistar Institute in 1938, shared very rare allele of $Es-4^\underline{a}$. Since this allele was only observed in these strains originated from the old Wistar rats, but was not observed in other 300 stains of rats so far tested in the world, it seems that SHR was originated from the old Wistar rats. It still remains a question whether WKY rats were also originated from the old Wistar rats. In order to clarify this question, a broad classification of strains by a comparison of major histocompatibility complex (MHC; designated as RT1 in rat) was performed. RT1 loci are composed of highly polymorphic genes encoding class I and class II transplantation antigens. Since RT1 region includes not only genes for transplantation-related antigens, but also susceptible genes responsible for the hypertensive effects in SHR rats (Pravenec et al., 1989), it is important to identify the RT1 haplotypes.

MATERIALS AND METHODS

A total of 44 rat strains of SHR, SHRSP and WKY was screened for RT1 loci. RT1 class I antigen is expressed on all tissues including lymphocytes,

Table 1. RT1 class I and class II haplotypes in SHR, SHRSP and WKY strains

	Class I		Class II		RT1 haplotype
Strains	RT1A^l	RT1A^k	RT1B/D^l	RT1B/D^k	
SHR/Jim	−	+	−	+	k
SHR/NCrj	−	+	−	+	k
SHR/Kyo	−	+	−	+	k
SHR/NCrg	−	+	−	+	k
SHR/NCru	−	+	−	+	k
SHR/NCr	−	+	−	+	k
SHR/NCrf	−	+	−	+	k
SHRC/Okj	−	+	−	+	k
SHRB2/Okj	−	+	−	+	k
SHR/NCri	−	+	−	+	k
SHR/Shi	−	+	−	+	k
SHR/Ta	−	+	−	+	k
SHRSR/N	−	+	−	+	k
SHRSRCL/Izm	−	+	−	+	k
SHRSRB1/Izm	−	+	−	+	k
SHRSRB2/Izm	−	+	−	+	k
SHRSRCH/Izm	−	+	−	+	k
SHRSP/Jim	−	+	−	+	k
SHRSP/Hos	−	+	−	+	k
SHRSP/N	−	+	−	+	k
SHRSP/Ta	−	+	−	+	k
SHRSP/German	−	+	−	+	k
SHR(SP)/Rm	−	+	−	+	k
SHRSPAsb/Okj	−	+	−	+	k
SHRSP/Shi	−	+	−	+	k
SHRSPA1/Izm	−	+	−	+	k
SHRSPA3/Izm	−	+	−	+	k
SHRSPA3H/Izm	−	+	−	+	k
SHRSPA4/Izm	−	+	−	+	k
WKY/Jim	−	+	NT	NT	k
WKY/Hos	−	+	NT	NT	k
WKY/Izm	−	+	−	+	k
WKY/N	+	−	NT	NT	l
WKY/NCrj	+	−	+	−	l
WKY/Cpb	+	−	+	−	l
WKY/NCru	+	−	+	−	l
WKY/Shi	+	−	+	−	l
WKY/Ta	+	−	+	−	l
WKY/Okj	+	−	+	−	l
WKY/OkjKrm	+	−	+	−	l
WKY/NagKrm	−	−	−	−	b?
W/Hok	−	+	−	+	k
W/Shi	−	+	−	+	k
WI/Iar	−	+	−	+	k

while RT1 class II antigen is expressed on B-lymphocytes and macrophages. Lymphocytes were prepared by gently pressing the lymph nodes with the bottom of syringe in PBS containing 0.1% BSA. Lymphocytes were stained with allospecific monoclonal antibodies (mAbs), followed by flow cytometric analysis.

RESULT AND DISCUSSION

As shown in Table 1, RT1 class I and class II haplotypes in many substrains and sublines of SHR, SHRSP, WKY and W rats were determined. This result clearly showed that every SHR, SHRSP and the old Wistar strains, W/Hok, W/Shi, and WI/Iar strains carried $RT1^k$ haplotype. On the other hand, WKY strains were classified into three groups having $RT1^k$, $RT1^l$ and probably $RT1^b$ haplotypes. Namely, WKY/Izm, WKY/Jim, and WKY/Hos carried $RT1^k$ haplotype, while the other WKY strains except WKY/NagKrm showed $RT1^l$ haplotype. WKY/NagKrm had neither $RT1^k$ nor $RT1^l$ haplotype ($RT1^b$?), suggesting that a contamination might have happened in this strain.

It is very important that SHR and some WKY strains shared $RT1^k$ haplotype, since the $RT1^k$ haplotype is very rare case in inbred strains of rats so far tested. In fact, it is so hard to find a strain having $RT1^k$ haplotype in the world except in Japan. This clearly suggests the close relationship between SHR and WKY strains with respect to their origin. This strongly supports the fact that SHR was developed from WKY colony. W/Hok, W/Shi, and WI/Iar strains, which were developed from the old Wistar stock in University of Tokyo, had $RT1^k$ haplotype, while other Wistar strains originated from the other Wistar stock showed $RT1^l$ or $RT1^u$ haplotype. This result is reasonable for the fact that WKY rats were originated from W/Hok in 1957 from Hokkaido University.

It is concluded that the old Wistar rats and WKY rats had heterozygous alleles of $RT1^k$ and $RT1^l$ in nearly 1960. It is interesting that only strains having $RT1^k$ haplotype were segregated into hypertensive rats, despite that the original WKY rats had both alleles. It may be suggested that $RT1^k$ haplotype is linked to one of the genes related to hypertension. Indeed, Pravenec et al. (1989) showed a linkage association between high blood pressure and $RT1^k$ haplotype. WKY rats having $RT1^k$ haplotype because of similarity to SHR and SHRSP must be suitable for a control strain of SHR and SHRSP rather than those having $RT1^l$ haplotype, though most WKY rats distributed from NIH have $RT1^l$ haplotype. It should be emphasized that full strain names of WKY strains as well as SHR and SHRSP lines should be described in the paper to avoid such a confusion.

REFERENCES

Hilbert, P., Lindpaintner, K., Beckmann, J. S., Serikawa, T., Soubrier, F., Dubay, C., Cartwright, P., De Gouyon, B., Julier, C., Takahashi, S., Vincent, M., Ganten, D., Georges, M., and Lathrop, G. M. (1991): Cromosomal mapping of two genetic loci associated with blood-pressure regulation in hereditary hypertensive rats. Nature 353: 521-529.
Matsumoto, K., Yamada, T., Natori, T., Ikeda, K., Yamada, J., and Yamori, Y. (1991): Genetic variability in SHR(SHRSR), SHRSP and WKY strains. Clin. Exp. Hypertension (In press).
Pravenec, M., Klir, P., Kren, V., Zicha, J., and Kunes, J. (1989): An analysis of spontaneous hypertension in spontaneously hypertensive rats by means of new recombinant inbred strains. J. Hypertension 7: 217-221.

ACKNOWLEDGMENTS. We thanks Drs. U. Ganten, T. Suzuki, K. Ikeda, A. Nagaoka, S. Makino, Y. Noda, menbers of Rijksinstituut and Charles River Co. groups for providing the rats.

Search for genetic determinants of environmental susceptibility in hypertension: effect of heat, immobilization stress and endotoxin

Jaroslav Kunes [1], Michal Pravenec [1], Vladimir Kren [2], Pavel Klir [1], Detlev Ganten [3], John J. Mullins [3], Johanne Tremblay and Pavel Hamet

Centre de Recherche Hôtel-Dieu de Montréal, Université de Montréal, 3850, rue Saint-Urbain, Pavillon Marie-de-la-Ferre, Montréal, Québec, Canada H2W 1T8; [1] Institute of Physiology, Czechoslovak Academy of Sciences, Prague; [2] Institute of Biology, Charles University, Prague, Czechoslovakia; [3] German Institute for Hig Blood Pressure Research, Heidelbeg, Germany

SUMMARY We demonstrated an increased susceptibility to different environmental stimuli in several genetic models of hypertension. At least two traits, thermosensitivity in mice (coded by the *Tms* locus) and differential susceptibility to endotoxin in rats (determined by a gene linked to the RT1 complex), may represent primary events associated with the pathogenesis of hypertension, since these two Mendelian traits have been shown to correlate with blood pressure in genetically segregating populations.

INTRODUCTION Spontaneously hypertensive rats (SHR) and mice (BPH) are highly sensitive to environmental temperature (Wright et al., 1978; Schlager, 1981; McMurthy and Wexler, 1981; McMurthy and Wexler, 1983; Malo et al., 1989). SHR exhibit enhanced stress-induced hyperthermia when compared to normotensive controls. We previously showed in spontaneously hypertensive mice that thermosensitivity *locus* (*Tms*) is associated with blood pressure (Malo et al., 1989). Our objective was to evaluate the genetic components of these anomalies. Therefore, in the present study, we tested the body temperature response to heat, immobilization stress and endotoxin in several inbred strains, RT1 congenic strains (with *k* haplotype of SHR on a normotensive background, BN.lx.1K, and conversely, with *n* haplotype of normotensive BN strain on hypertensive background, SHR.1N), and transgenic rats with mouse renin gene [TGR (mRen-2^d)27] (Pravenec et al., 1989; Mullins et al., 1990).

ANIMALS AND METHODS Ten- to fifteen-week old male rats or mice of the following strains were used: SHR - Charles River, Taconic Farms and the Institute of Physiology, Czechoslovak Academy of Sciences, Prague; Wistar-Kyoto (WKY) - Charles River and Taconic Farms; BN.lx and BN.lx.1K, referred to as BN and BN.1K - Institute of Biology, Faculty of Medicine, Charles University, Prague; SHR.1N - Institute of Physiology, Czechoslovak Academy of Sciences, Prague; TGR - University of Heidelberg; Sprague-Dawley (SD) outbred stock - Charles River and Harlan Sprague-Dawley; spontaneously hypertensive mice (BPH) and their normotensive controls (BPL) - obtained from Dr G. Schlager, Kansas, kept in the Centre de Recherche Hôtel-Dieu de Montréal Hospital.

For the determination of basal body temperature, the animals were quickly removed from the holding room and placed in plastic restraint cages for core temperature (Tco) measurement with an electronic probe inserted to 6 cm beyond the anus. Tco was monitored for 30 sec. "Stress-induced" hyperthermia was recorded under the same conditions but the probe was secured at the base of the tail and Tco was automatically registered for at least 20 min. The body temperature response to endotoxin was determined from values obtained before and after endotoxin injection (Lipopolysaccharide, serotype 055:B5, 500 µg/kg, i.p. Sigma). Mortality after heat stress was tracked in some strains of rats and mice. These animals were anesthetized with pentobarbital (30 - 40 mg/kg) and immersed up to their forelimbs in a water bath heated to 44 ± 0.1 °C. Heating was stopped when Tco reached 43 °C.

RESULTS AND DISCUSSION Basal body temperature was practically the same in all rats strains studied except for SD in which it was lower, there was no significant difference between normotensive and hypertensive animals. This is in contrast to the situation in mice. We observed previously significantly lower basal body temperatures in spontaneously hypertensive mice than in their normotensive controls (Malo et al., 1989).

Figure 1 illustrates the rate of body temperature increase in response to immobilization stress. A significantly higher rate of body temperature increase was observed only in SHR while no significant difference was noted for all other strains as compared to their respective controls. Since SHR and normotensive BN animals are progenitors of recombinant inbred strains (Pravenec et al., 1989), future studies will test this intermediate phenotype in recombinant inbred strains to determine its mode of inheritance and possible association with hypertension. Furthermore, it can be seen that there was no significant difference in the rate of body temperature increase in response to immobilization stress in TGR despite the relatively high degree of hypertension in these transgenic animals. However, when thermosensitivity was directly tested by immersion of the animals into a water bath of 44 °C under anesthesia, although the same degree of the Tco was reached in SD and TGR (43 °C), only the SD recovered with a decrease of body temperature. In the TGR, body temperature remained elevated and mortality was 100%. Higher mortality was also observed previously in BPH exposed to the same type of heat stress. In the F2 (BPHxBPL) population, we found that this trait is in large part under the control of a single gene (*Tms*) and moreover, that it is associated with a significant increase of blood pressure (Malo et al., 1989).

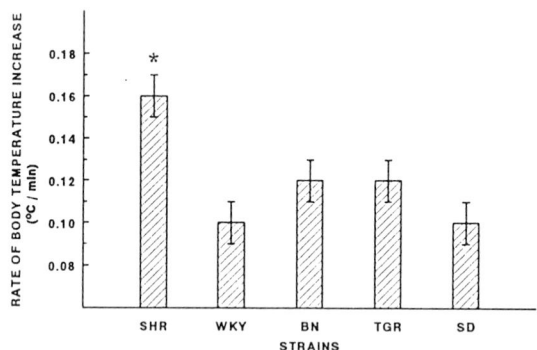

Fig. 1. Rate of body temperature increase in response to immobilization stress. Data expressed as mean ± SEM in °C/min of temperature increase recorded over 20 min in a restriction cage in various strains, as described in Methods. $p < 0.01$ as compared with either WKY or BN normotensive strains.

Changes in body temperature after endotoxin treatment were strain-specific. Differences observed in the congenic strains showed that a part of endotoxin sensitivity is determined by a gene within the RT1 complex although other genetic factors may also be important. Table 1 summarizes these overall results.

TABLE 1

Parameter	Rats	Mice
a) Basal body temperature	SHR=WKY=SHR.1N=BN.1K=BN=TGR>SD	BPL>BPH
b) Decrease in body temperature after endotoxin	BN.1K>BN=SHR.1N>SHR TGR>SD	
c) Mortality	TGR>SD	BPH>BPL

TGR, transgenic rats [mRen-2^d(27)]; SD, Sprague-Dawley stock; BPL, normotensive mice; BPH, hypertensive mice; all differences are significant at $p < 0.05$.

Endotoxin is a potent agonist of *TNFα* gene expression. Recently, we mapped *TNFα* to the RT1 complex close to *hsp70* (Pravenec et al., 1991a). Both genes are potentially involved in the regulation of responses to the environment (Pravenec et al., 1991b). We have previously demonstrated an increased expression of *hsp70* in hypertensives (Hamet et al., 1990a), and our parallel studies have revealed a polymorphism in both *hsp70* and *TNFα* in hypertension (Hamet et al., 1990b; Hamet et al., 1991). Further investigations analyzing a possible genetic link of their abnormal structure and/or expression with the pathogenesis of hypertension are in progress.

In summary, the results reported here extend the previous observation that genetically hypertensive animals are highly sensitive to environmental stimuli. Abnormalities seen in transgenic rats suggest that part of the phenotypic difference may be due to the renin-angiotensin system and/or may be secondary to high blood pressure. However, at least two traits of environmental susceptibility have proven to be Mendellian traits: 1. thermosensitivity in mice (*Tms* locus); and 2. sensitivity to endotoxin determined by RT1 *locus*, both significantly associated with blood pressure. These traits may, therefore, represent important primary events in the pathogenesis of spontaneous hypertension in mice and rats.

ACKNOWLEDGEMENTS These studies were supported by grants from the Medical Research Council of Canada and the Dairy Bureau of Canada. Johanne Tremblay is a scholar from Fonds de la Recherche en Santé du Québec. Drs Jaroslav Kunes and Michal Pravenec are visiting professors, supported by Servier Canada. The authors thank Monique Poirier and Régis Tremblay for their technical assistance throughout these investigations, Louise Chevrefils for preparing and Ovid Da Silva for editing this manuscript.

REFERENCES

Hamet, P., Malo, D., Hashimoto, T., Tremblay, J. (1990a): Heat stress genes in hypertension. *J Hypertens* 8 (Suppl. 7):S47-S52.

Hamet, P., Malo, D., Tremblay J. (1990b): Increased transcription of a major stress gene in spontaneously hypertensive mice. *Hypertension* 15:904-908.

Hamet, P., Kong, D., Pravenec, M., Kunes, J., Kren, V., Klir, P., Sun, Y.L., Tremblay, J. (1991): RFLP of a *hsp70* gene, localized in the RT1 complex, is associated with hypertension in SHR. *Hypertension* submitted.

Malo, D., Schlager, G., Tremblay, J., Hamet, P. (1989): Thermosensitivity, a possible new locus involved in genetic hypertension. *Hypertension* 14:121-128.

McMurthy, J.P. and Wexler, B.C. (1981): Hypersensitivity of spontaneously hypertensive rats (SHR) to heat, ether, and immobilization. *Endocrinology* 108:1730-1736.

McMurthy, J.P. and Wexler, B.C. (1983): Hypersensitivity of spontaneously hypertensive rats to heat and ether before the onset of high blood pressure. *Endocrinology* 112:166-171.

Mullins, J.J., Peters, J., Ganten, D. (1990): Fulminant hypertension in transgenic rats harbouring the mouse Ren-2 gene. *Nature* 344:541-544.

Pravenec, M., Klir, P., Kren, V., Zicha, J., Kunes, J. (1989): An analysis of spontaneous hypertension in spontaneously hypertensive rats by means of new recombinant inbred strains. *J Hypertens* 7:217-222.

Pravenec, M., Kong, D., Klir, P., Kren, J., Tremblay, J., Hamet, P. (1991a): A new extensive polymorphism in the rat TNFα gene: its mappint close to RT1 genes and identification of a unique allele in the *k* haplotype of spontaneously hypertensive rats. *J Exp Med* submitted.

Pravenec, M., Sun, Y.L., Kunes, J., Kong, D., Kren, V., Klir, P., Tremblay, J., Hamet, P. (1991b): Environmental susceptibility in hypertension: potential role of *hsp* and *tnfα* genes. *J Vasc Med Biol* submitted:

Schlager, G. (1981): The genetically hypertensive mouse. *New Trends in Arterial Hypertension* 17:321-331.

Wright, G., Knecht, E., Toraason, M. (1978): Cardiovascular effects of whole-body heating in spontaneously hypertensive rats. *J Appl Physiol* 45:521-527.

Dissociation of hypertension and abnormal activation of [K+, Cl-] cotransport in SHR erythrocytes

Rossella Rota *, Corinne Nazaret, Monique Santarromana **, Jean Georges Henrotte **, Ricardo Garay and Pascale Guicheney

*INSERM, Pharmacologie des Régulations Cardiovasculaires, Hôpital Necker, 75015 Paris, France, * Clinical Pathology, University of Medicine, 67100 L'Aquila, Italy, and ** CNRS, Faculté de Phamacie, Paris, France*

INTRODUCTION

Numerous alterations of red blood cells have been described to be associated to hypertension by studies on rats or humans. A decreased red cell volume has been observed in spontaneously hypertensive rats (SHR) (Sen et al., 1972; Bruschi et al., 1986) and in human hypertensives (Bruschi et al., 1986; Postnov et al., 1988). This may be due to some structural change in cell membrane and/or in the cytoskeleton inducing an alteration of ion transport systems such as $[K^+, Cl^-]$ (Arrazola et al., 1990) or $[Na^+, K^+, Cl^-]$-cotransports (Duhm & Göbel, 1984; Postnov et al., 1988). Nevertheless, two recent studies do not support the hypothesis of a negative association between erythrocyte volume and blood pressure in humans (Strazzullo et al., 1990; Cirillo and Laurenzi, 1989). The respective roles of $[Na^+, K^+, Cl^-]$ and of $[K^+, Cl^-]$-cotransport systems in regulation of erythrocyte volume is not well defined (Haas, 1989; Garay et al., 1988). The $[K^+, Cl^-]$-cotransport system is involved in cell volume regulation in erythrocytes (Kregenow, 1971) and several other cells (Arrazola et al, 1990). Under basal conditions the cotransport is quiescent and becomes activated by cell swelling thus extruding KCl and water. In SHR erythrocytes, the system is abnormally activated under physiologic conditions (Arrazola et al., 1990). This trait has been observed in other cell types such as thymocytes or vascular smooth muscle cells suggesting that it is genetically determined. In order to assess whether $[K^+, Cl^-]$-cotransport is linked to high blood pressure, we measured the activity of this system in 8 adult F1 and in 61 F2 hybrid rats derived from crossbreeding of female SHR and male WKY. $[Na^+, K^+, Cl^-]$-cotransport activity was also studied to determine the possible co-variation of the two systems.

METHODS

The SHR and normotensive Wistar-Kyoto rats (WKY) were obtained from Janvier Breeding Laboratories (Le Genest, France). Eight female SHR were crossed with eight male WKY. Fourteen couples of F1 rats were formed after randomization. 73 males were obtained in the F2 hybrid (SHR x WKY) generation. F2 rat blood pressures, measured by tail plethysmography in conscious animals on at least three separate occasions between 14-16 weeks of age, ranged from 120 to 190 mmHg. At 15-17 weeks of age, all rats were sacrificed. Rats were anesthetized with pentobarbital and blood was withdrawn by cardiac punction and immediately processed. Outward $[K^+, Cl^-]$-cotransport was measured according to a previously published protocol (Garay et al., 1988), slightly modified. Briefly, fresh erythrocytes were incubated in isotonic (305 ± 5 mOsm) or hypotonic saline medium (183 ± 5 mOsm) where Rb^+ replaced K^+. K^+ efflux was measured after 30 min of incubation at 37°C, in the presence and absence of 86 µM of DIOA (dihydroindenyloxyalkanoic acid), an inhibitor of the $[K^+,Cl^-]$-cotransport system. Outward $[K^+,Cl^-]$-cotransport was equated to DIOA-sensitive K^+ efflux. The activity of $[Na^+,K^+,Cl^-]$-cotransport was determined by measuring the bumetanide-sensitive Rb^+ influx, according to previously published protocol (Saitta et al., 1987). Briefly, fresh erythrocytes were incubated in Ringer-Rb medium where Rb^+ replaced K^+. Rb^+ influx was measured after 45 min of incubation at 37°C in the presence and absence of bumetanide (50 µM), an inhibitor of the $[Na^+,K^+,Cl^-]$-cotransport. Inward $[Na^+,K^+,Cl^-]$-cotransport was equated to bumetanide-sensitive Rb^+ influx. Fresh hearts were weighted after blotting on filter paper. They were dried at 80°C for 8 days, and maintained under vacuum (<15 mmHg) to reach constant values. Water weight was obtained by difference between fresh and dry weight, and expressed as percent of fresh weight. Statistical significance was estimated by using a Student's t test. Values were expressed as mean ± SEM.

RESULTS

Male SHR and WKY systolic blood pressures (BP) were: 173.7 ± 3.5 and 121.4 ± 2.9 (mmHg), respectively (n = 12). In isotonic medium, the mean DIOA-sensitive K^+ efflux was 2.66 ± 0.34 and 0.00 ± 0.10 (mmol/l. cells x h) in SHR and WKY erythrocytes. SHR and WKY values, in hyposmotic medium, were 10.2 ± 0.9 and 5.2 ± 0.6. Male F1 hybrid rats (mean BP: 151.5 ± 2.7 mmHg; n=8), presented a $[K^+,Cl^-]$-cotransport system activity very similar to WKY erythrocyte one in isotonic as well as in hypotonic medium (0.09 ± 0.06 and 2.64 ± 0.75 mmol/l. cells x h).

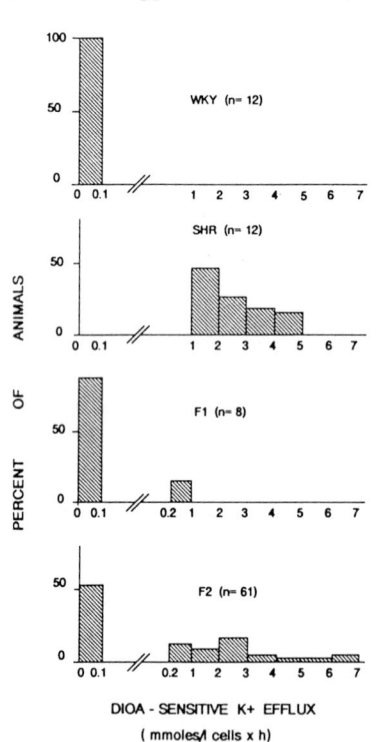

DIOA - SENSITIVE K+ EFFLUX
(mmoles/l cells x h)

The DIOA-sensitive K^+ efflux was determined for 61 F2 hybrid rats in isotonic and hypotonic media. No correlation was observed between BP levels and K^+ effluxes in isotonic medium (r = 0.054; n = 61). Figure 1 gives the frequency distribution of $[K^+,Cl^-]$-cotransport activity in SHR, WKY, F1 and F2 rat erythrocytes. In F2 rats the distribution was clearly bimodal. The system was activated in 29 rats and it was silent in the other 32, allowing to define two phenotypes: "High KCl group" and "Low KCl group". The mean K^+ effluxes were respectively: 2.30 ± 0.30 and 0.002 ± 0.002 (mmol/l cells x h; p < 0.001). Mean BP, heart/body weight ratios and heart water contents were identical for the two groups: 147.5 ± 2.2 (mmHg), 2.56 ± 0.04 (mg/g), 76.5 ± 0.12 (%) ("High KCl group") and 147.9 ± 2.6 (mmHg), 2.58 ± 0.04 (mg/g), 76.6 ± 0.20 (%) ("Low KCl group"). In contrast, heart weights and body weights were slightly lower in the "High KCl group" versus "Low KCl group" (1047 ± 21 mg, 408.9 ± 7.2 g, p<0.001 and 1112 ± 19 mg, 431.6 ± 7.7 g, p<0.001). No variation was observed in $[Na^+,K^+,Cl^-]$-cotransport activity between SHR and WKY (1.072 ± 0.097 and 1.138 ± 0.062 mmol/l cells x h) nor between the "High KCl" and "Low KCl" groups (0.846 ± 0.056 and 0.702 ± 0.053 mmol/l cells x h).

DISCUSSION

In WKY erythrocytes, the $[K^+,Cl^-]$-cotransport system was totally silent under basal conditions while it was clearly activated in the SHR. Moreover, the stimulation induced by hyposmotic medium was enhanced in SHR. The $[K^+,Cl^-]$-cotransport activity of the "High KCl group" was very close to the SHR one, while the "Low KCl group" was close to the WKY one. It appeared that the phenotypic character "High KCl" did not co-segregate with high blood pressure nor with cardiac hypertrophy. The lower heart weights of the "High KCl group" were not due to a water lost since the mean heart water contents were similar between the two groups. Other transport systems probably regulated water content and volume in cardiac cells. No difference in $[Na^+,K^+,Cl^-]$-cotransport activity was observed between the segregating phenotypes "High KCl" and "Low KCl" nor between the parents. This clearly shows that $[K^+,Cl^-]$ and $[Na^+,K^+,Cl^-]$-cotransport systems are independently regulated in erythrocytes. Numerous conflicting results concerning the $[Na^+,K^+,Cl^-]$-cotransport activity has been reported both for SHR and WKY erythrocytes (De Mendonca et al, 1982; Saitta et al, 1987; Feig et al., 1985; Duhm et al., 1984) and vascular smooth muscle cells (O'Donnell & Owen, 1988; Tokushige et al. 1986). It is difficult to know whether these discrepancies are due to differences in methodology, to the genetic heterogeneity of the WKY strains (Kurtz et al., 1989), or to physiologic factors regulating the activity of the system (Haas, 1989). In conclusion, the "High KCl" character observed in SHR is due to a genetic drift and is not involved in the developement of hypertension or cardiac hypertrophy.

REFERENCES

Arrazola, A., Rota, R., Soler Diaz, A., Hannaert, P.A., Nazaret, C., Beuzard, Y., Cragoe, E.J. Jr., Garay, R.P.(1990): Derepression and hyperactivation of a DIOA-sensitive $[K^+,Cl^-]$-cotransport system in spontaneously hypertensive rats (SHR). *Clin. & Exp. Hypertension* A12 (7), 1282.

Bruschi, G., Minari, M., Bruschi, M.E., Tacinelli, L., Milani, B., Cavatorta, A., Borgetti, A. (1986): Similarities of essential and spontaneous hypertension. Volume and number of blood cells. *Hypertension* 8, 983-989.

Cirillo, M., Laurenzi, M. (1989): Erythrocyte and platelet volume in human hypertension. The Gubbio Study Collaborative Group. *J. Hypertens.* 7(suppl 6), S168-S169.

De Mendonca, M,. Knorr, A., Grichois, M.L., Ben-Ishay, D., Garay, R.P., Meyer, P. (1982): Erythrocytic sodium ion transport systems in primary and secondary hypertension of the rats. *Kidney Int.* 21(suppl1), S69-S75.

Duhm, J., Göbel, B.O. (1984): Role of the furosemide Na+/K+ transport system in determining the steady-state Na^+ and K^+ content and volume of human erythrocytes in vitro and in vivo. *J. Membrane Biol.* 77, 243-254.

Feig, P.U., Mitchell, P.P., Boylan, J.W.(1985): Erythrocyte membrane transport in hypertensive humans and rats. Effect of sodium depletion and excess. *Hypertension* 7(3), 423-429.

Garay, R.P., Nazaret, C., Hannaert, P.A., Cragoe, E.J. Jr. (1988): Demonstration of a $[K^+,Cl^-]$-cotransport system in human red cells by its sensitivity to [(dihydroindenyl)oxy]alkanoic acids: regulation of cell swelling and distribution from the bumetanide-sensitive $[Na^+,K^+,Cl^-]$-cotransport. *Mol. Pharmacol.* 33, 696-701.

Haas, M. (1989): Properties and diversity of (Na-K-Cl)-cotransporters. *Annu. Rev. Physiol.* 51, 443-457.

Kregenow, F.M. (1971): The response of duck erythrocytes to nonhemolytic hypotonic media. *J. Gen. Physiol.* 58, 372-395.

Kurtz, T.W., Montano, M., Chan, L., Kabra, P. (1989): Molecular evidence of genetic heterogeneity in Wistar-Kyoto rats: implications for research with spontaneously hypertensive rat. *Hypertension* 13, 188-192.

O'Donnell, M.E., Owen, N.E. (1988): Reduced $[Na^+,K^+,Cl^-]$-cotransport in vascular smooth muscle cells from spontaneously hypertensive rats. *Am. J. Physiol.* 255, C169-C180.

Postnov, Y.V., Kravstov, G.M., Orlov, S.N., Pokudin, N.I., Postnov, I.Y., Kotelevtsev, Y.V. (1988): Effect of protein kinase C on cytoskeleton and cation transport in human erythrocytes. *Hypertension* 12, 267-273.

Saitta, M., Hannaert, P.A., Rosati, C., Meyer, P., Garay, R.P. (1987): A kinetic analysis of inward Na^+,K^+ cotransport in erythrocytes from spontaneously hypertensive rats. *J. Hypertens.* 5(suppl 5), S285-S286.

Sen, S., Hoffman, G.C., Stowe, N.T., Smeby, R.R., Bumpus, F.M. (1972): Erythrocytosis in spontaneously hypertensive rats. *J. Clin . Invest.* 51, 710-714.

Strazzullo, P., Cappuccio, F.P., Iacoviello, L., Cipollaro, M., Varriale, V., Giorgione, N., Farinaro, E., Mancini, M. (1990): Erythrocyte volume and blood pressure in a cross-sectional population-based study. *J. Hypertens.* 8 (2), 179-83.

Tokushige, A., Kino, M., Tamura, H., Hopp, L., Searle, B.M., Aviv, A. (1986): Bumetanide-sensitive sodium-22 transport in vascular smooth muscle cell of the spontaneously hypertensive rat. *Hypertension* 8, 379-385.

Is cardiovascular hypertrophy in young SHR the result of a recessive gene ?

Stephen B. Harrap, Glenn A. Mitchell and Tracey L. Norman

Genetic Physiology Unit, University of Melbourne, Department of Medicine, Austin Hospital, Heidelberg, Victoria 3084, Australia

Introduction:

Cardiovascular hypertrophy in young SHR (Gray 1984, Lee 1985) may indicate a primary genetic abnormality of growth in this strain. Hypertrophy might contribute to the development of hypertension by amplifying other genetic components of the SHR hypertensive process (Folkow 1989), or by a primary increase in cardiac output (Friberg & Nordlander 1990) or peripheral vascular resistance (Lever 1986).

Previous evidence has suggested that heart size is under genetic control, independent of blood pressure (Tanase et al 1982). The aim of this study was to investigate the inheritance of cardiovascular structure by comparing young spontaneously hypertensive rats (SHR), inbred normotensive Donryu (DRY) rats and their F1 hybrid.

Methods:

Only male rats were studied in these experiments. Inbred SHR and DRY colonies are maintained in the Genetic Physiology Unit by strict brother-sister mating, and the F1 hybrids were derived in equal number by crossing either male SHR with female DRY or male DRY with female SHR. All experiments were approved by the Austin Hospital Animal Welfare Committee.

Between 8 and 10 weeks of age body weight and systolic blood pressure (Model 12-28 BP system, IITC Life Science, California, USA) were measured in SHR (n=25), DRY (n=26) and F1 rats (n=60).

Cardiovascular structure was assessed at 9 weeks of age in separate groups of SHR (n=18), DRY (n=10) and F1 rats (n=23). For these studies rats were anaesthetised with pentobarbitone (50mg/kg, intraperitoneally) so that the bowel and mesenteric vasculature could be excised intact. Small arteries of between about 150-350 µm in external diameter were then selected for morphological study. The details of these methods using the Mulvany-Halpern small vessel myograph have been published previously (Harrap et al 1990). Medial cross-sectional area, lumen diameter, thickness of the media and the media-lumen ratio were determined. Hearts were removed at the time of sacrifice and weighed fresh.

Longitudinal systolic blood pressure and weight data were compared between groups using repeated measures analysis of variance (MANOVA, SPSS/PC+). Cross-sectional comparisons were made initially by oneway analysis of variance, followed by Student Newman Keuls range test for individual group comparisons.

Results:

F1 rats were heavier (MANOVA between 8 and 10 weeks of age: $F_{2,108}=47.7$, $P<0.0001$) than either parental strain (table 1), consistent with hybrid vigour.

Between 8 and 10 weeks of age, the systolic blood pressures of SHR were significantly higher (MANOVA between 8 and 10 weeks of age: $F_{1,47}=213$, $P<0.0001$) than DRY (table 1). The blood pressures of the F1 rats were intermediate and significantly different (MANOVA between 8 and 10 weeks of age: F1 vs DRY - $F_{1,86}=161$, $P<0.0001$; F1 vs SHR - $F_{1,83}=141$, $P<0.0001$) to the two parental strains (table 1).

	SHR		F1		DRY
Body weight (g)	221±3	*	255±4	*	206±3
Systolic blood pressure (mmHg)	190±2	*	170±1	*	144±3
Heart weight/ body weight (g/kg)	3.65±0.05	*	3.00±0.06		2.87±0.14
Lumen diameter (µm)	275±14		290±9		264±25
Media thickness (µm)	12.6±0.9	*	8.7±0.5		8.1±0.9
Media cross-sectional area (µm^2)	11973±1377	*	8394±579		7462±1492
Media/lumen ratio (%)	4.54±0.21	*	3.02±0.15		3.06±0.15

Table 1: Characteristics of young SHR, DRY and their F1 hybrids. Body weight and systolic blood pressure were calculated from the average of three readings in each rat between 8 and 10 weeks of age. Structural characteristics of the heart and mesenteric resistance vessels (lumen diameter, media thickness and cross-sectional area and media/lumen ratio) were measured at 9 weeks of age. Values are mean ± SEM, * indicates $P<0.05$ by Student Newman Keuls range test between adjacent groups.

The 9 week old SHR showed evidence of cardiovascular hypertrophy compared to the DRY (table 1). Not only was the heart weight/body weight ratio greater in SHR, but the mesenteric resistance vessels showed evidence of thickened media and increased media/lumen ratio (table 1).

However, the heart weight/body weight ratio and the estimates of resistance vessel structure were also significantly greater in the SHR compared with F1 rats (table 1). There were no statistically important differences in cardiovascular structure observed between the F1 and DRY rats (table 1).

Discussion:

These studies confirm that increased systolic pressure and hypertrophy of the heart and mesenteric resistance arteries are present in young SHR. Although the systolic blood pressure of the F1 rats was significantly higher than that of the DRY parents, there was no evidence of cardiovascular hypertrophy in the F1 hybrids.

Our observations suggest that factors other than blood pressure may be important determinants of structure in these young animals and that primary genetic factors may be relevant. The qualitative structural differences between SHR on one hand, and the DRY and F1 rats on the other is consistent with the effects of a genetic locus that determines cardiovascular growth and structure, at which the SHR is homozygous for a putative recessive "hypertrophic" allele. However, further studies of structure in young members of genetically segregating crosses (Harrap 1986) of SHR and DRY are necessary to test this hypothesis.

References:

Folkow B (1989): The structural cardiovascular factor in primary hypertension - pressure dependence and genetic reinforcement. J Hypertension 4(suppl 3): S51-S56

Friberg P, Nordlander M (1990): Influence of left ventricular and coronary vascular hypertrophy on cardiac performance. J Hypertension 8: 879-889

Gray SD (1984): Spontaneous hypertension in the neonatal rat Clin Exp Hypertens [A] 6:755-781

Harrap SB (1986): Genetic analysis of blood pressure and sodium balance in the spontaneously hypertensive rat. Hypertension 8:572-582

Harrap SB, Van der Merwe WM, Griffin SA, Macpherson F, Lever AF (1990): Brief ACE inhibitor treatment in young spontaneously hypertensive rats reduces blood pressure long-term. Hypertension 16: 603-614

Lee RMKW (1985): Vascular changes at the prehypertensive phase in the mesenteric arteries from spontaneously hypertensive rats. Blood Vessels 22: 105-126

Lever AF (1986): Slow pressor mechanisms in hypertension: A role for hypertrophy of resistance vessels. J Hypertens 4:515-524

Tanase H, Yamori Y, Hansen CT, Lovenberg W (1982): Heart size in inbred strains of rats. Part I. Genetic determination of the development of cardiovascular enlargement in rats. Hypertension 4: 864-872

The role of adrenal renin in steroid metabolism and development of hypertension in transgenic rats TGR (mREN2)

Jörg Peters, Maike Sander, Klaus Münter, Min Ae Lee, Behrus Djavidani, Michael Bader, Christiane Maser-Gluth, Paul Vescei, Detlev Ganten, and John J. Mullins

German Institute for High Blood Pressure Research and Department of Pharmacology, University of Heidelberg, Im Neuenheimer Feld 366, D-6900 Heidelberg, Germany

The dynamic interactions of primary pathophysiological changes and secondary regulatory mechanisms make it difficult to elucidate the role of a single factor in primary hypertension. Since the primary information, determining cell and whole body function, reside within the genes, their analysis is a major goal in hypertension research. Many genes involved in cardiovascular regulation have now been cloned and characterized, including the genes of the renin angiotensin system (RAS).

To overcome the difficulties in analyzing a complex genetic background, we generated a new monogenetic hypertensive rat model, the TGR(mREN2)27. By introducing an additional gene, the mouse ren2d renin gene into the germline of rats, hypertensive animals were established, in which the genetic basis of hypertension for the first time is exactly defined (1228). TGR(mREN2)27 develop hypertension at 5 weeks of age, reaching stably elevated blood pressure of 220 mmHg at 10-12 week of age. The TGR(mREN2)27 are very sensitive to low dose of Captopril, underlining the relationship between RAS- stimulation and hypertension. Interestingly, although the basic defect is an additional renin gene, plasma and kidney renin as well as plasma angiotensin I and II are suppressed. Instead, we detected a 20-fold elevated plasma prorenin and strong overexpression of the transgene in several extrarenal tissues.

Fig. 1 and 2 demonstrate the analysis of mouse renin gene expression by northern blot (Fig.1) and a RNAse protection Assay for mouse renin (Fig.2).

Fig. 1 : Northern blot analysis of renin mRNA

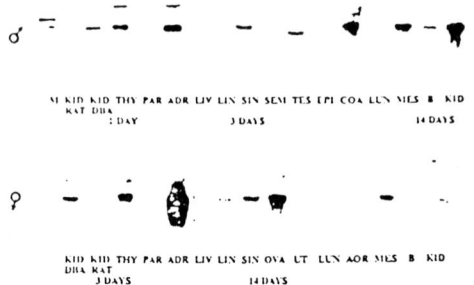

Fig. 1 : Northerm blot analysis. Northern blot analysis was performed on total RNA samples from tissues of transgenic animals as follows : In each lane 50 µg RNA was loaded, with the exceptions of adrenal gland (5 µg) and DBA/2 kidney (20 µg).

Abr. : M : kid : kidney, THY : thymus, PAR : parotis, ADR : adrenal gland, LIV : liver, LIN : large intestine, SIN : small intestine, SEM : seminar vesicle, TES : testis, COA : coagulation gland, LUN : lung, MES : mesenteric vessels.

Fig. 2 : RNAse protection assay of mouse renin mRNA

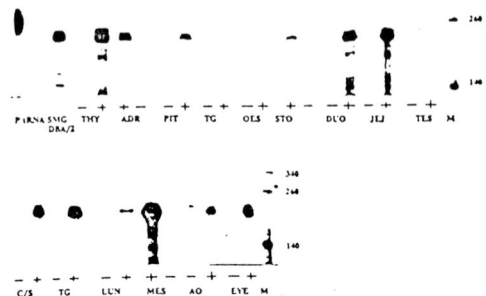

Fig. 2 : Ren-2 mRNA specific RNAse protection assay. The assay was performed using total RNA isolated from the respective tissues of transgenic and nontransgenic male rats. 50 µg of total RNA was hydrized, except SMG, DBA/2 and ADR : 0.5 µg. Exposure times ranging between 12 hours and 3 weeks.

B : brain, OVA : ovary, Ut : uterus, PIT : pituitary gland, TG : thyroid gland, OES : esophagus, STO : stomach, DUO : duodenum, JEJ : jejunum, C/S : cerebral cortex/septum, AO : aorta.

The RNAse protection assay specificly discriminates mouse renin mRNA from endogeneous rat renin mRNA, while the northern blot analysis controls the correct length of the transcript. The figures therefore demonstrate the presence of mouse specific renin mRNA with the expected length. The adrenal gland expresses the transgene by far at the highest level, the mouse renin gene being three orders of magnitude higher expressed than endogeneous rat renin in the adrenal. Using In situ hybridization and immunohistochemical analysis, transgene expression was mainly localized to the adrenal cortex, suggesting a role in adrenal steroid metabolism (Kidney international, Vol 41, 1992, in press). To determine, whether the adrenal RAS might be involved in the hypertensive process of TGR(mREN2)27, we investigated the activity of the adrenal RAS and correlated it with adrenal function. Mouse renin and prorenin in adrenal glands of TGR was found to be 30 times higher compared to control Sprague Dawley rats.

Additionally, the release of prorenin and active renin was strongly enhanced. The ratio of active renin content of adrenal cells to renin release was 40:1, that of adrenal cell prorenin to release was 10:1. This suggests different secretion mechanisms. Bilateral adrenalectomy, was followed by a significant drop of blood pressure (210±13 mmHg vs.163±23 mmHg) and a significant decrease of plasma prorenin (318±79 ng ANGI/ml*hr vs. 70 ±43 ng ANGI/ml*hr). In controls, blood pressure and plasma prorenin remained unchanged.

These results demonstrate, that the adrenal gland is a major source of circulating prorenin in the transgenic rats, TGR(mREN2)27. The role of prorenin in the development of hypertension awaits further studies. To investigate, whether an activated adrenal RAS has an impact on steroid metabolism, we analysed urinary steroid excretion in TGR(mREN2)27. Compared to SD controls, 24h- urinary deoxycorticosterone, corticosterone, aldosterone and its direct precursor 18-OH-corticosterone were significantly elevated at the age of 6 and 18 weeks, whereas in adult animals these steroids were back to controls. The elevation of both, mineralocorticoids and glucocorticoids, in the young transgenic rats parallels the development of blood pressure.

In conlcusion, we have found, that 1) the mouse renin transgene in TGR(mREN2)27 is expressed in a tissue specific manner and maintains specific regulatory control, 2.) the transcript is translated into a functional, biologically active protein in the adrenal gland, leading to a significantly stimulated adrenal renin 3.) the adrenal gland is a major source of plasma prorenin in TGR(mREN2)27 and 4.) the adrenal steroid metabolism in TGR(mREN2)27 is markedly stimulated, resulting in enhanced mineralo- and glucocorticoid excretion in young animals, which parallels the development of hypertension.

TGR(mREN2)27 are thus a model of low plasma renin hypertension, in which local tissue renin angiotensin systems might be of functional importance and they offer the opportunity to further detailed studies.

Kidney function and renin processing in transgenic rats (TGR mRen2-27)

Eberhard Hackenthal, Klaus Münter and Sybille Fritsch

Department of Pharmacology, University of Heidelberg, Germany

Renin secretion from the kidney is accompanied by the release of inactive prorenin. It is still unclear, whether prorenin secretion is of the constitutive or the regulated type, (see Hackenthal et al.,1990 for review), whether prorenin in the circulation or the interstitium can contribute to the activity of the renin-angiotensin-system either by its peripheral activation to renin, or by an enzymatic function of it`s own (see Sealey & Rubatto,1990 for review).
The recently established strain of transgenic rats carrying the mouse ren2-gene (Mullins et al.,1990) is a suitable experimental model to study some of these questions, because these animals develop fulminant hypertension despite normal plasma renin and angiotensin II concentrations. Interestingly, plasma prorenin is very high in these rats and seems to vary with blood pressure. We have therefore examined some functional properties of kidneys isolated from these rats, including the pattern of renin and prorenin secretion both for the rat and mouse enzyme in comparison to plasma concentrations of prorenin and renin.

METHODS

Animals. Male transgenic rats carrying the mouse ren2 gene (TGR mRen 2-27)(Mullins et al.,1990) were obtained from the breading facilities of the Dep.of Pharmacology through the courtesy of Dr.Ganten. They were reared on standard lab chow and tap water, and received no treatment (TG+) or treatment with captopril (10 mg/kg/day with the drinking water) starting from the 4th week of life until the experiment in the 7th week (TG/Cap). Blood pressure (tail plethysmography) and body weights were monitored at intervals. Transgen-negative animals (TG-) from the same breeding stock were used as controls.

Kidney perfusion. Kidneys were taken for isolated perfusion as described previously (Hackenthal et al., 1987). Briefly, kidneys were perfused at constant pressure (100 mm Hg) with a synthetic Krebs-Henseleit medium containing 25g/l bovine serum albumin (BSA) and 30g/l hydroxyethylstarch (HES) as oncotics. For prorenin secretion experiments HES was omitted and BSA reduced to 1g/l. Renal perfusate flow, glomerular filtration rate, and sodium excretion were measured as described (Hackenthal et al.,1987).

Analytical procedures. Renin in plasma and perfusate was estimated by radioimmunoassay of angiotensin II generated from an excess of rat angiotensinogen (Hackenthal et al.,1987). Prorenin was measured following activation with trypsin (Glorioso et al.,1983). Mouse renin and prorenin were differentiated from rat renin and prorenin by absorption of glycosylated rat renin to concanvallin-A-sepharose (Pharmacia), whereas mouse renin, which is not glycosylated remains unbound. Mouse renin was identified by immunoprecipitation with a mouse renin specific monoclonal antibody (kindly donated by Dr. Celio, Fribourg).

RESULTS AND DISCUSSION

Body weight, kidney weight, blood pressure.
Body weight in transgene-positive rats (TG+) in the 7th week was 199±4g, in transgene-negative controls (TG-) 240±4g and in captopril-treated transgene-positive rats (TG/cap) 187±4g. Kidney weights paralleled body weights, and were 842±21, 896±24 and 780± 24mg in TG+, TG- and TG/cap rats respectively. Blood pressures in the 7th week, immediately before kidney perfusion, were 194±20, 130±14, and 133±16 mmHg for the three groups, respectively. Thus, captopril-treatment had the intended effect of normalizing blood pressure in transgenic rats.

Kidney function.
Kidneys were perfused at constant pressure (100mm Hg). Perfusate flow rates (RPF) were 11.6±0.4 and 12.7±0.6 ml/min in TG+ and TG- kidneys, whereas in TG/cap rats RPF was significantly ($p < 0.05$) higher than in controls (14.6±0.5 ml/min). Significant differences were also observed with respect to GFR (0.43±0.04; 0.81±0.05; 0.71 ±0.03 ml/min in TG+; TG-; and TG/cap rats, respectively), filtration fraction and urine volume (not shown), as well as fractional sodium reabsorption (84.3±0.5; 60.1±1.3; and 60.7±0.5%, respectively).
Since in the isolated perfused kidney neither innervation, pressure changes, nor humoral factors are present to influence renovascular resistance and tubular function, it can be assumed that in transgenic as well as in captopril-treated rats stable adaptational changes occur, either morphological, functional, or both, which persist or become unmasked, when the kidneys are isolated from systemic regulatory mechanisms.
It remains to be clarified whether these changes in TG-positive rats are the consequence of chronic hypertension (however, such changes are not present to the same extent in other hypertensive models, e.g.in SHR), or of other functional alterations induced by the expression of the mouse renin transgene.

Kidney renin content.
As evident from Table 1, the total renin content of kidneys from TG+ rats is less than 5% of that in kidneys from TG- rats, whereas in spontaneously hypertensive rats, kidney renin content, at comparable blood pressures, is between 50 and 80% of that in control WKY rats (e.g. Morton et al.,1990). Captopril treatment completely restored the renin content of TG+ rats to control levels.

Table 1. Contribution of rat and mouse renin to kidney renin content in TGRmRen2-27 rats

	total renin ng ANGI/h/ kidney	% of renin unglycosylated	% of renin reacting with antibody to mouse renin
TG-negative(5)	903 ± 36	4.7 ± 0.3	0.7 ± 2.5
TG-positive(6)	36 ± 5	16.7 ± 1.9	16.7 ± 2.3
TG/capto(4)	1057 ± 71	5.1 0.3	6.3 ± 1.4

Most interestingly, stored renin in TG-positive and TG-captopril-treated rats is predominantly rat renin, as demonstrated both by the glycosylation status and the reactivity with a mouse renin antibody (Table 1). It should be noted that concavallin A-binding of glycosylated rat renin tends to underestimate rat renin, since even authentic rat renin does escape con A-binding by a few percent, as seen in TG- rats (Table 1). It has also to be considered that, mouse renin has a somewhat higher reaction rate with rat angiotensinogen than rat renin (about 50%, unpublished observations). This would also tend to overestimate the contribution of mouse renin. In any case, storage of mouse renin in TG-positive kidneys must be very low, particularly in captopril-treated rats. As rat and mouse renin mRNA are found in about equal concentrations in TG-positive kidneys (M.Paul, personal communications), rat and mouse renin can be assumed to be synthetized in about equal quantities. It therefore appears that these kidneys are unable to store mouse renin to the same extent as they store rat renin.

Kidney renin secretion.
Renin release from the isolated perfused kidney in TG-positive rats is about 35% of that in TG-negative

rats (see Table 2), which contrasts with the extremely low renin content in TG-positive kidneys (table 1). Captopril treatment of TG-positive rats raises the rates of renin secretion to that in control rats.

Table 2. Renin and prorenin release from isolated kidneys of transgenic rats (TGR mRen2-27)

	renin release			prorenin release		
	release ng ANGI per h/min	% glyco-sylated	% rat renin	release ng ANGI per h/min	% glyco-sylated	% rat renin
TG-negative(12)	19±8	87±7	100	12±3	87±8	100
TG-positive(11)	7±2	n.d.	80±8	20±4	45±2	72±8
TG/captopril(11)	18±5	80±8	71±7	124±8	34±3	33±10

Surprisingly, about 30% of the secreted renin represents mouse renin (antibody precipitation) whereas only 5% of kidney renin is mouse renin (Table 2). This discrepancy is even more pronounced in the pattern of prorenin secretion. Total prorenin release is not different between TG-positive and TG-negative rats and of the same magnitude as active renin secretion. In captopril-treated TG-positive rats, however, prorenin secretion is about 10fold that of controls in spite of a similar renin content of the kidneys, and about 65% of the secreted prorenin represent mouse renin. Data on the relative contribution of mouse and rat renin mRNA in kidneys of TG/cap rats are not available. However, total renin mRNA (mouse plus rat) in these kidneys is comparable to rat renin mRNA in TG-negative rats (unpublished observations), which is in accordance with a similar total renin content (see Table 1).

SUMMARY and CONCLUSIONS

Two important aspects emerge from the present study: First, rats from transgenic rats exhibit several differences as control rats in kidney function, in particular a significantly higher fractional sodium reabsorption, which is difficult to explain exclusively on the basis of the hypertensive state in these animals. Possibly, some other consequences of the mouse renin transgene are involved. Second, the kidney of transgenic rats seems to store preferentially rat renin, and the contribution of rat renin to total renin release is also high in transgene-positive rats whether treated with captopril or not. Prorenin secretion from captopril-treated rats, however, is predominantly mouse prorenin.
These data are compatible with the hypothesis that mouse prorenin synthetized in juxtaglomerular cells of the rat kidney is much less effectively sequestered into renin storage vesicles than rat prorenin, probably because it lacks glycosylation and thus a prerequisite for targeting. Therefore, less mouse prorenin is activated to renin, and more is released by constitutive secretion as such. The transgenic rat used in our studies is obviously a good model to further probe this hypothesis.

REFERENCES

Glorioso,N., Madeddu,P., Dessi Fulgheri,P., Fois,G., Meloni,F., Bandiera,F., Tonolo,G., and Rappelli A. (1983) Trypsin-activable inactive renin in rat plasma. Clin Sci 64: 137-140
Hackenthal,E., Aktories,K., Jakobs,K.H., and Lang,R.E. (1987) Neuropeptide Y inhibits renin release by a pertussis toxin sensitive mechanism. Am J Physiol 252: 543-F550
Hackenthal,E., Paul,M., Ganten,D., and Taugner,R. (1990) Morphology, physiology, and molecular biology of renin secretion. Physiol Rev 70: 1067-1116
Morton.J.J., Beattie,E.C., Griffin,S.A., MacPherson,F., Lyall,F., and Russo,D. (1990) Vascular hypertrophy, renin and blood pressure in the young spontaneously hypertensive rat. Clin Sci 79: 523-530
Mullins,J.J., Peters,J., and Ganten,D. (1990) Fulminant hypertension in transgenic rats harbouring the mouse Ren-2 gene. Nature 344: 541-544
Sealey,J.E., and Rubattu,S. (1989) Prorenin and renin as separate mediators of tissue and circulating systems. Am J Hypertens 2: 358-366

Sexual dimorphism of blood pressure in transgenic rats TGR(mREN2)27 harboring the murine *Ren-2* gene

Jürgen Bachmann, Ursula Ganten *, Frank Zimmermann, John J. Mullins, Günter Stock and Detlev Ganten *

*German Institute for High Blood Pressure Research and Department of Pharmacology, University of Heidelberg, W-6900 Heidelberg and * Max-Delbrück-Center for Molecular Medicine, O-1115 Berlin-Buch, Germany*

Male exhibit higher blood pressure than female genetically hypertensive rats (Cambotti et al. 1984; Ganten et al. 1989), and the prevalence of human hypertension is higher in men. To date, there is no conclusive explanation for this gender discrepancy. Experiments performed in spontaneously hypertensive rats (SHR) have shown that female SHR treated with testosterone during the neonatal period showed blood pressure values which were comparable to those of untreated male SHR. On the other hand, blood pressure of neonatally castrated male SHR was in the range of untreated female SHR (Cambotti et al. 1984). These results relate the sexual dimorphism with regard to hypertension to organizational effects of gonadal steroids on brain areas involved in blood pressure control during the neonatal period. These observations were confirmed and extended by Ganten et al. (1989) who showed that castration or treatment of newborn male SHR or SHRSP by the androgen receptor antagonists flutamide or cyproterone acetate kept blood pressure in later life at the level of female rats. The same treatment also effectively reduced blood pressure when it was performed in male SHR or SHRSP during the developmental phase of hypertension at nine weeks of age. These results indicate that in SHR, circulating testosterone affects the sexual dimorphism with regard to hypertension not only by its effects on the central nervous system at the neonatal stage, but also via different direct hormone receptor-mediated mechanisms.

A new monogenetic hypertensive rat model is the transgenic rat TGR(mREN2)27 harboring the murine *Ren-2* gene (Mullins et al. 1990). These rats develop severe hypertension. Preliminary data indicated that male TGR(mREN2)27 develop significantly higher blood pressure than female rats. This gender discrepancy supports the hypothesis of the renin gene being involved in the sexual dimorphism with respect to blood pressure. Testosterone stimulates renin mRNA in mice (Metzger et al. 1988). Since it was the murine DAB/*Ren-2* gene which was introduced into the transgenic rats, we treated young and adult female TGR(mREN2)27 with dihydrotestosterone and castrated young male TGR(mREN2)27 and recorded the effect of these treatment regimens on blood pressure.

MATERIALS AND METHODS

1. Animals:
TGR(mREN2)27 were progeny of the hypertensive founder number 27 which was generated by introduction of the murine *Ren-2* gene into the genome of Sprague Dawley rats by microinjection as described earlier (Mullins et al. 1990). Sprague Dawley rats (SD) obtained from the Central Institute for Laboratory Animal Breeding in Hannover (Germany) served as controls. Rats were kept under identical conditions, had free access to food and tap water, and were housed in temperature-controlled rooms (20-22°C) under a 12h light/dark cycle.

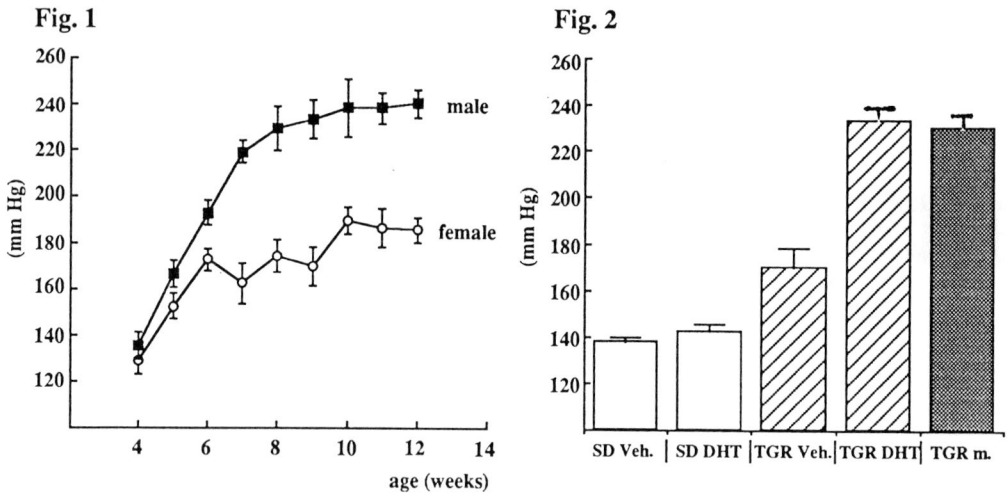

Fig. 1: Blood pressure development of male and female TGR(mREN2)27 from 4 to 12 weeks of age. p<0.05 between males and females between 6 and 12 weeks of age.

Fig. 2: Blood pressure of 10 weeks old female TGR(mREN2)27 (TGR) or Sprague Dawley rats (SD) after five weeks of treatment with 3 mg per day dihydrotestosterone (DHT) or vehicle (Veh.). Male TGR(mREN2)27 (TGR m.) were vehicle-treated, too. p<0.01 between TGR Veh., TGR DHT and TGR m.

2. Experimental protocols:
We performed four different types of experiments. Each experimental group consisted of 8 to 10 rats. All control animals were either sham-treated (drug vehicle) or sham-operated. Blood pressure was determined weekly by tail plethysmography carried out under light ether anesthesia as reported previously (Dietz *et al.* 1982).

1. Systolic blood pressure was determined in untreated male and female TGR(mREN2)27 from 4 to 12 weeks of age.
2. 5 weeks old intact female TGR(mREN2)27 or SD were treated with 3 mg dihydrotestosterone (DHT) (Merck, Darmstadt, Germany) dissolved in 0.2 ml vehicle administered daily by subcutaneous injection for 5 weeks. Vehicle consisted of castor oil benzylbenzoate (ratio 8:2). Blood pressure was measured weekly in DHT-treated and in control female TGR(mREN2)27 and SD and in a control group of male TGR(mREN2)27.
3. 39 weeks old intact female TGR(mREN2)27 were treated with DHT as described above for three weeks.
4. 4 weeks old male TGR(mREN2)27 were orchidectomized. Blood pressure was recorded for 8 weeks.

Statistics:
Results are expressed as mean±sem. Significant differences were evaluated by ANOVA followed by non-parametric rank tests (Kruskal-Wallis and Mann-Whitney tests). The null hypothesis was rejected when p<0.05.

RESULTS

1. Blood pressure in male and female TGR(mREN2)27
Fig. 1 shows the blood pressure development in male and female TGR(mREN2)27 at 12 weeks of age. Blood pressure is significantly higher in males compared to females.

2. Treatment of young female TGR(mREN2)27 with 3 mg/d DHT resulted in a significant increase in blood pressure (Fig.2). Blood pressure of female rats treated with DHT was in the range of male TGR(mREN2)27. There was no significant effect of DHT treatment on blood pressure in female SD.
3. Blood pressure of adult female TGR(mREN2)27 did not change significantly during DHT treatment (data not shown).
4. Orchidectomy of male TGR at four weeks of age resulted in a significant reduction of blood pressure compared to sham-operated animals by about 40 mm Hg (data not shown).

DISCUSSION

Male TGR(mREN2)27 manifest significantly higher blood pressure than females (Fig.1). This gender discrepancy was completely abolished by dihydrotestosterone treatment of young female TGR(mREN2)27, since DHT elevated blood pressure in females to the level of males (Fig.2). The development of hypertension in male TGR(mREN2)27 was delayed and reduced after orchidectomy. On the other hand, DHT did not have any effect on blood pressure in adult TGR(mREN2)27. These data indicate that testosterone has an important effect on the development of the sexual dimorphism with regard to blood pressure in young TGR(mREN2)27 but not on its maintenance in old TGR(mREN2)27.

It has been shown that renin content and renin mRNA in the salivary gland of mice are responsive to testosterone (Wilson et al. 1981; Catanzaro et al. 1985). Experiments performed in our laboratory showed that dihydrotestosterone treatment of NMRI mice enhanced renin mRNA levels in brain, submandibular gland, adrenal gland and heart (Metzger et al. 1988). Interestingly, different tissues showed a different time course with regard to the stimulation of renin mRNA by testosterone: In the adrenal gland, renin mRNA increased already two hours after DHT administration, whereas in the brain, a significant elevation of renin mRNA was found after 21 days of DHT treatment. A possible explanation for these observations is that local renin-angiotensin systems respond in a tissue-specific manner to testosterone with respect to time, mechanism and magnitude of renin stimulation. Since it is this murine *Ren-2* gene which was introduced into the transgenic rats TGR(mREN2)27 and which produced severe hypertension, the results of this study support the assumption that the renin gene and the stimulatory effect of testosterone on its expression are in part responsible for the higher blood pressure in males compared to females. An interaction of gonadal hormones with other components of the renin-angiotensin system (RAS), e.g. angiotensinogen, or with other systems involved in blood pressure control, e.g. the sympathetic nervous system, may contribute to the influence of gender on blood pressure. The transgenic rats TGR(mREN2)27 which differ from normotensive rats only by the additional renin gene are an excellent model to study the interactions between gonadal steroids and components of the RAS as a presumably important mechanism for the development of the sexual dimorphism with regard to hypertension.

REFERENCES

Cambotti, L.J., Cole, F.E., Gerall, A.A., Frohlich, E.D., and MacPhee, A.A. (1984): Neonatal gonadal hormones and blood pressure in the spontaneously hypertensive rat. *Am. J. Physiol.* 247, 258-264.

Catanzaro, D.F., Mesterovic, N., and Morris, B.J. (1985): Studies of the regulation of mouse renin genes by measurement of renin messenger ribonucleic acid. *Endocrinology* 117, 872-878.

Dietz, R., Schömig, A., Rascher, W., Strasser, R., Lüth, J.B., Ganten, U., and Kübler, W. (1982): Contribution of the sympathetic nervous system to the hypertensive effect of a high sodium diet in stroke-prone spontaneously hypertensive rats. *Hypertension* 4, 773-781.

Ganten, U., Schröder, G., Witt, M., Zimmermann, F., Ganten, D., and Stock, G. (1989): Sexual dimorphism of blood pressure in spontaneously hypertensive rats: effects of anti-androgen treatment. *J. Hypertens.* 7, 721-726.

Metzger, R., Wagner, D., Takahashi, S., Suzuki, F., Lindpaintner, K., and Ganten, D. (1988): Tissue renin-angiotensin systems: aspects of molecular biology and pharmacolog. *Clin. Exp. Hypertens. [A]* 10 (suppl.1), 1227-1238.

Mullins, J.J., Peters, J., and Ganten, D. (1990): Fulminant hypertension in transgenic rats harbouring the mouse *Ren-2* gene. *Nature* 344, 541-544.

Wilson, C.M., Cherry, M., Taylor, B.A., and Wilson, J.D. (1981): Genetic and endocrine control of renin activity in the submaxillary gland of the mouse. *Biochem. Genet.* 19, 509-523.

Animal models

Modèles animaux

Primary hypertension and the renin angiotensin system : from the laboratory experiment to clinical relevance

Michael Bader, Reinhold Kreutz, Jürgen Wagner, Karin Zeh, Manfred Böhm, Martin Paul and Detlev Ganten *

*German Institute for High Blood Pressure Research and Department of Pharmacology, University of Heidelberg, W-6900 Heidelberg, * Max-Delbrück-Center for Molecular Medicine, O-1115 Berlin-Buch, Germany*

INTRODUCTION

The pathogenetic mechanisms leading to human primary hypertension and their genetic background are complex. Several systems generating peptides which are active in cardiovascular regulation like the renin-angiotensin system (RAS) are considered to be involved in these processes. The investigation of these systems in humans has limitations for practical and ethical reasons. Most of these studies have been confined to the measurement of the plasma components of the RAS and their response to physiological and pathophysiological stimuli. With the evolving concept of local RAS, the investigation of the tissue-specific gene expression of its components has become increasingly important. The opportunities to study the action of these genes in humans are rare, since viable human tissue is only accessible from surgery specimens (Bruneval et al., 1988) or biopsy samples (Wagner et al., 1991), which provide only very small amounts of tissue.

To overcome this setback, animal models with genetic hypertension have successfully been developed e.g. the spontaneously hypertensive rat (SHR) and transgenic rats like TGR(mREN2)27 (Mullins et al., 1990), which show characteristics similar to human hypertension (Ganten, 1987). Alternatively, animal model systems for hypertension and other cardiovascular disorders have been produced by surgical interventions, for example by aortic banding or the ligation of coronary arteries to investigate the regulation of target genes. In addition, the establishment of cell culture systems, e.g. of vascular smooth muscle cells, allows studies of the cellular effects of peptides like angiotensin II (ANG II). The following sections will present examples of how these and other model systems can be used to elucidate the role of the RAS in the pathogenesis of hypertension and its genetic background and to develop new, more specific therapeutic methods to treat this disease in human beings.

THE RAS IN CARDIOVASCULAR TISSUE: CULTURED CELLS AND ANIMAL MODELS

In its classical definition, the RAS is an endocrine system, regulating blood pressure through its effector peptide, ANG II, which acts as a direct vasoconstrictor and stimulates aldosterone release from the adrenal cortex. Both mechanisms play an important role in the acute responses in the regulation of cardiovascular homeostasis. Later studies demonstrated that the actions of ANG II can go beyond the endocrine pathway, and it has been postulated that ANG is also active on the cellular level, exerting paracrine or even autocrine actions (Dzau, 1984). In addition, it was demonstrated that ANG biosynthesis can occur in the tissues themselves, leading to the concept of organ-based local RAS (Paul *et al.*, 1991). The functionality of these systems has been established in a number of tissues such as the kidney, adrenal gland, brain, heart and vasculature. Evidence that these tissue RAS act independently of the plasma system can be found in numerous studies investigating the chronic effects of angiotensin converting enzyme (ACE) inhibitors on blood pressure (Unger *et al.*, 1983). The reports demonstrated that the antihypertensive effects of these substances were predominantly correlated with the inhibition of ACE in the tissues and not in the plasma. In addition, new and interesting actions of ANG II were discovered which corroborated a functional role of the RAS going beyond blood pressure control. Specifically, the trophic actions of ANG II suggesting its role as a growth factor or modulator and the described angiogenic actions of the peptide point to a possible importance of the RAS in cardiovascular hypertrophy, vascular remodeling and myocardial injury or repair, which may have important implications for the treatment of cardiovascular disease (Paul and Ganten, 1991; Schelling *et al.*, 1991).

What is the evidence that the RAS has such functions in cardiovascular organs? The trophic actions of ANG II were first described by Schelling et al. (1978), who found that ANG II increased the cell number of cultured mouse fibroblasts. The effect was dose-dependent and could be blocked by the ANG II receptor antagonist, saralasin. These findings were later confirmed and expanded by other authors (for review see: Paul and Ganten, 1991; Schelling *et al.*, 1991). The stimulation of smooth muscle cells in culture by ANG II, however, had somewhat controversial effects. Whereas some authors also described hyperplastic effects of ANG II on vascular smooth muscle cells (Cambell-Boswell and Robertson, 1981), other studies detected a hypertrophic response only (Geisterfer *et al.*, 1988; Berk *et al.*, 1989). This apparent discrepancy can possibly be explained by species variability and differences in the experimental conditions.

Further evidence that ANG II is involved in growth phenomena can be derived from experiments showing its stimulatory effect on protoöncogenes in vascular smooth muscle cells. These genes play a role in the development of the cardiovascular structure and are normally not expressed in mature cells but can be expressed again under pathological conditions such as cardiovascular hypertrophy (Schneider and Parker, 1991). Indeed, several investigators (Taubman *et al.*, 1989; Naftilan *et al.*, 1989a; 1989b; 1990) were able to demonstrate that the peptide increased the expression of the protoöncogenes *c-fos*, *c-myc*, and *c-jun* as well as of the platelet derived growth factor (PDGF) in a dose-dependent manner. The direct link between ANG II and the hypertrophic changes was clearly demonstrated by experiments showing that antisense inhibition of *c-fos* (Rainer *et al.*, 1990) or PDGF (Itoh *et al.*, 1990) was able to block the positive effects of ANG II on DNA and protein synthesis in smooth muscle cells. Despite this it should be pointed out that the studies were all performed in cultured cells, and it remains to be determined whether or not there is an interaction between ANG II and protoöncogene activation in vivo and in hypertension.

Nevertheless, it has been shown that the RAS is activated in cardiac disorders such as cardiac hypertrophy and myocardial infarction (Lindpaintner and Ganten, 1991). Studies investigating the chronic phase of pressure overload hypertrophy of rat hearts induced by aortic banding showed an increased rate of conversion of ANG I to ANG II (Schunkert *et al.*, 1990). This coincided with a significant 3-fold increase in the ACE mRNA level in these hearts as determined by the polymerase chain reaction (Paul *et al.*, 1990). The regulation of the RAS in experimental myocardial infarction was investigated, among others, by Hirsch et al. (1991). These authors focussed on ACE expression in the chronic phase after experimental ligation of the A. coronaria sinistra in rats and found that both ACE mRNA level and enzyme activity were significantly elevated in the heart, whereas the activity of the RAS in the plasma and other organs remained unchanged. Taken together, these studies point to an important role for the local cardiac ANG synthesis in cardiovascular disease and might help to explain the beneficial effects of ACE inhibition in patients with cardiac hypertrophy or heart failure. It is still unclear, however, whether an increased activity of the cardiac ANG system is a primary or secondary factor for cardiac hypertrophy. Despite the fact that aortic banding can induce cardiac protoöncogene expression (Izumo *et al.*, 1988), ANG II is unable to induce the expression of the protoöncogenes *c-fos* and *c-myc* in the heart of rats subjected to aortic banding (Moalic *et al.*, 1991). More studies investigating different time periods, other species and other growth factors are needed to elucidate this question further. The fact remains that ACE inhibition reduces cardiac hypertrophy even at doses which do not lower the blood pressure, suggesting that it also influences local mechanisms independent of hemodynamics (Linz et al., 1989). In this context, it should also be pointed out that the beneficial effects of ACE inhibitors in the heart could at least in part be due to their action on the bradykinin system in which ACE plays an important role. This was also suggested by recently published studies (Linz et al., 1990; Wiemer et al., 1991). The use of specific inhibitors of the RAS and the bradykinin system should make it possible to dissect out their relative participation in the clinical actions of ACE inhibitors.

THE RAS IN HYPERTENSION: TRANSGENIC ANIMALS

Another way to discriminate the effects caused by the RAS from those by other peptide systems is to modulate its activity exclusively by incorporating the gene of one of its components into the genome of a normal animal, i.e. to produce a transgenic mouse or rat with one of the genes of the RAS. These animals enable investigators to study the effects of a single additional gene via a dysregulated RAS on the cardiovascular system. This is especially interesting when the gene is derived from humans in whom studies about the physiological effects of the RAS are difficult to perform. In addition, these animal model systems allow the testing of drugs that specifically interfere with the RAS like ANG II receptor antagonists and renin inhibitors, which are currently under intensive investigation. Two recently developed transgenic rat strains are described in the following sections.

The introduction of the *Ren-2* gene of the DBA/2 mouse into the genome of rats by microinjection techniques has led to the generation of the transgenic rat model TGR(mREN2)27 (Mullins et al., 1990). These rats develop fulminant hypertension, beginning at 4 weeks and reaching a maximum at 9 weeks of age. Although they exhibit dramatically high blood pressure levels (230-265 mmHg), the active components of the circulating RAS, namely renin, angiotensinogen and ANG II, are suppressed. The prorenin level is markedly raised in the plasma of transgenic animals, but the functional significance of this finding is still unclear.

The transgenic renin gene is expressed in various tissues, like the kidney, brain, heart, blood vessels, and thymus and at very high levels in the adrenal gland, leading to an overexpression of renin in most of these tissues (Peters et al., 1991). Only in the kidney, is rat renin gene expression suppressed compared with control Sprague-Dawley (SD) rats. This decrease of the endogenous renin mRNA might be caused partly by the high blood pressure and partly by a regulatory mechanism of the intrarenal RAS, i.e. a negative feedback regulation by ANG II on renin gene expression.

The adrenal gland exhibits the highest transgene expression in TGR(mREN2)27. This probably leads to a stimulated local adrenal RAS and increased local ANG II levels. Besides the other important functions of ANG II, it is well-known as a potent stimulator of adrenal steroid synthesis. This might explain the significantly enhanced urinary gluco- and mineralocorticoid excretion in TGR(mREN2)27 compared with SD rats up to an age of 18 weeks (Sander et al., 1991). These findings support the importance of the local tissue RAS, e.g. in the adrenal gland, and its effector peptide ANG II in the pathogenesis of hypertension in TGR(mREN2)27.

If the activity of the transgenic renin (most likely via increased tissue ANG II levels) is responsible for the development of hypertension in these animals, inhibitors of the RAS should normalise the blood pressure. In fact, the ACE inhibitor captopril (Mullins et al., 1990) reduces the blood pressure to approximately normotensive levels in TGR(mREN2)27. However, this effect might be due to the interference of this drug with the bradykinin system (see above). Therefore, we tested the action of the specific ANG II receptor type I antagonist, losartan (DuP 753). Four TGR(mREN2)27 each were treated with 0.5 and 10 mg/kg body weight daily of losartan by adding the potassium salt of the drug to the overnight drinking water for 4.5 weeks. After this period, the treatment was stopped. Blood pressure monitoring was continued for an additional 3 weeks.

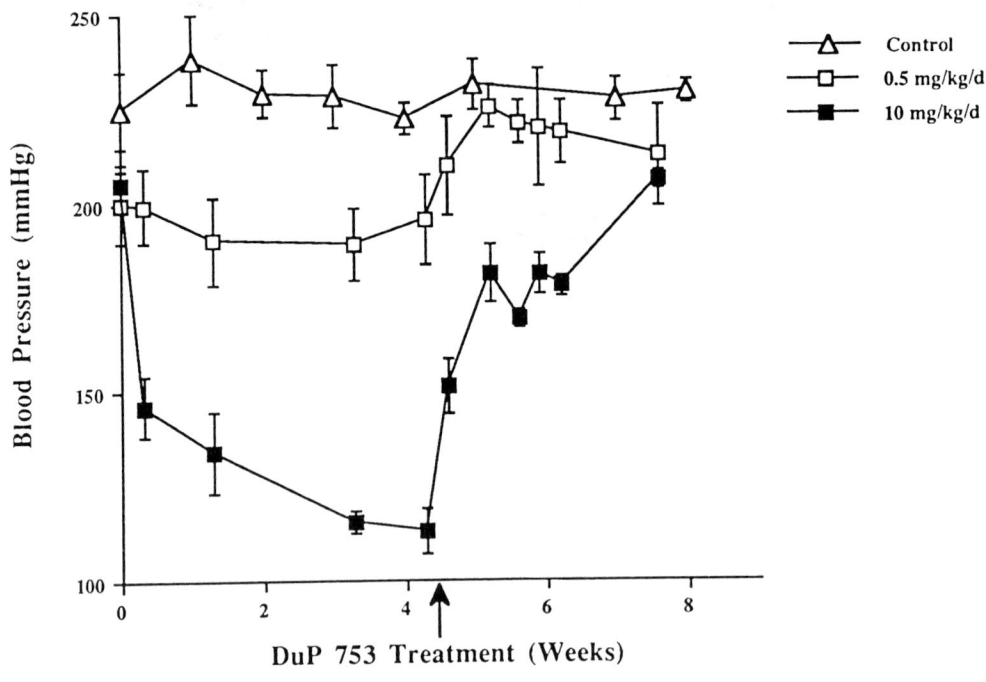

FIGURE 1:
Blood pressure values after losartan treatment of TGR(mREN2)27.
Eight heterozygous, male TGR(mREN2)27 were treated for 4.5 weeks with the ANG II receptor antagonist losartan (DuP 753), 4 animals at a dose of 0.5 and 4 animals at a dose of 10 mg/kg daily. Blood pressure was measured by tail plethysmography at the indicated time points before and during treatment and after withdrawal of the drug and compared with the values of 10 untreated, age-matched, male TGR(mREN2)27 (upper line).

The blood pressure was reduced drastically with 10 mg/kg daily and reached normotensive values after about 3 weeks (Fig. 1). After the cessation of treatment, the blood pressure rapidly increased again, reaching starting point levels after another 3 weeks. The lower dose of losartan resulted only in a slight reduction of blood pressure (Fig. 1).

In addition, the drinking behaviour was affected by losartan treatment: 10 mg/kg daily reduced the drinking volume after 10 days by about 50% (47.2±7.2 vs. 25.6±4.5 ml/d). This effect might be due to the blockade of central ANG II effects.

The plasma renin activity was elevated 13-fold and the plasma ANG II level 15-fold in the high-dose compared with the low-dose group after 4 weeks of treatment and returned to control values after the cessation of treatment, while the plasma prorenin concentration did not change significantly under losartan therapy. This observed upregulation of the plasma renin concentration is probably due to the blocked negative feedback mechanism of ANG II on the kidney renin secretion and, in addition, to the decline in blood pressure, which also regulates renin production by the kidney (Kurtz et al., 1990). The fact that the plasma prorenin concentration did not change significantly points to a blood pressure- and ANG II-independent regulation of its secretory pathway.

Thus, TGR(mREN2)27 show a sensitive response to ANG II receptor antagonists indicating the ANG II dependence of blood pressure in these animals. The relatively long periods to reach constant normotensive values at the beginning of treatment as well as the starting point levels after the cessation of treatment, and the already suppressed plasma RAS suggest an involvement of the local tissue RAS in the action of losartan.

Human primary hypertension is mostly not accompanied by a high activity of the plasma RAS but can be effectively treated by ACE inhibitors. This exhibits an interesting parallel to TGR(mREN2)27 and strengthens the validity of this rat strain as a low renin hypertension model for the testing of drugs which interfere with the RAS.

THE HUMAN RAS IN A RAT: TGR(hAOGEN)

The particular species-specificity of the human renin substrate reaction prevents enzymatical cross-reaction of rat renin with human angiotensinogen or human renin with rat angiotensinogen. As a consequence, even though they are unique models for the investigation of cardiovascular regulation, rats cannot be used for the development and testing of drugs interfering specifically with the human RAS, e.g. renin inhibitors.

In order to study the gene expression of human angiotensinogen and the species-specific kinetics of the human RAS as a model system for the testing of renin inhibitors, we generated transgenic rats harbouring the complete human angiotensinogen gene, TGR(hAOGEN). The construct comprised 1.1 kb of 5'-flanking sequences, five exons, four introns and 2.4 kb of 3'-flanking sequences with an overall size of 16.3 kb (Fukamizu et al., 1990).

From the founder animals which transmitted the transgene to their progeny, one line named TGR(hAOGEN)1663 expressed and secreted human angiotensinogen into the plasma at a concentration of 465.3 ± 44.9 µg/ml as measured by enzyme-linked immunosorbent assay using a human-specific monoclonal antibody. This exceeds the normal angiotensinogen level measured in human plasma (Gardes et al., 1982) as well as in rat plasma by approximately 7 times. The production of human angiotensinogen in the transgenic rats did not interfere with the level of rat plasma angiotensinogen, since no significant difference was found between transgenic and non-transgenic littermates.

As a reflection of the species-specificity of human angiotensinogen, similar levels of ANG II were demonstrated in TGR(hAOGEN) and control animals, indicating that rat renin does not cross-react with human angiotensinogen even in the presence of excess human substrate to form ANG I. Consequently, TGR(hAOGEN) are normotensive compared with transgene-negative controls.

However, the infusion of recombinant human renin rapidly raised the blood pressure in conscious, unrestrained TGR(hAOGEN) by 38% from normotensive values up to 198 mmHg systolic. The blood pressure response was paralleled by a corresponding increase in ANG II levels (data not shown). In the presence of the human-specific renin inhibitor, RO 425892, the hypertensive response to human renin infusions as well as the rise in plasma ANG II could be completely inhibited (Fig. 2). This indicates that (a) the interaction of human renin with human angiotensinogen is the sole cause of ANG II formation, (b) the transgenic human angiotensinogen gene product shows functional integrity, and (c) human renin does not interact with rat angiotensinogen.

When rat renin is infused in TGR(hAOGEN), eliciting an equipressor response compared with i.v. human renin, the addition of RO 425892 does not lower the blood pressure. Thus, in this case, the rise in blood pressure is due to the interaction of rat renin with rat angiotensinogen.

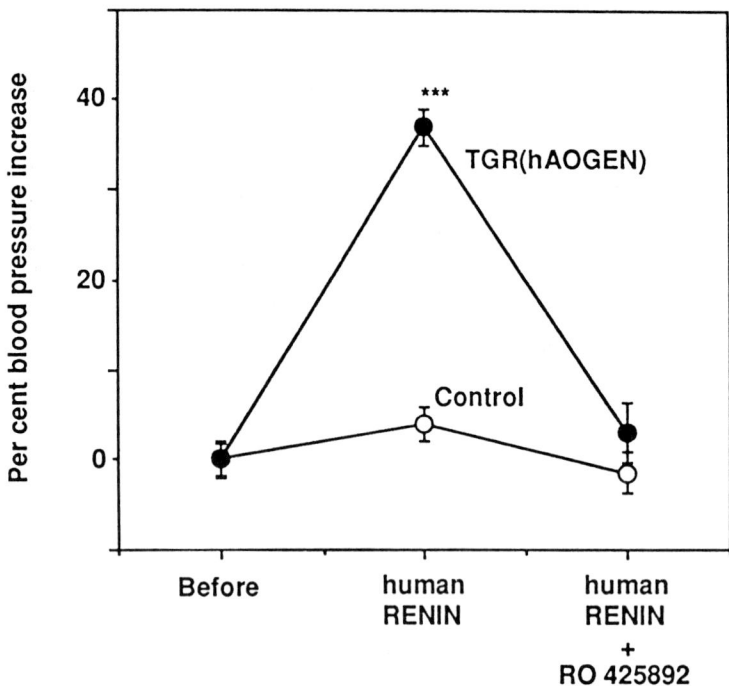

FIGURE 2:
In vivo species-specificity of the human renin-angiotensinogen reaction and of the human renin inhibitor RO 425892 in TGR(hAOGEN) rats.
The per cent increase of systolic steady-state blood pressure was determined in individual, conscious, unrestrained TGR(hAOGEN) rats (closed circles) or transgene-negative littermates (open circles) after infusion of human renin (5 µg ANG I/mlxh as i.v. bolus over 5 min). The human-specific inhibitor, RO 425892 (1000 µg/kg body weight i.v.) was infused 30 min after the human renin and normalised the blood pressure to pretreatment values.

Transgenic mice harbouring the mouse or rat angiotensinogen genes have been reported (Miller et al., 1989; Ohkubo et al., 1990; Kimura et al., 1992), but these constructs react with the host RAS or carry heterologous promotors. Using transgenic animals harbouring the human angiotensinogen gene under its own natural promotor offers an opportunity to study the regulation of the human gene in an animal model at the tissue level. Since these transgenic rats are accessible to haemodynamic or endocrinological investigations, human-specific drugs may be tested without the limitations of a primate model.

Finally, the generation of transgenic rats harbouring both the human renin and angiotensinogen genes may in the future serve as a model of human hypertension in rats characterised by the specific action of the human genes.

THE RAS IN THE MOLECULAR GENETICS OF HYPERTENSION: SHR

Several decades ago, researchers tried to bypass the difficulties of studies in human subjects with respect to the identification of the primary causes of arterial hypertension by developing strains of genetically hypertensive rats. It has been a general belief that the most considerable advantage of using inbred rats instead of human subjects is the homogeneity they provide. Nevertheless, it has been known for many years that a major problem of all research with inbred strains exhibiting a certain phenotype of interest is the chance fixation of genetic or phenotypical markers which have no part in the pathogenesis of the disease the model mimics (Rapp, 1983; Ganten, 1987). Moreover, most of the studies which found certain differences between normotensive and hypertensive inbred strains in a number of physiological and biochemical parameters suffered from a serious drawback: alterations in these parameters found to be associated with hypertension may represent either primary phenomena or secondary ones, due to the elevated blood pressure. The differentiation between these two possibilities was mostly based on speculation, and the discussion has been stimulated by evidence that the blood pressure might already be elevated in the SHR at birth (Gray, 1984). In two recent reports (St.Lezin et al., 1992; Johnson et al., 1992), additional information has been provided that a surprisingly high genetic dissimilarity in the DNA sequence between genetically hypertensive and control rats may account for a significant part of the interstrain differences in intermediate phenotypes which have been noted during the past few years. Therefore, the scientific value of these results with regard to the identification of the primary causes and pathomechanisms of arterial hypertension may be further impaired.

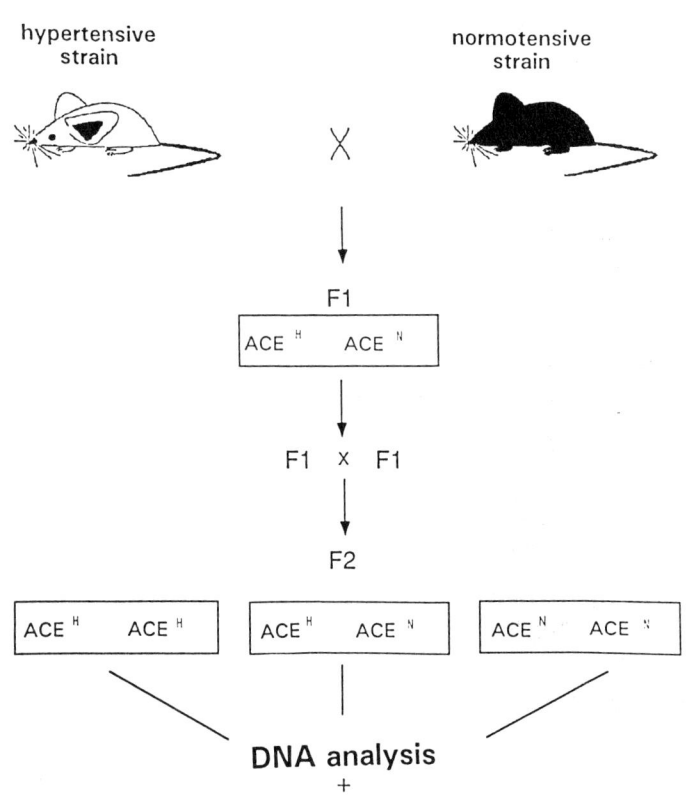

FIGURE 3:
Typical scheme of a cosegregation study in genetically hypertensive rats. A F2 cohort is generated by intercrossing F1 offspring derived from a hypertensive strain and a normotensive strain. The F2 animals are assayed for a given genotype and phenotype. In this case, it was determined whether the ACE allele of a hypertensive rat (ACE^H) has a greater influence on blood pressure (cosegregation) than that of a normotensive rat (ACE^N). To this purpose the blood pressure of the F2 rats that inherit the ACE^H allele is compared with the blood pressure of the F2 animals that inherit the ACE^N allele.

Research on the DNA level, in contrast, provides two major advantages. (1) It elucidates the primary, molecular genetic causes of hypertension. (2) Any DNA alteration found between the hypertensive and normotensive strains is independent of differences in the blood pressure or any other intermediate phenotype in these animals. In this respect, today's feasibility of molecular biological techniques have undoubtedly led to new exciting possibilities for hypertension research. Especially in the field of experimental hypertension, the advent of these methods has already led to deep insights into the molecular genetics of this disorder. The first molecular genetic studies in experimental hypertension investigated DNA markers in candidate genes thought to be involved in the development and maintenance of primary hypertension. In these studies, restriction fragment length polymorphisms (RFLPs) identified by the presence or absence of a restriction enzyme cleavage site allowed the distinction between the alleles of the hypertensive and normotensive animals at a certain candidate locus. Subsequently, the relevance of the RFLP for the hypertensive phenotype was assayed in classical crossbreeding experiments. These studies tested whether the DNA marker cosegregates with blood pressure in a F2 hybrid cohort derived from crossbreeding of the two parental (hypertensive and normotensive) strains (Fig. 3). Several cosegregation studies with RFLPs in the first intron of the renin gene acted as a paradigm for experiments with DNA markers in candidate genes and have, so far, produced controversial results which are discussed elsewhere (Kreutz et al., 1991).

The F2 animals studied by our group were derived from intercrosses between the stroke-prone SHR (SHRSP) and their normotensive controls the Wistar-Kyoto rats (WKY) in both reciprocal directions (SHRSP mothers with WKY fathers and SHRSP fathers with WKY mothers). Initially, we followed the candidate gene approach, in which the renin gene appeared to be an attractive candidate in SHRSP for several reasons but failed to show cosegregation with blood pressure (Lindpaintner et al., 1990).

These days, a profound improvement of the candidate gene strategy has become feasible by making use of a large number of randomly selected markers which distinguish between the alleles of the normotensive and hypertensive strains. This strategy, also termed the reverse genetic approach, applies DNA markers without prior knowledge of the gene or gene product involved in the pathogenesis of the disease under study. The principal advantage of this approach is that a multitude of loci dispersed across the genome leads to a fundamental increase in the chance of identifying the genes involved in a given disorder.

Using these more detailed linkage studies, two independent research groups identified an autosomal locus on chromosome 10 in the SHRSP genome which contributes to the variance of blood pressure in the set of our F2 hybrid animals (Hilbert et al., 1991; Jacob et al., 1991). The close linkage of this locus to the gene encoding the ACE led to the hypothesis that ACE is identical with the identified gene of this locus. Although ACE is a key enzyme in the RAS, renin rather than ACE had been believed to be the pivotal protein in this enzyme cascade so far. Therefore, ACE might become a new candidate gene in the genetic hypertension of SHRSP, as recognized by the reverse genetic approach, and its putative relevance will have to be substantiated or excluded by further, more refined, genetic or physiological studies. Finally, these investigations in experimental hypertension should complement studies in humans. We should keep in mind that the goal of all our efforts is to shed light on the causes of human primary hypertension rather than to unfold the molecular genetics of a specific animal model. In this respect, the identification of any gene and/or gene alteration which contributes to the development of high blood pressure in animal models will eventually provide a valuable guideline for molecular genetic studies of the human disease.

CONCLUSIONS

In the light of the molecular, cellular and genetic studies described above, the role of the RAS in hypertension and other cardiovascular diseases is becoming increasingly important, and the already developed animal and cell culture model systems will be of great value to investigate its cardiovascular effects in further detail. To achieve this goal, new model systems will be necessary, such as transgenic rats with other genes of the RAS or animals which overproduce genes of the RAS only in specific tissues. In addition, it will definitely be useful to "switch off" the activity of these genes in animals via antisense inhibition (Helene and Toulme, 1990) or homologous recombination in embryonic stem cells (Capecchi, 1991) in order to create new animal models which lack RAS activity partly or totally.

Despite this increasing importance, the RAS is only one of many systems involved in cardiovascular regulation and hypertension. The genetic studies are far from being complete, so that we may expect new interesting candidate genes, which point to other systems also involved in these processes. To evaluate their relevance for hypertension, one has to develop model systems, e.g. transgenic animals, for other peptides, such as endothelin, vasopressin or the atrial natriuretic factor (Steinhelper et al., 1990). The establishment of these animal strains and most of the results derived from them have been possible due to the rapid progress made in molecular biology and its use in medical research (Bader et al., 1992).

However, one has to be very careful in transferring the results obtained in animals and cell cultures to the human situation since species differences are especially marked in cardiovascular regulation. If this is kept in mind, the described experimental approaches will be valuable tools in the investigation and treatment of primary hypertension.

REFERENCES

Bader, M., Kaling, M., Metzger, R., Peters, J., Wagner, J., and Ganten, D. (1992): Basic methodology in the molecular characterization of genes. *J. Hypertens.* (In Press)

Berk, B.C., Vekstein, V, Gordon, H.M., and Tsuda, T. (1989): Angiotensin II-stimulated protein synthesis in cultured vascular smooth muscle cells. *Hypertension* 13, 305-314.

Bruneval, P., Fournier, J.G., Soubrier, F., Belair, M.F., DaSilva, J.L., Guettier, C., Pinet, F., Tardivel, I., Corvol, P., Bariety, J., and Camilleri, J.-P. (1988): Detection and localization of renin messenger RNA in human pathologic tissues using in situ hybridization. *Am. J. Pathol.* 131, 320-330.

Cambell-Boswell, M. and Robertson, A.L. (1981): Effects of angiotensin II and vasopressin on human smooth muscle cells in vitro. *Exp. Mol. Pathol.* 35, 265-276.

Capecchi, M. (1991): Altering the genome by homologous recombination. *Science* 244, 1288-1292.

Dzau, V.J. (1984): Vascular renin-angiotensin: A possible autocrine or paracrine system in control of vascular function. *J. Cardiovasc. Pharmacol.* 6, S377-S382.

Fukamizu, A., Takahashi, S., Seo, M.S., Tada, M., Tanimoto, K., Uehara, S., and Murakami, K. (1990): Structure and expression of the human angiotensinogen gene. *J. Biol. Chem.* 265, 7576-7582.

Ganten, D. (1987): Role of animal models in hypertension research. *Hypertension* 9 (Suppl I), I-2-I-4.

Gardes, J., Bouhnik, J., Clauser, E., Corvol, P., and Ménard, J. (1982): Role of angiotensinogen in blood pressure homeostasis. *Hypertension* 4, 185-189.

Geisterfer, A.A.T., Peach, M.J., and Owens, G.K. (1988): Angiotensin II induces hypertrophy, not hyperplasia, of cultured rat aortic smooth muscle cells. *Circ. Res.* 62, 749-756.

Gray, D. (1984): Spontaneous hypertension in the neonatal rat. *Clin. Exp. Hypertens. [A]* 6, 755-781.

Helene, C. and Toulme, J.-J. (1990): Specific regulation of gene expression by antisense, sense and antigene nucleic acids. *Biochim. Biophys. Acta* 1049, 99-125.

Hilbert, P., Lindpaintner, K., Beckmann, J.S., Serikawa, T., Soubrier, F., Dubay, C., Cartwright, P., DeGouyon, B., Julier, C., Takahasi, S., Vincent, M., Ganten, D., Georges, M., and Lathrop, G.M. (1991): Chromosomal mapping of two genetic loci associated with blood-pressure regulation in hereditary hypertensive rats. *Nature* 353, 521-529.

Hirsch, A.T., Talsness, C.E., Schunkert, H., Paul, M., and Dzau, V.J. (1991): Tissue-specific activation of cardiac angiotensin converting enzyme in experimental heart failure. *Circ. Res.* 69, 475-482.

Itoh, H., Pratt, R.E., and Dzau, V.J. (1990): Antisense oligonucleotides complementary to PDGF mRNA attenuate angiotensin-II induced vascular hypertrophy. *Hypertension* 16, 325 (Abstract).

Izumo, S., Nadal-Ginard, B., and Mahdavi, V. (1988): Proto-oncogene induction and reprogramming of cardiac gene expression produced by pressure overload. *Proc. Natl. Acad. Sci. USA* 85, 339-343.

Jacob, H.J., Lindpaintner, K., Lincoln, S.E., Kusumi, K., Bunker, R.K., Mao, Y.-P., Ganten, D., Dzau, V.J., and Lander, E.S. (1991): Genetic mapping of a gene causing hypertension in the stroke-prone spontaneously hypertensive rat. *Cell* 67, 213-224.

Johnson, M.L., Ely, D.L., and Turner, M.E. (1992): Genetic divergence between Wistar-Kyoto and the spontaneously hypertensive rat. *Hypertension* (In Press).

Kimura, S., Mullins, J.J., Bunnemann, B., Metzger, R., Hilgenfeldt, U., Zimmermann, F., Jacob, H., Fuxe, K., and Kaling, M. (1992): High blood pressure in transgenic mice carrying the rat angiotensinogen gene. *EMBO J.* 11 (In Press).

Kreutz, R., Higuchi, M., and Ganten, D. (1991): Molecular genetics of hypertension. *Clin. Exp. Hypertens. [A]* 13 (In Press).

Kurtz, A., Scholz, H., and della Bruna, R. (1990): Molecular mechanisms of renin release. *J. Cardiovasc. Pharmacol.* 16 (suppl. 4), S1-S7.

Lindpaintner, K., Takahashi, S., and Ganten, D. (1990): Structural alterations of the renin gene in stroke-prone spontaneously hypertensive rats: examination of genotype-phenotype correlations. *J. Hypertens.* 8, 763-773.

Lindpaintner, K. and Ganten, D. (1991): The cardiac renin-angiotensin system - An appraisal of present experimental and clinical evidence. *Circ. Res.* 68, 905-921.

Linz, W., Schölkens, B.A., and Ganten, D. (1989): Converting enzyme inhibition specifically prevents the development and induces regression of cardiac hypertrophy in rats. *Clin. Exp. Hypertens. [A]* 11, 1325-1350.

Linz, W., Martorana, P.A., Groetsch, H., Qi, B.J., and Schoelkens, B.A. (1990): Antagonizing bradykinin (BK) obliterates the cardioprotective effects of bradykinin and angiotensin-converting enzyme (ACE) inhibitors in ischemic hearts. *Drug Devel. Res.* 19, 393-408.

Miller, C.C., Samani, N.J., Carter, A.T., Brooks, J.I., and Brammar, W.J. (1989): Modulation of mouse renin gene expression by dietary sodium chloride intake in one-gene, two-gene and transgenic animals. *J. Hypertens.* 7, 861-863.

Moalic, J.M., Bauters, C., Himbert, D., Bercovici, J., Mouas, C., Guicheney, P., Baudoin-Legros, M., Rappaport, L., Eamnoil-Ravier, R., Mezger, V., and Swynghedauw, B. (1991): Phenylephrine, vasopressin and angiotensin II as determinants of proto-oncogene and heat-shock protein expression in adult rat heart and aorta. *J. Hypertens.* 7, 195-201.

Mullins, J.J., Peters, J., and Ganten, D. (1990): Fulminant hypertension in transgenic rats harbouring the mouse Ren-2 gene. *Nature* 344, 541-544.

Naftilan, A.J., Pratt, R.E., and Dzau, V.J. (1989a): Induction of platelet-derived growth factor A-chain and *c-myc* gene expressions by angiotensin II in cultured rat vascular smooth muscle cells. *J. Clin. Invest.* 83, 1419-1424.

Naftilan, A.J., Pratt, R.E., Eldridge, C.S., Lin, H.L., and Dzau, V.J. (1989b): Angiotensin II induces *c-fos* expression in smooth muscle via transcriptional control. *Hypertension* 13, 706-711.

Naftilan, A.J., Gilliland, G.K., Eldridge, C.S., and Kraft, A.S. (1990): Induction of the proto-oncogene *c-jun* by angiotensin II. *Mol. Cell. Biol.* 10, 5536-5540.

Ohkubo, H., Kawakami, H., Kakehi, Y., Takumi, T., Arai, H., Yokota, Y., Iwai, M., Tanabe, Y., Masu, M., Hata, J., Iwao, H., Okamoto, H., Yokoyama, M., Nomura, T., Katsuki, M., and Nakanishi, S. (1990): Generation of transgenic mice with elevated blood pressure by introduction of the rat renin and angiotensinogen genes. *Proc. Natl. Acad. Sci. USA* 87, 5153-5157.

Paul, M., Schunkert, H., Allen, P., and Dzau, V.J. (1990): Widespread distribution of angiotensin converting enzyme mRNA in human tissues. *J. Hypertens.* 8 (Suppl.3), S36 (Abstract).

Paul, M., Bachmann, J., and Ganten, D. (1991): The tissue renin-angiotensin system: new roles for an old player. *Trends Cardiovasc. Med.* (In Press).

Paul, M. and Ganten, D. (1991): The molecular basis of cardiovascular hypertrophy: the role of the renin angiotensin system. *J. Cardiovasc. Pharmacol.* (In Press).

Peters, J., Bader, M., Ganten, D. and Mullins, J. (1991): Tissue Distribution of Ren-2 expression in transgenic rats. In: *Genetic approaches to coronary heart disease and hypertension*, edited by Berg, K., Bulyzhenkov, V., Christen, Y. and Corvol, P. Berlin, Heidelberg, New York: Springer-Verlag, pp. 74-80.

Rainer, R.S., Eldridge, C.S., Gilliland, G.S., and Naftilan, A.J. (1990): Antisense oligonucleotide to *c-fos* blocks the angiotensin-II stimulation of protein synthesis in rat aortic smooth muscle cells. *Hypertension* 16, 326 (Abstract).

Rapp, J.P. (1983): A paradigm for the identification of primary genetic causes of hypertension in rats. *Hypertension* 5 (supp I), I-198-I-203.

Sander, M., Bader, M., Djavidani, B., Lee, M., Ganten, U., Peters, J., Mullins, J., Vecsei, P., and Ganten, D. (1991): Characterization of the hypertensive transgenic rats (TGR): Role of the adrenal gland. *5th European Meeting on Hypertension, Milan, 7. -10. June, 1991* , 640 (Abstract).

Schelling, P., Ganten, D., Speck, G., and Fischer, H. (1978): Effects of angiotensin II and angiotensin II antagonist saralasin on cell growth and renin in 3T3 and SV3T3 cells. *J. Cell. Physiol.* 98, 503-514.

Schelling, P., Fischer, H., and Ganten, D. (1991): Angiotensin and cell growth: a link to cardiovascular hypertrophy? *J. Hypertens.* 9, 3-15.

Schneider, M.D. and Parker, T.G. (1991): Cardiac myocytes as targets for the action of peptide growth factors. *Circulation* 81, 1443-1456.

Schunkert, H., Dzau, V.J., Tang, S.S., Hirsch, A.T., Apstein, C.S., and Lorell, B.H. (1990): Increased rat cardiac angiotensin converting enzyme activity and mRNA expression in pressure overload left ventricular hypertrophy. *J. Clin. Invest.* 86, 1913-1920.

St.Lezin, E., Simonet, L., Pravenec, M., and Kurtz, T.W. (1992): Hypertensive strains and normotensive 'control' strains: How closely are they related? *Hypertension* (In Press).

Steinhelper, M.E., Cochrane, K.L., and Field, L.J. (1990): Hypotension in transgenic mice expressing atrial natriuretic factor fusion genes. *Hypertension* 16, 301-307.

Taubman, M.B., Berk, B.C., Izumo, S., Tsuda, T., Alexander, R.W., and Nadal-Ginard, B. (1989): Angiotensin induces c-fos mRNA in aortic smooth muscle:Role of Ca2+ mobilization and protein kinase C activation. *J. Biol. Chem.* 264, 526-530.

Unger, Th., Ganten, D., and Lang, R.E. (1983): Converting enzyme inhibitors: antihypertensive drugs with unexpected mechanisms. *Trends Pharmacol. Sci.* 4, 514-519.

Wagner, J., Paul, M., Ganten, D., and Ritz, E. (1991): Gene expression and quantification of components of the renin-angiotensin-system from human renal biopsies by the polymerase chain reaction. *J. Am. Soc. Nephrol.* 2, 421 (Abstract).

Wiemer, G., Schoelkens, B.A., Becker, R.H.A., and Busse, R. (1991): Ramiprilat enhances endothelial autacoid formation by inhibiting breakdown of endothelium-derived bradykinin. *Hypertension* 18, 558-563.

Résumé

Le but de cette revue est de montrer comment les modèles animaux peuvent être utilisés pour préciser le rôle du système rénine angiotensine (SRA) dans la physiopathologie de l'hypertension humaine et développer des thérapeutiques nouvelles et plus spécifiques. Un premier paragraphe concerne le rôle du SRA dans les tissus cardiaque et vasculaire tel qu'apprécié à l'aide des modèles animaux et des cultures de cellules. A cet égard une revue des arguments expérimentaux montrant le rôle de l'angiotensine II comme facteur de croissance et d'angiogénèse est présentée et les données animales sont comparées à celles de la clinique. Le deuxième paragraphe décrit l'utilité des animaux transgéniques pour évaluer l'importance du SRA dans l'hypertension, en insistant tout spécialement sur les rats TGR (mREN2) 27 qui possèdent le gène REN2 de la souris et les rats TGR (hAOGEN) qui expriment la totalité - promoteur inclus - du gène de l'angiotensinogène humain. Ces derniers, en levant les difficultés liées à la spécificité d'espèce de l'action de la rénine sur son substrat peuvent être utilisés pour tester l'efficacité de molécules inhibitrices de la rénine humaine. Enfin le dernier paragraphe est consacré à la génétique moléculaire de l'hypertension et à son approche utilisant les souches de rats génétiquement hypertendus. Après avoir rappelé qu'en se plaçant au niveau de l'ADN les anomalies causales de l'hypertension étaient enfin accessibles, les deux principales approches méthodologiques - gènes candidats ou génétique inverse - sont explicitées. La mise en évidence par deux groupes différents d'une anomalie, coségrégant avec l'hypertension, située sur le chromosome 10 à proximité du gène de l'enzyme de conversion renforce le rôle potentiel du SRA. De telles études réalisées, chez l'animal, doivent permettre de guider celles qui, nécessairement devront se faire chez l'Homme. Ainsi, pour le SRA comme pour d'autres systèmes de régulation, l'application des techniques de la biologie moléculaire à des modèles animaux permettra de mieux cerner leur rôle physiopathologique. Toutefois, compte tenu des spécificités d'espèce que présente la fonction cardiovasculaire, toute extrapolation à l'Homme devra rester prudente.

Obese SHR (Koletsky rat) : a model for the interactions between hypertension and obesity

Richard J. Koletsky and Paul Ernsberger

Division of Endocrinology and Hypertension, Saint Luke's Hospital and Case Western Reserve University School of Medicine, 11311 Shaker Boulevard, Cleveland, Ohio 44104, USA

INTRODUCTION

In the course of breeding SHRs of the Kyoto-Wistar strain, a genetic mutation causing obesity appeared after a female SHR was mated with a normotensive Sprague-Dawley male. The genetically obese hypertensive strain was established after several generations of selective breeding(Koletsky, 1972; 1975). The abnormal phenotype is thought to be due to a single recessive gene (fa^k) related to the Zucker Fatty trait (fa)(Bray & York, 1979). The obese SHR is a unique strain of rat with genetic obesity, hyperlipidemia (Type IV), hyperinsulinemia, glomerulopathy with proteinuria and spontaneous hypertension. Abnormalities are present in the endocrine pancreas, adrenal, kidney, and gonads. The animals die prematurely due to renal disease.

The hypothalamus contains critical centers implicated in the control of blood pressure(Oparil et al., 1989; Ernsberger et al, 1985), food intake(Leibowitz & Shor-Posner, 1986), and autonomic dysfunctions that contribute to genetic obesity(Bray & York, 1979). The obese SHR is a model to study hypothalamic functions controlling body weight and blood pressure. Thus, we sought to further explore hypothalamic activity by examining circadian rhythms, the hypothalamic-pituitary-adrenal axis, the regulation of food intake by neurotransmitters, and the contribution of the sympathetic nervous system to the maintenance of blood pressure.

METHODS

Obese SHRs have been maintained by continuous inbreeding in a closed colony for 20 years. Obese SHRs were housed in a separate room at 23°C with usual 12h dark/light cycles and were housed individually after 6wk of age. Food (Purina rat chow) and tap water were available ad lib unless noted. Both male and female animals aged 3-6 mo were used for studies. Lean sex matched littermates served as controls. We compared diurnal rhythms in obese and lean SHRs. Food intake, water intake, urine output and urine corticosterone levels were measured in 12h light or dark cycles. Urine corticosterone was determined by a modification of a previously described radioimmunoassay(Giordano et al, 1976). To further explore the hyperadrenalism in obese SHRs, dexamethasone suppression testing was performed. After a 4d baseline, dexamethasone, a potent synthetic glucocorticoid, was administered in drinking water at successive doses of .001, .01, 0.1, 1.0, 10 µg/kg/d to both obese and lean SHRs. Urine was collected on the fourth day of treatment with each dose for corticosterone assay.

The indirect serotonin agonist fluoxetine was administered to male obese and lean SHR to explore the mechanism of hyperphagia in this model. Rats were food deprived for 24h, then given fluoxetine (10mg/kg, sq) or vehicle 1h prior to refeeding. Food consumption was determined 1, 4 and 24h following drug administration. Each animal was given both vehicle and drug in a crossover design.

Baseline averages of systolic blood pressure and heart rate were determined in obese and lean SHRs by tail cuff(Ernsberger et al, 1985). Under urethane anesthesia (1 g/kg, ip), direct arterial blood pressure measurements were obtained via insertion of a polyethylene cannula into either the femoral or brachial artery. Mean arterial blood pressure was taken before and after ganglionic blockade with chlorisondamine (0.4 mg, ip). Autopsies were performed at age 7-10 mo. Adrenal, kidney, heart and body weights as well as left ventricular wall thickness were recorded for each rat.

Data are expressed as mean ± standard error. Statistical analysis was by analysis of variance (ANOVA) with repeated measures as required.

RESULTS

Both obese SHRs and their lean siblings exhibited diurnal variations in food intake, water intake and urine production. Both groups were metabolically more active at night. Day and night the obese SHR ate, drank and urinated proportionately more than its lean siblings (Fig. 1). Diurnal rhythms of corticosterone production were present in both lean and obese SHRs, but the obese animals produced more corticosterone both day and night. Overall, obese SHRs produced twice the amount of corticosterone daily as lean siblings (Fig. 1). Dexamethasone suppression testing (Fig. 2) revealed the corticosterone production in lean SHRs was maximally suppressed by 0.01 µg/kg while the obese SHRs corticosterone production was suppressed only at a dose of 10 µg/kg.

Following 24h food deprivation, acute fluoxetine administration decreased food intake in both lean and obese animals (Fig. 3). Obese animals overcame the effect of fluoxetine by 4h, sooner than lean animals. At 24h, there were no differences between any of the groups.

Systolic blood pressure measured in the conscious state by tail cuff was somewhat lower in obese SHRs than lean littermates (obese: 176±1 mmHg, N=30; lean: 190±3 mmhg, N=17). Heart rates were nearly identical in the two phenotypes (obese: 436±4 bpm, N=30; lean: 431±7 bpm, N=17). Direct mean arterial pressure (MAP) under urethane anesthesia confirmed the tail cuff data (Table). Lower MAP was not due to reduced sympathetic tone since ganglionic blockade with chlorisondamine failed to eliminate the difference. Autopsies at 7-10mo showed that adrenal weight was increased 37% in obese SHRs consistent with their hyperadrenalism. The kidneys were also significantly enlarged consistent with their kidney disease. The obese SHRs had cardiac hypertrophy with a 25% increase in heart weight and an increase in left ventricular (LV) wall thickness.

DISCUSSION

The obese SHR is a unique animal model wherein genetic obesity and spontaneous hypertension coexist. The multitude of metabolic abnormalities present in this animal including hyperinsulinemia, hyperlipidemia (Type IV), hyperadrenalism and glomerular kidney disease each have their parallel in human obese hypertension. Our studies focused on the hypothalamus, which plays a critical role in regulating metabolic and cardiovascular function. Circadian metabolic studies showed that while diurnal patterns were maintained, obese SHRs are hyperphagic, polydipsic and polyuric compared to lean siblings. The obese SHR also produced nearly twice as much corticosterone per day as lean siblings. Much higher doses of dexamethasone are needed to suppress daily corticosterone production. To investigate hypothalamic control of eating behavior, we studied various serotonergic agonists(Nash et al, 1988). These agents are active in suppressing food intake in obese as well as lean SHRs, but with different timecourses. Thus, the hypothalamus may contribute to the multiple abnormalities in genetic obesity.

Originally, about 50% of the animals developed atherosclerosis. However, this pathologic finding has disappeared over the past 9 years, despite persisting hypertension and endogenous hyperlipidemia (Type IV). The

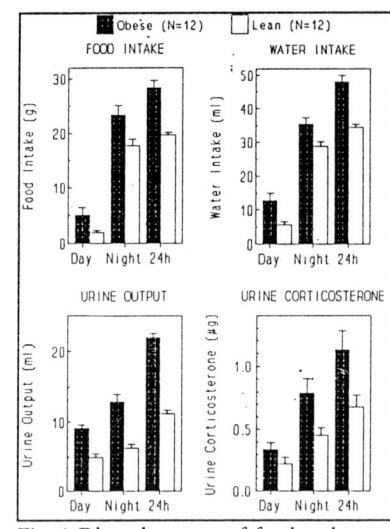

Fig. 1 Diurnal pattern of food and water intake, urine volume, and urine corticosterone in obese and lean SHR. Data were obtained during 12h light and dark cycles.

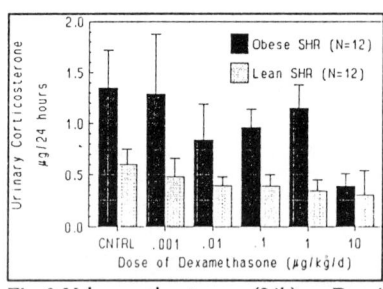

Fig. 2 Urine corticosterone (24h) on Day 4 of treatment with each cumulative dose of dexamethasone in obese and lean SHR.

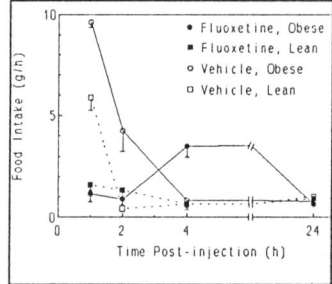

Fig. 3 Effect of fluoxetine (10 mg/kg, ip) on rate of food intake (g/h) following 24h food deprivation in obese (N=5) and lean (N=12) SHR.

TABLE

Strain (*p<.05, **p<0.01)	Body Wt, g	Adrenal Wt, mg	Kidney Wt, g	MAP (baseline)	MAP (+chlorisond.)	Heart Wt, g	LV Wall, mm
Lean (N=10)	300±25	42±3	2.1±.09	147±4	84±5	1.2±.09	3.6±.16
Obese (N=14)	575±22 **	58±4 **	2.9±.13 **	133±3 *	71±3 *	1.5±.05 **	4.0±.06 **

genetic defects that lead to hypertension and obesity may therefore be separate from the mutation that caused atherosclerosis.

Unlike the obese Zucker rat, which is normotensive according to most reports(Buñag & Barringer, 1988), the obese SHR is hypertensive. Obesity may not contribute to hypertension in this model. Lean siblings actually have higher blood pressure, whether measured by tail cuff or direct cannula. The obese phenotype may confer partial protection against spontaneous hypertension. The lower blood pressure in obese SHR persisted after ganglionic blockade, so it is probably not due to decreased sympathetic activity. Furthermore, cardiac ß-adrenergic receptors are unchanged in obese SHR relative to lean SHR(Ernsberger et al., 1991).

Treatment with a very-low-calorie diet for 12d fails to reduce hypertension in the obese SHR, although heart rate falls(Ernsberger et al., 1991). During refeeding blood pressure rises abruptly within 48h to reach or exceed the level in lean SHR. This refeeding hypertension(Ernsberger & Nelson, 1988) was due to increased sympathetic nervous activity, since it was reversed by ganglionic blockade with chlorisondamine and was associated with down-regulation of cardiac ß-adrenergic receptors(Ernsberger et al., 1991). Left ventricular wall thickness was further increased in obese SHR after refeeding. The harmful effects of refeeding were amplified in obese SHR relative to either lean SHR or to overfed obese Sprague-Dawleys(Ernsberger & Nelson, 1988).

The obese SHR (Koletsky Rat) with its multitude of metabolic problems remains an extremely important model to study the interactions of obesity and hypertension. Our studies suggest these animals have abnormalities in the hypothalamus. Further studies to characterize these abnormalities will lead to greater understanding of the relationship between and treatments for these two common conditions.

ACKNOWLEDGEMENTS

We thank Robert Voigt, Director of the Animal Resource Center at Case Western Reserve University for help in maintaining the colony. This work was supported by the Prentiss Foundation, St. Luke's Hospital.

REFERENCES

Bray, G.A. & York, D.A. (1979): Hypothalamic and genetic obesity in experimental animals: an autonomic and endocrine hypothesis. *Physiol. Rev.* 59, 719-809.

Buñag, R.D. & Barringer, D.L. (1988): Obese Zucker rats, though still normotensive, already have impaired chronotropic baroreflexes. *Clin. Exp. Hypertens. [A].* 10 Suppl 1, 257-262.

Ernsberger, P., Azar, S. & Azar, P. (1985): The role of the anteromedial hypothalamus in Dahl hypertension. *Brain Res. Bull.* 15, 651-656.

Ernsberger, P., Koletsky, R.J., Baskin, J.Z. & Foley, M. (1991): Refeeding hypertension in obese SHR. *Hypertension* 18, 422.

Ernsberger, P. & Nelson, D.O. (1988): Refeeding hypertension in dietary obesity. *American Journal of Physiology* 254, R47-R55.

Giordano, N.D., Koletsky, R.J. & Koletsky, S. (1976): Simultaneous determination of plasma aldosterone, corticosterone, 11-deoxycorticosterone, 18-hydroxydeoxycorticosterone, cortisol, and 11-deoxycortisol. *Am. J. Clin. Path.* 66, 588-597.

Koletsky, S. (1972): New type of spontaneously hypertensive rats with hyperlipemia and endocrine gland defects. *Spontaneous Hypertension: Its Pathogenesis and Complications*, ed. K. Okamoto, pp.194-197. Tokyo: Igaku Shoin Ltd.

Koletsky, S. (1975): Pathologic findings and laboratory data in a new strain of obese hypertensive rats. *Am. J. Pathol.* 80, 129-142.

Leibowitz, S.F. & Shor-Posner, G. (1986): Brain serotonin and eating behavior. *Appetite* 7(Suppl.), 1-14.

Nash, J.F., Bedol, C. & Koletsky, R.J. (1988): Effects of various serotonergic anorexic agents on deprivation-induced feeding in spontaneous obese hypertensive (Koletsky) rats. *Clin. Res.* 36, 358A.

Oparil, S., Yang, R.H., Jin, H.K., Wyss, J.M. & Chen, Y.F. (1989): Central mechanisms of hypertension. *Am. J. Hypertens.* 2, 477-485.

Pathophysiological characteristics of spontaneously hypertensive and hypercholesterolemic rats (hyper T-C rats)

Hiroyuki Ito, Tsuneyuki Suzuki and Kozo Okamoto

Department of Pathology, Kinki University School of Medicine, Osaka 589, Japan

SUMMARY

By brother-sister breeding of hybrids of M-SHRSP (malignant hypertensive rats) and SHC (hypercholesterolemic rats), inbred strain of spontaneously hypertensive and hypercholesterolemic rats (Hyper T-C rats) was established. In these rats, blood pressure is about 250mmHg and total cholesterol is 500mg/dl at 16 weeks of age. Moreover, these rats suffer severe renal failure (BUN 73 and creatinine 2.04). Histologically, both hypertension- and hypercholesterolemia-related changes were observed in arterial wall of many organs. Stroke lesion incidence rate was 40%. In particular, marked enlargement of kidney was found and histologically nephrotic gromerular changes were recognized. These rats must be a valuable model not only for hypertension and arteriosclerosis but also for renal failure.

INTRODUCTION

Both hypertension and hypercholesterolemia are major risk factors for cardiovascular and cerebrovascular diseases in humans. For the experimental study on the pathogenesis of such diseases, suitable animal model having both risk factors were required for long time. Using M-SHRSP (malignant or precocious SHRSP, Okamoto et al., 1985) and spontaneously hypercholesterolemic rats (SHC, Imai and Matsumura, 1973), Okamoto et al. (1989) tried to separate a new colony having both hypertension and hypercholesterolemia and established a inbred strain of Hyper T-C rat. These rats are keeping in our laboratory and reached at 34th generation. The aim of this experiment is to evaluate the characteristics of this special rat strain.

MATERIALS AND METHOD

1. Animals
   Hyper T-C rats were separated by brother-sister breeding of crossbred hybrid of M-SHRSP and SHC. In the present study, Hyper T-C rats from generation F28 to F32 were used. All rats were housed in air-conditioned room (22°C, and 50-70% humidity) and furnished tap water and stock chow diet (Funabashi SP, Funabashi Farm Ltd., Chiba, Japan) ad libitum. Chronological examination were performed for blood pressure, body weight and serum biochemistry. Comparative studies between Hyper T-C and SHRSP were carried out at 16 weeks of age.

2. Blood analysis
Blood were taken from jugular vein without anesthesia in every 2 weeks from 6 weeks of age. Blood analysis were performed using Coulter counter T-540. Serum were separated by centrifugation at 3000 rpm for 20 min. at room temperature. Serum analysis were carried out using TECHNICON SMAC III (C9100) system.

3. Pathological examination
All rats were autopsied after natural death or sacrifice and subjected to histopathological examination. Electronmicroscopical examinations were carried out for the kidneys by standard methods.

RESULTS

1. Blood pressure and body weight
Blood pressure of male Hyper T-C rats were already higher at 6 weeks of age, being around 160mmHg and then elevated to 200mmHg at 8 weeks and 250mmHg at 12 weeks of age. Female's blood pressure showed similar tendency, but slightly lower compared to that in male. Such elevation of blood pressure in Hyper T-C rats were slightly less in comparison with that in M-SHRSP, a parental strain.

Body weight increased from 6 to 12 weeks of age and then became plateau. Hyper T-C rats were heavier than those of M-SHRSP or SHRSP and similar to those of WKY. At 16 weeks of age, brain, heart, liver and adrenal grands were lighter but kidney was heavier in Hyper T-C rats than those in SHRSP or WKY.

2. Chronological changes in serum biochemistry
In Hyper T-C rats, serum albumin content were lower than in SHRSP after 12 weeks of age. As expected, total cholesterol increased dramatically after 10 weeks of age and similar changes were found in serum triglyceride, reaching to 700 mg/dl in the former and 900 mg/dl in the latter, respectively, whereas they were around 60 and 100 mg/dl in SHRSP. Furthermore, such tendency was also found in urea N and creatinine, but not in SHRSP. No significant difference was found in glucose. GOT and GPT were always lower in Hyper T-C rats than in SHRSP. For serum electrolytes, Na and CL were slightly lower and K and Ca were higher in Hyper T-C rats. Fe was markedly decreased after 8 weeks of age and was significantly lower from 12 to 16 weeks.

Comparison of some physical and biochemical parameters

	Hyper T-C	SHRSP	WKY	Anova*
Blood pressure (mmHg)	258.8 ± 7.15	250.6 ± 2.81	140.4 ± 4.52	$p < 0.01$
Body weight (g)	354.6 ± 13.5	264.8 ± 3.71	329.0 ± 9.3	$p < 0.01$
Brain (g/BW x100)	0.53 ± 0.02	0.69 ± 0.01	0.57 ± 0.01	$p < 0.01$
Heart (g/BW x100)	0.48 ± 0.03	0.53 ± 0.01	0.35 ± 0.01	$p < 0.01$
Kidney (g/BW x100)	0.81 ± 0.07	0.48 ± 0.01	0.32 ± 0.01	$p < 0.01$
Albumin (mg/dl)	3.41 ± 0.08	4.17 ± 0.03	3.72 ± 0.05	$p < 0.05$
BUN (mg/dl)	72.7 ± 14.60	18.3 ± 0.61	18.0 ± 0.29	$p < 0.01$
Creatinine (mg/dl)	2.04 ± 0.48	0.66 ± 0.02	0.64 ± 0.01	$p < 0.05$
t-Cholesterol (mg/dl)	503.7 ± 47.4	68.0 ± 2.6	81.6 ± 1.8	$p < 0.01$
Triglyceride (mg/dl)	371.3 ± 27.8	90.3 ± 6.3	72.4 ± 5.0	$p < 0.01$
Glucose (mg/dl)	125.0 ± 6.1	157.3 ± 4.1	127.2 ± 4.9	$p < 0.01$
Na (mEq/L)	158.3 ± 1.7	162.7 ± 1.7	160.0 ± 2.4	N.S.
K (mEq/L)	5.31 ± 0.23	4.23 ± 0.16	4.36 ± 0.04	$p < 0.01$
Ca (mEq/L)	11.09 ± 0.11	11.00 ± 0.18	10.16 ± 0.12	$p < 0.01$

* Anova one-way analysis of variance

3. Pathological examination

Average life span was about 130 days in males and 160 days in females, respectively. Stroke lesion incidence rate was 40% both in males and in females. Hypertensive vascular changes such as hyaline degeneration and/or angionecrosis were found in the brain, kidneys and heart in these rats, but incidence and degree of these changes were lower than in SHRSP. Marked enlargement of kidney was found in Hyper T-C rats. Histologically, glomerular changes compatible with nephrotic syndrome such as basement membrane thickening and fusion of podocyte processuss were recognized in these kidneys. Hypertensive arterial changes in kidney were less frequent compared to in SHRSP. In some rats, calcification in aortic wall was found, but not in SHRSP.

DISCUSSION

As summarized in Table, Hyper T-C rats have a unique characteristics which had never be seen in other strain. In addition to SHC, which are one of the original parents of Hyper T-C rats, several strains are used as animal models for hypercholesterolemia. Of these, hypercholesterolemia is accompanied by hypertension in the Lyon strain (Sassolas et al., 1981) and obese SHR (Koletsky, 1973), all of the other animals are normotensive. In comparison with Hyper T-C rats, Lyon strain show slightly milder hypertension and hypercholesterolemia and no stroke lesions were observed. Although obese SHR show similar cholesterol levels of about 500mg/dl, blood pressure level is slightly lower than in Hyper T-C rats. No hypertensive vascular changes or cerebral stroke lesions have been observed in this strain. Thant (1970) induced hyperlipemia by feeding SHR a high fat-cholesterol diet and Yamori (1977) has separated arteriopilidosis-prone rat (ALR) which develops real-time/reactive hyperlipidemia and fat deposition in arterial wall after receiving a HFC diet for a short period of time. Both showed hypertension and hyperlipidemia, but they required feeding of HFC diet. Hyper T-C rats show both sever hypertension and hypercholesterolemia without special treatment such as HFC.

Thus, this unique rats strain having both hypertension and hypercholesterolemia are established and characterized. These rats must be a valuable model not only for hypertension and arteriosclerosis but also for renal failure.

REFERENCES

Imai, Y. and Matsumura, H. (1973): Genetic studies on induced and spontaneous hypercholesterolemic rats. Atherosclerosis 18: 59-64.
Koletsky, S. (1973): Obese spontaneously hypertensive rat: a model for study of atherosclerosis. Exp. Mol. Pathol. 19: 53-60.
Okamoto, K., Higashizawa, T., Miyake, H., Ito, H. and Suzuki, T. (1989): Acta Med. Kinki Univ. 14: 211-227.
Okamoto, K,, Yamamoto, K., Morita, N. and Ohta, Y. (1985): Establishment and characteristics of rat with precocious and severe hypertension (M-SHRSP). Acta Med. Kinki Univ. 10: 73-95.
Sassolas, A., Vincent, M., Benzoni, D. and Sassad, J. (1981): Plasma lipid in genetically hypertensive rats of Lyon strain. J. Cardiovasc. Pharmacol. 3: 1008-1014.
Thant, M. (1970): Arteriosclerosis in spontaneously hypertensive rats on high fat diet. Jpn. Heart J. 34: 83-107.
Yamori, Y. (1977): Selection of arteriolipidosis-prone rats (ALR). Jpn. Heart J. 18: 602.

Nephropathy in the diabetic SHR: the effects of perindopril and triple therapy

Mark E. Cooper, Jon R. Rumble, Richard C. O'Brien, Terri J. Allen, George Jerums and Austin E. Doyle

Department of Medicine, Austin and Repatriation General Hospitals, University of Melbourne, 3084 Heidelberg, Australia

Abstract
The angiotensin converting enzyme inhibitor, perindopril and a conventional antihypertensive regimen [triple therapy: hydralazine, reserpine and hydrochlorothiazide] have been compared with respect to their effect on kidney function and albuminuria in hypertensive diabetic rats. Diabetes was induced with streptozotocin in spontaneously hypertensive rats (SHR) and they were randomised to receive no treatment, perindopril or triple therapy. There was a similar hypotensive effect with both drug regimens. Diabetes was associated with an increase in glomerular filtration rate but there was no difference among the three groups. Both drug regimens reduced albuminuria in the diabetic rats to a similar degree, apparently independently of their effects on the renin angiotensin system.

Introduction
Certain classes of antihypertensive agents have been reported to confer a specific benefit in retarding the progression of renal disorders such as diabetic nephropathy (Tolins & Raij, 1990). Previous studies by our group have suggested that hypertension is an important accelerator of both functional and structural features of diabetic nephropathy, the most sensitive marker of these changes being the dramatic increase in urinary albumin excretion observed in diabetic hypertensive rats (Cooper et al, 1988). The present study compares the effects of the ACE inhibitor, perindopril to triple therapy [hydralazine, reserpine and hydrochlorothiazide] on renal function and albuminuria over a 24 week period in diabetic SHR.

Research Design and Methods
Male spontaneously hypertensive rats [SHR, Okamoto strain] weighing between 200-250 grams, aged 8 weeks, were injected with streptozotocin intravenously (45mg/kg) after an overnight fast. Diabetic SHR receiving 2 units of Ultralente insulin per day, were randomised to receive either no treatment, perindopril (6mg/l in drinking water) or triple therapy [hydralazine 50mg/l, reserpine 4mg/l and hydrochlorothiazide 30mg/l all administered in drinking water]. Measurements of body weight, systolic blood pressure [indirect tail cuff plethysmography in conscious rats] and plasma glucose were performed at 4 weekly intervals. Plasma renin activity was measured by radioimmunoassay in diabetic SHR at 0, 1 and 16 weeks of diabetes. Plasma ACE activity was measured by a fluorometric technique in a subgroup of animals at week 1 (Jackson et al, 1986). Glomerular filtration rate (GFR) was measured by a single injection technique developed in our laboratory at 0, 4 and 12 weeks (Allen et al, 1990). Urinary albumin excretion was measured by radioimmunoassay at weeks 0, 8, 12, 16 and 24 (Cooper et al, 1988) and analysed after logarithmic transformation. Comparisons of normally distributed variables among the different groups over the study period were performed by analysis of variance using the Statview SE and Graphics Programme (Brainpower, Calabasas, California).

Results
Systolic blood pressure on treatment was significantly reduced in the perindopril (P) and triple therapy (TT) groups when compared to untreated (U) diabetic SHR [U 209±2, TT 145±1 and P 146±1

mmHg, p < 0.001]. There was no significant difference in blood pressure between the P and TT groups. There was no significant difference in serum glucose among the three groups [mean serum glucose on treatment; U 31.6±1.3, TT 31.2±1.3 and P 30.7±1.8 mM]. There was a modest reduction in body weight at week 24 in the P treated group (body weight, U 312±8, TT 323±7 and P 284±8g, p<0.05 P vs other groups).

After one week of diabetes there was a significant rise in plasma renin activity (PRA) in both the P and TT treated groups (Table 1). The increases in PRA in TT and P treated groups persisted over the study period. Plasma ACE activity was significantly reduced in the perindopril treated rats [U, 59 ± 7, n=8; TT, 49 ± 5, n=10; P, 25 ± 4 nmol histidyl-leucine/ml/min, n=13; p<0.01 versus other groups]. There was no significant difference in GFR among the three groups at week 0 or after induction of diabetes (Table 1). Induction of diabetes was associated with a significant increase in GFR in all groups. Both drug therapies reduced urinary albumin excretion when compared to untreated rats (Figure). There was no significant difference in albuminuria between P and TT treated rats.

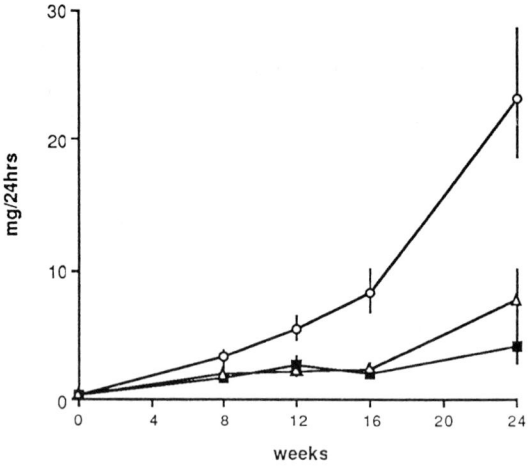

Geometric mean and tolerance factors shown for U (open circles), TT (open triangles) and P (closed squares).

Table 1 (Mean ± SEM are shown)

group	Plasma Renin Activity (ng/ml/hr)			GFR (ml/min)		
	week 0	week 1	week 16	week 0	week 4	week 12
U	7.5 ± 1.0	7.8 ± 1.2	8.0 ± 1.5	2.2 ± 0.1	2.7 ± 0.1†	2.9 ± 0.1†
TT	6.0 ± 0.8	19.1 ± 2.3*	20.2 ± 2.6**	2.2 ± 0.1	2.6 ± 0.1†	2.7 ± 0.1†
P	7.8 ± 1.0	21.5 ± 3.7*	18.3 ± 5.3*	2.2 ± 0.1	2.8 ± 0.1†	3.2 ± 0.2†

*p<0.05, **p<0.01 versus U; †p<0.01 versus week 0

Discussion

The present study extends findings observed in an initial project in which the combination of hydralazine and metoprolol was compared with the ACE inhibitor enalapril in diabetic SHR (Cooper et al, 1990). These two drug regimens were similar in effect on urinary albumin excretion and also reduced glomerular basement membrane thickness and glomerular volume. However, since metoprolol is a beta blocker which may itself suppress the renin angiotensin system (Antonaccio et al, 1986) it was difficult to determine from that study if the effects of the two treatments were related to their hypotensive action or to their action in suppressing the renin angiotensin system. The results of the present study indicate that the similarity in effect of triple therapy and the ACE inhibitor perindopril on albuminuria may be due to their actions as antihypertensive agents rather than via effects on the renin angiotensin system. Triple therapy stimulated the renin angiotensin system as detected by the rise in plasma renin activity. In contrast, perindopril acted to suppress the renin angiotensin system presumably by reducing angiotensin II levels through inhibition of the enzyme ACE. The rise in plasma renin activity with ACE inhibitor therapy probably represents a loss of feedback inhibition of angiotensin II on renin synthesis and secretion by juxtaglomerular cells.

Previous studies in this area have included comparisons between ACE inhibitors and other antihypertensive agents in various models of renal disease. In studies performed in normotensive streptozotocin diabetic Munich Wistar rats captopril was more effective than triple therapy in retarding the development of albuminuria and focal glomerulosclerosis over a 70 week study period (Anderson et al, 1989). The advantage of captopril over triple therapy was attributed to the ability of captopril to normalise the elevated glomerular capillary pressure in diabetic rats. A recent study by our own group comparing the ACE inhibitor, perindopril to triple therapy in diabetic Sprague-Dawley rats suggested a similar efficacy of both treatments with respect to preventing diabetes-associated increases in urinary albumin excretion (O'Brien et al, 1990). The differences between the two studies may relate to differences in rat strain since it has been previously shown that the Munich Wistar rat may be more susceptible to focal segmental glomerulosclerosis with ageing (Grond et al, 1986). It is therefore possible that some of the renoprotective effects of ACE inhibition may relate to glomerular injury unrelated to diabetes. Recent studies to determine if ACE inhibitors have a specific effect independent of their hypotensive action were performed by the administration of ramipril to uninephrectomised diabetic SHR in the setting of a normal and high salt intake (Fabris et al, 1991). Rats which received high salt intake and ramipril had no reduction in blood pressure and no effect on urinary albumin excretion, despite demonstrable ACE inhibition in the plasma and the kidney. In contrast, in animals with normal salt intake and ramipril therapy, blood pressure was decreased as was urinary albumin excretion. These findings suggest that in diabetic SHR the predominant effect of ACE inhibitors in reducing albuminuria is via their action as antihypertensive agents.

The mechanism by which antihypertensive agents ameliorate glomerular damage remains controversial. It has been suggested that glomerular hypertrophy *per se* may be an important determinant of progression of renal injury (Yoshida et al, 1989). In addition, glomerular hyperfiltration may itself be an important pathway for renal damage (Anderson et al, 1989). These two mechanisms could be relevant in diabetes in which there is evidence of both glomerular hypertrophy and increases in intraglomerular pressure and glomerular filtration rate.

At this stage, one must be cautious in applying the results of experimental studies to man. Furthermore, it should be noted that the present studies were performed in hypertensive animals and has recently extended to the role of antihypertensive agents in the normotensive situation. At present, many trials are in progress to determine the role of antihypertensive agents in both the normotensive and hypertensive context in patients with early and advanced diabetic renal disease. It should be noted that the findings observed in rodents, although not directly applicable to man, are very helpful in the initial evaluation of potential mechanisms and therapies for human diabetic renal disease.

Acknowledgements

These studies were supported by grants from the NH&MRC of Australia and Servier Laboratories.

References

Allen, T.J., Cooper, M.E., O'Brien, R.C., Bach, L.A., Jackson, B., Jerums, G.(1990): Glomerular filtration rate in the streptozocin diabetic rat: The role of exchangeable sodium, vasoactive hormones and insulin therapy. *Diabetes* 38; 1182-1190.
Anderson, S., Rennke, H.G., Garcia, D.L., Brenner, B.M.(1989): Short and long term effects of antihypertensive therapy in the diabetic rat. *Kidney Inter* 36; 526-536.
Antonaccio, M.J., High, J., DeForrest, J.M. and Sybertz, E.(1986): Antihypertensive effects of 12 beta adrenoreceptor antagonists in conscious spontaneously hypertensive rats: Relationship to changes in plasma renin activity, heart rate and sympathetic nerve function. *J Pharmacol Exp Ther* 238; 378-387.
Cooper, M.E., Allen, T.J., Macmillan, P., Clarke, B., O'Brien, R.C., Jerums, G., Doyle, A.E.(1988): Effects of genetic hypertension on diabetic nephropathy in the rat - Functional and structural characteristics. *J Hypertens* 6; 1009-1016.
Cooper, M.E., Allen, T.J., O'Brien, R.C., Papazoglou, D., Clarke, B., Jerums, G. and Doyle, A.E.(1990): Nephropathy in a Model Combining Genetic Hypertension with Experimental Diabetes: Enalapril versus Hydralazine and Metoprolol Therapy. *Diabetes* 39; 1575-79.
Fabris, B., Jackson, B. and Johnston, C.I.(1991): Salt blocks the renal benefits of ramipril in diabetic hypertensive rats. *Hypertension* 17; 497-503.
Grond, J., Beukers, J.Y.B., Schilthyis, M.S., Weening, J.J. and Elema, J.D.(1986): Analysis of renal structural and functional features in two rat strains with a different susceptibility to glomerular sclerosis. *Lab Invest* 54; 77-83.
Jackson, B., Cubela, R., Johnston, C.(1986): Angiotensin converting enzyme (ACE), characterization by 125I-MK351A binding studies of plasma and tissue ACE during variation of salt status in the rat. *J Hypertens* 4; 759-765.
O'Brien, R.C., Papozoglou, D., Allen, T. and Jerums, G.(1990): The effects of perindopril versus triple therapy on albuminuria in normotensive diabetic rats. *Kidney Inter* 38; 552-553, (Abstract).
Tolins, J.P. and Raij, L.(1990): Angiotensin converting enzyme inhibitors and progression of chronic renal failure. *Kidney Inter* 38 (Suppl 30): S118-S122.
Yoshida, Y., Fogo, A., Ichikawa, I.(1989): Glomerular hemodynamic changes vs. hypertrophy in experimental glomerular sclerosis. *Kidney Inter* 36; 654-660.

Hyperinsulinemia and decreased muscle deoxyglucose uptake in SHR but not in secondary hypertension

Michael Bursztyn, Drori Ben-Ishay and Alisa Gutman *

*Hypertension Unit, Department of Medicine, Hadassah University Hospital, Mount Scopus, P.O. Box 24035, Jerusalem 91240 and * Departement of Biochemistry, Hebrew University-Hadassah School of Medicine, Ein Karem, Jerusalem, Israel*

Epidemiologic and clinical research has recently intimated a link between essential hypertension and resistance to peripheral actions of insulin (DeFronzo and Ferannini, 1991). In SHR, the commonly utilized experimental counterpart of essential hypertenion, there is also increasing evidence of insulin resistance (Mondon and Reaven, 1988). There are numerous speculations as to how insulin resistance may relate to hypertension and, according to some of these, insulin might cause hypertension. Nevertheless, hypertension with its accompanying altered hemodynamics, microvascular rarefication, cell membrane alterations, increased cellular calcium and other hypertension-induced abnormalities may potentially affect sensitivity to insulin.

In an attempt to examine the possibility that hypertension may cause insulin resistance, we studied in vivo the muscle uptakes of [3H]-2-deoxyglucose (DOG) (Hom et al., 1981; Ferre et al., 1985; Kalderon et al., 1986) an undegradable glucose analogue and in vitro the epididymal uptake of [14C]-glucose in response to insulin (Kalderon et al., 1983; 1986) in SHR and WKY rats and in renovascular (RVH) and DOCA-salt (DOC) hypertensive rats and their respective normotensive controls (RVN and DCN).

METHODS

Male RVH and DOC rats were prepared by standard methods and were studied in the fasted state. Experiments were performed three weeks after induction of hypertension in DOC and RVH and their respective controls and at the age of eight weeks in male SHR and WKY rats. Blood pressure was recorded by the cuff tail method (Ueda Electronic Works, Osaka, Japan). Rats were briefly anaesthetized with ether and a tracer dose of [3H]-DOG, 2uCi/100 g body weight, was administered I.V. by the dorsal penile vein. Rats were awake within one to two minutes and tail blood was obtained for determination of plasma radioactivity at 2, 5 and 15 minutes. At 30 minutes rats were decapitated and blood was collected also for glucose and insulin levels, assayed by the glucose oxidase method and radioimmunoassay, respectively. Samples of heart, gastrocnemius muscle and spleen (as a non-insulin sensitive control) were frozen in liquid NO2. Epididymal fat pads were excised and immediately studied in vitro. In vivo uptake of DOG was determined as previously described (Hom et al. 1984, Kalderon et al. 1986) with minor modifications. A portion of frozen tissue was rapidly weighed, homogenized and boiled for two minutes in 2 ml of distilled water and centrifuged. The total [3H]-DOG radioactivity was determined in the supernatant. Separation of [3H]-DOG from [3H]-DOG phosphate was done as described by Ferre et al. (1985). Calculations of tissue incorporated label were corrected for vatiations in extrapolated radioactivity (from a logarithmic disappearance curve) at time zero.

In vitro uptake of 14C-glucose were performed on epididymal fat pad fragments incubated for two hours in a shaking bath at 37'C in 2 ml Krebs-Ringer bicarbonate buffer (pH 7.4) containing 1% bovine serum albumin and 14C-glucose (5.5 umole/ml, 0.02 uCi/umole) and 0, 10, 25 and 250 uU/ml of insulin. The medium was then acidified and CO_2 was collected on filter paper impregnated with hyamine hydroxide. Incorporation of 14C-glucose into triglycerides and glycogen was determined as previously described (Kalderon et al., 1983; 1986). Total uptake was calculated as the sum of incorporation into CO_2, triglycerides and glycogen.

Results are expressed as mean $\pm$ SE. The mean values of the hypertensive rats and their controls are compared by Student's t test for parametric, and the Mann-Whitney test for non-parametric values, respectively. P levels <0.05 are considered significant.

RESULTS

The blood pressure in RVH, DOC and SHR was 176 ± 2, 195 ± 5 and 181 ± 3 mmHg, respectively, significantly higher than that of RVN, DCN and WKY, 137 ± 4, 134 ± 2 and 135 ± 3 mmHg, respectively ($p<0.001$). Insulin levels were higher in SHR, 83.6 ± 8.4 vs. 51.5 ± 4.8 uU/ml in WKY, ($p<0.05$), and DOG plasma half life longer, 56 ± 13 minutes in SHR versus 27 ± 2 minutes in WKY ($p<0.05$). There were no such differences between RVH and RVN or DOC and DCN rats.

DOG uptake is shown in Table 1 and was significantly lower in heart and skeletal muscle of SHR compared with WKY.

Table 1

	No.	Spleen	[3H]-DOG cpm/g/1000 Heart	Muscle
SHR	8	1.1 ± 0.1	9.9 ± 1.5*	0.3 ± 0.03*
WKY	8	1.1 ± 0.1	17.1 ± 1.1	0.8 ± 0.2
DOC	14	0.4 ± 0.1	4.1 ± 1.4	0.4 ± 0.1
DCN	11	0.4 ± 0.1	3.8 ± 0.9	0.2 ± 0.1
RVH	12	2.3 ± 1.4	8.8 ± 1.5	0.5 ± 0.1
RVN	12	0.9 ± 0.3	8.9 ± 0.3	0.6 ± 0.2

* $p<0.02$

There were no significant differences in insulin stimulated 14C-glucose uptake by epididymal fat pad between any of the hypertensive rats and their respective controls (Figure 1). The incorporation of 14C-glucose into CO_2, triglyceride or glycogen was also not different between hypertensive and normotensive rats.

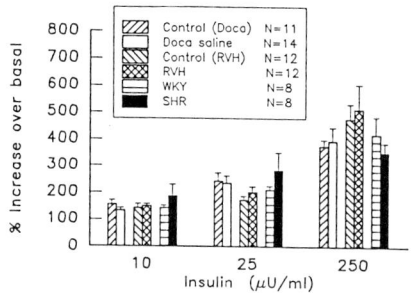

Figure 1: Insulin stimulated 14C–glucose uptake by epididymal fat pad of rats with primary and secondary hypertension.

DISCUSSION

The decreased DOG uptake by heart and skeletal muscles in SHR in the face of higher insulin and decreased DOG clearance strongly suggests insulin resistance relative to WKY and confirms the previous work of Mondon and Reaven (1988). However, we did not find evidence of resistance to insulin action in fat tissue. If, indeed, insulin resistance is confined to skeletal muscle, as our results suggest, then the resultant hyperinsulinemia in insulin sensitive tissues may activate the sympathetic nervous system, increase renal tubular sodium reabsorption or promote vascular hypertrophy, as recently reviewed (DeFronzo and Ferannini, 1991). The absence of any differences in either our *in vivo* or *in vitro* studies between either RVH or DOC and their normotensive controls suggests to us that insulin resistance is a primary and not a secondary phenomenon in hypertension.

REFERENCES

DeFronzo, R.A., and Ferannini, E. (1991): Insulin resistance, a multifaceted syndrome responsible for NIDDM, obesity, hypertension, dislipidemia and atherosclerotic cardiovascular disease. Diabetes Care 14, 173–194.

Ferre, P., Leturane, A., Burnol, A.F., Peincaud, L., and Girard, J. (1985): A method to quantify glucose utilization in vivo in skeletal muscle and white adipose tissue of the anaesthetized rat. Biochem. J. 228, 103–110.

Hom, F.G., Goodner, C.J., and Berrie, M.A. (1984): A [3H]–2–deoxyglucose method for comparing rates of glucose metabolism and insulin response among rat tissues in vivo: Validation of the model and the absence of an insulin effect on brain. Diabetes 33, 141–151.

Kalderon, B., Adler, J.H., Levy, E., and Gutman, A. (1983): Lipogenesis in the sand rat (psammomys obesus) Am. J. Physiol. 244, E480–E486.

Kalderon, B., Gutman, A., Levy, E., Shafrir, E., and Adler, J.H. (1986): Characterization of stages in the development of obesity. Diabetes syndrome in sand rat (psammomys obesus). Diabetes 35, 717–724.

Mondon, C.E., and Reaven, G.M. (1988): Evidence of abnormalities of insulin metabolism in rats with spontaneous hypertension. Metabolism 37, 303–305.

Effect of acute NaCl depletion on NaCl sensitive hypertension in borderline hypertensive rats

Gerald F. DiBona and Susan Y. Jones

Department of Internal Medicine, University of Iowa College of Medicine and Veterans Administration Medical Center, Iowa City, Iowa 52242, USA

INTRODUCTION

The borderline hypertensive rat (BHR) is the F_1 generation of a cross between a spontaneously hypertensive rats (SHR) and a normotensive Wistar-Kyoto (WKY) rat. Increased dietary NaCl intake (8 vs 1 % NaCl) produces hypertension in BHR and enhanced cardiovascular, renal sympathetic and functional responses to acute stress (DiBona & Jones, 1991a). We examined the effect of acute reduction in extracellular fluid (ECF) volume on arterial pressure and the cardiovascular, renal sympathetic and functional responses to acute stress in BHR fed 8 % NaCl.

METHODS

BHR were F_1 of crosses between female SHR and male WKY. They were weaned at 4 wks and randomly assigned to one of two groups, 1 or 8 % NaCl diet, from 4 to 16 weeks. They were anesthetized with methohexital and instrumented for measurement of mean arterial pressure (MAP), heart rate (HR) and efferent renal sympathetic nerve activity (ERSNA) and for inulin administration, blood sampling and collection of bladder urine. ECF volume was determined using inulin (Gaudino et al., 1948).

Study 1. ECF was determined in three groups of conscious BHR (N = 6 each): 1 % NaCl diet BHR, 8 % NaCl diet BHR and 8 % NaCl diet BHR that had received furosemide (F) 50 mg/kg bid i.p. for two days. Basal MAP, HR and urinary sodium excretion ($U_{Na}V$, μmol/min/gKW, gKW = gram kidney weight) were also determined.

Study 2. Responses to acute environmental stress (Koepke & DiBona, 1985) were determined in the three groups of conscious BHR. Consecutive 10 minute urine collection periods were made: two control periods preceded two acute environmental stress (air jet to head) periods which were followed by two recovery periods.

Urine volume was determined gravimetrically. Urine sodium concentration was measured by flame photometry. Urine and plasma inulin concentrations were determined by anthrone method (Fuhr et al., 1955). Statistical analyses were conducted with repeated measures analysis of variance (ANOVA) and post-hoc comparisons were done using the Newman-Keuls test (Wallenstein et al., 1980).

RESULTS

Study 1 (Table 1) Compared to 1 % NaCl BHR, 8 % NaCl BHR had increased body weight (BW), ECF, MAP and $U_{Na}V$ ($p < 0.05$). Furosemide administration restored ECF, MAP and $U_{Na}V$ to values not different from those in 1 % NaCl BHR.

Table 1

	1 % NaCl BHR	8 % NaCl BHR	8 % NaCl BHR-F
N	6	6	6
Body weight, gm	458 ± 9	433 ± 10	365 ± 15†
ECF, % BW	27.8 ± 1.8	35.1 ± 3.9*	26.4 ± 1.9
MAP, mm Hg	126 ± 4	148 ± 4*	121 ± 5
HR, bpm	405 ± 10	419 ± 15	423 ± 13
$U_{Na}V$, μmol/min/gKW	0.4 ± 0.1	1.6 ± 0.6*	0.2 ± 0.6

† $p < 0.05$ vs 1 % NaCl BHR and 8 % NaCl BHR; * $p < 0.05$ vs 1 % NaCl BHR and 8 % NaCl BHR-F.

Study 2 (Figure 1) Responses to air jet stress are absolute changes from the control period values (similar to the those in Table 1). Compared to 1 % NaCl BHR, 8 % NaCl BHR had greater ($p < 0.05$) pressor, tachycardiac, renal sympathoexcitatory and antinatriuretic responses to air jet stress. Furosemide administration decreased BW by 55 ± 3 gm (13.0 ± 6 %) from 424 ± 15 to 369 ± 14 gm in 8 % NaCl BHR-F. The pressor, tachycardic, renal sympathoexcitatory and antinatriuretic responses to air jet stress returned to values not different from those in 1 % NaCl BHR.

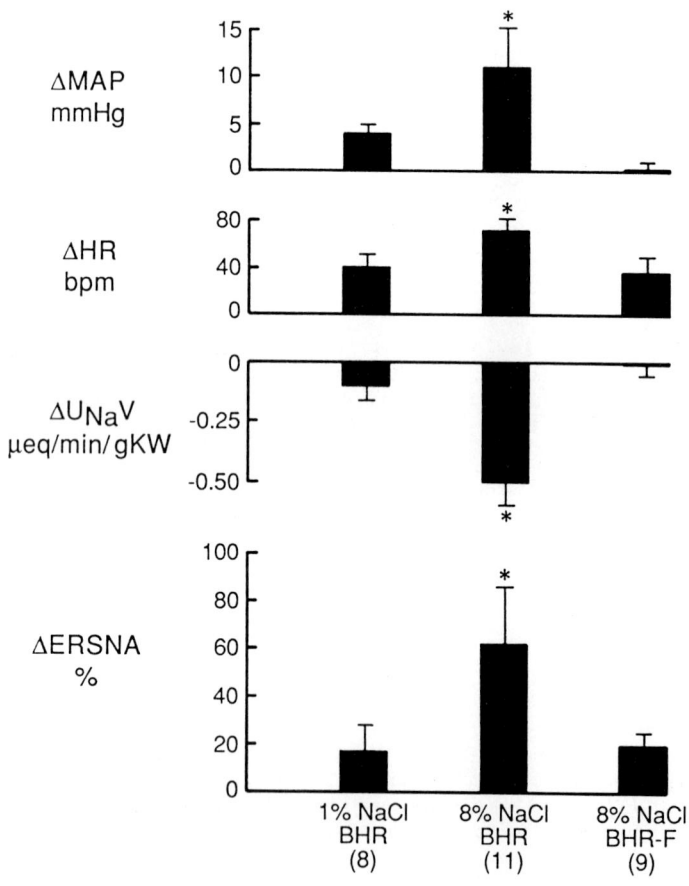

Figure 1. Responses to acute environmental stress. ( ) = number of rats, * $p < 0.05$ vs both 1 % NaCl BHR and 8 % NaCl BHR-F.

DISCUSSION

These studies demonstrate that acute NaCl depletion with reduction of ECF volume normalizes MAP and the pressor, tachycardic, renal sympathoexcitatory and antinatriuretic responses to acute stress in 8 % NaCl BHR.

Since NaCl induced hypertension in BHR persists after dietary NaCl intake is returned to normal (DiBona & Jones, 1991a), we explored the dependency of the hypertension and the augmented cardiovascular and renal responses to acute stress on the NaCl induced changes in ECF. Twelve wks of 8 % NaCl diet caused a significant increase in ECF which was reversed by furosemide administration. Normalization of ECF also returned the increased MAP and $U_{Na}V$ seen in 8 % NaCl BHR to the values observed in 1 % NaCl BHR. The augmented pressor, tachycardic, renal sympathoexcitatory and antinatriuretic responses to acute stress of 8 % NaCl BHR (compared to 1 % NaCl BHR) were also returned to levels observed in 1 % NaCl BHR when ECF was restored to normal with furosemide administration.

These results indicate that increased dietary NaCl intake, via a mechanism related to ECF volume and/or sodium, increases MAP and results in augmented cardiovascular and renal responses to acute environmental stress in BHR. Responses to acute environmental stress in SHR are abolished by administration of α-2 adrenoceptor agonists into the lateral cerebral ventricle (Koepke & DiBona, 1986) or the central amygdaloid nucleus (Koepke et al., 1987). Increased dietary NaCl intake increases the responsiveness of central nervous system α-2 adrenoceptors regulating ERSNA in both SHR (Koepke et al., 1988) and BHR (DiBona & Jones, 1991b). It is suggested that the alterations occurring in BHR consuming an increased dietary NaCl intake derive from a central nervous system effect via a mechanism(s) related to ECF volume and/or sodium.

ACKNOWLEDGEMENTS

This work was supported by National Institutes of Health grants DK 15843, HL 35163, HL 40222, HL 14388, HL 44546 and by grants from the American Heart Association-Iowa Affiliate and the Veterans Administration.

REFERENCES

DiBona, G.F. & Jones, S.Y. (1991a): Renal manifestations of NaCl sensitivity of borderline hypertensive rats. Hypertension 17, 44-53.

DiBona, G.F. & Jones, S.Y.(1991b): Central α-2 adrenoceptor responsiveness in borderline hypertensive rats. J. Hypertension 9, 543-547.

Fuhr, J., Kaczmarcyk, J. & Kruttgen, C.D. (1855): Eine einfache colorimetrische Methode zur Inulinbestimmung für Nierenclearanceuntersuchungen bei Stoffwechselgesunden und Diabetikern. Klin. Wochenschr. 33, 729-730.

Gaudino, M., Schwartz, I.L. & Levitt, M. (1948): Inulin volume of distribution as measure of extracellular fluid in dog and man. Proc. Soc. Exper. Biol. Med. 68, 507-509.

Koepke, J.P. & DiBona, G.F. (1985): High sodium intake enhances renal nerve and antinatriuretic responses to stress in conscious SHR. Hypertension 7, 357-363.

Koepke, J.P. & DiBona, G.F.(1986): Central adrenoceptor control of renal function in conscious hypertensive rats. Hypertension 8, 133-141.

Koepke, J.P., Jones, S. & DiBona, G.F.(1987): Alpha-2 adrenoceptors in amygdala control renal sympathetic nerve activity in conscious spontaneously hypertensive rats. Brain Res. 404, 80-88.

Koepke, J.P., Jones, S. & DiBona, G.F. (1988): Sodium responsiveness of central α-2 adrenoceptors in spontaneously hypertensive rats. Hypertension 11, 326-333.

Wallenstein, S., Zucker, C.L. & Fleiss, J.L. (1980): Some statistical methods useful in circulation research. Circ. Res. 47, 1-9.

The effect of certain anthypertensive drugs at several dose levels on hypertensive vascular lesions in M-SHRSP and SHRSP

Yoshio Ohta, Taka-Aki Chikugo and Kozo Okamoto

Department of Pathology, Kinki University School of Medicine, 377-2, Ohno-Higashi, Osaka-Sayama, Osaka 589, Japan

Introduction: Using M-SHRSP and SHRSP, animals which appear to be useful as models for studying human malignant hypertension, we have previously studied the histopathological effects of several antihypertensive drugs on the brains, the kidneys, and certain other organs (Okamoto et al., 1974, 1985, 1986). In this experiment, we examined the relationships among, and the antihypertensive effects of, different dosages of various antihypertensive drugs, as well as studied their healing effects in relationship to angionecrosis on the established, hypertensive vascular lesions found in these various organs.

Materials and methods: 11-week-old male M-SHRSP and 23-week-old male SHRSP were used. Angiotensin converting enzyme inhibitors (captopril or SQ 29,852) (Bristol-Myers Squibb, K. K. Tokyo), calcium antagonists (manidipine hydrochloride) (Takeda Chemical Industries, Ltd., Osaka) and AE0047 (Green Cross, Corp., Osaka) or a vascular smooth muscle relaxant (hydralazine hydrochloride) (CIBA-GEIGY Co., Ltd. Japan) were administered to various subgroups of M-SHRSP and SHRSP. SQ 29,852 or manidipine was administered orally in doses of 2, 5, 10, 20, 40, 60 or 80 mg/kg/day (mixed in Funabashi SP) to fourteen separate M-SHRSP subgroups. AE0047 was administered orally in doses of 10, 20, 40 mg/kg/day (mixed in Funabashi SP) to three additional M-SHRSP subgroups. Other subgroups of M-SHRSP were given combinations of SQ 29,852 and manidipine (20 or 40 mg/kg/day, each), AE0047 and SQ 29,852 (20 mg/kg/day, each) and AE0047 and manidipine (20 mg/kg/day, each), while others were given oral captopril, 40 mg/kg/day, (mixed in Funabashi SP) or hydralazine in drinking water (approximate dosage 15 mg/kg/day, or 80 mg/l). Further, SQ 29,852 (10, 40 or 80 mg/kg/day) or manidipine (20, 40 or 80 mg/kg/day) were administered to subgroups of SHRSP. M-SHRSP and SHRSP control subgroups were also maintained. Before and during treatment, body weights were measured daily and blood pressures (using the tail pulse pickup method without anesthesia) were measured every second day. All of the animals were autopsied and pathologically examined after sacrifice on the 1st to 10th, 15th, 20th, 30th days following the start of the experiment.

Results and discussion: Body weights gradually increased following treatment in all but the 2, 5, 80 mg/kg/day manidipine, the 40 mg/kg/day AE0047, and the AE0047 and manidipine combined subgroups. M-SHRSP given 2, 5, 10, 20 mg/kg/day SQ 29,852 separately showed only weak antihypertensive effects with blood pressures remaining over 250 mmHg. Angionecrosis was invariably observed in the kidneys and often found in the brain, heart and testes of the control 11-week-old M-SHRSP and/or 23-week-old SHRSP. Angionecrosis was recognized in the kidneys following administration of SQ 29,852 at 2 or 5 mg/kg/day for at least the first 30 days. However, with treatment levels at 10 or 20 mg/kg/day the angionecrosis disappeared within 20 days. Angionecrosis disappeared within 10, 10 or 4 days, respectively, in M-SHRSP given SQ 29,852 at 40, 60 or 80 mg/kg/day and all of these subgroups evidenced a moderate antihypertensive effect (blood pressures stayed above 210 mmHg). On the other hand, the separately treated manidipine subgroups, given doses of 2, 5 or 10 mg/kg/day showed only weak antihypertensive effects with blood pressures remaining high at over 250 mmHg and, although a weak healing effect of angionecrosis was found in 10 mg/kg/day group, with angionecrosis continuing to be recognized in all instances. For M-SHRSP given manidipine at a rate of 20 mg/kg/day, blood pressures dropped to around 200 mmHg and angionecrosis disappeared within 7 days. With manidipine treatment at 40 or 80 mg/kg/day, blood pressures lowered remarkably to around 170 mmHg and angionecrosis disappeared within 10 or 5 days, respectively. The blood pressures of subgroups treated with AE0047 only, in doses of 10, 20 or 40 mg/kg/day, dropped to around 180, 170 or 160 mmHg and angionecrosis disappeared within 11, 3 or 4 days, respectively. For combined SQ 29,852 and manidipine treatment at 20 or 40 mg/kg/day, blood pressures lowered to around 230 or 170 mmHg and angionecrosis disappeared within 5 or 2 days, respectively. For combined SQ 29,852 and AE0047, or AE0047 and manidipine at 20 mg/kg/day, blood pressures lowered to around 140 or 170 mmHg, respectively, and the disappearance of angionecrosis was recognized at least within 5 days. Blood pressures for the captopril treatment group remained around 250 mmHg, and angionecrosis disappeared within 18 days. Blood pressures for the hydralazine treatment group decreased slightly to around 240 mmHg, but angionecrosis did not disappear in all cases. For SHRSP given SQ 29,852 at 40 or 80 mg/kg/day, blood pressures lowered to around 240 or 230 mmHg and angionecrosis disappeared within 31 or 20 days, respectively. On the other hand, SHRSP given manidipine at 40 or 80 mg/kg/day evidenced marked antihypertensive effects with blood pressures decreased to around 180 or 160 mmHg, and angionecrosis disappearing within 30 or 10 days, respectively. The time course for disappearance of kidney and other organ angionecrosis was longer for SHRSP than for M-SHRSP. In this experiment, angionecrosis in the various organs was found only in the small arteries and/or arterioles, no angionecrosis was detected in the larger arteries. Furthermore, o the organs examined, the disappearance of angionecrosis in the kidneys seemed to be slowest. Some of the data (kidney angionecrosis over time) is summarized in Fig. 1. Angionecrosis is known to be one of the most important factors behind hypertensive vascular lesions and without appropriate treatment, rats with developed angionecrosis die rather quickly. However, we have previously shown that angionecrosis observed in various organs before treatment will disappear within a relative short time following administration of angiotensin converting enzyme inhibitors and life spans were greatly prolonged (Ohta et al., 1989, Okamoto et al., 1990, 1991). Okamoto et al. administered antihypertensive drugs to SHR and SHRSP, and noted no cerebrovascular lesions in treated rats wherein blood pressures were kept under 210 mmHg (Okamoto et al, 1975). On the other hand, Yamamot reported that a high incidence of angionecrosis was found in brain, kidney and other organs after blood pressures surpassed 220 mmHg (Yamamoto, 1989). However, our results with appropriate treatments did not agree with previous reports with regard to un-treated rats. Our results point to the following; 1) It it possible to heal hypertensive vascular lesions (angionecrosis) using SQ 29,852, captopril, manidipine or AE0047. 2) Their efficaciousness seems to be proportional to increases in dosage; furthermore, various combinations of these drugs may be more potent than that each of them separately. 3) Their effect upon SHRSP seems to be weaker than that upon M-SHRSP. 4) Under optimum doses of angiotensin converting enzyme inhibitors, favorable changes result in spite of continued high blood pressures. Finally, these results seems to indicate that the degree of antihypertensive effect does not correlate consistently with the disappearance of angionecrosis.

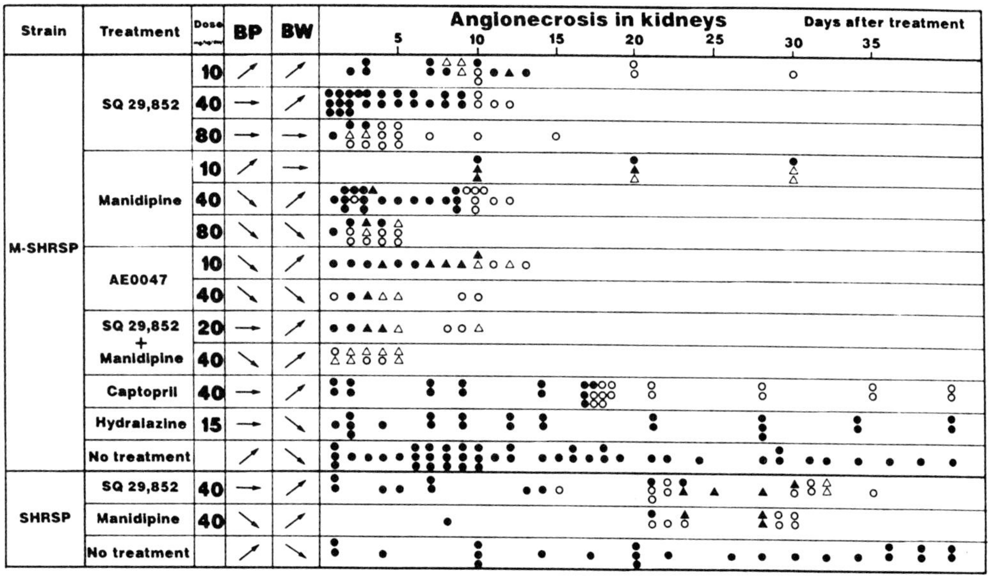

Figure 1. Angionecrosis time reference following treatment
BP: Blood pressure, ↗: BP>250 mmHg, →: 250>BP>210 mmHg, ↘: BP<210 at 10th day following treatment for M-SHRSP and at 30th day for SHRSP.
BW: Body weight, ↗: BW>110%, →: 110%>BW>100%, ↘: BW<100% at 10th day following treatment for M-SHRSP and at 30th day for SHRSP. (%: treated body weight/body weight just prior to treatment×100)
●: Angionecrosis was significant, ▲: Small Angionecrosis was found, △: Obscure angionecrosis was detected, ○: Angionecrosis was not detected

REFERENCES

Ohta, Y. et al., (1989): The therapeutic effects of several antihypertensive drugs and diet on M-SHRSP---Changes in life span, blood pressures, plasma hormones, fundus oculi and internal organs. Jpn Heart J. 30, 543-545.
Okamoto, K. et al., (1974): Establishment of the stroke-prone spontaneously hyper tensive rats (SHR). Circ Res. 34,35 (suppl), 143-153.
Okamoto, K. et al., (1975): Pathogenesis and prevention of stroke in spontaneously hypertensive rats. Science and Molecular Medicine. 48, 161s-163s.
Okamoto, K. et al., (1985): Establishment and characteristics of rat with preco cious and severe hypertension (M-SHRSP). Acta Med Kinki Univ. 10, 73-95.
Okamoto, K. et al., (1986): Establishment and use of the M strain of stroke-prone spontaneously hypertensive rat. J Hypertension. 4, 21-24.
Okamoto, K. et al., (1990): Therapy and prevention of hypertension of M-SHRSP. Clinical Experimental Hypertension. in press.
Okamoto, K. et al., (1991): Chronic treatment with captopril, SQ 29,852, hydra lazine and a 33% fish meal diet in M-SHRSP - malignant hypertensive rats. J Hypertension, accepted
Yamamoto, K. (1989): Characteristics of malignant hypertensive SHRSP (M-SHRSP) and normotensive WKY crossbred offspring (1): Establishment of 8 strains and their blood pressures and hypertensive vascular lesions incidence rates. Acta Med Kinki Univ. 14, 117-128.

Taurine improves cholesterol metabolism in stroke-prone spontaneously hypertensive rats (SHRSP) fed on hypercholesterolemic (HC) diets

Shigeru Murakami [1] [2], Masamichi Yamashita [2], Yasuo Nara [1] and Yukio Yamori [1]

[1] *Department of Pathology, Shimane Medical University, 89-1 Enya-Cho, Izumo 693 and* [2] *Research Center, Taisho Pharmaceutical Co. Ltd., 1-403, Yoshino-Cho, Omiya 330, Japan*

SUMMARY

Taurine was fed to SHRSP on an HC diet for 50 days and the effects of taurine on cholesterol metabolism were studied. The cholesterol levels in serum, liver, small intestine and aorta were markedly increased in rats on the HC diet. However, these increases were markedly attenuated by taurine treatment. Fat depositions of mesenteric arteries were also improved by taurine. Acyl CoA:cholesterol acyltransferase (ACAT) activity in the small intestine was significantly decreased by taurine, indicating a reduction of cholesterol absorption. These results demonstrated the hypolipidemic and anti-atherosclerotic effect of taurine, and a possible mechanism involved in these beneficial effects.

INTRODUCTION

Taurine (2-aminoethanesulfonic acid) is a sulfur-containing amino acid, that is widely distributed in various animal tissues. World-wide epidemiological studies (WHO CARDIAC Study, Nara et al., 1990) and investigations with animal models (Yamori et al., 1983; Yamauchi-Takihara et al., 1986; Petty et al., 1990) have suggested beneficial effects of dietary taurine on cardiovascular diseases. Since SHRSP easily develop hypercholesterolemia and arterial fat deposition in mesenteric, cerebrobasal and other small arteries within a few weeks after being HC diet (Yamori et al., 1976), cholesterol-loaded SHRSP is a suitable model for studying cholesterol metabolism in small animals. Here we investigated the effects of taurine on cholesterol metabolism by using SHRSP.

METHODS

Female SHRSP aged 3 months were used and were fed on an HC diet (20% suet, 5% cholesterol and 2% cholic acid mixed in a regular stock-chow diet, Funabashi SP) and water containing 1% NaCl for 50 days (HC diet group). A taurine-treated group (HC diet + taurine

---

Abbreviations: SHRSP, Stroke-prone spontaneously hypertensive rats; HC, hypercholesterolemic; ACAT, acyl CoA:cholesterol acyltransferase.

group) received the same diet containing 3% taurine. The taurine dose calculated from the diet consumption was approximately 2 g/kg/day. A control group received a regular stock chow diet and tap water. Blood samples were collected every 10 days. Serum total cholesterol was determined using an enzymatic method (Determiner TC555, Kyowa Medex Tokyo, Japan). Protein was determined by the method of Lowry et al. (1951). On the 50th day, the animals were sacrificed and their livers, small intestines, aortas and mesenteric arteries were quickly excised. One piece each of liver, small intestine and aorta was used for cholesterol determination (Folch et al., 1957) and another piece each of liver and small intestine was used for the preparation of microsomes to measure the ACAT activity. ACAT activity was assayed essentially as previously described (Helgerud et al. 1981). Mesenteric arteries were stained with Sudan III for the detection of fat deposition. The fat deposition in the whole free mesenteric arterial branches to the intestinal loop was evaluated by the following scores: 0 less than 20 fat deposits, 1 more than 20 fat deposits. Blood pressure was determined in conscious, restrained animals by a photo oscillometric method. The significance of differences was assessed by chi-square test (evaluation for fat deposition) or Student's t-test.

RESULTS AND DISCUSSION

There was no significant difference between the body weight of each group during the experiment period. Increased blood pressure caused by HC diet and NaCl was significantly reduced in the taurine-treated group ($p<0.01$). The liver weight of the HC group was about 80% higher than the normal group, while taurine significantly prevented the increase of liver weight by 44%. The serum cholesterol level was markedly increased in HC group (Table 1) and the increase was significantly reduced by taurine treatment. Cholesterol contents were also remarkably increased in liver ($p<0.001$), small intestine ($p<0.001$) and aorta ($p<0.01$) of the HC group, compared to the normal group. The increased cholesterol levels of liver, small intestine and aorta caused by HC diet were decreased by 18 ($p<0.01$), 37 ($p<0.05$) and 27% (not significant), respectively in the taurine-treated group. These results show that taurine reduced serum and tissue cholesterol levels in cholesterol-loaded SHRSP. Acyl CoA:cholesterol acyltransferase (ACAT) plays an important role in the absorption of cholesterol in the small intestine (Clark S.B. & Tercyak A.M. 1984). A significant decrease of ACAT activity in the small intestine by taurine was observed, which suggests decreased cholesterol absorption. The load of an HC diet to SHRSP for 50 days resulted in severe fa

Table 1 Effect of taurine treatment on serum cholesterol level

Treatment	Serum total cholesterol (mg/dl)				
	Day 0	Day 15	Day 25	Day 35	Day 45
Normal	52.0±3.7	68.7±3.5***	63.3±3.0***	74.7±3.2***	64.4±3.2***
HC diet	57.8±4.0	383.3±31.9	427.7±42.8	747.6±85.6	767.5±104.9
HC diet + Taurine	55.2±4.7	193.6±40.7**	225.5±46.0*	353.6±58.6**	365.6±58.6*

Values are mean ± SEM of 5-7 animals.
Significant difference from HC diet. *$p<0.05$, **$p<0.01$, ***$p<0.001$

deposition on mesenteric arteries as reported previously (Yamori et al. 1976). These fat depositions were significantly ($p<0.01$) improved by taurine treatment, suggesting an anti-atherosclerotic effect of taurine. Taurine has been reported to have a hypolipidemic effect in normotensive rats (Herrmann et al., 1959). Enhancement of cholesterol metabolism into bile acid through cholesterol 7α-hydroxylase is one possible mechanism for hypolipidemic action of taurine (Stephan Z.F. et al., 1987). This effect may be related to the improvement of cholesterol metabolism by taurine observed in cholesterol-loaded SHRSP together with the inhibition of cholesterol absorption from the small intestine.

REFERENCES

Clark, S.B. and Tercyak, A.N. (1984): Reduced cholesterol transmucosal transport in rats with mucosal acyl CoA: cholesterol acyltransferase and normal pancreatic function. *J. Lipid Res.* 25: 148-159.

Folch, J., Lees, M. and Sloane Stanley, G.H.(1957): A simple method for the isolation and purification of total lipids from animal tissues. *J. Biol. Chem.* 226: 497-509.

Helgerud, P., Saarem, K. and Norum, K.R. (1981): Acyl CoA:cholesterol acyltransferase in human small intestine: its activity and some properties of the enzymatic reaction. *J. Lipid Res.* 22: 271-277.

Herrmann, R.G. (1959): Effect of taurine, glycine and β-sitosterols on serum and tissue cholesterol in the rat and rabbit. *Circ. Res.* 7: 224-227.

Lowry, O.H., Rosebrough, N.J., Farr, A.L. and Randall, R.J. (1951): Protein measurement with the Folin phenol reagent. *J. Biol. Chem.* 193: 265-275.

Nara, Y., Zhao, G.S., Huang, Z.D., Li, Y.H., Mizushima, S., Mano, M., Zhang, H.X., Sun, S.F., Sato, T., Horie, R., Zhang, M.X., He, B.S., Mori, C., Hatano, S., Liu, L.S. and Yamori, Y. (1990): Relationship between dietary factors and blood pressure in China. *J. Cardiovasc. Pharmacol.* 16 (Suppl. 8): S40-S42.

Petty, M.A., Kintz, J. and DiFrancesco, G.F. (1990): The effects of taurine on atherosclerosis development in cholesterol-fed rabbits. *Eur. J. Pharmacol.* 180: 119-127.

Stephan, Z.F., Lindsey, S. and Hayes, K.C. (1987): Taurine enhances low density lipoprotein binding. *J. Biol. Chem.* 262: 6069-6073.

Yamauchi-Takihara, K., Azuma, J. and Kishimoto, S. (1986): Taurine protection against experimental arterial calcinosis in mice. *Biochem. Biophys. Res. Commun.* 140: 679-683.

Yamori, Y., Horie, R., Sato, M. and Fukase, M. (1976): Hypertension as an important factor for cerebrovascular atherogenesis in rats. *Stroke* 7: 120-125.

Yamori, Y., Wang, H., Ikeda, K., Kihara, M., Nara, Y. and Horie, R. (1983): Role of amino acids in the prevention and regression of cardiovascular diseases. In: *Sulfur amino acids: Biochemical and clinical aspects*, ed. K. Kuriyama, R.J. Huxtable & H. Iwata, pp.103-115. New York: Alan R. Liss, Inc.

Independent expressions of the sarcomeric α-actins in human and rat ventricles with development and aging : evidence of species dependent expressions

Lucie Carrier, Kenneth R. Boheler, Claudine Wisnewski and Ketty Schwartz

INSERM U.217, Hôpital Lariboisière, 41, boulevard de la Chapelle, 75010 Paris, France

Sarcomeric actin genes, α-cardiac and α-skeletal, are co-expressed in rodent and human hearts; however, their precise developmental pattern of expression was not known. Primer extension assays of total human and rat ventricular RNAs were performed using specific oligonucleotides for these gene products. In rat, we found that at 17-19 days *in utero*, both isoactins are co-expressed and that the α-skeletal actin mRNAs represent 28% of the total sarcomeric actin mRNA, which increased to 40% of the total at one week of age, remained constant until 3 weeks, and decreased to 5% of the total by age 2 months. In man, we found that the α-skeletal actin mRNAs accounted for 20% of the total in fetal ventricles, increased during the first decade of life to 48%, and further accumulated to 60% of the total in adults. These results indicate that the expression of the sarcomeric actin isogenes are species dependent and at least in man and in rat are regulated by different mechanisms.

INTRODUCTION

Actin is the major component of the thin filament of the sarcomere and it functions *in vivo* to activate myosin ATPase. In mammals, actin is encoded by a multigene family and 6 different isoforms are known to exist, two of which, α-skeletal and α-cardiac are found only in striated muscle (Vandekerckove and Weber, 1979). These two isoforms are almost identical, differing by only 4 amino acids over 375 residues. Two of the four differences are located at the amino terminus, the region where binding to myosin occurs during contraction. Because of the close similarity between the sarcomeric actin isoforms, and consequently the difficulty in measuring the abundance of these proteins in striated muscle, it has proven advantageous to study the relative accumulations of their isomRNAs. These mRNAs are the products of different genes which are located at different chromosomes and whose nucleic acid sequences are highly conserved excluding their 5' and 3' untranslated region which markedly differ. Taking into account these differences, it has been shown that the amounts of each isoactin vary with species, muscle type and development. However, most studies were conducted on the skeletal muscle and much less is known for cardiac muscle. From results published by Minty et al. (1983) and by Mayer et al. (1984), it was known that α-skeletal actin is present in neonate rat hearts, and Bishopric et al. (1987) estimated that it amounted to 50% of the total in one rat heart. In man, much less is known concerning the amount of the actin mRNAs present during development, with age or in disease states. Only two reports (Gunning et al., 1983; Bennetts et al., 1986) have shown that the two sarcomeric actins are co-expressed in the human ventricles and that the amount of both isomRNAs were nearly identical in the heart of a patient suffering from hypertrophic obstructive cardiomyopathy.

It was therefore the purpose of this study to precisely measure the amounts of the sarcomeric actins with ontogeny and aging in rat and human ventricles. To address this question, the proportions of the two sarcomeric actin transcripts in rat and in human ventricular RNAs have been measured by primer extension assays which simultaneously allow a precise quantification of each isomRNA.

MATERIAL AND METHODS

The relative proportions of α-skeletal and α-cardiac actin mRNAs were measured simultaneously in the same sample of rat or human RNA by the technique of primer extension. We have used two 18-base oligonucleotides complementary to a region of exon 2 (codons 31-37) and common to both α-skeletal and α-cardiac actin isogenes: one is specific to rat sarcomeric actins (Bishopric et al., 1987) and the other is specific to human actin genes (Boheler et al.,

1991). They were synthesized at the Pasteur Institute (Paris), purified on a 20% denaturing polyacrylamide gel, 5' end-labeled with [γ-^{32}P]ATP using T4 polynucleotide kinase for 1 h at 37°C. One picomole of the purified and labeled primer was then added to 10-13 µg of total RNA (prepared according to Chirgwin et al., 1979) in the reverse transcriptase reaction (M-MLV reverse transcriptase) and incubated exactly as described (Winegrad et al., 1990; Boheler et al., 1991). The precipitated and denatured (85% formamide) reaction products were loaded and separated on 6% (v/v) denaturing polyacrylamide/urea gels (1800 V for 2-3 h). The RNAs were analyzed several times on different gels to ensure the reproducibility of the results. The gel was then dried and exposed to X-Omat film at -70°C for several hours. Autoradiograms were scanned with a Shimadzu CS-9000 densitometer, and the relative densities of the bands determined. The data are reported as the percent of Skeletal/Sarcomeric α-actin mRNA. With rat heart RNA, two bands were detected of 186 and of 195 nucleotides which correspond to α-skeletal and α-cardiac actin mRNAs, respectively (Bishopric et al., 1987; Winegrad et al., 1990). With human heart RNA, the reverse transcriptase yields fragments of 222 and 174 nucleotides for α-skeletal and α-cardiac actin mRNAs, respectively (Boheler et al., 1991). The primer was specific for striated muscle RNAs because no signal was detected from liver RNA (not shown, see Boheler et al., 1991 and Winegrad et al., 1990). Results are expressed as means ± SD, and statistical significance between each group was evaluated by one-way analysis of variance and compared by Scheffe F-test. The threshold of significance was chosen as values of $p<0.05$.

RESULTS

To precisely determine the developmental regulation of actin isomRNA accumulations, the percentage of α-skeletal to sarcomeric actin mRNA in rat and human ventricles was quantitated by primer extension. Fig. 1 shows the results obtained with both rat and human ventricular RNAs:

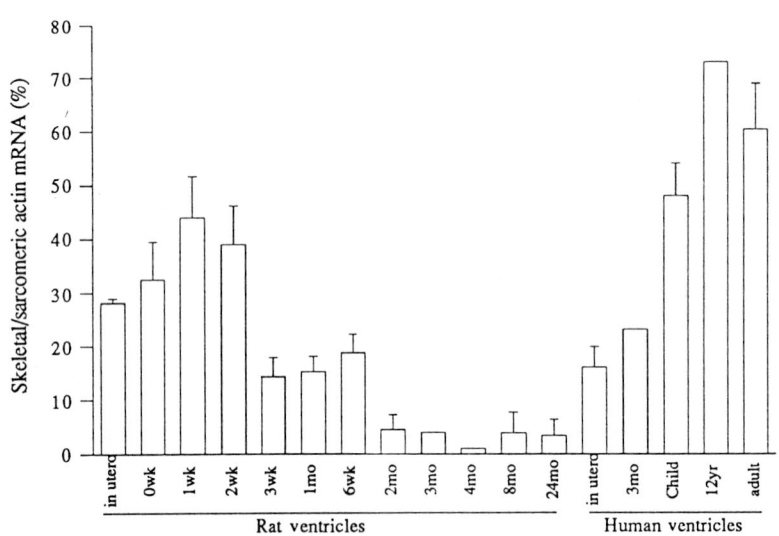

Fig. 1. *α-skeletal actin mRNA accumulations with development and aging.* Data for this graph were obtained from primer extension analysis of rat ventricular RNAs (left part of the graph) and of human ventricular RNAs (right part of the graph). The results are presented as the percentage of α-skeletal actin mRNA to total sarcoemric (α-cardiac + α-skeletal) actin mRNAs. Results are expressed as mean ± SD. *wk*, week; *mo*, months; *child*, children (3-8 years); *yr*, years.

In rat ventricles, the sarcomeric actins are always co-expressed, but the relative level of expression varied dramatically with age. At 17 and 19 days in utero, α-skeletal actin mRNAs represent 28.1±0.8% of the total, its proportion increases 8 days after birth to 44.0±7.6% (NS, p=0.15) and remains constant for 2 weeks, decreases by 3 weeks of age to 15.2±2.9%, and represents in aged rat ventricles only 3.4±3.0% of the total (Carrier et al., submitted). In human ventricles, the pattern of expression is opposed: α-skeletal actin is the minor component of the fetal ventricles (mean values 16.0±8.5%, n=3) and does not change markedly after birth (23%). It increases during the first decade of life (mean value 48.0±6.1%, n=3), and by 12 year of age a drastic reversal of the pattern is apparent. At this time, α-skeletal actin becomes the most abundant form (73%), and remains so in adult hearts (60.4±8.5%). The results have also been confirmed by dot blot analysis with cloned sequences specific for each actin isomRNA (Boheler et al., 1991).

DISCUSSION

We have determined the precise time course of expression of the α-cardiac and α-skeletal actin isogenes during ontogeny and aging. This study first confimed that the sarcomeric actin mRNAs are co-expressed in both rat and human ventricular RNAs. It is unknown why the sarcomeric α-actins are coexpressed or what functional differences if any exist between these two proteins. The co-expression could be explained by the fact that during certain periods of the development one isoform may not be sufficient for the synthesis of adequate quantities of actin; furthermore, the functional differences between the two isoactin have yet to be demonstrated, and experiments such as *in vitro* mobility assays could be used to resolve this issue.

In the rat heart, it is important to note that α-skeletal transcripts do not reaccumulate with aging. For the other major sarcomeric protein, it has been shown that the β-myosin heavy chain transcript accumulations decrease with development as that of the skeletal actin isomRNAs (Lompré et al., 1984) but it is re-accumulated with rat senescence (O'Neill et al., 1991). This suggests important differences in the regulation of the expression of the sarcomeric protein genes in the heart within the same species.

One of the main findings of the present study is that the sarcomeric actins are regulated in man in an apparently opposite manner to that seen in the rat heart. α-cardiac actin is the major isoform of the human fetal heart, whereas α-skeletal actin predominates in young and adult hearts. Man is the only species in which the α-skeletal actin mRNAs accumulate at higher levels than α-cardiac actin mRNAs in adult. We have also recently shown that the α-skeletal actin isomRNA remains the most abundant isoform with human heart failure (Boheler et al., 1991). The significance of this accumulation in both normal and failing heart is unknown. The role of the α-skeletal actin in human heart has to be clarified. Furthermore and as in the rat, the pattern of developmental expression of the β-myosin heavy chain genes in human ventricles (Bouvagnet et al., 1987; Mercadier et al., 1973) shows that this isomRNA is almost the exclusive form present at all stages of development and indicates a complete dissociation with the expression of the α-skeletal actin gene.

In conclusion, our results provide additional evidence of species dependent expression of the sarcomeric α-actin isogenes in the mammalian heart. Measurement of RNA accumulations alone are insufficient for one to determine at what level this multigene family is regulated. Transcriptional controls are undoubtedly involved but other levels of regulation could be involved and explained the complex regulations necessary for the coordinated expression of the functioning sarcomere.

REFERENCES

Bennetts, B.H., Burnett, L. & dos Remedios, C.G. (1986): Differential co-expression of α-actins genes within the human heart. *J. Mol. Cell. Cardiol.* 18, 993-996.
Bishopric, N.H., Simpson, P.C., & Ordahl, C.P. (1987): Induction of the skeletal α actin in α1 adrenoreceptor-mediated hypertrophy of rat cardiac myocytes. *J. Clin. Invest.* 80, 1194-1199.
Boheler, K.R., Carrier, L., de la Bastie, D., Allen, P.J., Komajda, M., Mercadier, J.J., & Schwartz, K. (1991): Skeletal actin mRNA increases in the human heart during ontogenic development and is the major isoform of control and failing human hearts. *J. Clin. Invest.* 88, 323-330.
Bouvagnet, P., Neveu, S., Montoya, M., & Léger, J.J. (1987): Developmental changes in the human cardiac isomyosin distribution: an immunohistochemical study using monoclonal antibodies. *Circ. Res.* 61, 329-336.
Chirgwin, J.M., Przybyla, A.E., MacDonald, R.J., & Rutter, W.J. (1979): Isolation of biologically active ribonucleic acid from sources enriched in ribonucleases. *Biochemistry 18, 5294-8299.*
Gunning, P., Ponte, P., Blau, H., & Kedes, L. (1983): α-skeletal and α-cardiac actin genes are co-expressed in adult human skeletal muscle and heart. *Mol. Cell. Biol.* 3, 1985-1995.
Lompré, A.M., Nadal-Ginard, B., & Madhavi, V.J. (1984): Expression of the cardiac ventricular α and β myosin heavy chain genes is developmentally and hormonally regulated. *J. Biol. Chem.* 259, 6437-6446.
Mayer, Y., Czosneck, H., Zeelon, P.E., Yaffe, D., & Nudel, U. (1984): Expression of the genes coding for the skeletal muscle and cardiac actins in the heart. *Nucl. Acid. Res.* 12, 1087-1100.
Mercadier, J.J., Bouveret, P., Gorza, L., Schiaffino, S., Clark, W.A., Zak, R., Swynghedauw, B., & Schwartz, K. (1973): Myosin isoenzymes in normal and hypertrophied human ventricular myocardium. *Circ. Res.* 53, 52-62.
Minty, A.J., Alonso, S., Caravatti, M., & Buckingham, M. (1982): A fetal skeletal actin mRNA in the mouse and its identity with cardiac actin mRNA. *Cell* 30, 185-192.
O'Neill, L., Holbrook, N., & Lakatta, E.G. (1991): Progressive changes from young adult age to senescence in mRNA for rat cardiac myosin heavy chain genes. *Cardiosciense* 2, 1-5.
Vandekerckove, J., & Weber, K. (1979): The complete amino acid sequence of actins from bovine aorta, bovine heart, bovine fast skeletal muscle, and rabbit slow skeletal muscle. *Differentiation* 14, 123-133.
Winegrad, S., Wisnewsky, C., & Schwartz, K. (1990): Effect of thyroid hormone on the accumulation of mRNA for skeletal and cardiac α-actin in hearts from normal and hypophysectomized rats. *Proc. Natl. Acad. Sci. USA* 87, 2456-2460.

Development of a new strain of rats with inherited stress-induced arterial hypertension

Arkady L. Markel

Institute of Cytology and Genetics, Russia Academy of Sciences, Siberian Branch, 630090, Novosibirsk 90, Russia

Rats with genetic arterial hypertension gained the status of experimental models for studying the mechanisms of essential hypertension in man. There exist extreme variants of genetic susceptibility to arterial hypertension allowing its spontaneous development (Okamoto & Aoki, 1963). Pathology, however, is, as a rule, the result of genotype-environment interaction. Thus, information concerning the mechanisms of human hypertension has been obtained from salt (Dahl et al., 1962) and DOCA-salt (Ben-Ishay et al., 1972) sensitive strains of rats. It is known that emotional stress underlies certain hypertensive reactions. This prompted us to use emotional stress as an inducer of arterial hypertension in a population of rats selectively bred for emotional stress responsiveness.

The newly developed strain designated as ISIAH rats (Inherited stress-induced, or stress-sensitive, arterial hypertensive rats) was derived from a randombred Wistar colony (Markel, 1985). Systolic arterial blood pressure (SABP) was measured by the tail-cuff method. The basal SABP was obtained under ether anesthesia to exclude the possible effect of psychological stress associated with the measurement procedure. The response of SABP to emotional stress was evaluated in conscious rats after 30 min restriction in small wire cages. Individual assignment to the hypertensive group was based on a cut-off value of 150 mm Hg. The mean basal SABP in the original population was 118 (males, n=158) and 112 (females, n=126) mm Hg. Restriction for 30 min produced an emotional stress slightly increasing the population mean for SABP to 128 (males) and 117 (females) mm Hg. However, in some rats stress-induced SABP rose to 150 mm Hg or higher. This allowed us to use these rats for developing a strain with inherited stress-sensitive arterial hypertension. The choice of rats for subsequent breeding was based on the evaluation of basal and stress-induced SABP levels. At present, we established two substrains of ISIAH rats: the first is not completely inbred, because brother-sister matings were avoided, and the second was started from the 15-th generation of outbred ISIAH rats with the aim of developing a completely inbred strain. There are now 14 generations of the second inbred sub-

strain. The mean SABP under stress increased by 29-th generation
of the first outbred strain to 208 (males) and 180 (females) mm Hg
and in the second inbred strain to 199 (males) and 175 (females)
mm Hg. There was an elevation in basal SABP, too. It reached 160
(males) and 143 (females) mm Hg in the outbred strain and 166
(males) and 149 (females) mm Hg in the inbred strain. This unpro-
voked rise in the basal SABP was unexpected because cumulative selection differential for basal SABP was very low. We reasoned as
follows: the lowering of the stress response threshold produced by
selection resulted in borderline spontaneous hypertension observed
as a slight rise in basal SABP.

A summary of our recent studies of ISIAH rats follows. Rat behavior was analysed in an open-field arena and spontaneous activity
was measured with a special device in the home cage (Markel, 1986)
The SHR were much more active in the open-field test and home cage
than the Wistar and ISIAH rats. However, the index of behavioral
reactivity (the ratio of locomotion before and after adaptation in
the open-field arena) in the ISIAH rats was 2.7 fold higher than
in Wistar or SHR strains. There was an agreement between the compared behavioral and hypertensive patterns: enhanced spontaneous
locomotion of the SHR was associated with spontaneous increase in
SABP, and the ISIAH rats showed high behavioral and SABP reactivity to stress.

Physiological markers of sympathetic nerve activity were studied.
The ISIAH rats showed increased activities of tyrosine hydroxyl-
ase and phenylethanolamine-N-methyltransferase, and also an increase in adrenaline concentration in the adrenals. Plasma immunoreactive insulin, liver glycogen content, and tolerance to glucose infusion in the ISIAH strain were all reduced (Shorin et al.,
1990). Subsequently, corticosterone plasma level in the ISIAH rats
was found to be lower after immobilization stress and higher after stress induced by a combination of stimuli (ether, blood sampling, novel situation) as compared to Wistar rats (Markel et al.,
1986). The ISIAH strain also showed a reduced plasma corticosterone response to intracerebroventricular injection of noradrenaline and the alpha-1-adrenoceptor agonist produced a marked response of the SABP, which decreased in Wistar and increased in the
ISIAH and SHR strains (Markel et al., 1987). A negative correlation was found between adrenocortical and blood pressure responses
to central adrenergic stimulation. It was concluded that the
changes of brain noradrenergic mechanisms may be responsible for
alteration in the central regulation of both SABP and adrenocortical function in the ISIAH rats.

We also studied the brain catecholaminergic system (Markel et al.,
1991). It was shown that the concentration and metabolic rate of
noradrenaline were decreased in certain brain areas. A distinct
attenuation of depressor reactions mediated by the brain beta-adrenergic mechanisms and a decrease in concentrations of beta-adrenoceptors in the medulla and alpha-adrenoceptors in hypothalamus of the ISIAH rats were observed. In contrast, the density of
alpha-1-adrenoceptors in the medulla was significantly higher
(Shishkina et al., 1991). Data supporting the crucial role of the
central noradrenergic mechanisms in the pathogenesis of stress-
sensitive hypertension came from following experiments (Naumenko
at al., 1990; Maslova et al., 1991). Injections of L-DOPA during

early postnatal life (21-25 days after birth) produced a persistent normalization of the SABP and adrenocortical responses to stress and intracerebroventricular noradrenaline injections.

In conclusion, it is hoped that the hypertensive ISIAH strain of rats would promote elucidation the genetic and physiological mechanisms of arterial hypertension.

REFERENCES

Ben-Ishay, D., Saliternik, R., and Welner, A. (1972): Separation of two strains of rats with inherited dissimilar sensitivity to DOCA-salt hypertension. Experientia, 28, 1321-1322.

Dahl, L.K., Heine, M., and Tassinari, L. (1962): Role of genetic factors in susceptibility to experimental hypertension due to chronic excess salt ingestion. Nature (London), 194, 480-482.

Markel, A.L. (1985): Experimental model of inherited arterial hypertension conditioned by stress (in Russian). Izvestia Acad. Nauk SSSR, Seria Biol., 3, 466-469.

Markel, A.L. (1986): Behavioral changes in rats with inherited arterial hypertension (in Russian). Zurn. Vish. Nervn. Deyat., 5, 956-962.

Markel, A.L., Dygalo, N.N., and Naumenko, E.V. (1986): Reactivity of hypothalamo-hypophyseal-adrenocortical system in rats with inherited arterial hypertension (in Russian). Bull. Exper.Biol. i Med., 101, 678-680.

Markel,A.L., Amstyslavski, S.Y., and Naumenko, E.V. (1987): The central adrenergic mechanisms of blood pressure regulation in rats with inherited arterial hypertension. Biogenic Amines, 4, 329-338.

Markel, A.L., Maslova, L.N., and Naumenko, E.V. (1991): Genetic arterial hypertension and brain catecholaminergic mechanisms. In Proc. Constituent Congr. Internat. Soc. for Pathophysiol. Moscow, May 28 - June 1. Abstracts, ed. G. Kryzhanovsky, p. 99. Kuopio (Finland): Suomen Graafiset Palvelut OY LTD.

Maslova, L.N., Markel, A.L., and Naumenko, E.V. (1991): Treatment with L-DOPA in early life restored pituitary-adrenocortical response to emotional stress in adult rats with inherited arterial hypertension. Brain Res., 546, 55-60.

Naumenko, E.V., Maslova, L.N., and Markel, A.L. (1990): Correction of arterial blood pressure in adult rats with inherited stress-induced arterial hypertension by enhancement of catecholamine metabolism in early postnatal period. Endocrinol. Experimentalis, 24, 241-248.

Okamoto, K., and Aoki, K. (1963): Development of a strain of spontaneously hypertensive rats. Jpn. Circ. J., 27, 282-293.

Shishkina, G.T., Markel,A.L., and Naumenko, E.V. (1991): Brain adrenoceptors in rats with inherited stress-sensitive arterial hypertension (in Russian). Genetika, 27, 279-284.

Shorin, Yu.P., Markel, A.L., Selyatitskaya, V.G., Palchikova, N.A. Grinberg, P.M., and Amstyslavski, S.Y. (1990): Endocrine-metabolic relations in rats with inherited stress-induced arterial hypertension (in Russian). Bull. Exper. Biol. i Med., 109, 575-576.

Intraretinal newly formed vessel in experimental hypertensive rat

Satoru Kimura, Hiroshi Yoshimoto and Shuichi Matsuyama

Department of Ophthalmology, Hirosaki University School of Medicine Hirosaki, 036, Japan

Introduction

Retinal newly formed vessel is considered to be one of the most charactistic features of vacular reaction to severe tissue ischemia and a main cause of visual disturbance following retinal vascular disorders. But the mechanism of its development has not been fully clarified. In this study, we experimentally produced severe hypertensive retinopathy using renal hypertensive rats to observe the developmental procedure and fate of intraretinal new vessels.

Methods

Renovascular hypertension was produced in 32 rats of Wistar-Kyoto strain by Goldblatt-Drury's method.[1] Blood pressure and ophthalmoscopic findings were monitered once a week. The eyeballs were enucleated and immersed in 1% gluthalaldehyde solution for 2 hours and in 2% OsO_4 solution as a post fixation later than 6 months of the duration of sustained high blood pressure over 200mmHg. Then the retina was served for light and electron-microscopic examination. All experimental procedures were carrided out under intraperitoneal anesthesia with pentobarbital sodium 20 mg/kg.

Results

Ophtalomoscopic changes and elevation of blood pressure are reported in previous studies [2]-[4]. On light microscopic observation, disorganization of the outer retinal layer progessed correlating with duration of severe hypertension. In several cases survived for more than 6 months, the pigment epithelial cell proliferation developed into the retina, but not into the vitreous cavity, accompaning with numerous abnormal microvessels.

On electronmicroscopy of these retinal vessels, 4 types of capillary were observed : (1) microvesssels with thickened basement membrane but no other morphological abnormalities compared with ordinary or normal capillaries, (2) ghost microvesssels with wall solely composed of basement membrane layer and lumen entirely occupied by glial elements, (3) microvesssels found in or around the tissues accompanied with proliferation of retinal pigment epithelial cells and showing the characteristics of immature newly formed vessels (Fig. 1, 3) and (4) microvessels which were considered to be newly formed but mature from the fea ures of wide lumia and well-developed basement membrane. Electron dense intraluminal plasma protein was often found in these vessels (Fig.4).

Discussion

Our previous reports [4],[5] revealed that prolonged severe hypertensive state induces disorganization of outer retina and intraretinal proliferation of pigment epithelial cell. Identification for newly formed vessel is also reported previously [5]. In present study, morphological changes of retinal capillaries are examined electronmicroscopically. Findings of abnormal vessels (both occluded vessels and newly formed vessels) are similar to that of human cases of ischemic retinal disease[6],[7]. Newly formed vessels can be divided into 2 types according to their morphological characteristics. One is the vessel of low maturity, which has large endothelial nuclei of rich organelles and slit-like narrowed lumia (Fig. 1,3). The other is the vessel of high maturity, which keeps wide lumina and well developed basement membrane (Fig 4). It is notable that abnormal strand-like structure of high electron density, which is thought to be condensation of plasma protein, is frequently observed in the lumina of mature newly formed vessels. This finding suggests to be an initial sign of re-occlusion probably due to intravascular fibrin formation. We conclude that developement and regression of newly formed vessels is simultaneously occur in ischemic retina.

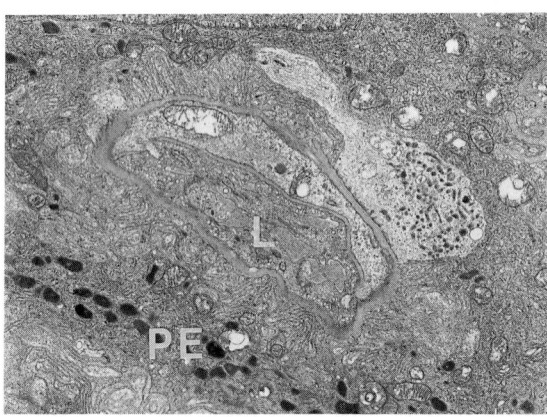

Figure 1. Newly formed vessel observed in pigment epithelial cell layer (PE) ; Basement membrane is surrounded by apical processes of pigment epithelial cell. Lumen (L) is poorly developed. (× 7,200)

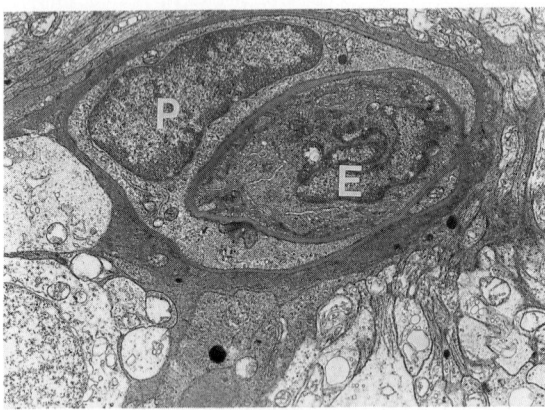

Figure 2. Immature newly formed vessel observed in nerve fiber layer ; Endothelial cell (E) has large nucleus and thin basement membrane is surrounded by pericyte (P). Lumen is unrecognizable. (× 14,000)

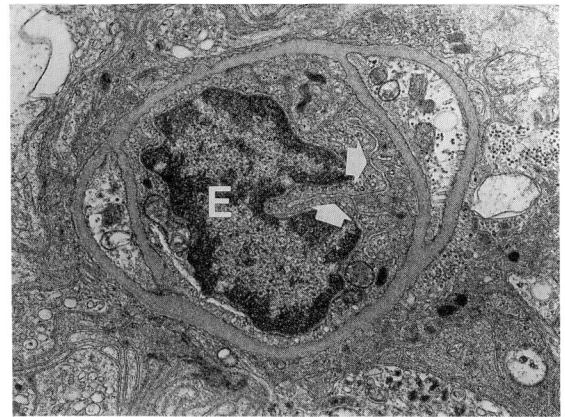

Figure 3. Immature newly formed vessel observed in innner plexiform layer ; Lumen (→) is extremely narrow. Endothelial cell (E) has lage nucleus. (× 7, 200)

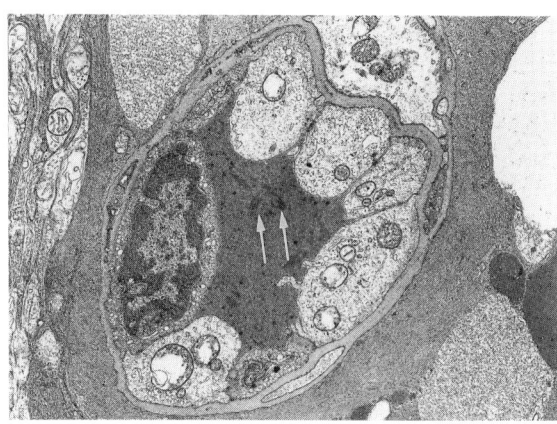

Figure 4. Mature newly formed vessel observed in outer nuclear layer ; Basement membrane is moderately thickened. High electron density strand (→) is observed in lumen. (× 10, 000)

Refferences

1) Drury D R : The production by a new method of renal insufficiency and hypertension. J Exp Med. 68 : 693-698, 1938.
2) Yoshimoto H : On the study of experimental renal hypertension : Ophthalmoscopic and lightmicroscopic observation. Acta Soc Ophthalmol Jap. 77 : 1951-1961, 1973.
3) Yoshimoto H : On the study of experimental renal hypertension : Electronmicron scopic observation. Acta Soc Ophthalmol Jap. 78 : 649-663, 1974.
4) Yoshimoto H and Matsuyama S : A histopathological study of late-phase severe retinochoroidopathy in experimental renovascular hypertensive rats. Acta Soc Ophthalmol Jap. 91 : 756-770, 1987.
5) Kimura S and Yosihmoto H : Intraretinal neovascularization in rats with experimental renovascular hypertension. Acta Soc Ophthalmol Jap. 94, 18-24, 1990.
6) Miller H et al. Diabetic neovascularization : permeability and ultrastructure. Invest Ophthalmol Visual Sci. 25, 1338-1342, 1984.
7) Kimura T. The cellular pathology of the occluded vessels of the human retina in hypertension and diabetes mellitus : Electron microscopic investigation. Folia Ophthalmol Jap. 24, 1211-1223, 1973.

Cataracta in hypertensive rats

Noboru Saito, Kousaku Noda [1], Yoshikazu Yamasaki [2], Kozo Matsubayashi, Teruhiko Okada [3] and Shoji Nishiyama [4]

Department of Geriatrics, [3] Department of Anatomy, [4] Department of Hygiene, Kochi Medical University, Nankoku-City, Kochi 783, Japan and [1] Department of Ophthalmology, [2] Department of Laboratory Phatology, Kochi Red Cross Hospital, Kochi-City, Kochi 780, Japan

There have been some reports about rat cataracta(Koch et al., 1977; Ichinohe et al., 1983), especially using spontaneously hypertensive rats(SHR). We found the occurrence of immature cataracta in old hypertensive rats of stroke-resistant SHR(SHRSR) and in very old normotensive rats of Wistar Kyoto rats(WKY)(Saito et al., 1989; Noda et al., 1989). Therefore, in this study we investigated the relationship between the occurrence of cataracta and aging or blood pressure level.

Methods   Rats of both sexes were used. As hypertensive rats 127 SHRSP(male 47%) were 1 to 17 months old and 93 SHRSR(male 50%) were 1 to 29 months old. As normotensive rats 114 Wistar Kyoto rats(WKY, male 43%) were 1 to 29 months old. These rats had been fed on ordinary chow and had drunk tap water ad libitum under constant temperature, humidity and 12-hour light in animal center of kochi Medical University. Systolic blood pressure of rats was measured by tail-cuff method(Narco PE-300).   The presence and grades of cataracta were determined after mydriasis with mydrin in rats without anesthesia using handsliplamp by a ophthalmologist(Noda,K.)   After anesthesia with urethan(1ml of 10% urethan per 100g body weight), the lens crystallina, corpus ciliare and the other tissues or organs were removed for microscopic specimens with Hematoxylin-Eosin staining.

Results   Systolic blood pressure was highest in SHRSP(195±21mmHg, M±SD), higher in SHRSR(168±14mmHg) and lowest in WKY(134+10mmHg).   All rats of three strains developed cataracta by aging, though the age of the occurrence of cataracta differed among three strains. The appearance of cataracta was found earliest in SHRSP and latest in WKY. The degrees of cataracta in rat eyes could be tentatively divided into 5 stages : 1) the stage without cataracta ; 2) the initial changes in posterior cortex ; 3) the slight turbidness in posterior subcortical regions(cataracta cupuliformis) ; 4) the severe turbidness in posterior subcortical regions ; and 5) the severe turbidness in posterior and anterior subcortical regions, indicating an immature or mature cataracta(Figs 1-2).   When the stages of cataracta more than the slight turbidness in posterior subcortical regions were adopted as cataracta, the presence of cataracta was 11.9% in SHRSP aged 2 to 5 months,93% in SHRSP aged 6 to 11 months, 100% in SHRSP aged 12 to 17 months, 50.4% in SHRSR aged 6 to 11 months, 94.1% in SHRSR aged 12 to 17 months, 100% in SHRSR aged 18 to 23 months, 0% in WKY aged 18 to 23 months and 100% of WKY aged 24 to 29 months(Fig 3).   The prevalence of cataracta according to the above 5 stages was shown in Figs 4a-c.   Concerning pathohistological findings the destruction of lens fiber in posterior subcortical regions, and the atrophy and hyalinization of ciliary process were observed microscopically(Table 1, Figs 5).

Discussion   Rat cataracta occurred by aging in 3 strains, earliest in SHRSP and latest in WKY, when systolic blood pressure was highest in SHRSP, higher in SHRSR and lowest in WKY, showing the tendency to be accelerated in hypertensive rats such as SHRSP or SHRSR. Aging process may be accelerated by hypertension. The pathohistological findings showed the atrophy and hyalinization of ciliary process, which might result in the alteration of aquous humor contents between the iris and lens, and in the occurrence of cataracta. Hypertension can accelerate the degenerated changes of ciliary process. Lens is an avascularture tissue, and consists of protein, water and so on. The increment of lens water may contribute partially to the occurrence of cataracta(Ichinohe, 1985). Furthermore, cholesterol synthesis is done locally in lens and may relate to membrane function of lens, of which synthesis was suppressed by administration of an inbibitor of HMG-CoA reductase(Mosley et al., 1989). It was estimated from the above results that hypertension could accelerate the occurrence of cataracta induced by aging. Further study is necessary for clarifying detailed mechanism of cataracta.

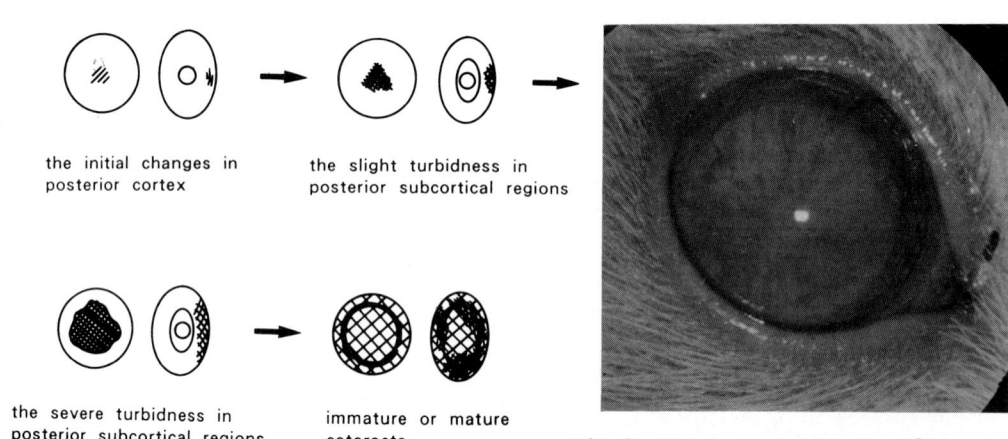

Fig 2 Immature cataracta of female SHRSR aged 27 months

Fig 1 **Progression of Cataracta in Rats**

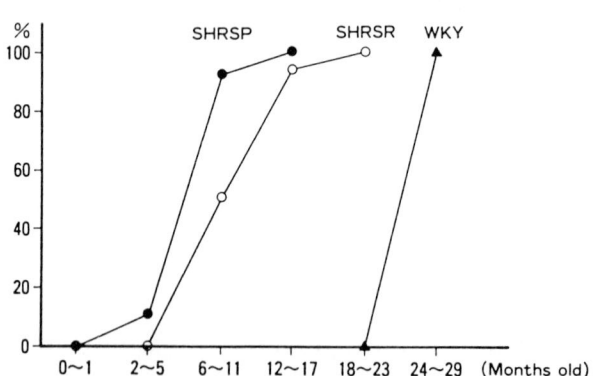

Fig 3 **Rat Cataracta** (the stages of more than slight turbidness in posterior subcortical regions)

Age	Total Cases	Male	Female	Ciliary Process					Damages of Lens structure (%)		
				Atrophy (%)		hyalinization (%)					
				−	+	−	±	+	−	±	+
SHRSP											
8.5 ± 4.0 M	6	3	3	83	17	33	50	17	50	33	17
20.8 ± 3.5 M	6	0	6	67	33	0	17	83	0	50	50
SHRSR											
10 ± 3.9 M	5	4	1	100	0	20	80	0	40	60	0
20.8 ± 4.0 M	8	0	8	38	62	0	0	100	0	0	100
WKY											
9.4 ± 3.2 M	6	4	2	100	0	67	0	33	100	0	0
19.7 ± 2.9 M	8	1	7	100	0	0	63	37	88	12	0

M : months

Table 1 Microscopic Findings of Ciliary Process and Lens

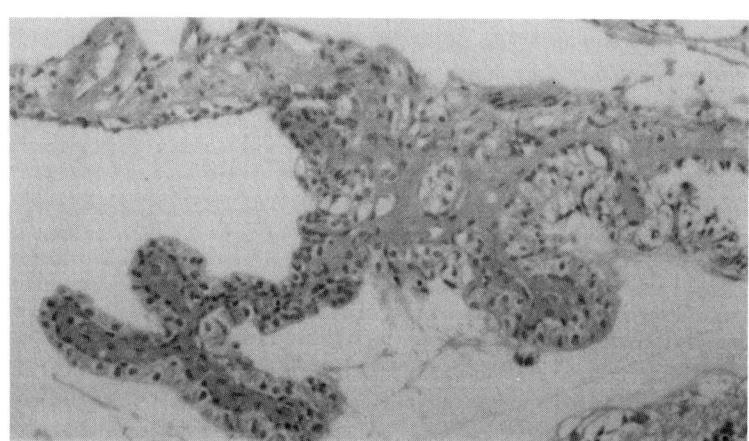

Fig 5 Hyalinoid material deposits of ciliary process in female SHRSP aged 17 months.

Summary 1. Concerning the degrees of rat cataracta, 5 stages were observed in this study, from the stage without cataracta to immature or mature cataracta.
2. Cataracta was shown in all cases of SHRSP aged 12 to 17 months, of SHRSR aged 18 to 23 months and of WKY aged 24 to 29 months, indicating the earliest occurrence of cataracta in SHRSP and the latest occurrence in WKY.
3. Microscopic findings of lens showed the destroyed structures and fibers in posterior subcortical regions, accompanying the degenerated changes of ciliary process.

References

Koch,H.R., Fisher,A. and Kaufman,H.(1977): Occurrence of cataracts in spontaneously hypertensive rats.　Ophthalmol. Res. 9:189-193.

Ichinohe,S., Yamagami,K., Yoshimoto,H. and Matsuyama,S.(1983): Cataract found in stroke-prone spontaneously hypertensive rats(SHRSP).　Folia Ophthalmol. Jpn. 34:10-15(in Japanese, but abstract in English).

Saito,N., Matsubayashi,K. and Noda,K.(1989): Retinal artery and cataracta in SHR. Jpn. Heart J. 30:576.

Noda,K., Ueno,H., Saito,N., Matsubayashi,K.and Yamasaki,Y.(1989): Cataracts in Wistar-Kyoto rats(WKY) and spontaneously hypertensive rats(SHRSP and SHRSR). J.Eye 6:1855-1858(in Japanese, but abstract in English).

Ichinohe, S.(1985): A morphological study on water distribution in the cataractous lens in stroke-prone spontaneously hypertensive rats(SHRSP). Folia Ophthalmol. Jpn. 36:470-477(in Japanese, but abstract in English).

Mosley,S.T., Kalinowski,S.S., Schafer,B.L.and Tanaka,R.D.(1989): Tissue-selective acute effects of inhibitors of 3-hydroxy-3-methylglutaryl coenzyme A reductase on cholesterol biosynthesis in lens.　J. Lipid Res. 30:1411-1420.

Effects of antihypertensive agents on osteoporosis in SHRSP

Satoru Tsuchikura [1] [3], Satoshi Fukuda [1], Haruzo Iida [1],
Katsumi Ikeda [2], Yasuo Nara [2] [3] and Yukio Yamori [2] [3]

[1] Division of Comparative Radiotoxicology, National Institute of Radiological Sciences, Anagawa 4-9-1, Chiba 260, [2] Shimane Institute of Health Sciences and [3] Department of Phatology, Shimane Medical University, Chioji 89-1, Izumo 693, Japan

SUMMARY: A long term administration of antihypertensive agents, nifedipine and hydralazine in SHRSP as a model of osteoporosis showed no significant affect on the process of osteoporosis, indicating severe hypertension was not the major cause of osteoporosis in SHRSP. Although bone volume was not increased, mineral apposition rate and bone formation rate were increased in nifedipine group.

We reported that SHRSP (Stroke-prone spontaneously hypertensive rat) developed spontaneously low turnover type osteoporosis with the process of aging as well as hypertension. SHRSP, therefore, is regarded as a good model for observing the effects of antihypertensive agents on osteoporosis. In the present study, we examined the effects of nifedipine and hydralazine on osteoporotic bone changes in SHRSP.

MATERIALS AND METHODS

SHRSP, 15 females in total, were divided into the following 3 groups at the age of 8 weeks. (1) Control group: Funabashi SP diet (FSPD), (2) Nifedipine group: Nifedipine of a daily dose of 30 mg/kg of body weight was added to FSPD. (3) Hydralazine group: Hydralazine of a daily dose of 18mg/kg body weight was added in water. Their blood pressure by tail-pulse pickup method and body weight were measured once weekly for 28 weeks. Prior to sacrifice, tetracycline and calcein were injected for double bone labeling to analyze bone dynamic as well as static parameters in an interval of 7 days. The femur and tibia were removed for bone analyses. Mechanical property (breaking force, displacement) of femur cortical bone was measured by a three point bending method using a bone strength measuring apparatus (Model MZ-500, Maruto Co., Ltd.). The femur used for test of mechanical property was weighed for the wet weight, and solved in nitric acid after incineration in an electric furnace. The concentration of calcium was measured by o-Orthocresolphtalein Complexone method. The ash and calcium contents were calculated as follows: ash weight (%) = ash weight / wet weight x 100, calcium weight (%) = calcium weight/wet weight x 100. Total calcium in serum was measured by an electrode method.
Undecalcified tibial proximal epiphysis was stained by Villanueva's bone stain (Villanueva and Mehr, 1977), dehydrated in alcohol and acetone and embedded in methylmethacrylate. Block was cut thin with an inner blade cutter (Maruto, Co., Ltd.). Thereafter, histological sections of 10-15 μm thickness were obtained with grinding with glass plates. Histomorphometric measurement on cancellous bone area (secondary spongiosa) of tibia was performed by a semiautomatic image analyzer (Kontron 64, Carl Zeiss Co.) using the "Osteoplan" software (Malluche et al., 1982).

RESULTS

The blood pressures were lowered significantly in nifedipine and hydralazine groups during the experiment, at the end, 180 ± 6 in nifedipine group, 152 ± 13 in nydralazine group, whereas 233 ± 19 in control. There were no significant differences in body weight between experimental groups and control group. No significant differences in breaking force and displacement (Table 1), ash and calcium contents (Table 2) of femur and bone volume and mean trabecular thickness (Table 3) were noted between experimental groups and control group (Table 1), but mineral apposition rate and bone formation rate were increased significantly ($p<0.05$) in nifedipine group (Table 3). The values of total and ionic calcium were shown in Table 4.

Table 1 Breaking force and displacement of femur in nifedipine, hydralazine and control groups, 28 weeks after treatment

	Breakin force(kgf)	Displacement(mm)
Control	17.50 ± 1.93	0.54 ± 0.11
Nifedipine	16.04 ± 1.04	0.53 ± 0.05
Hydralazine	15.97 ± 0.53	0.54 ± 0.11

Table 2 Ash and calcium contents of femur

	Ash (%)	Calcium (%)
Control	45.2 ± 0.4	24.7 ± 1.3
Nifedipine	44.8 ± 1.0	25.3 ± 0.6
Hydralazine	45.3 ± 0.5	25.6 ± 0.8

Table 3 Histomorphometric values of cancellous bone area of tibial metaphysis

	Control	Nifedipine	Hydralazine
Bone volume (%) (Volume trabecular bone/volume total bone)	167 ± 27	152 ± 50	153 ± 23
Mean trabecular thickness (μm) (Mean trabecular width)	114 ± 9	129 ± 15	112 ± 9
Mineral apposition rate (μm/day) (Mean distance/labeling interval)	0.528 ± 0.126	$0.903 \pm 0.238*$	0.504 ± 0.171
Bone formation rate (%/year) Volume referent (Mean label length x mineral apposition rate/mean trabecular area)	0.129 ± 0.09	$0.419 \pm 0.128*$	0.102 ± 0.089

*Significant differences from control. ($p<0.05$)

Table 4 Total calcium and ionic calcium in serum

	Control	Nifedipine	Hydralazine
Total calcium (mg/dl)	11.9 ± 1.01	0.4 ± 0.81	1.1 ± 1.4
Ionic calcium (mmol/l)	1.48 ± 0.03	1.45 ± 0.15	1.56 ± 0.05

DISCUSSION

Many investigators reported the possible cause and mechanism on hypertension in SHR and SHRSP might be related to abnormalities of calcium metabolism due to vitamin D-related intestinal absorption and renal leak of calcium, secondary hyperparathyroidism caused by hypocalcemia, primary hyperparathyroidism with increase of PTH and circulating hypertensive factor of parathyroid origin (Pang and Lewanczuk, 1989), and abnormality of cell membrane function related to calcium etc. All these alterations were closely related to bone metabolism, particularly development of osteoporosis. Present experiment eliminated that severe hypertension which might cause renal calcium leak was not the major cause of osteoporosis in SHRSP. Nifedipine, a calcium antagonist, is an antihypertensive drug to reduce total periheral resistance with a subsequent decrease of blood pressure and has multiple effects (Albers et al., 1991). Although antihypertensive treatment with nifedipine, typical Ca antagonist might supposedly affect bone metabolism, it was recently reported that nifedipine administered for three years had no effect on bone metabolism in male Caucasian including patients with osteoporosis so far observed by the measurement of bone mineral density. Our data obtained in this study indicated also both nifedipine and hydralazine had no remarkable effect on bone and calcium metabolism, but observed increases in mineral apposition rate and bone formation rate in nifedipine treated group were rather suggestive of the stimulation of osteoblast activity which should be related to a new bone formation. However, since no evidence for increased bone volume was obtained in nifedipine treated group, further study is needed for analyzing the detailed nifedipine effect on bone metabolism in hypertension.

It is concluded that chronic antihypertensive treatments by both nifedipine and hydralazine had no adverse effect on the development of osteoporosis in SHRSP.

REFERENCES

Albers, M. M., Johnson, W., Vivan, V., and Jackson, R. D. (1991); Chronic use of the calcium channel blocker Nifedipine has no significant effect on bone metabolism in men. *Bone.* 12, 39-42.

Malluche, H. H., Sherman, D., Meyer, W., and Massry, S. G. (1982) : A new semiautomatic method for quantitative static and dynamic bone histology. *Calcif. Tissue.* 34, 439-448.

Pang, P. T. and Lewanczvk, R. Z. (1989): Parathyroid origin of a new circulating hypertensive factor in spontaneously hypertensive rats. *Am. J. Hypertension* 2, 898-902.

Villanueva, A. R. and Mehr, L. (1977)): Modification of the Goldner and Gomori-step trichrome stains for plastic-embedded thin sections of bone. *Am. J. Med. Technol.* 34, 536-538.

Further study on osteoporosis in SHRSP: quantitative analyses by bone histomorphometry and serum biochemical constituents related to bone

Satoshi Fukuda [1], Satoru Tsuchikura [1][3], Haruzo Iida [1], Katsumi Ikeda [2], Yasuo Nara [2][3] and Yukio Yamori [2][3]

[1] Division of Comparative Radiotoxicology, National Institute of Radiological Sciences, Anagawa 4-9-1, Chiba 260, [2] Shimane Institute of Health Sciences and [3] Shimane Medical University, Chioji 89-1, Izumo 693, Japan

SUMMARY: As the characteristics of osteoporosis in SHRSP such as its age related changes, quantitative changes of bone volume after ovariectomy, and response to dietary factors, sodium loading and calcium supplementation were defined.

We reported that SHRSP (Stroke-prone spontaneously hypertensive rats) developed osteoporotic bone disorders spontaneously and could be utilized as its model for in man at the 6th International Symposium on Rats with Spontaneous Hypertention and Related Studies in 1989 (Yamori, et al., 1989). We further examined the characteristics of bone metabolism in detail by following experiments.

MATERIALS AND METHODS

Experiment I: SHRSP, 30 females and 30 males in total and 5 of each, were use at the age of 1, 2, or 3, 5, 7, 10 and 15 months to examine the age related changes in bone metabolism. Age matched normotensive Wistar Mishima rats and, in part, SHR were used as the control. Experiment II: Female of SHRSP and normotensive Wistar Kyoto rat (WKY), five of each were ovariectomized (OVX) and sacrificed 2 months later to examine the effects of the defect of sex hormones. Experiment III: Fifty females of SHRSP and 50 WKY, at the age of 3 months, were divided into two main groups of intact and OVX groups. Each group was again divided into the following five groups fed on: (1) a standard control diet (NaCl: 1%, Ca: 0.75%), (2) high NaCl: 4%, high Ca: 4.7% diet, (3) high NaCl, low Ca: 0.04% diet, (4) low NaCl: 0.2%, high Ca: 4% diet, (5) low NaCl, low Ca diet, for 2 months.
In each experiment, tetracycline and calcein were injected 11 and 4 days prior to sacrifice, respectively for bone labeling to analyze bone dynamic as well as static parameters in histomorphometry. The femur was used for the test of mechanical property (breaking force and displacement) by a three point bending method (Fig. 1) using a bone strength apparatus (Model MZ-500, Maruto, Co., Ltd.). Thereafter, the femur used in the test of mechanical property was weighted for the wet weight, incinerated in an electric furnace and solved in nitric acid. The concentration of calcium was measured by o-Cresolphthalein Complexone method. Calcium content of femur was calculated as a percent for the wet weight. Undecalcified tibial proximal epiphyses were stained with Villanueva's bone stain (Villanueva and Mehr, 1977), dehydrated in alcohol and acetone and embedded in methylmethacrylate. Thereafter histological section of 10-15 μm thickness were obtained by grinding with glass plates. Histomorphometric measurement was performed by a semiautomatic analyzer using "Osteoplan" software (Malluche et al., 1982).

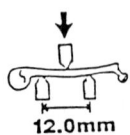

Fig.1 Three point bending method

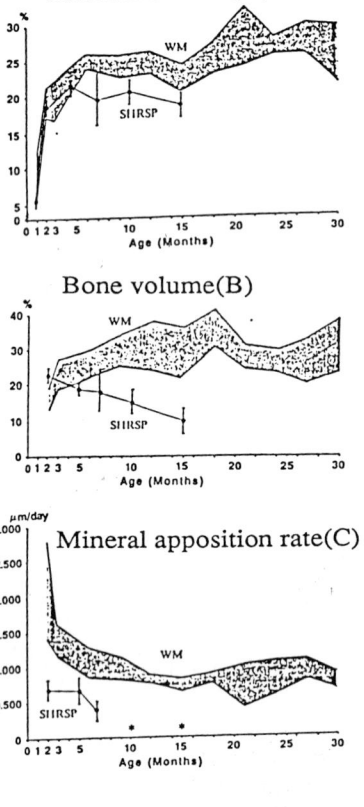

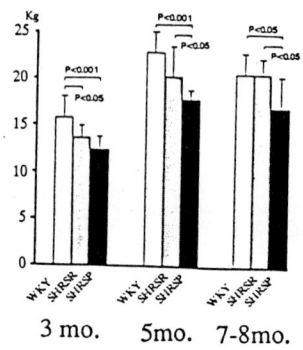

Fig.2 Breaking force of femur in male WKY, SHR and SHRSP

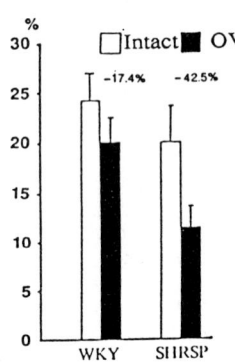

Fig.4
Decrease of bone volume in tibial proximal epiphysis in WKY and SHRSP 8 weeks after OVX.

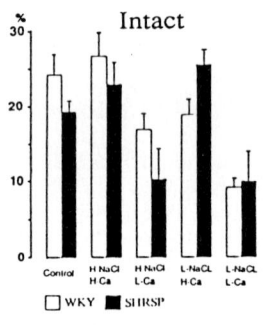
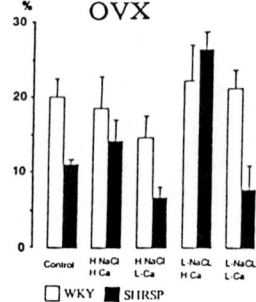

Fig.3
Age related changes in calcium content of femur(A), bone volume(B) and mineral apposition rate (C) in female SHRSP and normotensive Wistar Mishima(WM). Astaric marks (C) indicated the values could not be obtained because of too narrow space between double labelings.

Fig.5
Bone volume in each group fed on diets of different NaCl and Ca contents in intact and OVX groups of WKY and SHRSP.

RESULTS

In the experiment I, all data of the breaking force (Fig. 2) and calcium content (Fig. 3) of femur, bone volume (Fig. 3) and mineral apposition rates (Fig. 3) in SHRSP began to decrease after the bones developed normally up to the age of 3-5 months, whereas those in normotensive rats did not changes, or rather increased in the calcium content and bone volume. In the experiment II, remarkable decreases of bone volume in OVX-SHRSP were observed as compared to that of OVX-WKY (Fig. 4). In the experiment III, in both intact and OVX groups, unbalanced supplementation of high NaCl and low Ca decreased the bone volume in SHRSP than those in WKY, and the reduction was more marked in the OVX group than in the intact group (Fig. 5).

DISCUSSION

The data (Figs. 2 and 3) obtained in the experiment I demonstrated that a tendency to osteoporosis started in SHRSP when the blood pressure reached the level over 200 mmHg, after the bone developed normally during the blood pressure elevation up to the age of 3 months. This indicates may be some common factors and their interaction in the development of severe hypertension and osteoporosis. Remarkable decreasing of mineral apposition rates suggested that the decrease of bone volume in SHRSP was due to the difference in the accelerated bone resorption and decrease of bone formation, and indicated a low turnover type of senile osteoporosis. It is likely related to its abnormalities of calcium metabolism, either the low (Wright and Rankin, 1982) or high (Lau et al., 1984) level of serum calcium, and decrease of vitamin D metabolites in serum (Schedl et al., 1984) indicating a reduction of intestinal absorption of calcium as the cause of low level of calcium in serum in SHR. Besides, renal leak of calcium and secondary hyperparathyroidism (McCarron et al., 1981) caused by the reduced serum calcium suggest that the osteoporosis in SHRSP might be induced by abnormality of calcium metabolism, particularly due to decrease of serum calcium. Moreover, there remain other possible causes such as primary hyperparathyroidism. It may be speculated that these factors or mechanisms are commonly involved in both osteoporosis and hypertension. Results in the experiment II indicated that sex hormones such as estrogen and ovarial functions in SHRSP might be normal and not related to spontaneous loss of bone mass, because a high turnover type osteoporosis with postmenopuse was observed after OVX. Results in the experiment III indicated that the bone metabolism in SHRSP could functionally response to salt loading, calcium supplementation and probably various drugs.

In conclusion, osteoporosis in SHRSP is one of senile changes developed under genetic influence and its interaction with hormonal or dietary factors and therefore, SHRSP can be utilized as good models for basic and clinical studies on osteoporosis in man.

REFERENCES

Lau, K., Zilos, D., Spirnak, J., and Eby, B. (1984): Evidence for an intestinal mechanism in hypercalciuria of spontaneously hypertensive rats. Am. J. Physiol. 247, E625-E633.

Malluche, H. H. ,Sherman, D., Meyer, W., and Massry, S. G. (1982): A new semiautomatic method for quantitative static and dynamic bone histology. Calcif. Tissue. 34, 439-448.

McCarron, D. A., Yung, N. N., Ugoretz, B. A., Krutzik, S. (1981): Disturbances of calcium metabolism in the spontaneously hypertensive rat. Hypertention, suppl.I, 3,162-167.

Schedl, H. P., Miller, D. L., Pape, J. M., Horst, R. L., and Wilson, H. D. C. (1984): Calcium and sodium transport and vitamin D metabolism in the spontaneously hypertensive rat. J. Clin. Invet. 73, 980-986.

Villanueva, A. R. and Mehr, L. (1977): Modification of the Goldner and Gomori-step trichrome stains for plastic-embedded thin sections of bone. Am. J. Med. Technol. 34, 536-538.

Wright, G. L. and Rankin, G. O. (1982): Concentration of ionic and total calcium in plasma of four models of hypertension. Am. J. Physiol. H365-H370.

Yamori, Y., Fukuda, S., Tuchikura, K., Ikeda, K., Nara, Y., and Horie, R. (1989): Stroke prone SHR as a model for osteoporosis. Clin. Exp. Hypertension A13 (in press).

Beneficial effect of alacepril on glucose metabolism in both non-diabetic and diabetic spontaneously hypertensive rats

Toshiaki Sato, Yasuo Nara *, Yuzuru Kato and Yukio Yamori *

Departments of Internal Medicine and Pathology *, Shimane Medical University, Izumo, Japan

SUMMARY

Present studies were performed to explore the long-term effect of angiotensin-converting enzyme (ACE) inhibition with aracepril on glucose tolerance in non-diabetic and diabetic spontaneously hypertensive rats (SHR). Diabetes was developed in SHR by neonatal injection of streptozotocin (STZ). Twelve STZ-treated SHR (DM) and 14 non-treated SHR (C) at the age of two months were equally divided into two groups, respectively, as follows; C, C+alacepril, DM and DM+alacepril. Six months after treatment, alacepril not only lowered blood pressure (p<0.01) but also decreased proteinuria (p<0.01). Moreover, alacepril significantly improved glucose intolerance, hyperinsulinemia in C and hyperglycemia in DM. It is concluded that ACE inhibitor aracepril improves glucose tolerance in both non-diabetic and diabetic SHR in addition to the reported preventive effect on proteinuria.

INTRODUCTION

Hypertention, which is more common in diabetic patients than non-diabetics, contributes to their increased cardiovascular morbidity and mortality. Therefore, blood pressure as well as plasma glucose levels should be strictly controlled in diabetic patients. Many antihypertensive drugs are known to have adverse effects on glycemic control in diabetic patients. However, we previously revealed that effective treatment with an anti-hypertensive drug improved glucose tolerance in hypertensive diabetic rats (Sato et al., 1986), which were established by neonatal injection of STZ in SHR (Sato et al., 1987). The aim of the present study was to explore the long-term effect of ACE inhibition with alacepril on glucose tolerance in non-diabetic and diabetic SHR.

Abbreviations: SHR, spontaneously hypertensive rats; STZ, streptozotocin; ACE, angiotensin-converting enzyme

METHODS

Two-day-old SHR pups were subcutaneously injected with 100 mg/kg STZ in 0.05 mol citrate buffer as previously described (Sato et al., 1987). Controls were injected with the equivalent volume of citrate buffer. Twelve STZ-treated SHR (DM) and 14 non-treated SHR (C) at the age of two months were equally divided into two groups, respectively, and treated follows; 1) C, 2) C+alacepril (25 mg/kg p.o.), 3) DM and 4) DM+alacepril. Six months after treatment, the rats were individually housed in metabolic cages for collecting 24 hr urine Glycosuria and proteinuria were determined. Blood pressure (BP) was measured by indirect tail plethysmography. Then, oral glucose tolerance test (OGTT) was performed. At fasting 30, 60 and 120 min. after glucose administration (2 g/kg), blood was collected and plasma glucose (PG) and immunoreactive insulin (IRI) were determined. Urine glucose and PG were determined by a glucose-oxidase method. IRI was determined by a double-antibody radio immunoassay. Statistical differences among groups were evaluated by ANOVA, followed by Fisher's test for pairwise comparisons.

RESULTS and DISCUSSION

As shown in Table 1, BP was significantly lowered in alacepril treated groups which were accompanied by a significant decrease in proteinuria. We previously reported that suitable anti-hypertensive treatment reduced proteinuria in this animal model (Sato et al., 1987) Alacepril had beneficial effect on urinary protein excretion. ACE-inhibitors were shown decrease proteinuria in hypertensive diabetic patients with established nephropathy (Hommel al., 1986) as well as in normotensive diabetic patients with microalbuminuria (Marre al.,1987). In experimental diabetes, the ACE inhibitor, enalapril, was shown to prevent the development of albuminuria and glomerulosclerosis in both hypertensive and normotensive diabetic rats (Cooper et al., 1989).

Table 1. Body weight, blood pressure, proteinuria, plasma creatinine and blood urea nitrogen (BUN) after 6 months of alacepril treatment in non-diabetic SHR (C) and diabetic SHR (DM).

Type (n)	Body Weight (g)	Blood Pressure (mmHg)	Proteinuria (mg/day)	Creatinine (μmol/l)	BUN (mmol/l)
C (7)	204±6	185±3*	63±6*	46.9±2.7	6.96±0.39
C+Alacepril (7)	201±6	148±7	46±6	46.0±3.5	6.71±0.54
DM (6)	184±9*	177±4*	130±18*	43.3±6.2	10.96±0.75
DM+Alacepril (6)	197±14	158±4	82±10	46.9±6.2	10.53±1.96

Values are given as the mean ± SD. *p<0.01 vs treated group.

Fig. 1 shows PG and IRI responses to OGTT. Glucose tolerance, hyperinsulinemia in C group (Left, Top) and hyperglycemia in DM groups (Right, Top) were significantly improved alacepril treatment. Alacepril treatment also improved glucose tolerance in the non-diabetic SHR. ACE-inhibitors are becoming popular anti-hypertensive drugs because of their efficacy and low incidence of side effects. Acute and long-term studies suggested that ACE-inhibitor

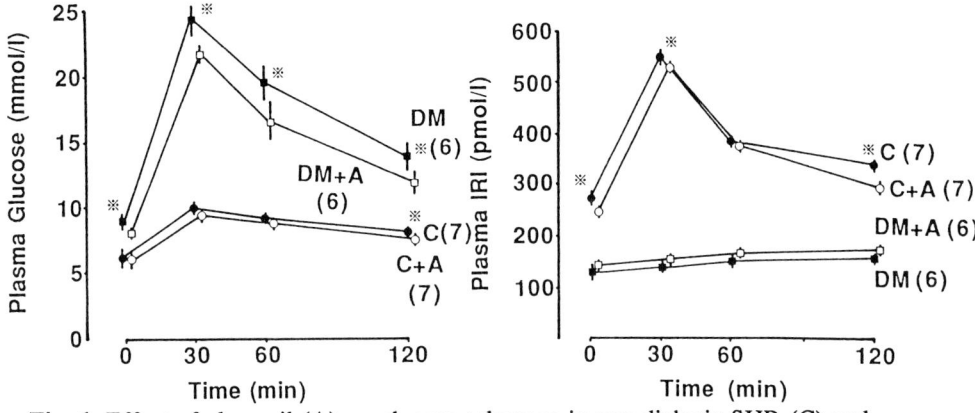

Fig. 1. Effect of alacepril (A) on glucose tolerance in non-diabetic SHR (C) and diabetic SHR (DM). Number of animals are shown in parentheses. Values are given as the mean ± SD. Significantly difference from treated group. (*p< 0.05)

ncrease peripheral insulin sensitivity in non-insulin dependent diabetes mellitus and essential hypertension, i.e. in two different types of insulin resistance (DeFronzo, 1988; Ferrannini et al., 1987). Several recent reports showed that SHR were insulin resistant and hyperinsulinemic (Reaven et al., 1989). Present study suggests that alacepril may improve insulin resistance in both groups.

These hypertensive diabetic rats can be regarded as good models to study the interaction between diabetes mellitus and hypertension and also the implication of anti-hypertensive treatment in diabetes.

REFERENCES

Cooper, M.E., Allen, T.J. et al. (1989): Enalapril retards glomerular basement membrane thickening and albuminuria in tha diabetic rat. *Diabetologia* 32, 326-328.

DeFronzo, R. (1988): The triumvirate: B-cell, muscle, liver. A collusion responsible for NIDDM. *Diabetes* 37, 667-687.

Ferrannini, E., Buzzigoli, G. et al. (1987): Insulin resistance in essential hypertension. *N. Engl. J. Med.* 317, 350-357.

Hommel, E., Parving, H.H. et al. (1986): Effect of captopril on kidney function in insulin-dependent diabetic patients with nephropathy. *Br. Med J.* 293, 467-470.

Marre, M., Leblanc, H. et al. (1987): Converting enzyme inhibition and kidney function in normotensive diabetic patients with persistent microalbuminuria. *Br. Med. J.* 294, 1448-1452.

Reaven, G.M., Chang, H. et al. (1989): Resistance to insulin-stimulated glucose uptake in adipocytes isolated from spontaneously hypertensive rats. *Diabetes* 38, 1155-1160.

Sato, T., Nara, Y. et al. (1986): Improved glucose metabolism in hypertensive diabetic rats by antihypertensive therapy. *J. Hypertension 4 (suppl. 6)*, 163-165.

Sato, T., Nara, Y. et al. (1987): New establishment of hypertensive diabetic animal models; Neonatally streptozotocin-treated spontaneously hypertensive rats. *Metabolism* 36, 731-737.

Sato, T., Nara, Y. et al. (1987): Effect of calcium antagonists on hypertension and diabetes in new hypertensive diabetic models. *J. Cardiovasc. Pharmacol. 10 (suppl. 10)*, 192-194.

Impairment of lipid metabolism in heart cell cultures from newborn spontaneously hypertensive rat

E. Millanvoye-Van Brussel *, J. Simon *, M.A. Devynck and M. Freyss-Béguin

INSERM, Département de Pharmacologie, CHU Necker, 156, rue de Vaugirard, Paris, France

Genetic hypertension appears associated with various functional or structural abnormalities of the cell membrane. Among them, alterations in lipid composition are believed to play a determinant role. Erythrocytes (Montenay-Garestier et al., 1981), platelets (Aragon-Birlouez et al.,1984) and smooth muscle cells (Tsuda et al.,1988) of hypertensive rats exhibit decreased membrane fluidity and reduced percentages of phospholipid-bound linoleic and arachidonic acids (Singer et al., 1983). Conversely, high linoleic acid intake and infusion are hypotensive (Reddy et al., 1989).

As regards heart tissue, relatively little information is now available on the nature of the cellular responses to hypertension and on the biochemical mechanisms mediating those responses. Previous studies have shown that genetic hypertension is associated, during the early neonatal development, with cardiac cell hyperplasia, hypertrophy and polyploidy (Clubb et al.,1987).

The present study was undertaken to determine whether lipid metabolism is altered in cultures of cardiac cells from genetically hypertensive newborn rat, even before the development of high blood pressure.

METHODS

We have compared the distribution of long chain fatty acids among phospholipids and neutral lipids in cultured heart myocytes from spontaneous hypertensive (SH, Okamoto-Aoki strains) and Wistar-Kyoto (WKY) newborn rats.

<u>Animal</u>: 3 day-old pups were taken from SH or WKY rats (CER Janvier, France). As evidenced by the increased heart to body weight ratio found in the SHR pups ($7.56 \pm 0.10 \; 10^{-3}$) compared to WKY pups ($5.98 \pm 0.14 \; 10^{-3}$), increased cardiac mass occured in SHR before development of blood pressure.

<u>Heart cell cultures</u>: Cell cultures were prepared as previously described (Freyss-Beguin et al. 1989). Cells were isolated by trypsinization and myoblasts were separated from fibroblasts by a differential attachment technique. The purity of beating myoblast cultures was maintained by addition of ß-D arabino-furanosyl-cytosine.

<u>Analysis of cellular fatty acids</u>: The cells were scrapped off and the lipids extracted according to Folch et al.,(1957). The lipids were fractionated by silicic acid column chromatography. Neutral lipids and phospholipids were subjected to BF_3 transmethylation. The acyl methyl esters formed were analyzed by capillary gas chromatography. The results are expressed as µg fatty acids/mg protein.

<u>Statistics</u>: Fatty acids pooled into saturated ($\Delta=0$), mono- and dienoic ($\Delta=1,2$) and polyunsaturated ($\Delta \geq 3$) groups (Fig 1) were compared by the Student paired t-test. Results are expressed as the differences between SHR and control cells.

RESULTS AND DISCUSSION

The present results reveal that newborn SHR heart myocytes contain less phospholipids than those from WKY rats on a protein basis. The mass of associated fatty acids was reduced when compared to WKY myocytes ($0.01<p<0.05$ for saturated and polyunsaturated fatty acids, $0.001<p<0.01$ for mono- and dienoic fatty acids) (Fig 1).

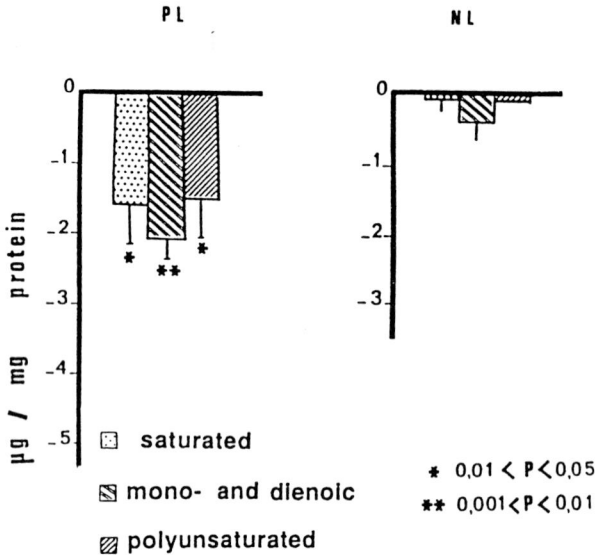

Fig.1: Reduction of the amounts of fatty acids incorporated into phospholipids (PL) and neutral lipids (NL) in SHR myocytes when compared to WKY myocytes.

With regard to the individual fatty acids incorporated into phospholipids (Fig.2), linoleic acid (C18:2) shows the most important reduction (-48%, $0.001<p<0.01$) followed by oleic acid (C18:1, -31%), arachidonic acid (C20:4, -24%) and docosahexaenoic acid (C22:6, -20%). In contrast, the individual fatty acids incorporated into cell neutral lipids were similar in both strains.

This phospholipid deficiency could induce a remodelling of cell structure, which may alter membrane fluidity and play a role in the functional disturbances of the SHR cell membrane. As shown by our preliminary experiments concerning the metabolic pathway of [^{14}C]- unsaturated fatty acids, the deficiency observed in SHR cells could result from an alteration of the phospholipid turnover, involving a decrease in their acylation due, at least in part, to a reduced uptake and/or an enhanced release. This latter is regulated by phospholipase A_2. Indeed an increased phospholipase A_2 activity has been already described in kidneys (Kawaguchi *et al.*. 1986) and aorta of adult SH rats (Limas *et al.*. 1981). Work is now in progress to specify the mechanisms involved.

These lipid alterations observed in newborn cultured heart myocytes suggest that intrinsic factors, probably genetically determined, are active as early as in the first days of life, in the absence of neurohumoral regulations and of hemodynamic stress.

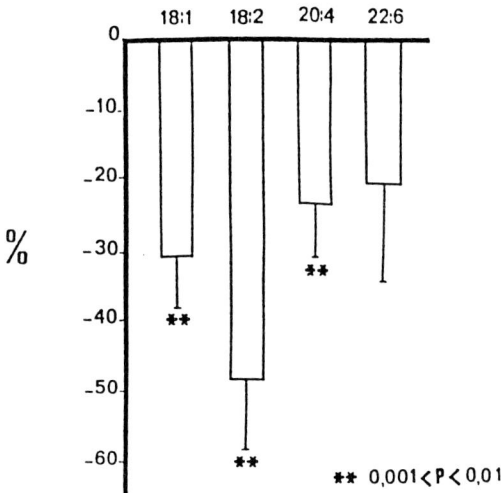

Fig.2: Individual unsaturated fatty acids associated to phospholipids. The results are expressed as the difference in % between SHR and WKY myocytes.

REFERENCES

Aragon-Birlouez, I., Montenay-Garestier, T., Devynck, M. A. (1984): Further analysis of cell membranes in genetic hypertension in rats by diphenyl-hexatriene fluorescence polarization. *Clin. Sci.* 66, 717-72

Clubb, F.J., Bell, P.D., Kriseman, J.D., Bishop, S.P. (1987): Myocardial cell growth and blood pressure development in neonatal spontaneously hypertensive rats. *Lab. Invest* 56, 189-197.

Folch, J., Lees, M., Stanley, G.H.S.(1957): A simple method for the isolation and the purification of total lipids from animal tissues. *J. Biol. Chem.* 226, 497-509.

Freyss-Beguin, M., Millanvoye-Van Brussel, E., Duval, D. (1989):Effect of oxygen deprivation on metabolism of arachidonic acid by cultures of newborn rat heart cells. *Am. J. Physiol.* 247, H444-H451.

Montenay-Garestier, T., Aragon, I., Devynck, M.A., Meyer, P., Helene, C.(1981): Evidence for structural changes erythrocyte in membranes of spontaneously hypertensive rats: a fluorescence polarization study. *Biochem. Biophys.Res Commun.* 160, 660-665.

Kawaguchi, H., Yaduda, H. (1986): Increased phospholipase A_2 activity in the spontaneously hypertensive rats. *J. Hypertension*, 4, S387-S38.

Limas C., Goldam, P., Limas, C. J. (1981): Aortic phospholipid deacylation-reacylation cycle in spontaneously hypertensive rats. *Am. J. Physiol.* 240, H33-H38.

Reddy S.R., Talwalkar, R., Downs, J., Koltchen, T.A. (1989): Effect of linoleic acid infusion on blood pressure in normotensive and hypertensive rats. *Am. J. Physiol.* 257, H611-H617.

Singer, P., Voigt, S., Moritz, V. (1983): Changes of polyunsaturated fatty acids in serum lipids of spontaneously hypertensive rats during the onset of high blood pressure. *Prost. Leuk Med.* 12, 399-408.

Tsuda, K., Tsuda, S., Minatogawa, Y., Iwahashi, H., Kido, R., Masuma, Y. (1988): Decreased membrane fluidity of erythrocytes and cultured vascular smooth muscle cells in spontaneously hupertensive rats: an electron spin resonance study. *Clin.Sci.* 75, 477-480.

Age-related changes in activities of rate-limiting enzymes in lipid metabolism of stroke-prone spontaneously hypertensive rats

Hiroshi Ogawa, Tomoyo Tanaka and Sukenari Sasagawa

Department of Hygiene, Kinki University School of Medicine, 377-2, Ohnohigashi, Osaka-Sayama City, Osaka 589, Japan

The rate-limiting enzymes in plasma lipoprotein metabolism, lipoprotein lipase (LPL) and hepatic triglyceride lipase (H-TGL), play a critical role in the catabolism of plasma lipoprotein. LPL, which is localized on the luminal surface of capillary endothelial cells, catalyzes the hydrolysis of triglycerides of chylomicron (CM) and very low density lipoprotein (VLDL) to their remnants (Nilsson-Ehle et al., 1980). H-TGL, which is located on the sinusoidal surface of the liver, appears to catalyze the hydrolysis of triglycerides and phospholipids constituents of intermediate density lipoprotein (IDL) (Murase & Itakura, 1981) and high density lipoprotein (HDL), especially HDL_2 subclass (Kinnunen, 1984). These two enzymes are released into the circulation as post-heparin plasma lipolytic activity (PHLA) after intravenous injection of heparin.

On the other hand, cholesterol 7α-hydroxylase (7α-hydroxylase) is also the rate-limiting enzyme in the catabolism of hepatic cholesterol and it catalyzes the introduction of a hydroxyl group in 7α-position of cholesterol which is the key step in the catabolism of cholesterol to bile acids in the liver (Myant & Mitropoulos, 1977).

These three kinds of rate-limiting enzymes are thought to be closely related to the development of atherosclerosis and coronary heart diseases. In the present report, we investigated age-related changes in the activities of these rate-limiting enzymes in stroke-prone SHR (SHRSP), to study possible relationship between hypertension and the development of atherosclerosis and to elucidate the characteristic lipid metabolism in SHRSP.

MATERIALS AND METHODS

Male SHRSP and the age-matched male Kyo:Wistar rats (WKY) at various ages until 12 months of age were used. The rats were housed in a polystyrene cage with a 12h/12h light/dark cycle with light on at 8:30 AM and given a stock chow (CE-2, Clea Japan Inc., Osaka). Post-heparin plasma samples were obtained between the hours of 10 and 11 AM from the jugular vein 3 min after intravenous injection of heparin (300 units/kg) under light ether anesthesia without fasting. H-TGL activity in the PHLA was selectively immunoprecipitated by the addition of anti-rat H-TGL antiserum (Ogawa et. al., 1991), and the residual LPL activity and PHLA were measured by RIA method according to the method of Nilsson-Ehle & Schotz (1976) using tri-$[1-^{14}C]$ Oleate as a substrate. H-TGL activity was estimated after subtracting LPL activity from PHLA.

In the case of the measurement of 7α-hydroxylase activity, the animals were killed between the hours of 10 and 11 AM by bleeding after fasting overnight, and their livers were perfused with saline and removed immediately. The hepatic microsomal fraction was separated by ultracentrifugation and suspended in 0.1M phosphate buffer (pH 7.4) containing 1 mM EDTA and used for the assay of 7α-hydroxylase. The enzyme assay was performed using HPLC according to the method of Ogishima & Okuda (1986).

The total lipids of the liver were extracted by the method of Folch et al. (1957) and the contents of cholesterol and phospholipid were enzymatically determined by commercially available kits (Cholesterol C-II test Wako and Phospholipid B test Wako, Wako Pure Chemical Industries, LTD., Osaka).

RESULTS AND DISCUSSION

Age-related changes in activities of plasma rate-limiting enzymes were shown in Fig. 1. LPL activity decreased with age until around 3-4 months of age in both strains. Thereafter, in WKY, the activity gradually increased with age until around 8 months of age, then it appeared to follow almost the same value. However, in SHRSP, the activity showed almost no change from 4 months of age until 12 months of age. The 3-4 months of age corresponds to the established-stage of hypertension in SHRSP. Accordingly, hypertension may secondly affect the LPL activity in SHRSP.

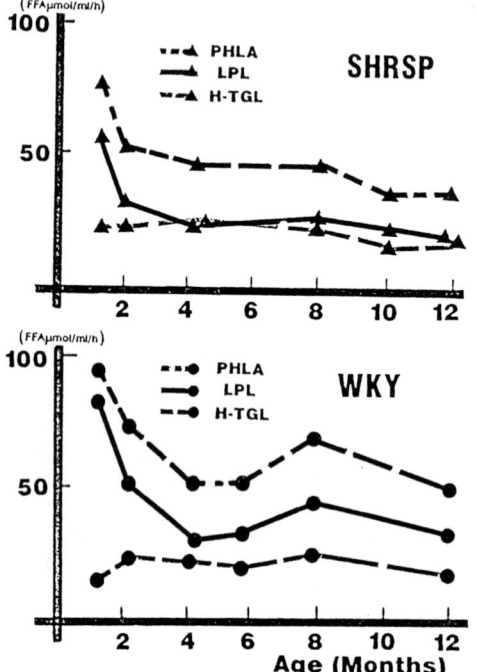

Fig. 1. Age-related changes in post-heparin plasma lipolytic activity (PHLA), and activities of lipoprotein lipase (LPL) and hepatic triglyceride lipase (H-TGL) in SHRSP and WKY.

Moreover, the LPL activity in SHRSP was significantly lower than that in WKY throughout the experimental period. This suggests that genetic factor may reflect the LPL activity in SHRSP. Nikkila et al. (1980) have reported that the HDL (HDL$_2$) particles are formed following the hydrolysis of VLDL triglycerides catalyzed by LPL, and the formation of HDL$_2$ depends on the LPL activity and is promoted under high VLDL turnover. Therefore, the lower activity of LPL in SHRSP indicates a decrease in production of HDL associated with decrease of VLDL turnover compared with WKY. This is in good accordance with our previous report (Ogawa et al., 1985) that HDL, especially apoE-rich HDL which may play an important role in reverse cholesterol transport, is significantly low in SHRSP compared with WKY.

On the other hand, H-TGL activity was not markedly affected by aging and showed almost constant value throughout the experimental period in both strains, and no significant difference was observed between SHRSP and WKY. Kuusi et al. (1982) have shown that the degradation of HDL (HDL$_2$) is enhanced by H-TGL, which catalyzes the hydrolysis of HDL phospholipids and triglycerides. Accordingly, our result suggests that there may be no significant difference in the hepatic uptake of remnants and the degradation of HDL between SHRSP and WKY.

Age-related change in the activity of 7α-hydroxylase was shown in **Fig. 2**. The 7α-hydroxylase activity gradually increased until around 8 months of age in both strains, except in SHRSP at the age of 2 months when the activity markedly increased. Further studies are needed to elucidate this marked increase in SHRSP. No similarity was observed between age-related change in 7α-hydroxylase activity and that in the content of hepatic cholesterol or phospholipid in both strains. However, the activity in SHRSP was significantly lower than that in WKY throughout the experimental period. This suggests that the catabolism of hepatic cholesterol is low in SHRSP compared with WKY, and indicates a rapid increase in hepatic cholesterol when fed a high-cholesterol diet.

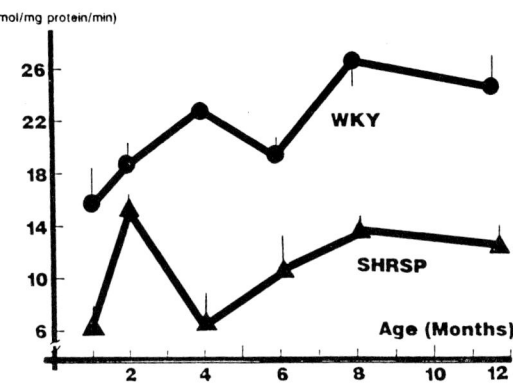

Fig. 2. Age-related change in cholesterol 7α-hydroxylase activity in SHRSP and WKY. The vertical bars indicate the standard error of the mean.

These results provide evidence that activities of LPL and 7α-hydroxylase are genetically low in SHRSP compared with WKY. In addition, they suggest a decrease of HDL production associated with low condition of VLDL turnover and a decrease of catabolism of hepatic cholesterol in SHRSP, resulting in a typical pattern that may be associated with atherosclerosis.

REFERENCES

Folch, J. et al. (1957): A simple method for the isolation and purification of total lipids from animal tissues. J. Biol. Chem. 226, 497-509.

Kinnunen, P.K.J. (1984): Hepatic endothelial lipase. In Lipases, ed. B.Borgstrom & H.L. Brockman, pp. 307-328. Amsterdam: Elsevier Science Publishers B.V..

Kuusi, T. et al. (1982): Function of hepatic lipase in lipoprotein metabolism. In Atherosclerosis VI, ed. G. Schettler, A.M. Gotto, Jr., G. Middelhoff, A.J.R. Hanicht & K.R. Jurutka, pp. 628-632. Berlin: Springer Verlag.

Murase, T. & Itakura, H. (1981): Accumulation of intermediate density lipoprotein in plasma after intravenous administration of hepatic triglyceride lipase antibody in rats. Atherosclerosis 39, 293-300.

Myant, N.B. & Mitropoulos, K.A. (1977): Cholesterol 7α-hydroxylase. J. Lipid Res. 18, 135-153.

Nikkila, E.A. et al. (1980): Lipoprotein lipase and hepatic endothelial lipase are key enzymes in the regulation of plasma HDL, particularly HDL_2. In Atherosclerosis V, ed. A.M. Gotto, Jr., L.C.Smith & B.Allen, pp. 387-392. New York: Springer Verlag.

Nilsson-Ehle, P. & Schotz, M.C. (1976): A stable, radioactive substrate emulsion for assay of lipoprotein lipase. J. Lipid. Res. 17, 536-541.

Nilsson-Ehle, et al. (1980): Lipolytic enzymes and plasma lipoprotein metabolism. Annu. Rev. Biochem. 49, 667-693.

Ogawa, H. et al. (1985): Studies on SHRSP fed on a high-fat and high-cholesterol diet--Alterations of lipo- and apolipoproteins. Jpn. J. Hyg. 40, 627-635.

Ogawa, H. et al. (1991): Effect of cholesterol feeding on the compositions of plasma lipoproteins and plasma lipolytic activities in SHRSP. Clin. Exper. Hypertension 13, in press.

Ogishima, T. & Okuda, K. (1986): An improved method for assay of cholesterol 7α-hydroxylase activity. Anal. Biochem. 158, 228-232.

Reproductive characteristics are modulated by genetic and oviductal uterine milieu after one-cell embryo transfer in spontaneously hypertensive and normotensive rats

Silvia H. Azar and Hugh Hensleigh
with the technical assistance of Elaine Matthys

Departments of Medicine, and Obstetrics and Gynecology, University of Minnesota Medical School, Box 736 UMHC, 516 Delaware Street Southeast, Minneapolis, Minnesota 55455, USA

INTRODUCTION

Several reproductive parameters in spontaneously hypertensive rats (SHR) differ [1] from normotensive Wistar Kyoto rats (WKY)--some of which, genetic factors could account for. But pregnant SHR show higher blood pressure (BP) values than WKY at all gestation stages, with significant reductions in BP [2,3] and utero-placental blood flow [3] prior to parturition--hemodynamic patterns temporally associated with high fetal BP [3]. Therefore adaptive responses must occur in maternal and fetal neuro-endocrine-cardiovascular systems that could alter factors that determine gestation length--besides fetal genotype--such as fetal growth and/or hormonal fetal/maternal communication that starts parturition [4]. SHR have longer gestation periods [1] and smaller litter size and pup body weight [1,5] than WKY. To test whether non-genetic factors contribute to this variability, we analyzed reproductive parameter data from studies which assessed the effects of oviductal-uterine and lactation milieus on pup BP in SHR and WKY [6].

METHODS

The hypothesis was that SHR reproductive patterns are altered by the environmental factors of oviductal-uterine milieu and genetics (SHR and WKY strains [6]). At 12-14 hours post-coitum, environmental manipulation occurred as 1-cell shr or wky homozygous embryos were transferred to SHR or WKY oviducts, reciprocally or homologously. End-points were ovulation and pregnancy rates, number of implanted embryos resulting in births, pregnancy length and body weight gain, litter size and weight, and percentage of small and normal litters.

First generation male and females (SHR/WKY) from Taconic Farms (Germantown, NY, USA), fed Rodent Chow (Ralston Purina, St Louis, MO, USA) ad libitum, were kept in a temperature, humidity and 14 Light/10 Dark controlled room. At 12-16 weeks, females were tested between 19:00-20:00 hours for receptive estrous by using behavioral responses to vasectomized males [8]. Donors and recipients were mated with fertile or vasectomized males respectively and embryo transfers were done 12-14 hours later, in sterile conditions. An assistant assessed body weight, gave anesthesia (methohexital 50mg per kg/body weight), did surgical incisions and kept records. An operator (H.H.) removed oviducts with eggs, put them in BWW media [9], released the embryos from the oviduct and kept them in an incubator [9] until transfer. SHR had fewer eggs, so an SHR donor was added per 2 recipients-as live births and litter survival [1] depend on the number of transplants. After surgery, rats were caged alone. Rats give birth during the day [4,8], so we watched them from day-20 about every 4 hours, from 07:00 to 19:00 hours. Data were analyzed with Student's t, 2-way ANOVA, and logistic regression tests.

RESULTS

Ovulation rates (number of embryos at time of transfer) were 14% higher in WKY (12.5±.3, n=89) than in SHR (11.1±.2, n=87), p<.001. Comparison of ovulation values to the behavioral estrous test's showed the latter was 94% successful for SHR (n=144) and 96% for WKY (n=137). Because of ovulation rate and body weight's direct relationship [1], and interstrain body weight (g) differences (SHR: 210±2; WKY:272±4, p=.0001), we estimated ovulation rates to body weight ratios and found SHR had 13% more embryos relative to body weight (.052±.001, n=144) than WKY (.046±.001, n=137), p<.01. Data means ± sem are shown next.

Reproductive variables: SHR/WKY with homozygous fetuses of homologous or reciprocal shr/wky strain.

Variables	sS	sW	wW	wS
Number of transferred embryos per dam:	12 ± .5 (32)	12 ± .5 (32)	13 ± .5 (28)	13 ±.5 (36)
% of transferred embryos born:	34 ± 6 (32)	43 ± 4 (32)	58 ± 4 (28)	47 ± 5 (36)
Pregnancy rate:	66% (32)	75% (32)	75% (28)	83% (36)
Pregnancy length, hours:	526 ± 2 (12)	515 ± 2 (16)	503 ± 4 (10)	524 ± 2 (17)
Time of birth (hours of light):	4 ± .04 (26)	6.8 ± .6 (24)	7 ± .6 (19)	6.2 ±.4 (29)
Litter size, born pups, live/dead, per litter:	6 ± .7 (21)	7 ± .6 (24)	8 ± .5 (21)	6 ± .4 (30)
% of litters with 6 or more pups:	48% (22)	84% (25)	82% (23)	58% (31)
Average pup body weight/litter:	5.3 ± .1 (22)	5.3 ± .1 (25)	5.9 ± .1 (23)	5.9 ± .1 (31)

Abbreviations. s and w: shr and wky embryo; S and W: SHR and WKY uterus; number of rats shown in parentheses; pregnancy length: day-1 (time of transfer:11:25±.07 hour,n=127) through day of birth.

ANOVA showed the number of transferred embryos, percent developing to term, and pregnancy rate were not affected by uterus or embryo strain--but for both variables, SHR had numerically lower values. Pregnancy length was longer in SHR (sS+wS, 524.5±1.6, n=29) than in WKY (wW+sW, 511.8±2.6, n=26), F=13.6, p=.0001. Parturition time was affected by both factors and their interactions. WKY uterus resulted in births at a more advanced light period (wW+sW, 6.86 ±.4, n=43) than SHR (sS+wS, 5.15±.3, n=55), F=15, p=.001, and an shr embryo shortened time of birth (sS +sW, 5.27±.4, n=50 vs. wW +wS, 6.7±.3, n= 48), F=10, p=.002. But with wky embryos, SHR's time of parturition was lengthened, while shr did not change WKY's, F=3.8, p=.05.

Litter size was not affected by uterus strain, but SHR and WKY with transfer procedures had smaller litters than non-manipulated WKY (11.3±.2, n=105) and SHR (9.4±.3, n=105) dams. A 2-way interaction showed SHR uterus reduced wky litter size, p=.05. Percentages of normal size litters were higher for WKY (wW+sW) than for SHR (sS+sW), F=5.2, p=.0001. Pup body weight was larger for wky (wW+wS) than for shr (sS+sW), F=6.4, p=.001.

DISCUSSION

This study shows oviductal-uterine and embryo strain factors are important determinants of reproductive variability in SHR. Uterus strain accounted for about 90 percent of pregnancy duration, almost two-thirds of time of birth and and about three-fourths of the percent of normal litter size variability. Pup body weight variability was almost entirely due to embryo strain.

Ovulation rate was higher in WKY and we transferred a similar number of embryos, but the average percentage developing to term was 38 for SHR and 52 for WKY, in contrast to non-manipulated SHR (85) and WKY (90). This indicates procedure-related embryo waste--with SHR milieu having a greater effect and WKY improving shr survival. To develop pregnancy after transfer, embryos must be synchronized with uterine events [4]. With optimal synchronization, Gray and Lawrence [1] produced 80 percent pregnancy rates in WKY--similar to our's, yet only 32 percent of their's developed to term compared to our 67. SHR's were even lower-these authors have respective rates of 22 and 34 percent for pregnancy and embryo survival, compared to our.

Our use of 1-cell embryos (they used 8 to 16-cell) could explain the differences (among other factors). It is unlikely that differences between manipulated and non-manipulated dams are due only to time-related synchronization factors as implants were done 12-14 hours after behavioral estrous (similar in both strains), and [unpublished data] shr and wky blastocysts implant at the same time. Some implanted embryos could have been faulty, as seen in 50 percent of human embryos which implant and are then lost. Perhaps synchronization factors levels also had an affect--e.g., anesthesia and surgery stresses alter factors which affect oviductal transport and development of embryos (oviductal fluid volume/composition hormones). Also, because of hyperactivity, SHR respond more to stress. Thus, whether early pregnancy loses were due to chromosomal aberrations and/or adverse maternal milieu and/or faulty implantation is unclear.

Gray and Lawrence found significantly higher embryo waste in wky, we found it in shr. Aside from embryo and donor age, we have no explanation for this. SHR uterine milieu was unfavorable to transferred embryos, suggesting strain-related factors (primary and/or secondary) that decrease embryo viability. At the late morula stage, embryos require a physiological signal to trigger blastocoele formation and expansion for implantation [10]. We found [unpublished data] smaller blastocyst to blastocoele ratios in shr when almost two-thirds of embryos had implanted (SHR: 66±3, n=7, WKY: 69±2, n=7-percentages). Perhaps deficiencies and/or excesses exist in SHR uterine secretions (hormonal, nutrients, electrolytes or others) that do not allow full expansion of the blastocysts at implantation, resulting in faulty implantation and then embryo waste. Improved pregnancy rates and pup numbers in shr with WKY support this possibility.

Within species, fetal genotype is pregnancy length's main determinant; yet, the manner of genotype expression varies. It starts with a surge of fetal corticosterone near birth. Then a maternal hormonal cascade leads to increased estrogen/progesterone ratio production, elaboration of prostaglandin F2 and luteolysis (antepartum decline in relaxin and progesterone), and other factors acting on myometrium, endometrium and cervix, ending with birth [4]. In our study--unexpected from non-polytocous species behavior--pregnancy duration was due to uterus strain with events occurring after implantation as expected. Time of parturition, a circadian event dependent on light cues, is postulated to be maternally determined. Our study showed both factors modulate it.

Number of fetuses may be associated to the luteolytic process and influence time of birth. In our study the differences between strains was not large enough to account for the changes. It has been suggested that there is an endogenous circadian luteolytic process in rats during the antepartum period. If so, its function is altered in SHR. Gestation duration in rats kept in dark is shorter, the interstrain differences in gestation observed by Gray and Lawrence was similar to ours, though they kept a 12 L /12 D cycle.

Thus, both uterus strain and embryo strain influenced reproduction in this model of hypertension.

REFERENCES

1. Gray SD, Lawrence CC. (1983): Reciprocal embryo transfer between spontaneously hypertensive and normotensive rat strains: Reproductive characteristics and transfer technique. Clin Exp Hypertens: Hypertens in Pregnancy B2(3),351-369.
2. Azar S, Sanchez Pena. (1991): Continuous blood pressure monitoring by radio-telemetry during pregnancy and lactation in spontaneously hypertensive and normotensive rats. In Hypertension in Pregnancy, pp119-122. Editors, Cosmi EV and Di Renzo GC. Monduzzi Editore, Bologna, Italy.
3. Azar S, et al. (1986): Umbilical blood pressures and utero-placental blood flow in spontaneously hypertensive rats. J. Hypertens. 4 (suppl 3), pp 369-371.
4. Liggins GC. (1982): The fetus and birth. In Embryonic and Fetal Development. Ed. CR Austin, RV Short, pp 135-141. Cambridge University Press.
5. Azar S, et al. (1991): Environmental factor(s) during suckling exert long-term effects upon blood pressure and body weight in spontaneously hypertensive and normotensive rats J. Hypertens. 9, pp 309-327.
6. Azar S, et al (1991): Oviductal uterine and nursing environment alter blood pressure development in spontaneously hypertensive and normotensive rats. J. Hypertens. (suppl) In press.
7. Okamoto K, Aoki K. (1963): Development of a strain of spontaneously hypertensive rats. Jpn. Circ. J. 27, 282-293.
8. Moore-Ede MC, et al. (1982): Circadian timing of physiological systems. In The Clocks That Time Us, pp. 278-294. Harvard University Press, Cambridge, Massachusetts.
9. Hogan B, et al. (1988): Culture media for preimplantation embryos. In Manipulating the Mouse Embryo. A Laboratory Manual pp. 249-257. Cold Spring Harbor Laboratory, N.Y.
10. Manajwala FM, et al. (1989): Blastocoele expansion in the preimplantation mouse embryo: role of the extracellular sodium and chloride and possible apical routes of entry. Developmental Biology. 133: 210-220.

Effect of hydralazine on the decline in force and fatigue resistance in skeletal muscles from spontaneously hypertensive rats

Sarah D. Gray, Richard C. Carlsen and Richard Atherley

Department of Human Physiology, School of Medicine, University of California, Davis, CA 95616, USA

SUMMARY

Hydralazine was administered to SHR and WKY via the drinking water to determine whether blood pressure per se is responsible for the decreased skeletal muscle performance previously noted in SHR. Blood pressure was lowered by the treatment and some improvement was noted in muscle properties. Nonetheless, aside from its blood pressure lowering propertie, hydralazine itself appears to depress muscle function in normotensive animals so it is difficult to determine the extent to which blood pressure is responsible for the muscle deficit.

INTRODUCTION

Several investigators have shown that, in addition to the well known cardiovascular changes, essential hypertension in humans (Frisk-Holmberg, 1983; Juhlen-Dannfelt, 1979) and spontaneous hypertension in rats (Carlsen & Gray, 1987) are both associated with significant alterations in skeletal muscle function. The human studies suggest that there is a hypertension-induced conversion of slow twitch to fast twitch fibers in mixed muscles. Performance tests in the same human studies suggest that the conversion of slow fibers to fast is correlated with the magnitude of the pressor response elicited by an isometric exercise test. Many skeletal muscle studies (Brown et al., 1976; Hudlicka et al., 1982) have shown that there is a strong positive correlation between fiber type and capillary supply. Conversion of fast to slow fiber types by chronic stimulation results in increased capillary density, along with the enzyme conversion to the highly oxidative profile which characterizes slow muscle. The implications of the human hypertension studies are that metabolic conversion of muscle fibers to the fast type may be associated with a decrease in the capillary supply to the muscle. It isn't clear whether hypertension per se induces the fiber metabolic changes which could then cause alterations in the vascular supply, or whether the hypertension causes a relative capillary ischemia which induces metabolic changes in the fibers. Although one group has reported evidence of slow to fast fiber conversions in SHR skeletal muscles (Ben Bachir-Lamrini, 1990), we found little evidence for altered fiber or capillary distributions in spontaneous hypertension, using histochemical analysis of the muscles (Gray, 1988). However, we did find severe deficits in muscle function in both fast and slow hindlimb muscles of 6 month-old spontaneously hypertensive rats (SHR) that were not found in younger animals (Carlsen & Gray, 1988). An SHR fast muscle, medial gastrocnemius (MG), displayed decreased twitch and maximal tetanic tensions and decreased potentiation (treppe) at the beginning of a fatigue test, when compared to normotensive WKY. SHR slow muscle, soleus (SOL), also showed functional deficits, with a decrease in force generation, as well as a significant decrease in fatigue resistance during a 4 minute fatigue test. The present study is an attempt to determine whether long-term reduction in blood pressure to the normotensive range by administration of hydralazine could ameliorate the muscle deficits noted in SHR.

METHODS

The 8 week antihypertensive regimen was as follows: SHR and WKY rats were given 1% hydralazine in the drinking water from the age of 16 weeks to 24 weeks when the physiological assessment of muscle function was performed. Blood pressure was measured weekly by tail cuff plethysmography. In the acute experiments (see Carlsen and Gray, 1987 for details of the technique), animals were anesthetized with ketamine (85 mg/kg) and xylazine (12 mg/kg) and the distal tendon of either the medial gastrocnemius or soleus muscles isolated, divided and attached to a Grass FT03 force transducer by 1-0 suture. The sciatic nerve was exposed in the popliteal fossa and the sural and common peroneal nerve branches isolated and transected; the tibial nerve was exposed and placed over bipolar platinum hook electrodes and covered with petroleum jelly. Muscle temperature was maintained at 34-35° C by radiant heat. Stimulation parameters for a 4 minute fatigue test were: for MG, 50 Hz for 330 ms, 1 train/sec; for SOL, 40 Hz for 330 ms, 1 train per sec. Muscle lengths and weights were recorded at the end of the experiment.

RESULTS

The hydralazine treatment was effective in lowering the blood pressure. Mean systolic pressure (mm Hg) in untreated animals was: WKY = 119 and SHR = 171; in hydralazine treated it was: WKY = 108 and SHR = 121.

TABLE 1: Comparison of Untreated and Hydralazine-treated Muscle Function Parameters in WKY and SHR (Mean + SE)

	BWt (g)	MWt (g)	BPs (mm Hg)	dPo/dt (g/ms)	Pt (Nx10-2)	Pt/CSA (N/cm2)	Po (Nx10-2)	Po/CSA (N/cm2)	Pt/Po
SOLEUS									
UNTREATED:									
SHR (17)	393 ± 4 *	.167 .003 *#	201.2 3.0 *	5.2 .35	30.2 2.2 #	.51 .05	202.3 11.3	3.47 0.23	.15 .01
WKY (16)	534 ± 12 *	.209 .01 *#	114.3 .8 *	5.7 .3	46.0 2.5 #	.64 .03 #	278.9 11.5	3.95 .19 #	.17 .01
TREATED:									
SHR (11)	399 ± 8 *	.196 .10 *#	120.7 3.3 *	3.3 0.25	39.8 1.7 *#	.57 .04	196.7 10.3	2.76 .12	.21 .01
WKY (9)	525 ± 9 *	.274 .02 *#	107.2 1.0 *	4.4 0.3 *#	48.4 4.7	.51 .042	289.6 20.9 #	3.10 .24 #	.17 .01
MEDIAL GASTROCNEMIUS									
UNTREATED:									
SHR (12)	393 ± 4 *	.967 .02 *	201.2 3.0 *	34.8 1.3	151.4 13.69 *	.531 .048	1066.3 121.1	3.75 .44	.15 .01
WKY (13)	534 ± 12 *	1.36 .06 *#	114.3 .8 *	45.9 3.0	238.6 19.2	.711 .042 #	1383.7 123	4.14 .23 #	.17 .01
TREATED:									
SHR (9)	399 ± 8 *	1.04 .08 *	120.7 3.3 *	34.8 1.3	194.8 11.2	.58 .02	1217.0 45	3.65 .19	.16 .01
WKY (9)	525 ± 9 *	1.64 .11 *#	107.2 1.0 *	39.5 4.3	242.5 14.6	.58 .06 #	1240.0 71.3	2.95 .32 #	.18 .01

ABBREVIATIONS:
BWt = body weight
MWt = muscle weight
BPs = systolic blood pressure
Pt = twitch tension
dPo/dt = rate of rise of tetanus tension
n = ( )
Po = maximum tetanus tension
Pt/Po = twitch-tetanus ratio
Pt/CSA = twitch tension normalized to muscle x-sec A
Po/CSA = tetanus tension normalized to muscle x-sec A
Significance: All * and # <.01
  * = significant difference between strains in the same group
  # = significant difference in treated and untreated of same strain

Hydralazine treatment caused a decrease in blood pressure and an increase in muscle weight. Untreated, absolute and normalized twitch and tetanic tensions were lower in SHR than in WKY. Treated, absolute twitch tension in SHR SOL was increased, but when normalized to x-sec area it was not different; tetanus tension decreased. Treatment decreased both absolute and normalized tetanus tension in WKY soleus. IN MG, normalized twitch and tetanus tension remained unchanged in SHR after treatment, whereas both values declined in WKY.

Figure 1 illustrates the effect of hydralazine on soleus muscle fatigue resistance. Fatigue resistance of untreated SHR soleus was more variable and generally lower than that of WKY soleus. Hydralazine treatment tended to improve fatigue resistance in SHR muscles and did not affect WKY.

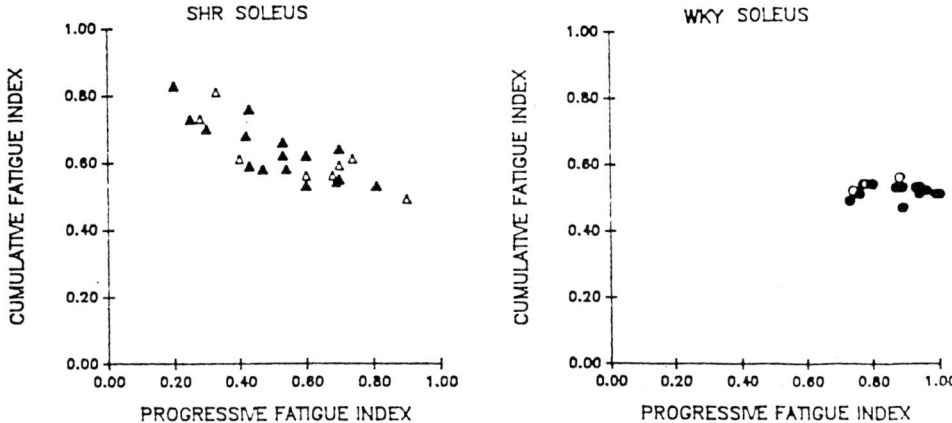

O = open symbols indicate hydralazine treatment
● = filled symbols indicate untreated muscles

DISCUSSION

Although hydralazine was effective in lowering blood pressure to the normotensive range, its effect on muscle performance was not so straightforward. Fatigue resistance was slightly improved in SHR soleus muscle. Functional parameters like twitch and tetanus tension were differentially affected in SHR and WKY. Muscle wet weight was increased in SOL and MG in both strains following treatment with hydralazine. Since absolute contractile force did not increase proportionately with the increase in wet weight, normalized tension actually decreased following hydralazine treatment. This suggests that the increase in wet weight is not the result of muscle hypertrophy, but rather may be a result of a drug-induced increase in intracellular fluid. Although pressure lowering by hydralazine has a slight ameliorative effect on fatigue resistance, the drug appears to have a direct effect on muscle which tends to decrease muscle performance, so that treated muscles may actually be slower and weaker.

ACKNOWLEDGMENT   Supported by NIH grant HL 42463.

REFERENCES

Ben Bachir-Lamrini, L., Sempore, B., Mayet, M-H. & Favier, R. (1990): Evidence of a slow-to-fast fiber type transition in skeletal muscle from spontaneously hypertensive rats. Am. J. Physiol. 258:R352-R357.

Brown, M.D., Cotter, M.A., Hudlicka, O. & Vrbova, G. (1976): The effects of different patterns of muscle activity on capillary density, mechanical properties and structure of slow and fast rabbit muscles. Pfluger's Arch. 361:241-250.

Carlsen, R.C. & Gray, S.D. (1987): Decline of isometric force and fatigue resistance in skeletal muscles from spontaneously hypertensive rats. Exper. Neurol. 95:249-264.

Frisk-Holmberg, M., Essen, B., Fredrikson, M., Strom, G. & Wibell, L. (1983): Muscle fibre composition in relation to blood pressure response to isometric exercise in normotensive and hypertensive subjects. Acta Med. Scand 213:21-26.

Gray, S.D. (1988): Histochemical analysis of capillary and fiber-type distributions in skeletal muscles of spontaneously hypertensive rats. Microvasc. Res. 36:228-238.

Hudlicka, O., Dodd, L., Renkin, E.M. & Gray, S.D. (1982): Early changes in fiber profile and capillary density in long-term stimulated muscles. Am. J. Physiol. 243:H528-H535.

Juhlen-Dannfelt, A., Frisk-Holmberg, M., Karlsson, J., & Tesch, P. (1979): Central and peripheral circulation in relation to muscle-fibre composition in normo- and hyper-tensive man. Clin. Sci. 56:335-340.

Kidney function and renal factors

Facteurs rénaux

Renal factors involved in the pathogenesis of genetic forms of hypertension

Giuseppe Bianchi and Patrizia Ferrari

Chair of Nephrology, University of Milan, Department of Nephrology Dialysis and Hypertension, S. Raffaele Hospital, Via Olgettina 60, Milano 20132, (Italy) and Prassis Sigma Tau Research Institute, Via Forlanini 3, Settimo Milanese 20019, Milano, Italy

SUMMARY

The renal function studies carried out in four rat models of genetic hypertension, namely Dahl, Lyon, Milan Hypertensive Strain (MHS) and Spontaneously Hypertensive Rat (SHR), are described here in an attempt to identify similarities or differences among them. This attempt is hampered by methodological differences and the genetic heterogeneity within at least two of these strains. However, even with these provisos, some conclusions may still be drawn. In three of these strains (Dahl, MHS and SHR) where kidney cross transplantation experiments were performed, the kidneys of the hypertensive strains caused higher blood pressure than those of their appropriate normotensive control strains, independently of the recipient. This effect also occurred at the pre-hypertensive stage. In the Lyon, Dahl and SHR strains, GFR tended to be lower and renal vascular resistance higher, while the opposite pattern occurred in MHS, where a marked increase in tubular reabsorption was also observed, together with higher interstitial hydrostatic pressure at the pre-hypertensive stage. A renal sodium retention occurring during the development of hypertension, and an increase in a ouabain-like or pressor humoral factor have been detected in those strains that were measured (MHS, Dahl and SHR). A rightward shift of the pressure natriuresis curve was observed at kidney level in all four strains. In conclusion, a primary clear cut abnormality has been detected in Dahl, MHS and SHR strains, even though the cellular mechanisms underlying such an abnormality may differ in these three strains of rats.

INTRODUCTION

The evaluation of renal mechanisms in genetic hypertension is hampered by the interrelationships between renal function and many other physiological functions such as blood pressure, body fluids and electrolytes with all their regulatory hormones, sympathetic drive to the kidney etc. In fact, it is almost impossible to establish whether a given kidney abnormality detected in the whole animal arises from a primary renal alteration or is secondary to some other extrarenal factor. On the other hand, the usefulness of the animal models of genetic hypertension in the detection of the primary genetic-molecular mechanisms responsible for "genetic" or "essential" types of human hypertension also depends upon our ability to dissect, within the complex arrays of the whole body's physiological interrelationships, those peculiar functions which are directly affected by the primary genetic mechanism responsible for hypertension. Therefore, in our discussion we shall attempt to separate primary from secondary renal alterations. We shall also try to illustrate, in at least one strain, the methodological problems involved in the detection of the biochemical-cellular events responsible for the primary renal alteration. Consequently, our discussion will focus upon the following three points:

1) - Effect of renal transplantation on blood pressure;

2) - Different types of renal pressor mechanisms at work in the different strains of rats evaluated by: a) studies on isolated kidneys, with special regard to the pressure-natriuresis curve; b) studies on the whole animal.

3) - Biochemical-cellular mechanisms underlying renal mechanisms in at least one of these strains.

Because of space limitations we can only consider here the findings obtained in four strains, namely Dahl, Lyon, SHR and MHS, which are also the best studied strains with regard to their kidney function.

RENAL TRANSPLANTATION

For the reasons given in the introduction, it is clear that the most straightforward experiment for the evaluation of a primary pressor role of the kidney is its cross-transplantation between genetic hypertensive rats and their appropriate controls. In this case also, secondary kidney modifications can interfere with the interpretation of the results. However, transplantation at the prehypertensive stage or between animals whose blood pressure has been kept at a normal level with antihypertensive treatment, can eliminate this type of interference.

Dahl strain. There are two strains of Dahl rats one (DS/Jr) that is fully inbred and the other (DS) that seems not yet fully inbred (O'Dowd & Rapp 1991). Unfortunately, kidney cross-transplantation experiments have only been carried out in the second strain (Dahl et al 1972, Dahl et al 1974, Dahl & Heine 1975, Morgan et al 1990). Because of the peculiarity of these rats, which develop hypertension only when fed with a high salt diet (Dahl et al 1968), the pressor secondary kidney changes could be excluded. So far, the results of two research groups are available (Dahl et al 1972, Dahl et al 1974, Dahl & Heine 1975, Morgan et al 1990) and they consistently show that: on low salt diet DS rats (which develop hypertension on high salt diet) had lower blood pressure when they received a kidney from a DR rat (which remains normotensive on a high salt diet) than when they received a DS kidney, and vice versa, the blood pressure of DR rats increased when given a DS kidney. That is, DS kidney caused higher (aprox. +10 mmHg) levels of BP, irrespective of the recipients. On high salt diet DR rats developed hypertension only when transplanted with a DS kidney, while DS rats developed hypertension independently of the type of transplanted kidney (DS or DR), even though DS rats receiving a DS kidney showed slightly higher BP levels than when receiving a DR kidney. Therefore, beside the primary renal mechanism some other extrarenal mechanisms must be at work in DS rats receiving a high salt diet.

SHR strain. Three research groups carried out kidney cross-transplantation between SHR and Wistar Kyoto (WKY) rats (Coburn et al 1972, Kawabe et al 1979, Rettig et al 1990A, Rettig et al 1990B). The genetic heterogeneity of these two strains of rats has been subsequently shown (Nabika et al 1991) however, after the preliminary negative results obtained by Coburn et al (1972), the other two groups (Kawabe et al 1979, Rettig et al 1990A, Rettig et al 1990B) showed that the kidney removed from SHR caused a higher level of blood pressure in F_1 than the kidney removed from WKY. Furthermore, Rettig et al (1990B), in a very detailed and carefully conducted study, demonstrated that a very significant portion of the blood pressure difference between a substrain of SHR (the stroke prone SHR developed in Heidelberg) and its control WKY strain was due to a primary kidney alteration, even though other extrarenal mechanisms could contribute to the blood pressure difference between the two strains.

MHS strain. Kidney cross-transplantation between adult MHS and their controls, the Milan normotensive strain (MNS), showed that the kidney of MHS caused higher blood pressure in the recipient than the kidney of MNS (Bianchi et al 1974). This difference was also noted when transplantation was carried out at a very young age, where only a small difference in blood pressure between the two strains was found and very similar results were obtained (Fox and Bianchi 1976).

Lyon strain. to our knowledge kidney cross-transplantation has not been carried out yet in this strain.

In conclusion, in all the three strains where kidney cross transplantation has been carried out a significant pressure effect of the kidney removed from the hypertensive strains has been found and this effect has been attributed to a primary kidney dysfunction.

STUDIES ON ISOLATED KIDNEYS AND COMPARISONS WITH THE KIDNEY FUNCTION *IN VIVO*.

The comparisons among the different strains is hampered by the differences in the methods used to study the function of isolated kidneys and by the genetic heterogeneity of the SHR and Dahl strains. However, we may try to overcome these problems by selecting those results which have been obtained under comparable experimental conditions. For instance, the results obtained with isolated kidneys perfused with artificial medium plus albumin or of whole blood will be discussed separately.

Dahl strain. In artificial perfusion medium the function (GFR, RBF, Na and H_2O excretion) of kidneys removed from DS and DR rats, kept on low or high salt diet, did not seem to differ with the exception of vascular resistance which was higher in DS kidney (Steele & Challoner-Hue 1988). When perfused with whole blood both *in vitro* (Tobian *et al* 1978) or *in situ* (Roman 1986), but with a particular experimental set up which allowed the influence of extrarenal hormonal or nervous factors to be minimized (Roman 1986), the function of the DS kidney differed from that of the DR kidney. In fact, GFR and Na excretion were lower while renal vascular resistance was higher in DS when perfused at the same hydrostatic pressure of DR. The kidneys from animals on high salt diet, showed greater differences in function than the kidneys from animals on low salt diet (Roman 1986). Kidney function differences were also seen in the whole animal when measured in Dahl rats purchased from Brookhaven (DS) as compared to Dahl rats inbred by John Rapp (DS/Jr) (Roman & Kaldunski, In press). In fact, the GFR of the latter was definitely lower (-39%), compared to its control (DR/Jr), while this difference was less (-25%) when GFR of DS was compared to GFR of DR. This small difference was due to the high variability of the DS values. In some DS animals GFR was reduced by 50% (as in DS/Jr strain), in some DS animals GFR was identical to the values observed in the DR/Jr rats. This may reflect the genetic heterogeneity of the DS rats produced in Brookhaven (O'Dowd 1991).

The marked decrease of total GFR in DS/Jr rats, together with a much greater heterogeneity of single nephron GFR, may be due to the progressive glomerular disease described by Sterzel *et al* (1988). This glomerulopathy may also account for the proteinuria of DS/Jr rats and for the clear-cut increased values of BP on low salt diet of DS/Jr rats compared to DR/Jr rats (151± 4 vs 130 ± 5 mm Hg) (Roman & Kaldunski 1991). Probably the minor differences in the change in single nephron function observed by Azar *et al* (1978) in the DS rats from Brookhaven was due to the relatively lesser degree of inbreeding occurring in the rats used by these AA.

A careful study of the **pressure-natriuresis** relationship was carried out on the kidney perfused *in situ* with blood and under well controlled hormonal and nervous influences (Roman & Kaldunski, in press). This study showed that on low salt diet both in DS and DS/Jr rats, the slope of the relationship curve was lower as compared to those of DR and DR/Jr rats, the slope in DS/Jr rats being slightly lower than DS. In other words, both DS and DS/Jr kidneys required higher renal perfusion pressure to excrete the same amount of sodium. On a high salt diet, a shift towards the right of the pressure-natriuresis curve of DS/Jr rather than a change in the slope was observed. The same changes were observed for GFR, while RBF was not statistically different in the four strains at all the perfusion pressures and was well autoregulated on the low salt diet while on the high salt diet RBF tended to be lower in DS/Jr than in DR/Jr. The same AA, using basically the same techniques, studied the excretion of Na, Cl and H_2O handling in the different portions of the nephron (Roman & Kaldunski 1991). Proximal tubular and collecting duct reabsorption was found to be lower while loop of Henle reabsorption was higher in DS/Jr as compared to DR/Jr. When DS were compared with DR the same changes were observed but they reached the statistical significance only for the Henle's loop data.

The above studies (Roman 1986, Roman & Kaldunski, in press) were carried out in denervated kidneys, the rats were adrenalectomized, and the plasma levels of aldosterone, norepinephrine, hydrocortisone and vasopressin were kept constant. **Cortical and papillary blood flow** and **renal interstitial pressure** were similar in DR/Jr and DS/Jr on low salt diet at all the perfusion pressures (Roman & Kaldunski, in press). On high salt diet papillary flow and renal interstitial pressure were lower in DS/Jr than in DR/Jr when the kidney perfusion pressure was increased. Therefore, on low salt diet the decrease in the pressure-natriuresis slope of the DS/Jr was not accompanied by any change in the above mentioned hormonal or physical factors. Conversely, a lower increase in renal interstitial pressure in DS/Jr rats may contribute to this rightward shift of the pressure-natriuresis curve.

In view of these findings, which demonstrate an impairment of the DS kidney's ability to excrete Na^+ (rightward shift of the pressure-natriuresis curve, increased tubular Na^+ reabsorption), it has been suggested that this intrinsic renal defect may trigger the release of a saluretic substance able, on the one hand, to normalize the Na handling but, on the other hand, responsible for the systemic increase of vascular resistance (de Wardener & MacGregor 1980). The first experiment, using parabiotic techniques, supported this hypothesis (Dahl *et al* 1967), demonstrating that when DR and DS rats, on high Na diet, were joined by parabiosis, DR developed a marked hypertension while DS showed BP levels lower than those of single DS or DS + DS rats (Dahl *et al* 1967). More direct measurements of such a substance have not as yet been performed in DS and DR rats, but its analogy with the circulating ouabain-like factor detected in various forms of genetic (de Wardener *et al* 1987, Wauquier *et al* 1988) and essential hypertension (MacGregor *et al* 1981, Hamlyn *et al* 1982), is very likely.

In conclusion, the most clear-cut abnormalities in DS/Jr kidney are: 1) a reduction of the overall glomerular filtration rate which may be secondary to the glomerular morphological abnormalities described by Sterzel *et al* (1988) and 2) a decrease in fractional Na, Cl and H_2O excretion, which seems to be secondary to an increased reabsorption along the Henle's loop (Roman & Kaldunski 1991). This increased tubular reabsorption also seems to be due to a primary change in tubular handling of Na and Cl since no difference between DS/Jr and DR/Jr in medullary flow or renal interstitial pressure was detected, at least on the low salt diet.

The body fluids and hemodynamic changes occurring in DS and DR when salt intake was increased were consistent with a volume dependent hypertension. In fact, the same degree of plasma volume expansion occurred both in DS and DR rats, however, the blood pressure of DS was approximately 25 mm Hg higher after 24h of high salt diet, implying a right-shift in the pressure-natriuresis curve (Greene *et al* 1990). Moreover, the prevention of volume expansion on high salt diet, blocked the development of hypertension in DS (Greene *et al* 1990).

Lyon strain. Liu *et al* (1991) evaluated the function of isolated kidney removed from genetically hypertensive Lyon (LH) rats, normotensives (LN) and low blood pressure (LL) controls. Kidneys were perfused with an artificial medium (Krebs-Henseleit) containing a gelatin derivative as an oncotic agent. Under basal conditions GFR and urinary Na excretion were lower while vascular resistance was higher in LH compared to LN and LL values and the excretion of prostanoid metabolites (TxB_2, 6-keto-$PGF1\alpha$, $PGF2\alpha$, and PGE_2) were not statistically different in the three strains. During norepinephrine or phenylephrine infusion prostanoid excretion increased in all the three types of kidneys but the magnitude of TxB_2 increase was significantly greater in the LH kidneys. The slope of the pressure-natriuresis curve was significantly lower in LH kidney compared to the other two and the infusion of a thromboxane antagonist enhanced this slope only in LH kidney.

Studies in the whole animal showed that the turnover of norepinephrine was elevated in the kidney of LH rats (Sautel *et al* 1988) and the urinary excretion of 6-Keto-$PGF1\alpha$ and of TxB_2 was markedly increased in LH (Geoffroy *et al* 1986). Taken together, these results seem to indicate that the elevated prostanoid renal excretion is secondary to an increased sympathetic drive to the kidney in LH. These kidney hormonal changes may be relevant to the pathogenesis of hypertension since the treatment of LH with a thromboxane synthetase antagonist (OKY 046) or a thromboxane A_2 receptor blocker (AH 23848) almost normalized blood pressure (Geoffroy *et al* 1990). Interestingly, these two compounds given at 3 weeks of age required another 3 weeks of delay to exhibit their antihypertensive action and the effect persisted 1 more week after cessation of the treatment with AH 23848 (Geoffroy *et al* 1990).

In conclusion, the most significant difference between LH kidneys and the kidneys of the other strains LN and LL are: increased vascular resistances, noradrenalin turnover and TxB_2 production in LH kidneys which also display, when perfused *in vitro*, a lower GFR and urinary sodium excretion with a reduced slope of the pressure-natriuresis curve under norepinephrine infusion.

SHR Strain. The function of the isolated kidneys of adult SHR and WKY rats was measured using an artificial medium with and without albumin at different perfusion pressures (Firth *et al* 1989). At any pressure, SHR kidney perfused with albumin showed lower values of plasma flow, GFR, urinary sodium and FENa and FELi (fractional excretion of lithium as an estimation of proximal tubular resorption) while the fractional handling of Na and H_2O at the distal sites of the nephron (based on the assumption that Li was handled only in the proximal tubules) was similar in the two kidney strains at all pressures. When albumin was omitted from the perfusion, there was a marked increase in urinary Na in the kidneys of the two strains (more than 20 times the values in presence of albumin) and the values of SHR kidney were higher than those of WKY. GFR was also higher in SHR kidney while the FENa was similar and FELi tended to be lower than that seen in presence of albumin, however, the difference was small. When the same study was repeated in young (4 weeks old) SHR and WKY rats, the only detectable differences between the two types of kidneys were an increased vascular resistance and a higher FENa at any pressure, and a type of leftward shift of the pressure-natriuresis curve in SHR kidneys. FELi was not measured at this age (Salvati *et al* 1987A).

Roman (1987) studied the function of isolated SHR and WKY kidneys perfused *in situ* with blood (described for Dahl rats in the previous paragraph) to minimize nervous and hormonal differences between the two strains. In young (3-5 weeks old) animals GFR and RPF were similar at any pressure while the excretion of Na and H_2O were shifted towards the right in SHR as pressure increased. (Roman 1987). The same study carried out in adult rats (10-20 week old) gave basically the same results with a greater shift and a lower slope of the **pressure-natriuresis** curve in SHR (Roman & Cowley 1985). While no difference in GFR, RBF or peritubular and glomerular capillary pressures were detected. In spite of the similar changes in whole renal and cortical blood flow, the increase of **papillary blood flow** with increasing perfusion pressure was not as high in SHR as in WKY (42). This phenomenon was present both in young (3-5 week old) and adult rats, where it was more marked.

A lower papillary blood flow would explain the decrease of the medullary interstitial hydrostatic pressure. This reduction in medullary pressure, in presence of the renal capsule, would be transmitted to the whole kidney. Because of the well documented positive relationship between kidney interstitial hydrostatic pressure and tubular reabsorption, Roman (1990) & Cowley (in press) proposed that the lower kidney interstitial hydrostatic pressure for any given kidney perfusion pressure could be responsible for the rightward shift of the pressure-natriuresis curve in SHR. As the medullary blood flow derives exclusively from the perfusion of the juxtamedullary nephrons, it was logical to study the pressure-diameter relationship of the preglomerular vasculature of the adult SHR and the WKY juxtamedullary nephrons, under controlled conditions and after blockade of the vascular tone with a low calcium solution. The tone in SHR preglomerular vessels was greater than that in WKY (Gebremedhim et al 1990). Low calcium solution abolished this difference while indomethacine had no effect. This study was carried out on the isolated kidney perfused with a physiological salt solution (Gebremedhim et al 1990).

Arendshorst et al (Arendshorst 1979, Dilley & Arendshorst 1984, Dilley et al 1984, Arendshorst et al 1990) studied the role of the kidney in the pathogenesis of hypertension in SHR. Their major findings were:

1) In the whole animal, as compared to WKY, 6 week old SHR were moderately hypertensive and had reduced GFR, RBF and an increased renal vascular resistance (Dilley et al 1984). At 12-14 week of age when hypertension is fully developed in SHR, GFR and RBF were similar in the two strains (Dilley & Arendshorst 1984, Arendshorst & Beierwaltes 1979). The reduction of GFR at young age seemed to be due to enhanced tubuloglomerular feed-back, reduced ultrafiltration coefficient and glomerular plasma flow (Dilley & Arendshorst 1984).

2) The renal vascular tone in young SHR was more dependent on angiotensin converting enzyme activity than in WKY (Arendshorst et al 1990). The vascular reactivity to Angiotensin II was enhanced in SHR and indomethacin abolished the strain difference in the renal response to Angiotensin (Chatziantoniou et al 1990).

3) Exaggerated salt and water renal retention occurred during the development of hypertension in young SHR in relation to age-matched WKY (Beierwaltes et al 1982).

These findings have been confirmed by other investigators (Harrap & Doyle 1986, Harrap et al 1986) under more or less different experimental conditions, but without minimizing the influence of nervous or hormonal influences to the kidney as did Roman & Cowley (1985). In particular, Harrap & Doyle (1988) showed that the reduction of renal blood flow and GFR in young SHR was associated with the development of hypertension, even though with genetic cosegregation studies a genetic association could not be demonstrated between blood pressure and the total exchangeable body sodium (Harrap 1986). The major discrepancy between the results obtained by Arendshorst et al in the whole animal (Arendshorst 1979, Arendshorst et al 1990, Dilley & Arendshorst 1984, Dilley et al 1948) and those obtained by Roman (Roman 1987, Roman & Cowley 1985) with isolated kidney in situ are the differences in RBF and GFR between young SHR and WKY. As discussed above, the latter groups of AA failed to find a reduced RPF and GFR in young SHR and, according to their results, the shift in the pressure-natriuresis curve was due to a greater tubular reabsorption of Na and water (Roman 1987). However, according to Roman et al (1988) the greater tubular reabsorption in SHR was secondary to a lower renal interstitial pressure which, in turn, was due to a lower papillary blood flow. Therefore, in this case also, the increase in the preglomerular vascular tone of the juxtamedullary nephrons could be the primary cause of the shift of the pressure-natriuresis curve.

<u>In conclusion,</u> the overall body of data so far obtained by studying the renal function of SHR support the notion that the most likely intrarenal major cause responsible for the shift of the pressure-natriuresis curve and for the pressure effect of the kidney after transplantation is an increased tone of the preglomerular vessels even though a primary difference in tubular handling of Na and H_2O between SHR and WKY may not be entirely excluded. The enhanced renal vascular tone in SHR may certainly be influenced by the sympathetic drive to the kidney and could partly explain the discrepancy between the data obtained from the whole animals and those obtained from the isolated kidney.

Kallikrein, renin, different arachidonic acid metabolites, mineralocorticoid hormones, and catecholamine may all have an influence on both the vascular tone and the tubular reabsorption of Na and H_2O (Cowley, et al, 1991). As synthesis and activity of these substances in SHR and WKY kidneys have been shown to be different, at least during some phases of hypertension or under particular experimental circumstances (Shibouta et al 1981, Sinaiko & Mirkin 1974, Berecek et al 1980), to our knowledge, it is not possible to establish whether the shift of the pressure-natriuresis curve in SHR is due to some primary alteration of one of the pathways responsible for the production of these substances or if it is due to some primary alteration of the function of those cells directly involved in the pressure-natriuresis curve such as: tubular, vascular muscle, or glomerular cells. Whatever the primary mechanism is, the experiments of kidney transplantation clearly indicate that it must be an intrarenal mechanism.

MHS strain. When the function of **isolated kidneys** from young (4 weeks old) MHS and MNS was studied *in vitro* by using an artificial medium (Krebs-Heinseleit) plus albumin and 1 mM Ca^{++} the following results were obtained (Salvati et al 1984, Salvati et al 1987B). GFR, urinary flow, overall tubular sodium reabsorption and Kidney O_2 consumption were greater while vascular resistance was lower in the MHS kidney. These differences were influenced by the concentration of Ca in the perfusate, in fact, raising the concentration to 1,25 mM, the differences in GFR, tubular Na reabsorption and O_2 consumption disappeared while the difference in urinary flow increased and an impairment of concentrating ability appeared in MHS kidney (Salvati et al 1987B).

The **pressure-natriuresis** curves expressed as the relation between perfused pressure and fractional excretion of Na (Salvati et al 1987A) were similar in young MHS and MNS, however it must be noticed that, because of the much higher level of GFR in MHS, the tubular Na load was much higher in MHS than in MNS (102 vs 52 mmol/min/g kidney weight) in order to achieve the same urinary Na excretion (2 mmol/min/g kidney weight). Kidneys removed from adult animals showed almost the same functional differences except vascular resistances which were similar in the two strains and the pressure-natriuresis curve (expressed as the relation between perfusion pressure and fractional excretion of Na) that was shifted toward the right in MHS (Salvati et al 1987A). Taken together, these results support the notion that a primary increase of tubular reabsorption in MHS may cause both the renal functional changes observed *in vitro* and the greater pressure effect after kidney transplantation. To gain further information about the mechanisms underlying tubular reabsorption in MHS the effects of three diuretics amiloride, hydrochlorothiazide and bumetanide were tested on the same isolated kidney preparation using kidneys removed from young MHS and MNS (Salvati et al 1990). The tubular effect of bumetanide in MHS kidneys was much greater and it appeared at a lower concentration as compared to the effect of bumetanide in the MNS kidney or to the effect of the other two diuretics in the MHS kidney. Also the natriuretic effect of ouabain (10^{-3} M) was much greater in MHS than in the MNS isolated kidney (Foulkes et al, in press), however, this difference appeared only when ouabain was given to kidneys after 75 minutes of *in vitro* perfusion, but it was not present when ouabain was given after only 15 minutes of perfusion. It must be noted here that the natriuretic response to hydrochlorothiazide is similar in MHS and MNS at the two time-intervals of perfusion. Therefore, it was likely that perfusion *in vitro* of isolated MHS kidneys removed some factors which prevent the full tubular action of ouabain (Foulkes et al, in press). Consistent with these findings, there is other evidence supporting the presence of higher levels of circulating ouabain-like factors in MHS than in MNS. In particular, Holland et al (1987) found, by a cytochemical assay, a big increase of the plasma inhibitory activity on the Na-K ATPase both of young and adult MHS, as compared to MNS. Furthermore, MHS hypothalamus contained 2-3 fold more ouabain-like factor than MNS (Ferrandi et al 1991).

The **studies on the whole animals** may be summarized as follows: GFR and urinary flow were greater while plasma and renal renin were lower in young MHS than in MNS of the same age and these differences tended to disappear as hypertension was fully developed in MHS (Bianchi et al 1975, Ferrari et al 1982). Balance studies showed a renal Na retention in MHS during the development of hypertension (Bianchi et al 1975). Micropuncture studies in young MHS and MNS showed that the single nephron GFR was greater in MHS which also show a greater whole kidney GFR, a blunted tubuloglomerular feed back mechanisms and an increased renal interstitial hydrostatic pressure (Boberg & Persson 1986). After few days, when a 20 mmHg blood pressure difference between MHS and MNS was present, the renal interstitial pressure difference became similar in the two strains, glomerular tubular feedback became more activated in MHS and the difference in the whole and single nephron GFR tended to disappear.

COMPARISONS AMONG THE FOUR STRAINS

As underlined in the introduction there are many problems when trying to compare the different strains of rats because of: 1) differences in the methods and experimental conditions used for measuring renal function 2) difficulties in dissecting primary from secondary kidney function changes and in selecting those experimental results which better reflect the function of the kidney in its body environment 3) genetic heterogeneity in the SHR and Dahl strains. However, in spite of these provisos, in Table 1 we have tried to summarize the results discussed so far. When contrasting results were found (for instance the question of GFR and RPF in the prehypertensive stage of SHR) we included in the table those results that were obtained under the experimental conditions that were closer to the *in vivo* conditions and the reader should consult the comprehensive and balanced view of this aspects in the previous paragraphs. From the data on Table 1, some general statements can be made; findings which are common to all the strains where the appropriate experiment has been performed:

1) by kidney transplantation it is possible to "transplant" hypertension or a significant portion of it; 2) a renal retention of Na has been found during the development of hypertension; 3) a right-ward shift of the pressure-natriuresis curve with an increased tubular reabsorption in at least a portion of the nephron; 4) an increase of a ouabain-like or pressor plasma factor.

Table 1. Comparisons among the four strains of rats. (more detailed comparisons and limitations explained in text).

	Dahl	Lyon	MHS	SHR
1) Pressor effect of the kidney after transplantation				
- prehypertensive stage	↑		↑	↑
- hypertensive stage	↑ or =		↑	↑
2) Pressure-Natriuresis curve				
- prehypertensive stage	RS			RS
- hypertensive stage	RS and ↓ S	↓ S	RS	RS and ↓ S
3) Tubular Na reabsorption				
- prehypertensive stage	↑		↑	↑
- hypertensive stage	↑		↑	↑
4) Ouabain-like or pressor plasma factors at the hypertensive stage	↑		↑	↑
5) Renal Na retention during the development of hypertension	↑		↑	↑
6) GFR - prehypertensive stage	↓		↑	↓
- hypertensive stage	↓↓	↓	=~↑	=
7) Renal vascular resistances				
- prehypertensive stage	↑		↓	↑
- hypertensive stage	↑	↑	=	↑
8) Renal interstitial hydrostatic pressure				
- prehypertensive stage	=		↑	↓
- hypertensive stage	↓		=	↓

RS = Rightward shift of the Pressure-Natriuresis curve
S = Slope of the Pressure-Natriuresis curve
↑ = ↓ (increased, equal or decreased in the hypertensive strain as compared to its appropriate control)

As far as renal vascular resistance and GFR are concerned, two functional patterns have been found. In Dahl, SHR and Lyon rats renal vascular resistance are increased and GFR is reduced while in MHS the opposite change occurs. It is interesting to note that also in offspring of hypertensive patients these different patterns of renal function have been found (Bianchi et al 1983, Van Hooft et al 1991). In MHS there is also an increase of renal interstitial pressure while in SHR there is a decrease of this variable and in Dahl rats no significant change, at least in the prehypertensive phase. These data demonstrate:

1) the central role of the kidney in different types of genetic hypertension as suggested by Guyton many years ago (Guyton & Coleman 1969);

2) different pathophysiological patterns of renal abnormalities may occur in different strains;

3) increased renal vascular tone and reduced GFR as the most clear-cut renal function abnormalities in those strains (SHR, LH and Dahl) where increased sympathetic drive seems to contribute to the pathogenesis of hypertension (Bianchi et al 1990). In particular, the opposite effect on blood pressure was found when the influence of acute mental stress was studied in parallel in MHS and SHR (increase in SHR and decrease in MHS) (Hallback et al 1977, Hallback & Folkow 1974).

BIOCHEMICAL-CELLULAR MECHANISMS

With the provisos underlined above, we may try to define those types of cells whose alterations may be responsible for the renal dysfunction of each strain. From the previous discussion, it would seem that vascular smooth muscle or glomerular cells in Dahl, SHR and LH and tubular cell in MHS are the cells that should be used for detecting the primary genetic-molecular mechanisms. In Dahl, SHR and LH nervous cells, particularly the sympathetic nerve endings, should also be considered in this respect. For MHS the only way in which we can explain the greater pressor effect after transplantation of a kidney, which displays *in vitro* increased GFR and tubular reabsorption together with a lower vascular resistances, is to postulate that the primary cause of hypertension consists of an increased tubular reabsorption of sodium and water.

Again, space limitations and the lack of some crucial data do not allow an integrated discussion which could include the available data at cellular-biochemical levels in SHR, Dahl and LH strains, in an attempt to identify a genetic molecular mechanism responsible for the above described renal functional changes. In fact, if we admit that genetic factors are responsible for an important portion of the blood pressure difference between these hypertensive strains and their appropriate controls, we have to conclude that some molecular-biochemical difference may underlie these physiological differences. We may summarize the data (in this regards) so far accumulated in the MHS, to illustrate the type of problems we have to face in order to accomplish this task and the usefulness of identifying a precise pathophysiological link between organ dysfunction and cellular dysfunction for the detection of the genetic molecular mechanisms.

The faster Na transport across the tubular cells of MHS detected in the isolated kidney perfused *in vitro* was confirmed when isolated luminal membranes or tubuli were studied (Ferrandi *et al* 1990, Hanozet *et al* 1985) (74,75). In fact, it was shown that the Na/H countertransport in brush border vesicles (Hanozet *et al* 1985) (75), the Na-K cotransport in luminal membrane of the tick ascending limb (Ferrandi *et al* 1990) and the Na-K ATPase of the proximal and ascending limb portions of the tubuli (Melzi *et al* 1989) were all working at a faster rate in MHS preparations than in MNS preparations. However, at this step, it was not possible to distinguish between intrinsic cellular abnormalities leading to a faster rate of ion transport and extracellular abnormalities such as increased tubular load or abnormal hormonal tissue systems (Renin, prostaglandin, kallicrein, etc.) which may influence tubular reabsorption *in vivo* and their effect may persist on the cell membrane studied in vitro. Based on the assumption that a genetic cellular abnormality may also be present in other cells, which may not be affected by the same extracellular influences of the renal cells we have studied erythrocytes. MHS erythrocytes and MHS tubular cells when compared to the same type of MNS cells, present the following common pattern of changes: a faster Na-K cotransport, a lower volume and intracellular Na content Ferrari *et al* 1987), a lower calpastatin activity and Vmax of the Ca pump (Vezzoli *et al* 1986, Pontremoli *et al* 1986). Therefore, the same genetic abnormality may be present in both MHS cell types. With bone marrow transplantation (Bianchi *et al* 1985) we demonstrated that these erythrocyte abnormalities were present in the stem cells and were not due the extracellular influences. With genetic co-segregation studies we demonstrated a genetic association between erythrocytes abnormalities and the level of blood pressure in F_2 hybrids (Bianchi *et al* 1985). Therefore, erythrocytes may be considered an appropriate cell to study the molecular abnormalities responsible for these cellular dysfunctions which underlie renal abnormality in MHS. Applying different types of cell manipulation, we concluded that the network of membrane skeleton proteins which is below the cell membrane lipid bilayer, may be responsible for the Na-K cotransport and cell volume differences between MHS and MNS erythrocytes (Ferrari *et al* 1991). A difference in the finger print of cytoskeletal protein patterns after digestion with proteolytic enzymes have been found for two of these cytoskeletal proteins. 70% of the sequence of the gene coding for one of these two proteins has been determined and a point mutation has been detected (Salardi *et al* 1989, Tripodi *et al* 1991).

At present, many studies are in progress to evaluate the relationship between this point mutation and the abnormality in ion transport across the membrane, the renal dysfunction and the development of hypertension. We do not know yet whether these studies will furnish the proof of a genetic link between the mutation within one of these proteins and the renal dysfunction responsible for hypertension. However, we believe that this type of methodological approach may be one of the most appropriate for studying the genetic-molecular mechanisms underlying organ dysfunction in genetic hypertension and it may be applied to other genetic rat models of hypertension. Furthermore, should the link between a given gene mutation and a given physiological abnormality be demonstrated, at some future time, in a genetic animal model of hypertension, then we may evaluate whether in man also such a link is at work.

REFERENCES

Arendshorst, W.J. (1979): Autoregulation of renal blood flow in spontaneously hypertensive rats. *Circ. Res.* 44, 344-349.

Arendshorst, W.J. and Beierwaltes, W.H. (1979): Renal and nephron hemodynamics in spontaneously hypertensive rats. *Am. J. Physiol.* 236(Renal Fluid Electrol. Physiol. 5), F246-F251.

Arendshorst, W.J., Chatziantoniou, C., and Daniels, F. (1990): Role of angiotensin in the renal vasoconstriction observed during the development of genetic hypertension. *Kid. Int.* 38(suppl 30), S92-S96.

Azar, S., Johnson, M.A., Iwai, J., Bruno, L., and Tobian, L. (1978): Single-nephron dynamics in "post-salt" rats with chronic hypertension. *J. Lab. Clin. Med.* 91, 156-166.

Beierwaltes, W.H., Arendshorst, W.J., and Klemmer P.J. (1982): Electrolyte and water balance in young spontaneously hypertensive rats. *Hypertension* 4, 908-917.

Berecek, K.H., Schwertschlag, U., and Gross, F. (1980): Alterations in renal vascular resistance and reactivity in spontaneous hypertension of rats. *Am. J. Physiol.* 238(Heart Circ. Physiol. 7), H278-H293.

Bianchi, G., Fox, U., DiFrancesco, G.F., Giovanetti, A.M., and Pagetti, D. (1974): Blood pressure changes produced by kidney cross-transplantation between spontaneously hypertensive rats and normotensive rats. *Clin. Sci Mol. Med.* 47, 435-488.

Bianchi, G., Baer, P.G., Fox, U., Duzzi, L., and Pagetti, D. (1975): Changes in renin, water balance and sodium balance during development of high blood pressure in genetically hypertensive rats. *Circ. Res.* 36&37(suppl I), 153-161.

Bianchi, G., Cusi, D., Barlassina, C., Lupi, G.P., Ferrari, P., Picotti, G.B., Gatti, M., and Polli, E. (1983): Renal dysfunction as a possible cause of essential hypertension in predisposed subjects. *Kidney International* 23, 870-875.

Bianchi, G., Ferrari, P., Trizio, D., Ferrandi, M., Torielli, L., Barber, B.R., and Polli, E. (1985): Red blood cell abnormalities and spontaneous hypertension in the rat: a genetically determined link. *Hypertension.* 7, 319-325.

Bianchi, G., Ferrari, P., Barber, B.R. (1990): Lessons from Experimental Genetic Hypertension: in *Hypertension: Pathophysiology, Diagnosis and Management.* eds J.H. Laragh and B.M. Brenner, pp.901-922. Raven Press Ltd.

Boberg, U. and Persson, E.G. (1986): Increased tubuloglomerular feedback activity in Milan hypertensive rats. *Am. J. Physiol.* 16(Renal Fluid Electrol. Physiol. 19), F967-F974.

Chatziantoniou, C., Daniels, F.H., and Arendshorst, W.J. (1990): Exaggerated renal vascular reactivity to angiotensin and thromboxane in young genetically hypertensive rats. *Am. J. Physiol.* 259(Renal Fluid Electrol. Physiol. 28), F372-F382.

Coburn, R.J., Manger, W.M., and Dufton S. (1972): Absence of renal participation in genesis of hypertension in spontaneously hypertensive rats. *Clin. Res.* 20, 589.

Cowley Jr., A.W., Roman, J.R., and Kreiger, J.E. (1991): Pathways linking renal excretion and arterial pressure with vascular structure and function. *Clin. Exp. Pharmacol. hysiol.* 18, 21-27.

Cowley Jr. (in press): Long-term control of arterial blood pressure. *Phys. Rev.*

Dahl, L.K., Knudsen, K.D., Heine, M., and Leitl, G. (1967): Effects of chronic excess salt ingestion. Genetic influence on the development of salt hypertension in parabiotic rats. Evidence for a humoral factor. *J. Exp. Med.* 126, 687-699.

Dahl, L.K., Knudsen K.D., and Heine, M. (1968): Effects of chronic excess salt ingestion: Modification of experimental hypertension in the rat by variations in the diet. *Circ. Res.* 22, 11-18.

Dahl, L.K., Heine M., and Thompson K. (1972): Genetic influence of renal homografts on blood pressure of rats from different strains. *Proc. Soc. Exp. Biol. Med.* 140, 852-856.

Dahl, L.K., Heine M., and Thompson K. (1974): Genetic influence of the kidneys on blood pressure: Evidence from chronic renal homografts in rats with opposite predispositions to hypertension. *Circ. Res.* 34, 94-101.

Dahl, L.K. and Heine, M. (1975): Primary role of renal homografts in setting chronic blood pressure levels in rats. *Circ. Res.* 36, 692-696.

de Wardener H.E. and MacGregor G.A. (1980): Dahl's hypothesis that a salt uretic substance may be responsible for a sustained rise in arterial pressure: its possible role in essential hypertension. *Kid. Int.* 18, 1-9.

de Wardener, H., Millett, J., Holland, S., MacGregor, G.A., and Alaghband-Zadeh, J. (1987): Ouabain-like Na^+,K^+-ATPase inhibitor in the plasma of normotensive and hypertensive humans and rats. *Hypertension* 10(suppl 1), 52-56.

Dilley, J.R. and Arendshorst, W.J. (1984): Enhanced tubuloglomerular feedback activity in rats developing spontaneous hypertension. *Am. J. Physiol.* 247(Renal Fluid Electrol. Physiol. 16), F672-F679.

Dilley, J.R., Steir, C.T., and Arendshorst, W.J. (1984): Abnormalities in glomerular function in rats developing spontaneous hypertension. *Am. J. Physiol.* 246(Renal Fluid Electrol. Physiol. 15), F12-F20.

Ferrandi, M., Salardi, S., Parenti, P., Ferrari, P., Bianchi, G., Braw, R. and Karlish, S.J.D. (1990): $Na^+/K^+/Cl^-$-cotransporter mediated Rb+ fluxes in membrane vesicles from kidneys of normotensive and hypertensive rats. *Biochim. Biophys. Acta.* 1021, 13-20.

Ferrandi, M., Minotti, E., Salardi, S., Florio, M., Bianchi, G., and Ferrari, P. (1991): The hypothalamic ouabain-like factor in the Milan hypertensive rat (MHS). *Abstracts of 5th Eur. Soc. Hypertens. Meeting*, Milan, Italy.

Ferrari, P., Cusi, D., Barber, B.R., et al (1982): Erythrocyte membrane and renal function in relation to hypertension in rats of the Milan hypertensive strain. *Clin. Sci.* 63, 61s-64s.

Ferrari, P., Ferrandi, M., Torielli, L., Canessa, M., and Bianchi, G. (1987): Relationship between erythrocyte volume and sodium transport in the Milan hypertensive rat and age-dependent changes. *J. Hypertens.* 5, 199-206.

Ferrari, P., Torielli, L., Cirillo, M., Salardi, S., and Bianchi, G. (1991): Sodium transport kinetics in erythrocytes and inside-out vesicles from the Milan rats. *J. Hypertens.* 9, 703-711.

Firth, J.D., Raine, A.E.G., and Ledingham, J.G.G. (1989): Sodium and lithium handling in the isolated hypertensive rat kidney. *Clin. Sci.* 76, 335-341.

Foulkes, R., Ferrario, R.G., Salvati, P., and Bianchi, G. (In press): Differences in ouabain-induced natriuresis between isolated kidneys of Milan hypertensive rats. *Clin. Sci.*

Fox, U. and Bianchi, G. (1976): The primary role of the kidney in causing the blood pressure difference between the Milan Hypertensive strain (MHS) and the normotensive rats (MNS). *Clin. Exp. Pharmacol. Physiol.* Suppl 3, 71-74.

Gebremedhim, D., Fenoy, F.J., Harder, D.R., and Roman, R.J. (1990): Enhanced vascular tone in the renal vasculature of spontaneously hypertensive rats. *Hypertens.* 16, 648-654.

Geoffroy, J., Benzoni, D., Vincent, M., and Sassard, J. (1986): Urinary prostaglandins and thromboxane B_2 in genetically hypertensive rats of the Lyon strain. *J. Hypertens.* 4(suppl 3), S37-S39.

Geoffroy, J., Benzoni, D., Vincent, M., and Sassard, J. (1990): Thromboxane A_2 and development of genetic hypertension in the Lyon rat strain. *Hypertension* 16, 655-661.

Greene, A.S., Yuan Yu, Z., Roman, R.J., and Cowley, Jr., A.W. (1990): Role of blood volume expansion in Dahl rat model of hypertension. *Am. J. Physiol.* 258(Heart Circ. Physiol. 27), H508-H514.

Guyton, A.C., and Coleman, T.G. (1969): Quantitative analysis of the pathophysiology of hypertension. *Circ. Res.* 24(suppl. 1), 1-19.

Hallback, M. and Folkow B. et al (1974): Cardiovascular responses to acute mental "stress" in spontaneously hypertensive rats. *Acta. Physiol. Scanda.* 90, 684-698.

Hallback, M., Jones, J.V., Bianchi, G., and Folkow, B. (1977): Cardiovascular control in the Milan strain of spontaneously hypertensive rat (MHS) at "rest" and during acute mental "stress". *Acta. Physiol. Scanda.* 99, 208-216.

Hamlyn, J.M., Ringel, R., Schaeffer, J., et al (1982): A circulating inhibitor of Na^+,K^+-ATPase associated with essential hypertension. *Nature.* 300, 650-652.

Hanozet, G.M., Parenti, P., and Salvati, P. (1985): Presence of a potential-sensitive Na^+ transport across renal brush-border membrane vesicles of the Milan Hypertensive strain. *Biochim. Biophys. Acta.* 819, 179-186.

Harrap, S.B. (1986): Genetic analysis of blood pressure and sodium balance in spontaneously hypertensive rats. *Hypertension* 8, 572-582.

Harrap, S.B., Nicolaci, J.A., and Doyle, A.E. (1986): Persistent effects on blood pressure and renal haemodynamics following chronic angiotensin converting enzyme inhibition with perindopril. *Clin. Exp. Pharmacol. Physiol.* 13, 753-765.

Harrap, S.B. and Doyle, A.E. (1986): Renal haemodynamics and total body sodium in immature spontaneously hypertensive and Wistar-Kyoto rats. *J. Hypertens.* 4(suppl 3), S249-S252.

Harrap, S.B. and Doyle, A.E. (1988): Genetic co-segregation of renal haemodynamics and blood pressure in the spontaneously hypertensive rat. *Clin. Sci.* 74, 63-69.

Holland S., Millett, J., Alaghband-Zadeh, J., de Wardener, H., Ferrari, P., and Bianchi, G. (1987): Cytochemically assayable Na^+,K^+ ATPase inhibition by Milan hypertensive rat plasma. *Hypertension* 9, 498-503.

Kawabe, K., Watanabe, T.X., Shione, K., and Sokabe, H. (1979): Influence on blood pressure of renal isografts between spontaneously hypertensive and normotensive rats, utilizing the F1 hybrids. *Jpn. Heart J.* 20, 886-894.

Liu, K.L., Aissa, A.H., Laréal, M.C., Benzoni, D., Vincent, M., and Sassard, J. (1991): Adrenergic stimulation of renal prostanoids in the Lyon hypertensive rat. *Hypertension* 17, 296-302.

MacGregor, G., Fenton, S., Alaghband-Zadeh, J., Marakandu, N., Roulston, J.E., and de Wardener, H. (1981): Evidence for a raised concentration of a circulating sodium transport inhibitor in essential hypertension. *Br. Med. J.* 283, 1355-1357.

Melzi, M.L., Bertorello, A., Fukuda, Y., Muldin, I., Sereni, F., and Aperia, A. (1989): Na,K-ATPase activity in renal tubule cells from Milan hypertensive rats. *Am. J.. Hypertens.* 2, 563-566.

Morgan, D.A., DiBona G.F., and Mark A.L. (1990): Effects of interstrain renal transplant on NaCL-induced hypertension in Dahl rats. *Hypertension* 15, 436-442.

Nabika, T., Nara, Y., Ikeda, K., Endo, J., Yamori, Y. (1991): Genetic heterogeneity of the spontaneously hypertensive rat. *Hypertension* 18, 12-16.

O'Dowd, B.F., and Rapp J.P. (1991): Heterogeneity of renin alleles in outbred Dahl salt-sensitive (Brookhaven) rats. *Hypertension* 18, 9-11.

Pontremoli S., Melloni, E., and Salamino, F. (1986): Decreased level of calpain activity in red blood cells from Milan hypertensive rats. *Biochem. Biophys. Res. Commun.* 138, 1370-1375.

Rettig, R., Folberth, C.G., Stauss, H., Kopf, D., Waldherr, R., Baldauf, G., and Unger T. (1990A): Hypertension in rats induced by renal grafts from renovascular hypertensive donors. *Hypertension* 15, 429-435.

Rettig, R., Folberth, C.G., Stauss, H., Kopf, D., Waldherr, R., and Unger T. (1990B): Role of the kidney in primary hypertension: a renal transplantation study in rats. *Am. J. Physiol.* 258(Renal Fluid Electrol. Physiol 27), F606-F611.

Roman, R.J., and Cowley Jr., A.W. (1985): Abnormal pressure-diuresis-natriuresis response in spontaneously hypertensive rats. *Am. J. Physiol.* 248(Renal Fluid Electrol. Physiol. 17), F199-F205.

Roman, R.J., (1986): Abnormal renal hemodynamics and pressure-natriuresis relationship in Dahl salt-sensitive rats. *Am. J. Physiol.* 251(Renal Fluid Electrol. Physiol 20), F57-F65.

Roman, R.J. (1987): Altered pressure-natriuresis relationship in young spontaneously hypertensive rats. *Hypertension* 9(suppl III), 130-136.

Roman, R.J., and Kaldunski, M.L. (1988): Renal cortical and papillary blood flow in spontaneously hypertensive rats. *Hypertension* 11,(6 part 2) 657-663.

Roman, R.J., (1990): Alterations in renal medullary hemodynamics and the pressure natriuresis response in genetic hypertension. *Am. J. Hypertension* 3, 893-900.

Roman, R.J., and Kaldunski, M. (1991): Enhanced chloride reabsorption in the loop of Henle in Dahl salt-sensitive rats. *Hypertension* 17, 1018-1024.

Roman, R.J., and Kaldunski, M. (in press): Pressure natriuresis and cortical and papillary blood flow in inbred Dahl rats. *Am. J. Physiol.*

Salardi, S., Saccardo, B., Borsani, G., Modica, R., Ferrandi, M., Tripodi, G., Soria, M., Ferrari, P., Baralle, F.E., Sidoli, A., and Bianchi, G. (1989): Erythrocyte adducin differential properties in normotensive and hypertensive rats of the Milan strain. *Am. J. Hypertens.* 2, 229-237.

Salvati, P., Pinciroli, G.P., and Bianchi, G. (1984): Renal function of isolated perfused kidneys from hypertensive (MHS) and normotensive (MNS) rats of the Milan strain at different ages. *J. Hypertens.* 2(suppl 3), 351-353.

Salvati, P., Ferrario, R.G., and Bianchi, G. (1987A): Natriuretic capacity in isolated kidneys of rats of the Milan strain before and after the development of hypertension: comparison with spontaneously hypertensive rats. *J. Hypertens.* 5(suppl 5), S235-S237.

Salvati, P., Ferrario, R.G., Parenti, P., and Bianchi, G. (1987B): Renal function of isolated perfused kidneys from hypertensive (MHS) and normotensive (MNS) rats of the Milan strain: Role of calcium. *J. Hypertens.* 5, 31-38.

Salvati, P., Ferrario, R.G., and Bianchi, G. (1990): Diuretic effect of bumetanide in isolated perfused kidneys of Milan hypertensive rats. *Kid. Int.* 37, 1084-1089.

Sautel, M., Saquet, J., Vincent, M., and Sassard, J. (1988): NE turnover in genetically hypertensive rats of the Lyon strain. II. Peripheral organs. *Am. J. Physiol.* 255(Heart Circ. Physiol. 24), H736-H741.

Shibouta, Y.Z., Terashita, Z., Inada, Y., Nishikawa, K., and Kikuchi, S., (1981): Enhanced thromboxane A_2 biosynthesis in the kidney of spontaneously hypertensive rats during development of hypertension. *Eur. J. Pharmacol.* 70, 247-256.

Sinaiko, A. and Mirkin B. (1974): Ontogenesis of the renin-angiotensin system in spontaneously hypertensive and normal Wistar rats. *Circ. Res.* 34, 693-696.

Steele, T.H. and Challoner-Hue, L. (1988): Increased vascular response to calcium channel agonist by Dahl S rat kidney. *Am. J. Physiol.* 254(Renal Fluid Electrol. Physiol 23), F533-F539.

Sterzel, R.B., Luft, F.C., Gao, Y., Schnermann, J., Briggs, J.P., Ganten, D., Waldherr, E., Schnabel, R., and Kritz, W. (1988): Renal disease and the development of hypertension in salt-sensitive Dahl rats. *Kid. Int.* 33, 1119-1129.

Tobian, L., Lange, J., Azar, S., Iwai, J., Koop, D., Coffee, K., and Johnson, M.A. (1978): Reduction of natriuretic capacity and renin release in isolated, blood-perfused kidney of Dahl hypertension-prone rats. *Circ. Res.* 43(Suppl I), 192-197.

Tripodi, G., Piscone, A., Borsani, G., Tisminetzky, S., Salardi, S. Sidoli, A., James, P., Pongor, S., Bianchi., G., and Baralle, F.E. (1991): Molecular cloning of an adducin-like protein: evidence of a polymorphism in the normotensive and hypertensive rats of the Milan strain. *Biochem. Biophys. Res. Comm.* 177, 939-947.

Van Hooft, I.M., Grobbee, D.E., Derkx, F.H. and de Leeuw, P.W. (1991): Renal hemodynamics and the renin-angiotensin-aldosterone system in normotensive subjects with hypertensive and normotensive parents *New Engl. J. Med.* 324, 1305-1311.

Vezzoli, G., Elli, A., Tripodi, M.G., Bianchi, G., and Carafoli, E. (1985): Calcium ATPase in erythrocytes of spontaneously hypertensive rats of the Milan strain. *J. Hypertens.* 3, 645-648.

Wauquier, I., Pernollet, M.G., Grichois, M.L., Lacour, B., Meyer, P., and Devynck, M.A. (1988): Endogenous digitalis-like circulating substances in spontaneously hypertensive rats. *Hypertension* 12, 108-116.

Résumé

Les études des fonctions rénales menées dans quatre modèles d'hypertension génétique chez le Rat : les souches de Dahl, Lyon, Milan (MHS) et la souche japonaise (SHR) sont résumées ici dans le but de mettre en évidence leurs similarités ou leurs différences. Cette tentative est rendue difficile par l'utilisation de méthodes diverses et par l'hétérogénéité génétique qui existe dans au moins deux de ces souches. Toutefois, malgré ces difficultés un certain nombre de conclusions peuvent être tirées. Dans trois de ces souches (Dahl, MHS et SHR) des transplantations rénales ont été réalisées montrant que les reins de la souche hypertendue élevaient plus la pression artérielle que ceux de la souche normotendue contrôle et ce quel que soit le receveur. Cette action était observée même au stade de pré-hypertension. Dans les souches de Lyon, Dahl et SHR la filtration glomérulaire tendait à être plus basse et les résistances vasculaires rénales plus hautes, alors que c'est l'inverse qui était observé chez les MSH où une élévation importante de la réabsorption tubulaire était aussi observée en association avec une élévation de la pression hydrostatique interstitielle au stade de pré-hypertension. Une rétention rénale de sodium pendant le développement de l'hypertension et une élévation dans un facteur humoral "ouabaine-like" ou presseur ont été détectées dans toutes les souches où elles ont été recherchées (MHS, Dahl et SHR). Un déplacement vers la droite de la courbe de pression-natriurèse a été démontré au niveau rénal dans les quatre souches. En conclusion une franche anomalie primitive a été mise en évidence dans les souches de Dahl, MHS et SHR et ceci bien que les mécanismes cellulaires provoquant cette anomalie puisse différer dans ces trois souches de rats.

Adrenal renin, angiotensinogen and angiotensin in stroke-prone spontaneously hypertensive rats

Shokei Kim, Masayuki Hosoi, Toyokazu Takada * and Kenjiro Yamamoto

*Department of Pharmacology, Osaka City University Medical School, Osaka 545, Japan and * Central Research Laboratories, Santen Pharmaceutical Co., Ltd., Osaka 533, Japan*

Various extrarenal tissues, including the adrenal gland, brain, heart, and blood vessels possess the endogenous renin-angiotensin(Ang) system, independently of the circulating system(Dzau et al., 1988). Stroke-prone spontaneously hypertensive rats(SHRSP), established by Okamoto et al., develop cerebrovascular and renal vascular lesions, hence are a useful animal model of human malignant hypertension(Okamoto et al., 1974). In the present study, we measured renin, angiotensinogen and Ang contents in the adrenal gland of SHRSP.

MATERIALS AND METHODS

Animals: Twenty-five week-old SHRSP and Wistar-Kyoto rats(WKY) were used. All animals were killed by decapitation, both adrenal glands were rapidly removed and frozen in liquid nitrogen until use.
Extraction of adrenal glands: For the measurement of Ang II, one adrenal gland of each animal was boiled in 0.5 ml distilled water for 5 min, then homogenized in 0.05N HCl. The supernatant, obtained by centrifugation was applied to Sep-Pak C_{18} cartridges, as described below. For the measurement of renin and angiotensinogen concentration, the contralateral adrenal gland of each animal was homogenized in 50 mM sodium phosphate buffer/pH 7.0/0.15 M NaCl/5 mM Na_2EDTA/2 mM phenylmethanesulfonyl fluoride/2 mM potassium tetrathionate(20% homogenate). The supernatant was obtained by centrifugation at 30,000 X g for 1 h at 4 °C.
Determination of plasma and adrenal Angs: Measurement of Ang II was carried out by reverse phase high performance liquid chromatography(HPLC) combined with specific radioimmunoassay(RIA). Briefly, the samples of adrenal extracts(about 1 ml) were applied to Sep-Pak C_{18} cartridge columns. The column was washed with 10 ml 0.1% TFA and 10 ml of the mixture of methanol/water/TFA(10/89.9/0.1, vol/vol). The Ang II, retained by the cartridge, were eluted with 4 ml of the mixture of methanol/water/TFA(80/19.9/0.1, vol/vol). The eluates were dried in a vacuum centrifuge evaporator(CC-180, TOMY SEIKO, Japan) and dissolved in 250 μl 10 mM phosphoric acid/pH 3.4, and chromato-

graphed on an ODS-80TM C_{18} reverse phase HPLC column(4.6 mm X 25 cm, Tosoh, Japan). The separation of Angs were effected by using a linear gradient of methanol concentration from 30 to 75% in 10 mM phosphoric acid/pH 3.4 over a period of 20 min at the flow rate of 1.0 ml/min. Fractions of 0.3 ml were collected into bovine serum albumin(BSA)-coated polypropylene tubes, dried in a vacuum centrifuge evaporator. The fractionated samples were dissolved in RIA buffer(70 mM sodium phosphate/pH 7.1/50 mM $NaCl/2$ mM $Na_2EDTA/100$ M diisopropylfluorophosphate/0.3% BSA) and subjected to RIA of Ang II.

Measurement of prorenin: Prorenin in the adrenal extracts was measured by trypsin activation, as described(Kim et al., 1991a).

Assay of angiotensinogen: Angiotensinogen in the adrenal extracts was indirectly measured by enzymatic assay using pure rat renal renin(Kim et al., 1991b).

Determination of plasma aldosterone: The plasma aldosterone concentration was determined by RIA using a commercially available kit(SORIN BIOMEDICA S.p.A, Italy).

RESULTS AND DISCUSSION

In 25 wk-old SHRSP with malignant hypertension, the adrenal Ang II concentrations were about 5-fold higher than those of WKY, accompanied by a 4-fold increase in the adrenal renin(Kim et al., 1991c). Prorenin was not detected in the adrenal gland of SHRSP or WKY, being in agreement with the fact that prorenin is rapidly released without storage. To determine whether the elevated adrenal Ang II levels in SHRSP are due to an increase in the local generation or in uptake of circulating Ang II, the effects of bilateral nephrectomy on the adrenal Ang and renin levels were examined. The adrenal Ang II content in SHRSP did not decrease 24 h after nephrectomy and was 10-fold higher than that in nephrectomized control WKY(Kim et al., 1991c). These results suggest that the adrenal Ang II derives mainly from a local generation rather than from uptake of circulating Ang II and that the production of Ang II may be increased in the adrenal gland of SHRSP with malignant hypertension. As there were about 3-fold higher concentrations of plasma aldosterone in nephrectomized SHRSP than nephrectomized WKY(Kim et al., 1991c), the increased adrenal Ang II may contribute to increases in the release of aldosterone. In addition, adrenal Ang II may stimulate the release of adrenal catecholamine. We postulate that elevation of Ang II in the adrenal gland of SHRSP likely contributes to acceleration of malignant hypertension in these animals.

Interestingly, angiotensinogen was not detected in the adrenal gland of SHRSP or WKY, in contrast to the high concentrations of adrenal renin, thereby indicating that the amount of angiotensinogen synthesized in the adrenal tissue is small. These observations suggest that the limiting factor for the generation of Ang II in the adrenal gland may be angiotensinogen rather than renin.

REFERENCES

Dzau, V.J.(1988): Circulating versus local renin-angiotensin system in cardiovascular homeostasis. Circulation. 77(Suppl I), 1-4.

Kim, S., Hosoi, M., Nakajima, K., and Yamamoto, K. (1991a): Immunological evidence that kidney is primary source of circulating inactive prorenin in rats. Am. J. Physiol. 260, E526-E536.
Kim, S., Hosoi, M., Nakajima, K., and Yamamoto, K. (1991b): Amino-terminal amino acid sequence and heterogeneity in glycosylation of rat renal renin. J.Biol.Chem. 266, 7044-7050.
Kim, S., Hosoi, M., Shimamoto, K., Takada, T., and Yamamoto, K. (1991c): Increased production of angiotensin II in the adrenal gland of stroke-prone spontaneously hypertensive rats with malignant hypertension. Biochem. Biophys. Res. Commun. 178, 151-157.
Okamoto,K., Yamori, Y., and Nagaoka, A. (1974): Establishment of the stroke-prone spontaneously hypertensive rat(SHR). Circ.Res. 34(Suppl I), I-143-I-153.

Abolished DA-1 receptor-mediated inhibition of renal tubular Na+, K+-ATPase in spontaneously hypertensive rats

Chang J. Chen, Subhash J. Vyas, Joseph Eichberg [1], Robert E. Beach [2] and Mustafa F. Lokhandwala

Departments of Pharmacology and [1] Biochemical and Biophysical Sciences, University of Houston, Houston, TX and [2] Division of Nephrology, University of Texas Medical Branch, Galveston, TX, USA

There is evidence which suggests that an abnormality of renal dopaminergic system in spontaneously hypertensive rats (SHR) might be involved in impaired renal sodium excretion in this model of hypertension. It is demonstrated that in young SHR renal tissue and/or urinary dopamine (DA) excretion is elevated, yet renal sodium excretion is less in the SHR than WKY rats (Kambara et al., 1987). The renal responses to exogenously administered DA receptor agonists are diminished in the adult SHR (Felder, 1990). It is also reported that the DA receptor adenylate cyclase coupling is less efficient in the renal proximal tubules of adult SHR compared to WKY rats (Kinoshita et al., 1989).

It is known that one of the mechanisms by which DA produces natriuresis is via activation of renal tubular DA-1 receptors located on the basolateral membrane (BLM) and the cellular signalling processes involve activation of phospholipase C (PLC) with subsequent inhibition of Na^+,K^+-ATPase, leading to an inhibition of tubular sodium reabsorption (Felder et al., 1989). The objective of our study was to determine DA-induced activation of PLC using renal cortical slices and DA-induced inhibition of Na^+,K^+-ATPase using the BLM of renal proximal tubule both in the SHR and WKY rats of 10-12 weeks of age.

METHODS

<u>Measurement of Phospholipase C Activity</u>: The animals were anesthetized with pentobarbital (50 mg/kg, i.p.) and the kidneys were removed and immersed in ice-cold Krebs-Ringer-Bicarbonate Buffer (KRB). The outer renal cortex was removed and chopped to 500 µ slices, which were incubated at 37°C in aerated KRB (0.6 ml) containing 25 µCi/ml of [^{3}H]-inositol for 2 hours, followed by washing 4 times with ice-cold KRB to remove unbound activity. The slices were distributed among tubes, to which various concentrations of DA (1, 3 and 10 mM) were added and incubated for 60 minutes. In separate groups of experiments, the relative involvement of DA-1 receptors and α-adrenoceptors in DA-induced activation of PLC was assessed by incubating slices with selective DA-1 receptor antagonist SCH 23390 (30 µM) and non-selective α-adrenoceptor blocker phentolamine (10 µM) respectively, for 20 minutes before addition of DA.

The slices were then homogenized and centrifuged. The supernatant containing inositol phosphates (IPs) were separated by ion exchange chromatography using ACCELL QMA anion exchange Sep-Paks (Water Associates, Milford, MA) with ammonia formate based solutions (Wreggett and Irvine, 1987). The activity in the fractions was measured using a scintillation counter (Beckman LS 7500, Irvine, CA) and expressed as dpm. The lipids (total) in the cortical slices were extracted from the pellet.

The phospholipase C activity is expressed in terms of fractional release of combined inositol phosphates described as follows:

$$\text{Fractional release} = \frac{\text{dpm IPs}}{\text{dpm IPs} + \text{dpm TL}} \times 100$$

where $IPs = IP_1 + IP_2 + IP_3$ and TL = total lipids.

Measurement of Na^+,K^+-ATPase Activity: BLMs from rat cortex were prepared by the method of Sacktor et al. (1981) as modified by Schwab, Klahr and Hammerman (1984). In brief, homogenized renal cortex was centrifuged for 15 minutes at 4500 revolutions per minute (rpm). The supernatant was recentrifuged for 20 minutes at 14,000 rpm and the pellet resuspended. Percoll was added to the sucrose solution in a volume ratio of 1.0 ml Percoll per 11.5 ml sucrose solution. The mixture was centrifuged at 17,000 rpm for 35 minutes. The top, cloudy membrane band was separated from the dense pellet, resuspended in KCl solution and centrifuged twice at 17,000 rpm for 30 minutes.

Na^+,K^+-ATPase activity was determined by the method of Quigley and Gotterer (1969) on 100 μl of membrane suspension, following permeabilization by rapid freezing in dry ice/acetone and thawing, with absorbance determined at 740 nM (Beckman Model 25 Spectrophotometer, Fallerton, CA). The reaction was initiated by the addition of 4 mM Tris-ATP in the presence of 5 mM ouabain or an equal volume of deionized water. After 15 minutes at 37°C the reaction was terminated by addition of 50 μl cold 50% trichloroacetic acid. Na^+,K^+-ATPase activity was measured as the difference between total ATPase and ouabain-insensitive ATPase activities and was expressed as nMol pi per mg·protein per minute.

RESULTS

Dopamine-Induced Activation of Phospholipase C: Dopamine (1, 3 and 10 mM) produced concentration-related increases in inositol phosphates release in both renal cortical slices of WKY and SHR. In WKY rats, DA produced 38±6%, 71±9% and 106±22% increases over basal level at the respective concentrations. However, in the SHR, the same range of DA concentrations only produced 13±6%, 49±6% and 50±16% increases over basal, which were significantly less than those seen in the WKY rats (Table 1). It was also noted that the basal activity of PLC was significantly higher in the SHR. The experiments with antagonists showed that in WKY rats approximately 50% of DA-stimulated IP production was blocked by DA-1 receptor antagonist SCH 23390 and 50% was blocked by α-adrenoceptor antagonist phentolamine. In contrast, in the SHR, DA-1 receptor antagonist SCH 23390 did not have any significant effect on DA-induced activation of PLC and furthermore approximately 70% of DA-stimulated IP production in the SHR was blocked by phentolamine (data not shown).

Table 1: Effect of dopamine on renal cortical PLC activation in adult SHR and WKY rats

	Basal Activity (%)	Dopamine Concentration (mM, % increase over the basal activity)		
		1	3	10
SHR	7.36±0.32†	13±6	49±6*†	50±16*†
WKY	5.61±0.27	38±6*	71±9*	106±22*

Data are represented as mean ± SEM for 2-3 experiments performed in quadruplets. *p < 0.05, significant difference within the group as compared with the basal activity; † p<0.05, significant difference between SHR and WKY rats.

Dopamine-Induced Inhibition of Na^+,K^+-ATPase: Dopamine (10^{-7}, 10^{-8} and 10^{-9}M) inhibited Na^+,K^+ATPase in a concentration-dependent manner in WKY rats (Table 2). However, in the SHR, DA failed to cause significant inhibition in all concentrations employed. There were no differences in basal Na^+,K^+-ATPase activity between the SHR and WKY rats. In separate group of WKY rats, DA-induced inhibition of Na^+,K^+-ATPase was attenuated by selective DA-1 receptor antagonist SCH 23390 in a concentration-related manner (data not shown), indicating the involvement of tubular DA-1 receptor. In addition, SCH 23390 alone did not have significant effect on Na^+,K^+-ATPase activity.

DISCUSSION

The present study clearly shows that: 1) DA-induced activation of PLC, which is linked to both α-adrenoceptor and DA-1 receptor, was significantly diminished in renal cortical slices of SHR as compared to WKY rats. 2) The diminished DA-induced activation of PLC in the SHR was due,

Table 2: Effect of dopamine on Na^+,K^+-ATPase in the basolateral membrane of proximal tubule from the SHR and WKY rats

	Basal Activity	7	8	9 (-Log Dopamine M)
		(nMolPi/mg.protein/min)		
SHR	426±43	372±45	343±64	358±78
WKY	452±55	214±52*	269±50*	333±62

Data are represented as mean ± SEM. N=10 animals per group. *p < 0.05, significant difference within the group as compared with the basal activity.

mainly, if not entirely, to an impaired DA-1 receptor function. 3) DA, which inhibited Na^+,K^+-ATPase in the WKY rats in a concentration-dependent manner, had no significant effect in the SHR. The functional significance of diminished DA-induced PLC activation and the possible link between the diminished DA-induced PLC activation and abolished DA-mediated inhibition of Na^+,K^+-ATPase in the SHR remain to be further investigated.

It is known that intrarenally produced DA increases renal sodium excretion mainly via activation of tubular DA-1 receptor, which is coupled to both adenylate cyclase and PLC. It is reported that activation of adenylate cyclase following occupation of DA-1 receptor is linked to an inhibition of Na^+-H^+ exchange whereas DA-1 receptor-mediated activation of PLC is followed by protein kinase C activation with subsequent inhibition of Na^+,K^+-ATPase (Felder, et al. 1989). Inasmuch as both pathways are involved in overall DA-induced natriuresis, it is highly possible that a defect in either one or both of these pathways might contribute to the abnormal renal sodium excretion in the SHR. Indeed, it is recently reported that DA receptor adenylate cyclase coupling process is less efficient in the adult SHR (Kinoshita, et al. 1989). The observations of this study that DA-1 receptor mediated activation of PLC was diminished and DA-induced inhibition of Na^+,K^+-ATPase was abolished in the SHR strongly suggest that DA-1 receptor coupled PLC signal transduction pathway is also impaired in the SHR. Although the final regulation of renal sodium excretion occurs mainly in the distal nephron, sodium delivery to the distal nephron, which is determined largely by the functional status of Na^+,K^+-ATPase in the proximal tubule, has a great impact on overall urinary sodium excretion. Therefore, loss or reduced influence of renal DA on this enzyme may potentially lead to abnormal renal sodium handling in the SHR, thus contributing to development and/or maintenance of high blood pressure in this model of hypertension.

REFERENCES

Felder, R. A., Felder, C. C., Eisner, G. M. and Jose, P. A. (1989): The dopamine receptor in adult and maturing kidney. Am. J. Physiol. 287: F315-F327.
Felder, R. A., Seikaly, M. G., Cody, P., Eisner, G. M. and Jose, P. A. (1990): Attenuated renal response to dopaminergic drugs in spontaneously hypertensive rats. *Hypertension* 15: 560-569.
Kambara, S., Yoshimura, M., Takahashi, H. and Ijichi, H. (1987): Enhanced synthesis of renal dopamine and impaired natriuresis in spontaneously hypertensive rats. *Jpn. Heart J.* 28: 594.
Kinoshita, S., Sidhu, A. and Felder, R. A. (1989): Defective dopamine-1 receptor adenylate cylcase coupling in the proximal convoluted tubules from the spontaneously hypertensive rats. *J. Clin. Invest.* 84: 1849-1859.
Quigley, J. P. and Gotterer, G. S. (1969): Distribution of (Na^+,K^+)-stimulated ATPase activity in rat intestinal mucosa. *Biochem. Biophys. Acta.* 173: 456-468.
Sacktor, B. L., Rosenbloom, I. L., Liang, C. T. and Cheng, L. (1981): Na^+-gradient and sodium plus potassium gradient-dependent glutamate uptake in renal basolateral membrane vesicles. *J. Membr. Biol.* 60: 63-71.
Schwab, S. J., Klahr, S. and Hammerman, M. R. (1984): Na^+-gradient Pi uptake in basolateral membrane vesicles from dog kidney. *Am. J. Physiol.* 246: F663-F669.
Wreggett, K. A. and Irvine, R. F. (1987): Rapid separation method for inositol phosphates and their isomers. *Biochem. J.* 245: 655-660.

Effect of converting enzyme inhibitor, perindopril, on angiotensin peptides in plasma and kidney of the rat

Duncan J. Campbell, Anne C. Lawrence, Amanda Towrie, Athena Kladis and Anthony J. Valentijn

St. Vincent's Institute of Medical Research, 41 Victoria Parade, Fitzroy, Victoria 3065, Australia

Converting enzyme inhibitors (CEI) are valuable antihypertensive agents, but the mechanism of their hypotensive effect is not fully understood. The acute hypotensive effect of CEI may be of much longer duration than the apparent inhibition of angiotensin converting enzyme (ACE), as determined by measurement of plasma ACE activity or the pressor response to angiotensin I (Ang I) (Chen et al., 1984; Cohen & Kurz, 1982; Di Nicolantonio & Doyle, 1985; Sweet et al., 1981; Unger et al., 1985). Moreover, these drugs have only a transient effect on circulating levels of angiotensin II (Ang II), with levels returning towards normal within 24 h, despite a maintained hypotensive response (Juillerat et al., 1990; Mento et al., 1989; Mento & Wilkes, 1987). This dissociation between the hypotensive effect of CEI and their effect on plasma levels of Ang II has led to the proposal that the hypotensive effect is dependent upon an effect on Ang II levels in tissue rather than in plasma (Chen et al., 1984; Cohen & Kurz, 1982; Di Nicolantonio & Doyle, 1985; Sweet et al., 1981; Unger et al., 1985). This proposal is in accord with increasing evidence that tissue angiotensin systems play a more important role in blood pressure regulation than the circulating renin angiotensin system (Campbell, 1985; Admiraal et al., 1990). Various tissues, including kidney, show a prolonged suppression of ACE activity which parallels the prolonged suppression of blood pressure during and following cessation of CEI administration (Chen et al., 1984; Cohen & Kurz, 1982; Unger et al., 1985). Evidence that inhibition of renal ACE may be important for the antihypertensive effect of CEI includes the reduction in antihypertensive effect following bilateral nephrectomy (Antonaccio et al., 1979; Sweet et al., 1981). Moreover, the prolonged reduction in blood pressure of spontaneously hypertensive rats following short term treatment with CEI is associated with correction of the elevated renal vascular resistance in these rats (Harrap et al., 1986).

In the present study we investigated the effects of the CEI, perindopril, on components of the renin angiotensin system in plasma and kidney of rats. Using high performance liquid chromatography-based radioimmunoassays we quantified 8 angiotensin peptides in plasma and kidney: Ang-(1-7), Ang II, Ang-(1-9), Ang I, Ang-(2-7), Ang III, Ang-(2-9), and Ang-(2-10). In addition, we measured renin and angiotensinogen levels in plasma and kidney, renin mRNA levels in kidney, and angiotensinogen mRNA levels in kidney and liver. Full details of the methodology are described elsewhere (Campbell et al., 1991).

In plasma, the highest dose of perindopril reduced ACE activity to 11% of control, increased renin 200-fold, and reduced angiotensinogen to 11% of control. Renal angiotensinogen levels fell to 12% of control. Kidney renin mRNA levels increased 12-fold, but renal renin content, and angiotensinogen mRNA levels in kidney and liver were not influenced by perindopril treatment.

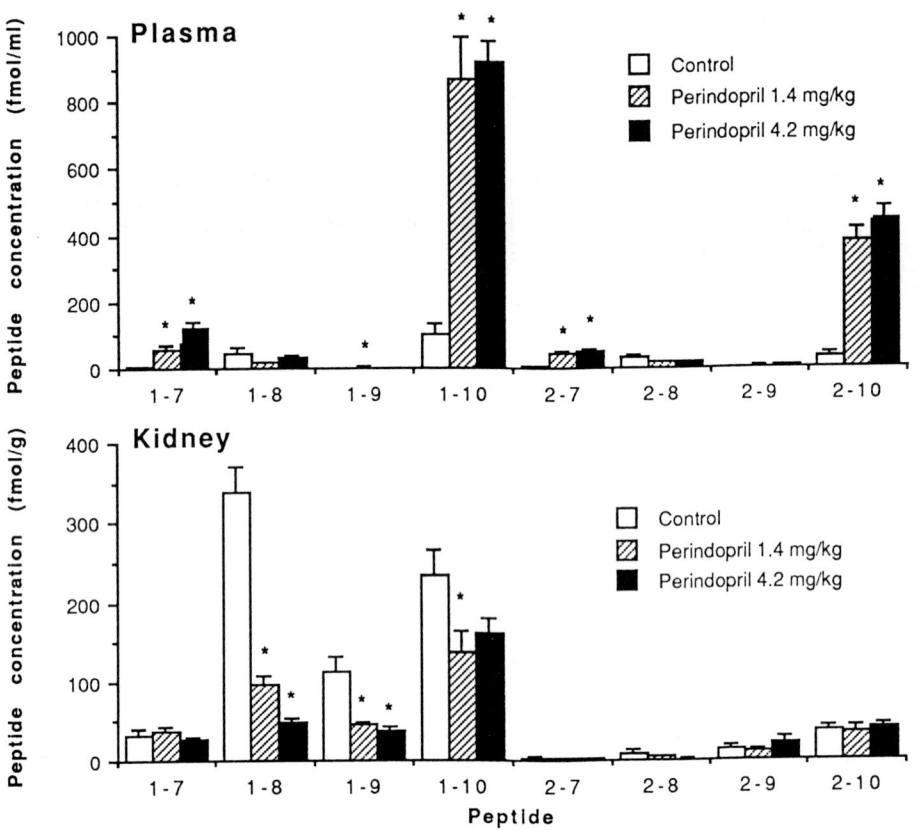

Fig. 1. Angiotensin peptide levels in plasma and kidney of rats administered either 0, 1.4 or 4.2 mg/kg perindopril in their drinking water for 7 days. 1-7, angiotensin-(1-7); 1-8, angiotensin II; 1-9, angiotensin-(1-9); 1-10, angiotensin I; 2-7, angiotensin-(2-7); 2-8, angiotensin III; 2-9, angiotensin-(2-9); 2-10, angiotensin-(2-10). Data are presented as means ± SEM, n = 6. *, $p < 0.05$, compared with control.

Angiotensin peptide levels in plasma and kidney are shown in Fig. 1. The levels of Ang-(1-7), Ang II, Ang-(1-9) and Ang I in kidney were higher than plasma levels, consistent with their local production in kidney. Perindopril had markedly different effects on angiotensin peptide levels in plasma and kidney. In plasma, the highest dose of perindopril increased Ang-(1-7), Ang I, Ang-(2-7), and Ang-(2-10) levels 25-, 9-, 10-, and 13-fold, respectively. Plasma levels of Ang II and Ang III did not show any significant change from control for either dose of perindopril. In contrast to plasma, renal levels of Ang II showed a marked decrease to 14% of control levels for the higher dose of perindopril, and Ang I, Ang-(2-10), and Ang-(1-7) levels did not increase. Both plasma and kidney showed evidence of inhibition of conversion of Ang I to Ang II, as indicated by the fall in Ang II:Ang I ratio which occurred.

These results demonstrate a differential regulation of angiotensin peptides in plasma and kidney. Although acute administration of CEI causes a fall in plasma Ang II levels in rats (Mento & Wilkes, 1987), chronic administration is associated with normal plasma Ang II levels (Mento et al., 1989), as shown in the present study, or elevated plasma Ang II levels (Mento & Wilkes, 1987). Similarly, in man, plasma Ang II levels return to normal within 24 h of CEI administration despite a maintained inhibition of ACE (Juillerat et al., 1990). The return of plasma Ang II levels to normal despite continued inhibition of ACE can be accounted for by the marked elevation of circulating renin and Ang I levels, sufficient to overcome the effects of CEI (Juillerat et al., 1990). The failure of renal Ang I levels to increase with perindopril administration is of considerable importance, given that circulating renin levels, and thus renal renin secretion rate, were increased 200-fold. Analogous to the argument proposed for the maintenance of plasma Ang II levels during perindopril administration, it can be argued that the failure of renal Ang I levels to increase was a critical determinant of the degree to which renal Ang II levels fell with perindopril administration. These data provide direct support for the hypothesis that the hypotensive action of CEI is dependent on an effect on Ang II levels in tissue rather than in plasma, and also provide support for the proposal that inhibition of renal ACE is important for the antihypertensive effect of CEI.

CEI administration was associated with marked increases in circulating renin, with consequent consumption of angiotensinogen. The fall in plasma levels of angiotensinogen had an important rate limiting effect on Ang I production, as shown by the 10-fold increase in plasma Ang I levels, compared with a 200-fold increase in circulating renin levels. The failure of kidney Ang I levels to increase with perindopril treatment, taken together with the fall in kidney angiotensinogen levels, suggest that angiotensinogen may be a major rate limiting determinant of angiotensin peptide levels in the kidney.

REFERENCES

Admiraal, P.J.J., Derkx, F.H.M., Danser, A.H.J., Pieterman, H. & Schalekamp, M.A.D.H. (1990): Metabolism and production of angiotensin I in different vascular beds in subjects with hypertension. *Hypertension* 15, 44-55.

Antonaccio, M.J., High, J.P., Rubin, B. & Schaeffer, T. (1979): Contribution of the kidneys but not adrenal glands to the acute antihypertensive effects of captopril in spontaneously hypertensive rats. *Clin. Sci.* 57, 127s-130s.

Campbell, D.J. (1985): The site of angiotensin production. *J. Hypertens.* 3, 199-207.

Campbell, D.J., Lawrence, A.C., Towrie, A., Kladis, A. & Valentijn, A.J. (1991): Differential regulation of angiotensin peptide levels in plasma and kidney of the rat. *Hypertension* (in press).

Chen, X., Pitt, B.R., Maolli, R. & Gillis, C.N. (1984): Correlation between lung and plasma angiotensin converting enzyme and the hypotensive effect of captopril in conscious rabbits. *J. Pharmacol. Exp. Ther.* 229, 649-653.

Cohen, M.L. & Kurz, K.D. (1982): Angiotensin converting enzyme inhibition in tissues from spontaneously hypertensive rats after treatment with captopril or MK-421. *J. Pharmacol. Exp. Ther.* 220, 63-69.

Di Nicolantonio, R. & Doyle, A.E. (1985): Comparison of the actions of the angiotensin-converting enzyme inhibitors enalapril and S-9490-3 in sodium-deplete and sodium-replete spontaneously hypertensive rats. *J. Cardiovasc. Pharmacol.* 7, 937-942.

Harrap, S.B., Nicolaci, J.A. & Doyle, A.E. (1986): Persistent effects on blood pressure and renal haemodynamics following chronic angiotensin converting enzyme inhibition with perindopril. *Clin. Exp. Pharmacol. Physiol.* 13, 753-765.

Juillerat, L., Nussberger, J., Ménard, J., Mooser, V., Christen, Y., Waeber, B., Graf, P. & Brunner, H.R. (1990): Determinants of angiotensin II generation during converting enzyme inhibition. *Hypertension* 16, 564-572.

Mento, P.F., Holt, W.F., Murphy, W.R. & Wilkes, B.M. (1989): Combined renin and converting enzyme inhibition in rats. *Hypertension* 13, 741-748.

Mento, P.F. & Wilkes, B.M. (1987): Plasma angiotensins and blood pressure during converting enzyme inhibition. *Hypertension* 9(Suppl III), III-42-III-48.

Sweet, C.S., Gross, D.M., Arbegast, P.T., Gaul, S.L., Britt, P.M., Ludden, C.T., Weitz, D. & Stone, C.A. (1981): Antihypertensive activity of N-[(S)-1-(ethoxycarbonyl)-3-phenylpropyl]-L-Ala-L-Pro (MK-421), an orally active converting enzyme inhibitor. *J. Pharmacol. Exp. Ther.* 216, 558-566.

Unger, T., Ganten, D., Lang, R.E. & Scholkens, B.A. (1985): Persistent tissue converting enzyme inhibition following chronic treatment with Hoe498 and MK421 in spontaneously hypertensive rats. *J. Cardiovasc. Pharmacol.* 7, 36-41.

Hemodynamic and fluid and electrolyte changes associated with the development of one-kidney, figure-8 renal wrap hypertension during constant sodium intake

Joseph R. Haywood and Paula Guerra

Department of Pharmacology, The University of Texas Health Science Center, 7703 Floyd Curl Drive, San Antonio, TX 78284-7764, USA

INTRODUCTION

Reduced renal function, retention of sodium and a direct relationship between the level of sodium intake and arterial pressure are considered hallmarks of sodium-dependent hypertension (Ganguli et al., 1979; Greene et al., 1990). These events are thought to lead to an expansion of body fluid volume and a subsequent increase in cardiac output as the initiating mechanism for hypertension (Coleman & Guyton, 1969). The one-kidney, figure-8 renal wrap model of hypertension is associated with impaired renal function (Lozano & Haywood, 1987), and arterial pressure is sodium sensitive (Haywood et al., 1985). However, previous studies of animals on *ad lib* sodium intake have not indicated a net positive sodium balance or increase in cardiac output during the onset of this model of hypertension (Haywood & Mutchler, 1980; Hinojosa & Haywood, 1986). The purpose of the present study was to determine the effect of a fixed sodium intake on body fluid and electrolyte regulation, arterial pressure and cardiac output.

METHODS

Two groups of male Sprague-Dawley rats (300-325 gm) were used in these studies. In the first study, animals were prepared with femoral vascular catheters while anesthetized with methoxyflurane. The rats were then placed in metabolic cages and tethered to a swivel system. Sodium intake was maintained at 2.4 meq/day by infusing isotonic saline intravenously at a rate of 0.7 ml/hr. Urine volume and urinary sodium concentration were measured daily. Fluid balance was determined as the difference between the fluid intake (infused volume plus *ad lib* water intake) minus urine volume. Sodium balance was estimated as the difference between infused sodium minus urinary sodium excretion. A three day baseline period was conducted in which arterial pressure and heart rate were measured for a 1 to 2 hour period and daily metabolic collections were taken. Then, the rats were randomly subjected to one-kidney, figure-8 renal wrap procedure or sham wrap (unilateral nephrectomy). Daily arterial pressure and heart rate measurements and metabolic collections were continued for an additional five days.

The same protocol was used in a second study. However, the rats were prepared with electromagnetic flowprobes on the ascending aorta for measurement of cardiac output. After recovery from surgery, arterial pressure, heart rate and cardiac output were measured daily. Total peripheral resistance was calculated from the arterial pressure and cardiac output measurements.

All data are expressed as mean ± SEM. Comparisons between groups over time were made using a two-way analysis of variance with repeated measures. Based on the results of the two-way analysis, appropriate post-hoc tests were performed. Significance was taken at the $p<0.05$ level.

RESULTS

Following the renal wrap procedure, mean arterial pressure rose from 110±2 mm Hg to 148±4 mm Hg on day 1 post-wrap and remained significantly elevated through the five days of observation (Fig. 1). Heart rate rose significantly only on day 2 post-wrap. In the sham operated rats, neither

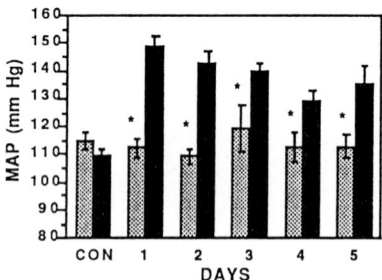 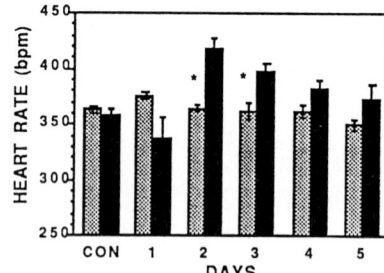

Fig. 1. Mean arterial pressure (MAP) and heart rate in sham operated (stipled bar) and renal wrapped (solid bar) animals through the five day study.
* denotes differences between groups.

mean arterial pressure or heart rate changed throughout the study. Fluid intake (i.e., water intake) increased during the post-wrap period from a control intake of 37±2 ml/day to a peak of 56±7 ml/day on day 4. Urine volume, on the other hand, decreased initially after the induction of hypertension (28±3 ml/day to 22±4 ml/day), then rose to a peak of 52±3 ml/day on day 2 and remained elevated through the rest of the study. As a result, fluid balance increased sharply on day 1 post-wrap (Fig. 2). Since sodium intake was constant and sodium excretion fell from 2.3±0.1 meq/day to 1.1±0.2 meq/day the day after the induction of hypertension, sodium balance increased significantly. The sham operated rats experienced no significant change in fluid or sodium balance throughout the study.

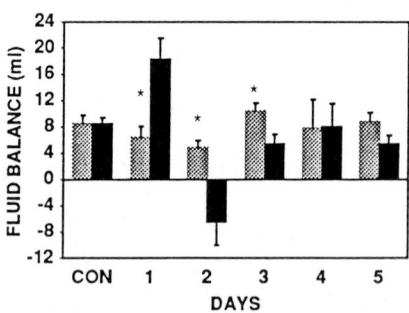 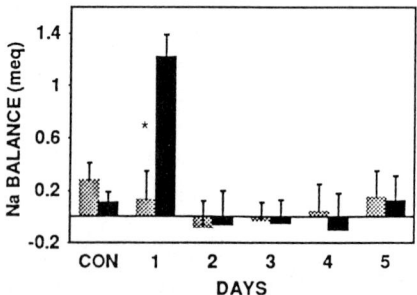

Fig. 2. Daily fluid balance and sodium balance in sham operated (stipled bar) and renal wrapped (solid bar) animals through the five day study.
* denotes differences between groups.

In the hemodynamic experiment, cardiac index increased from 25.2 ± 0.7 ml min^{-1} 100gm^{-1} to 27.7 ± 1.5 ml min^{-1} 100gm^{-1} (N.S.) on the second day of the hypertension and then receded to pre-wrap levels. Total peripheral resistance index, however, rose from 4.3 ± 0.1 mm Hg/ml min^{-1} 100gm^{-1} to 5.0 ± 0.4 mm Hg/ml min^{-1} 100gm^{-1} ($p<0.05$) on day 1 and remained elevated throughout the study. The sham operated animals did not experience any change in any hemodynamic parameter.

DISCUSSION

The positive sodium and fluid balance are common traits of sodium-dependent hypertension (Ganguli et al.,1979). In one-kidney, figure-8 renal wrap animals, there is a 50% reduction in renal blood flow, glomerular filtration rate and sodium excretion indicating a sodium retaining state (Lozano & Haywood, 1987). However, in previous studies with this model of hypertension, no change or a negative sodium balance was observed (Haywood & Mutchler, 1980). The animals attempted to regulate body sodium by a homeostatic reduction in the ingestion of sodium by reducing food intake. In the present study, infusion of sodium was used to maintain a constant sodium intake. Since the animals were unable to compensate for the renal retention of sodium by altering intake, the positive sodium and fluid balance occurred.

The rise in arterial pressure in these animals was similar to increases observed at this stage of hypertension in animals with *ad lib* sodium intake (Haywood & Ball, 1987). Therefore, the positive sodium and fluid balance did not cause a further increase in the level of blood pressure. The sodium and volume retention and rise in arterial pressure was not associated with an elevation in cardiac output as has been observed in other models of sodium-dependent hypertension (Ganguli et al., 1979). However, it is possible that an increase in cardiac output occurred during the first 24 hours without being detected since measurements were not made until day 1 post-wrap. The hypertension was associated with a 16% rise in total peripheral resistance index. This increase was similar to the change observed in *ad lib* normal and high sodium fed rats following renal wrapping (Hinojosa & Haywood, 1986; Haywood & Ball, 1987). Thus, the positive sodium balance and expansion of fluid volume resulted in a vasoconstrictor-mediated hypertension.

REFERENCES

Coleman, T.G. & Guyton, A.C. (1969): Hypertension caused by salt loading in the dog. III. Onset transients of cardiac output and other circulatory variables. *Circ. Res.* 25, 153-160.

Ganguli, M.L., Tobian, L. & Iwai, J. (1979): Cardiac output and peripheral resistance in strains of rats sensitive and resistant to NaCl hypertension. *Hypertension* 1,3-7.

Greene, A.S., Yu, Z.Y., Roman, R.J. & Cowley, A.W. (1990): Role of blood volume expansion in Dahl rat model of hypertension. *Am. J. Physiol.* 258, H508-H514.

Haywood, J.R. & Ball, N.A. (1987): Hemodynamic changes during the onset of normal sodium one-kidney, figure-8 renal wrap hypertension. *Fed. Proc.* 46, 523.

Haywood, J.R., Brennan, T.J. & Hinojosa, C. (1985): Neurohumoral mechanisms of sodium-dependent hypertension. *Fed. Proc.* 44, 2393-2399.

Haywood, J.R. & Mutchler, T.L. (1980): Sodium metabolism in one-kidney Grollman renal hypertension. *Fed. Proc.* 39, 496.

Hinojosa, C. & Haywood, J.R. (1986): Hemodynamic changes during onset of high-sodium one-kidney figure-8 renal hypertension. *Am. J. Physiol.* 251, H908-H914.

Lozano, S.C. & Haywood, J.R. (1987): Alterations in renal function during the onset of one-kidney, figure-8 renal wrap hypertension. *Fed. Proc.* 46, 523.

Plasma and tissue angiotensin converting enzyme variability in Wistar Kyoto and spontaneously hypertensive rats

Bruno Michel [1], Michèle Grima, Corinne Welsh, Catherine Coquard, Mariette Barthelmebs [1] and Jean-Louis Imbs [1]

[1] *Institut de Pharmacologie, URA DO 589 CNRS, Faculté de Médecine and Hypertension Clinique, CHR, Université Louis Pasteur, 67000 Strasbourg, France*

INTRODUCTION

Spontaneously hypertensive rats (SHR) and normotensive Wistar Kyoto (WKY) rats are frequently used in experimental studies. Although both strains of SHR and WKY rats have been assumed to be fully inbred, recent data have revealed that between animals of both strains from different commercial sources, there are biological and genetic variations (Kurtz et al., 1987; Kurtz et al., 1989; Louis et Lowes, 1990). To investigate the possibility that angiotensin converting enzyme (ACE) could be affected by this variability, we obtained SHR and WKY rats from three commercial suppliers in France and measured plasma and tissues ACE action in these rats under identical conditions.

MATERIALS AND METHODS

Animals

Eight week-old male SHR and WKY rats were bought from three different suppliers in France : Iffa Credo, l'Arbresle; Charles River, Cléon; Janvier, le Genest Saint Isle. Before the start of study, the rats (three per strain and per supplier) were kept in our laboratory for one week and maintained on a standard diet (normal salt diet, 0.4% sodium) and tap water ad libitum. The rats were studied under the same environmental conditions.

Plasma and tissue sampling

The rats were exsanguinated under ether anaesthesia by puncturing the abdominal aorta. The blood was collected in a heparinized syringe and centrifuged at 2000 g for 10 min (+4°C) to separate the plasma, which was stored at -20°C. Fragments of lung (right apex), heart (apex) and kidney (cortex and medulla) were removed and rinsed in 0.9% NaCl solution. These tissue samples were stored at -20°C. After defreezing, the organs were homogenized in Triton X-100 (0.3%) and the suspensions were centrifuged (11500 g for 20 min) after sonication. The supernatants were diluted in Triton X-100 (0.3%) for fluorimetric determination of ACE activity.

Determination of ACE activity

ACE activity was determined according to Unger et al. (1982) on the plasma and tissues samples using an artificial substrate, Cbz Phe-His-Leu. To ensure that a linear relationship was maintained between ACE activity and protein content, the protein concentration in the assay was maintained at less than 2 mg/ml (tissue) or 20 mg/ml (plasma) (Welsch et al., 1989). The protein concentration was assessed by the method of Lowry et al. (1951).

Statistics

The results are expressed as the mean ± SEM and compared with a two factor analysis of variance to test for an interaction between suppliers and strain. As an interaction was identified, for each tissue the differences between rats from the different suppliers were compared by analysis of variance followed by localisation of differences (Scheffé's test). Differences between SHR and WKY rats were analyzed using Student's t test; $p < 0.05$ was considered significant.

RESULTS

Comparison between suppliers

We found that WKY rats from one commercial source differed from those of the others with respect to both plasma and tissue ACE activities. Similarly, significant variations in SHR from the different sources were recorded (Table I).

Table I. Angiotensin converting enzyme activities (nmol His-Leu/min/mg protein) in plasma and various tissues from Wistar Kyoto (WKY) and spontaneously hypertensive (SHR) rats obtained from three commercial suppliers : Iffa Credo, Janvier, Charles River.

Tissue	Strains	Suppliers		
		Iffa Credo	Janvier	Charles River
LUNG	WKY	489 ± 48	339 ± 10	427 ± 8
	SHR	481 ± 69	386 ± 17	385 ± 11
PLASMA	WKY	6.53 ± 1.1	2.66 ± 0.4	2.69 ± 0.2
	SHR	3.08 ± 0.04	4.86 ± 0.8	2.45 ± 0.2
HEART	WKY	3.97 ± 0.5	2.64 ± 0.1	2.90 ± 0.2
	SHR	3.36 ± 0.4	4.14 ± 0.4	2.59 ± 0.2
RENAL CORTEX	WKY	2.13 ± 0.3	4.03 ± 1.4	0.35 ± 0.01
	SHR	0.75 ± 0.1	4.71 ± 0.9	0.34 ± 0.02
RENAL MEDULLA	WKY	3.97 ± 0.5	2.64 ± 0.1	1.16 ± 0.5
	SHR	3.36 ± 0.4	4.14 ± 0.4	2.15 ± 0.1

Data are means ± SEM. *$p < 0.05$, **$p < 0.01$ (n = 3)
Comparison between suppliers : ANOVA + Scheffe's test
Comparison between WKY and SHR rats : Student's t test

Comparison of WKY rats and SHR provided by the same supplier

Table I shows that plasma and tissue ACE activities were similar in the two strains from Charles River (with the exception of the lung) but not in the strains from Janvier and Iffa Credo. In the case of the last two commercial suppliers, plasma and tissue ACE activities were either higher (Janvier) or lower (Iffa Credo) in the SHR than in WKY rats.

CONCLUSION

Our results confirmed the existence of biological variations among WKY rats as supported by Kurtz et al. (1987) and showed a similar variation among SHR from the three suppliers. Since human plasma ACE level is under genetic control which seems to account for half of the variation of ACE levels (Rigat et al., 1990), we suggest that these results reflect genetic heterogeneity among the SHR strains and the WKY rat strains from the different suppliers and confirm the problem of how to interpret studies comparing SHR and WKY rats. This study also shows that the level of ACE activity does not seem to be a determining factor in the development of hypertension in SHR.

REFERENCES

Kurtz, TW. and Curtis Morris, JR. (1987): Biological variability in Wistar Kyoto rats. Hypertension 10: 127-131.
Kurtz, TW., Montano, M., Chan, L. and Kabra, P. (1989). Molecular evidence of genetic heterogeneity in Wistar-Kyoto rats : implications for research with the spontaneously hypertensive rats. Hypertension 13: 188-192.
Louis, WJ. and Lowes, LG. (1991): Genealogy of the spontaneously hypertensive rat and Wistar-Kyoto rat strains : implications for studies of inherited hypertension. J. Cardiovasc. Pharmacol. 16(suppl. 7): S1-S5.
Lowry, OM., Rosebrough, NJ., Lewis Farr, A. and Randall, RJ. (1951): Protein measurement with the folin phenol reagent. J. Biol. Chem. 193: 265-275.
Rigat, B., Hubert, C., Alhenc-Gelas, F., Cambien, F., Corvol, P. and Soubrier, F. (1990): An insertion/deletion polymorphism in the angiotensin I-converting enzyme gene accounting for half the variance of serum enzyme levels. J. Clin. Invest. 86: 1343-1346.
Unger, T., Schöll, B., Rascher, W., Lang, R.E. and Ganten, D. (1982): Selective activation of the converting enzyme inhibition MK 421 and comparison of its active diacid form with captopril in different tissues of rat. Biochem. Pharmacol. 31: 3063-3070.
Welsch, C., Grima, M., Giesen, EM., Helwig, JJ., Barthelmebs, M., Coquard, C. and Imbs, JL. (1989): Assay of tissue angiotensin converting enzyme. J. Cardiovasc. Pharmacol. 14(suppl. 4): S26-S31.

H-pump and Na-H exchange in isolated single proximal tubule and cortical collecting duct of spontaneously hypertensive rats

Georges Dagher and Claude Sauterey

Laboratoire de Physiologie cellulaire, Collège de France, 11, place Marcellin Berthelot, 75005 Paris, France

There is convincing evidence to suggest a permissive role to the kidney in the development and maintenance of hypertension (Guyton et al, 1980). Balance studies in hypertension revealed a mild acidosis (Lucas et al, 1988) and a reduced ability to excrete sodium and water (Beierwaltes et al,1982). Recent observations suggested that an intrinsic difference in the tubular function of SHR could contribute to the enhanced Na^+ reabsorption. Fractional Na^+ and water excretion was significantly lower in SHR as compared to WKY (Roman & Cowley,1985). The activity of the Na^+-H^+ exchanger (Morduchowicz et al,1989) and that of the Na^+-K^+-ATPase (Garg et al, 1985) was found to be increased in brush border membranes and proximal segments from SHR rats.

The proximal tubule plays a vital role in acid-base homeostasis by reabsorbing filtered bicarbonate and regenerating bicarbonate when required. It is also implicated in the reabsorption of NaCl. These processes are accomplished by a variety of transport pathways. Most of bicarbonate reabsorption occurs in the first millimiters of the proximal tubule and is dependent on proton secretion coupled to sodium reabsorption via the Na^+-H^+ exchanger and to a lesser extent, mediated by a H^+ pump (Alpern,1990).

In this study, we wished to examine the activity of two transporters the Na^+-H^+ exchange and the H^+ pump in the superficial proximal tubule of SHR as compared to WKY controls. In order to assess the contribution of these pathways to Na^+ reabsorption and H^+ secretion along this tubule, we have determined their activities in single isolated segments dissected at different locations along the PCT.

METHODS

Spontaneously hypertensive rats (SHR) and Wistar Kyoto (WKY) were obtained from Janvier Laboratories. The rats were studied at two ages 5 wks and 9 wks. Superficial single proximal tubules and cortical collecting ducts were isolated from collagenase treated kidneys. S1 segments were selected within the initial portion of the tubule (first mm) and S2 segments within the portion located at distance > 1.5 mm from the glomerulus. Cells were loaded with (BCECF). The tubule was fixed on a glass cover slip which was then glued to a steel chamber mounted on an inverted Leitz Diavert microscope. pHi was determined by alternately exciting the dye at 450 and 500 nm while measuring the fluorescence emissionat 530 nm.

RESULTS

One commonly used approach for studying proton extrusion mechanisms is to acutely load the cells with acid, and monitor the subsequent recovery of cellular pH towards its initial level (Roos & Boron,1981). In the present study, single isolated segments were acid loaded by transiently exposing the cells to 30 mM ammonium chloride. pHi spontaneously recovers from this acid load as a result of one or more acid extrusion mechanisms located in the luminal and basolateral cell membranes. The activity of the NEM-sensitive H$^+$ pump was assayed by following pH recovery from an acid load in the absence of external sodium. The activity of the Na$^+$-H$^+$ exchanger was assayed by following pH recovery from an acid load in the presence of external sodium and NEM.

H extrusion mechanisms in S1 segments from SHR as compared Wistar Kyoto rats.

We have examined the Na independent and Na dependent pH recovery mechanisms in S1 segments from young and adult WKY and SHR. The activity of the Na-independent pathway in this segment varied between 0.1 and 0.4 pH unit/min.

The first rates of the Na$^+$-dependent pathway in young and adult rats was assessed at comparable cell pH of 6.8±0.05. In young rats, before the development of hypertension, the Na$^+$-dependent pathway had a significantly higher activity in SHR with a mean±SE of 0.22 ± 0.06 pH units/min, (n=15) as compared to WKY (0.10±0.02,n=13, p≤0.025). In adult rats the tendency of a higher activity of this pathway was observed in SHR (0.16±0.03,n=13) but was not statistically significant when compared to adult WKY(0.10±0.01,n=14). In this study we have assumed that cellular Na$^+$ was uniformly low as the tubule was exposed to NMG medium before the addition of external sodium.

H -extrusion pathways in S2 segments in SHR as compared to WKY

The activity of the Na$^+$ independent H extrusion mechanism was assessed in 68 S2 segments from WKY and SHR. In adult rats, the activity of this pathway is markedly increased in the WKY(0.29±0.08,n=12) as compared to SHR (0.03±0.01,n=20, p≤0.001), while in the young rats (5wks) no significant difference could be observed between the two strains (0.03±0.01vs 0.03±0.01). On the other hand, it should be noted that in the WKY strain the activity of the Na$^+$- independent pathway increases markedly with age, while in the SHR the activity of this transporter in adult rats is similar to that observed in young animals. These results strongly suggest an impaired maturation of the Na$^+$-independent H$^+$ efflux mechanism in the SHR strain.

The initial rate of the Na$^+$-dependent H$^+$ efflux was assessed in 73 S2 segments. No difference could be observed in the activity of this pathway between both strains either in the young or adult groups (0.22 pHunit/min). Similarly the activity of the Na-H exchanger was not significantly different between S1 and S2 segments in each of the strains.

H Pump and Na-H exchange in cortical collecting duct.

No significant difference in either the H pump activity or the Na-H exchange could be observed between SHR (n=5)and control rats (n=5). Similarly the buffering capacity was not different between the two strains.

Discussion

The proximal tubule plays a vital role in acid base homeostasis by reabsorbing filtered bicarbonate and regenerating required bicarbonate. These processes are accomplished by luminal H$^+$ secretion. A number of studies have established that a Na$^+$-H$^+$ exchanger accounts for most of luminal acidification, and recent reports suggested a role for a NEM sensitive H$^+$ pump in this segment . On the other hand sodium reabsorption in this segment is mediated on the apical membrane by a number of transport processes among them the Na$^+$-H$^+$ exchanger. On the basolateral side, the Na$^+$-K$^+$ pump is largely responsible for sodium extrusion from the cell (Alpern, 1990). Our results show an increase in the activity of the Na$^+$-H$^+$ exchanger in S1 segment from young SHR. This is in accord with a previous report showing an increase in the activity of this transporter in BBM vesicles from young SHR (Morduchowicz et al,1989). On the other hand Garg et al (1985) reported an increased Na$^+$-K$^+$-ATPase activity in PCT of a 5 wks old SHR compared to WKY. Thus an enhanced activity of these two pathways could account for the reduced ability to excrete sodium observed in young SHR (Beierwaltes et al,1982). On the other hand in the adult rats we did not observe any difference of the Na$^+$-H$^+$ exchanger in either the S1 or S2 segment between the two strains. This could be consequent to morphological modifications in the cell's features with age, or to modulation of the activity of this transporter by haemodynamic or hormonal factors, further investigations are needed to answer this question. Interestingly the Na^+-K^+-ATPase activity was not modified in the adult SHR (Garg et al,1985) and Na^+ excretion was found to be normal (Beierwaltes et al,1982).

A number of observations suggested the presence of an electrogenic H^+ pump in the PCT that contributes to bicarbonate reabsorption (Alpern,1990).The present study shows that the activity of the NEM-sensitive H^+ pump is about 5 times higher in the S1 segment as compared to that observed in the S2 segment of young rats. This is in accord with an axial heterogeneity in apical H^+ secretion previously reported in the rat PCT (Maddox & Gennari,1987). Interestingly in the S2 segment, the activity of this pathway increases markedly with age in the WKY, while in the SHR the H^+ pump activity in both young and adult rats is almost unsignificant. These results suggests an impairment in the maturation process of the H^+ pump in the S2 segment of the hypertensive strain.

In summary, the present study provides evidence for an increase in the Na^+-H^+ exchanger activity in S1 segment from young SHR and an impaired maturation of the H^+ pump in the S2 segment of adult hypertensive rats. Several studies has related the inability of the kidney of SHR to excrete sodium to an excessive tubular reabsorption. In the proximal tubule, Na^+ reabsorption is known to be regulated by hormonal factors and to be dependent on variations of luminal solute concentrations and transepithelial P.D along the tubule. An increase in the Na^+-H^+ exchanger and an an impairment in the H^+ pump activity would induce a modification in solute profile along the proximal tubule. As a consequence Na reabsorption is most likely to be increased in this segment, the reabsorption of other ions in particular bicarbonate, is more difficult to predict and requires futher investigations.

REFERENCES

ALPERN R. J. Cell mechanisms of proximal tubule acidification, 1990. Physiol. Rev. 70: 79-109.

BEIERWALTES, W.H., W.J. ARENDSHORST, AND P.J. KLEMMER,1982. Electrolyte and water balance in young spontaneously hypertensive rats. Hypertension, 4: 908-915

COWLEY, A. W., Jr., and R. J. ROMAN,1983. Renal dysfonction in essential hypertension-implications of experimental studies. Am. J. Nephrol, 3 : 59-72.

GARG, L.C., N. NARANG, and S. Mc ARDLE,1985. Na, K ATPAase in nephron segments of rats developing spontaneous hypertension. Am. J. Physiol, 249 (Renal Fluid Electrolyte Physiol. 18) : F863-F869.

GUYTON A.C., T. G. COLEMAN, D. B. YOUNG, T. E. LOHMEIER, and J. W. DECLUE,1980. Salt balance and long-terme pressure control. Annu. Rev. Med, 31 : 15-27.

LUCAS. P., B. LACOUR, L. COMTE, and T. DRUEKE, 1988. Pathogenesis of abnormal acid-base balance in the young spontaneously hypertensive rat. Clin. Sci. 75 : 29-34.

MADDOX D.., and J.F. GENNARI,1987. The early proximal tubule: a high capacity delivery responsive site. Am. J. Physiol. 252: F573-F584.

MORDUCHOWICZ G.A, D. SHEIKH-HAMAD, O.D. JO, E. NORD, D. LEE, and N. YANAGAWA,1989. Increased Na/H antiport activity in the renal brush border membrane of SHR. Kid. International, 36: 576-581.

ROMAN R.J. and A.W. COWLEY,1985. Abnormal pressure diuresis natriuresis response in spontaneously hypertensive rats . Am. J. Physiol. 248, (Renal Fluid Electrol. Physiol. 17): F199-F205,.

ROOS, A., and W.F. BORON,1981. Intracellular pH. Physiol. Rev. 61 : 296-434.

A modeling study of alterations in transport processes along rat proximal tubule in hypertension : implications in solute reabsorption

S.R. Thomas and G. Dagher

INSERM U.383, Faculté de Médecine Necker and Laboratoire de Physiologie Cellulaire, Collège de France, Paris, France

One ubiquitous aspect of hypertension is the diminished ability of the kidney to excrete sodium. This decrease is thought to result, in part, from an intrinsic defect in tubular sodium absorption. Recent studies comparing proximal tubules from spontaneously hypertensive rats (SHR) to those of normotensive WKY rats showed alterations in certain parameters, such as increased Na/H exchange (Morduchowicz et al., 1989), increased Na/K pump (Garg et al., 1985), and decreased GFR. To gain insight into possible implications of these observations for global solute balance, we have investigated their effects using a computer model developed by us which faithfully reproduces many aspects of normal PCT function.

Thanks to detailed studies of most of the individual transport systems in the renal proximal tubule in the last few years, there is now a general consensus concerning kinetic mechanisms for most of them and experimental estimates of their transport parameters. It thus now becomes possible to incorporate this new membrane-level information into a global tubule model in order to simulate luminal solute reabsorption.

Model description

On the cellular level, we modeled individual transport systems in both apical and basolateral membranes and also included the paracellular pathway.

The apical cell membrane includes the asymmetric, neutral Na/H antiport and an active proton pump as well as a co-transport of organic solutes with sodium. There are also passive diffusional pathways for CO_2, protons, and K^+. In the basolateral membrane, we included Na-$3HCO_3$ co-transport, K-Cl co-transport, the Na/K ATPase, and passive diffusion of glucose, CO_2, protons, and K^+. Flows of each species are subject to the constraints of mass balance and macroscopic electroneutrality.

This steady state cellular model, formulated as a system of space-centered, finite-difference equations, was then integrated along the length of the proximal tubule to a distance of 5 mm in steps of 0.1mm or less. Intracellular and luminal concentrations and electrical potential along the tubule were left free to evolve as a function of transport. Water absorption was considered to result simply from the transepithelial hydroosmotic driving force, which, given the high hydraulic filtration coefficient, leads naturally to quasi-isosmotic transport with a very slightly hypotonic lumen. Apart from the various parameters that define the transport rates, the only fixed inputs to the model were peritubular solute concentrations, initial luminal concentrations and SNGFR. In our basic model, we considered that all transport parameters were constant along the whole length of the tubule except for proton secretion, which was allowed to decrease exponentially as a function of distance.

RESULTS OF MODEL SIMULATIONS

Control simulations:

With this configuration, the predicted longitudinal profiles of luminal solute concentrations fit nicely with control experimental data in Sprague-Dawley animals. Fig. 1 depicts the profiles of Na^+, Cl^-, HCO_3^-, and glucose concentrations (expressed as a fraction of their entering values) and for water reabsorption from a typical simulation of the model.

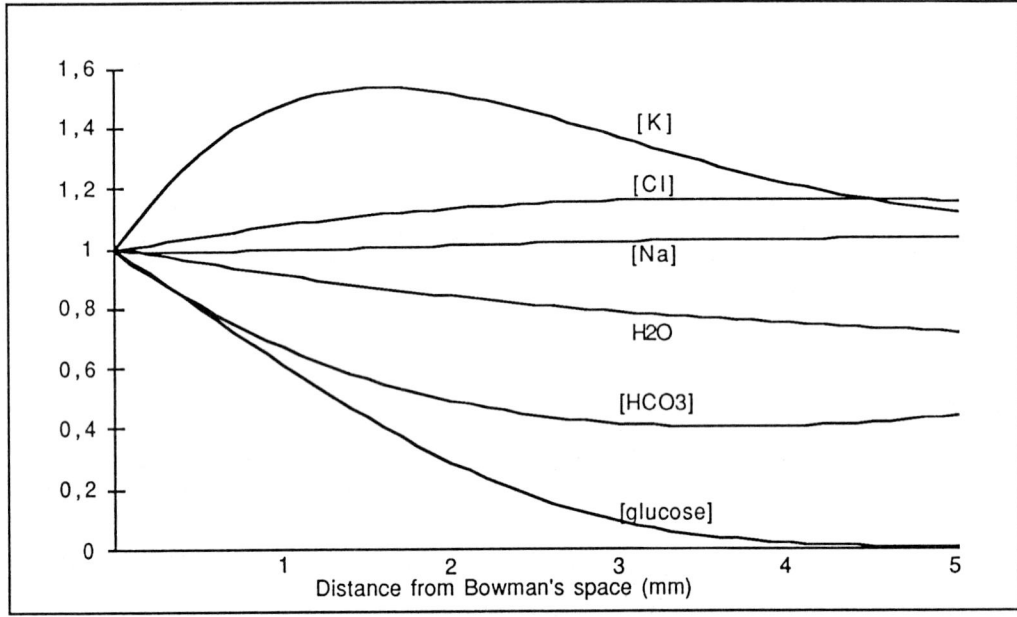

Figure 1. Longitudinal profiles of solute concentrations and volume flow expressed as a fraction of their values at the beginning of the tube.

Simulations with altered transport parameters:

Since to our knowledge no measurements of either the solute profiles or the kinetic transport parameters in proximal tubules of SHR have been reported, we were obliged to simulate the expected changes by appropriate modification of parameters in a model based on normal rats.

A doubling of sodium-proton exchanger activity in the model predicts a 40% stimulation of Na/K pump activity at the beginning of the tubule and a 70% increase in bicarbonate and, as can be seen in Table 1, a 46% increase in water reabsorption in the first mm of the PCT.

Because of the prolonged 'contact time' and despite reduced delivery rate, decreasing GFR by 30% predicts increased (143%) fractional bicarbonate reabsorption in the first mm. Similarly, fractional glucose and volume reabsorption were also predicted to increase by 38% and 50%, respectively, whereas there was virtually no change in their absolute reabsorption.

Table 1. Fractional and absolute reabsorption as % of control values at 1 mm

	Bicarbonate		Glucose		Volume Flow	
	fractional	absolute	fractional	absolute	fractional	absolute
Decreased GFR	143%	95%	138%	92%	150%	102%
Double Na/H	170%	170%	102%	102%	146%	146%

On the other hand, a 25% increase in the maximal velocity (Vmax) of Na/K pump did not modify the profile of solute reabsorption in the model, suggesting that the pump is working well below its maximal rate and that therefore modifications of its Vmax might be less important than changes in the affinities for the substrates.

These results demonstrate the utility of modeling studies for obtaining qualitative information on the possible implications of these changes in solute reabsorption in the PCT of SHR, and may therefore contribute to a better understanding of the pathogenesis of hypertension.

REFERENCES

GARG, L.C., N. NARANG, and S. Mc ARDLE (1985): Na, K ATPAase in nephron segments of rats developing spontaneous hypertension. *Am. J. Physiol, 249 (Renal Fluid Electrolyte Physiol. 18)* : F863-F869.

MORDUCHOWICZ G.A, D. SHEIKH-HAMAD, O.D. JO, E. NORD, D. LEE, and N. YANAGAWA (1989): Increased Na/H antiport activity in the renal brush border membrane of SHR. *Kid. International* 36: 576-581.

Biphasic effects of an adenosine analogue on the cyclic AMP formation in isolated rat glomeruli

Yuhong Liu, Satoshi Umemura, Nobuhito Hirawa, Yoshiyuki Toya, Minoru Kihara, Tamio Iwamoto, Shuichi Hayashi, Kazuyoshi Takeda, Shunsei Young and Masao Ishii

Second Department of Internal Medicine, Yokohama City University, 3-9, Fukuura, Kanazawa-Ku, Yokohama, 236, Japan

Many studies have focused on the structure, function and mechanism of action of adenosine A 1 (A_1) and adenosine A 2 (A_2) receptors in vaious tissues. In the kidney, up to now, adenosine receptors have been found in glomeruli (Abboud, 1983; Freissmuth, 1987; Palacio, 1987), vascular tissues (Freissmuth, 1987; Murray, 1987), medullary thick ascending limbs of Henle and cortical collecting tubules (Arend, 1987; Palacio, 1987). It has been reported that adenosine can regulate renal blood flow, glomerular filtration rate (Hall,1986; Hall, 1985), renin secretion (Churchill, 1987; 1985; Murray, 1984) and angiotensin-II formation (Hall, 1985; 1986) and affect urinary flow and electrolyte excretion (Churchill, 1985; Hall, 1985; Miyamoto, 1988). These results suggest the important roles of adenosine receptors in the kidney.

The goal of the present study is to investigate whether A_1 and/or A_2 receptors are present in glomeruli of rat kidneys by measuring cyclic AMP (cAMP) which is a key substance of the second messenger system of these receptors.

Materials and Methods: Fifteen male Wistar-Kyoto rats (WKY) were used in the study. They were devided into 2 groups. One group (n=9) was used to examine the effect of NECA (5-N-ethylcarboxamidoadenosine: adenosine receptor agonist) on the basal production of cAMP and the other group (n=6) to examine the effect of NECA on the parathyroid hormone (PTH)-induced production of cAMP. The left kidney was removed after perfusion, sliced and treated with a collagenase solution. Glomeruli (G) were isolated under a stereomicroscope in an ice cold-buffer solution containning RO 20-1724 (10^{-4}M), a phosphodiesterase inhibitor. Four glomeruli were transfered to a tube containing 20 µl of the buffer solution. Following 5 min of preincubation at 37°C, NECA at defferent concentrations was added to the tubes with or without PTH (3.05 µ g/ml) and incubated with the glomeruli at 37°C for 2 min. The reaction was terminated by adding 10% trichloroacetic acid. The cAMP production by glomeruli was measured by radioimmunoassay. The data were analyzed with the Student's paired t-test.

Results: NECA, an adenosine receptor agonist, showed a biphasic effect on the PTH-induced production of cAMP in rat glomeruli (Fig.1). NECA at a high concentrtion (5×10^{-5}M) displayed an A_2 receptor stimulating effect, since it increased cAMP production from 0.10 ± 0.63 to 0.54 ± 0.08 pmol/4G (n=9; p<0.01) as showed in Fig. 1. Furthermore, NECA at this concentration stimulated the glomerular production of cAMP in the presense of PTH from 0.35 ± 0.06 to 0.80 ± 0.22 pmol/4G (n=6; p<0.05). On the contrary, NECA at a low concentration (5×10^{-9}M) inhibited the PTH-induced production of cAMP in glomeruli from

0.35 ± 0.06 to 0.22 ± 0.05 pmol/4G (n=6, p<0.05) (Fig. 1), suggesting that NECA at this concentration activates A_1 receptors. However, NECA at the low concentration did not decrease significantly the basal production of cAMP (0.10 ± 0.03 vs. 0.06 ± 0.03 pmol/4G, n=9, ns) (Fig. 1).

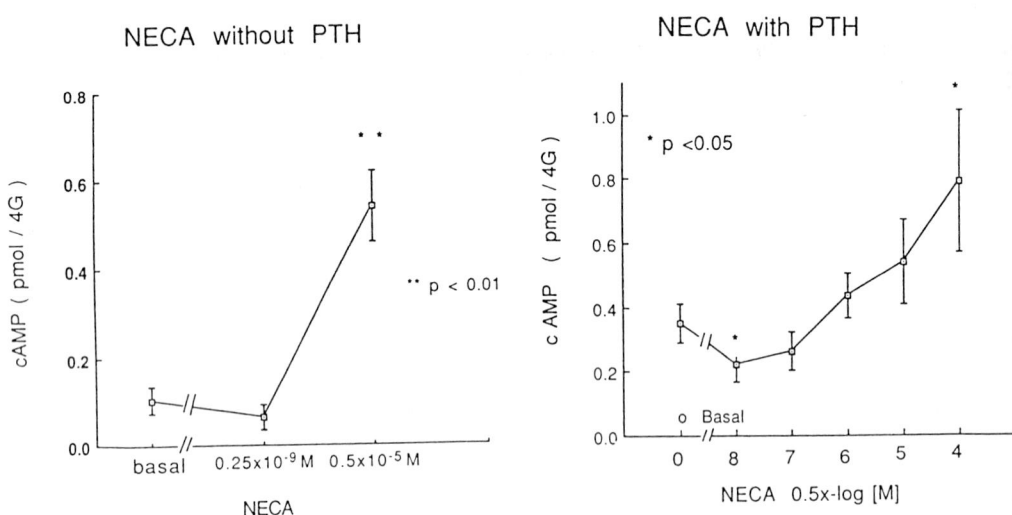

Fig. 1. Effect of NECA on the production of cAMP in rat glomeruli in the absence (left) and in the presence (right) of PTH.

Discussion and Conclusion: It is well known that one of the intracellular signal transduction systems of adenosine receptors is the adenylate cyclase-cAMP sytem. Stimulation of A_1 receptors decreases cAMP production, while stimulation of A_2 receptors increases it. It has been demonstrated that NECA affects both A_1 and A_2 receptors in respect to the cAMP production and that the mode of action of the agent varies depending on its concentration (Arend, 1987). The present study showed that NECA at low and high concentrations resulted in different effects; inhibiting and stimulating the glomerular cAMP production, respectively. These results suggest that there exist both A_1 and A_2 receptors in isolated rat glomeruli. These findings seem to be consistent with those of the previous reports which, although their methods were different from those used in the present study, showed that glomeruli contained A_1 and/or A_2 receptors in rats (Abboud, 1983), rabbits (Freissmuth, 1987) and human (Palacio, 1987). As well, the results of the present study seem to contribute to understanding the mechanisms of action of adenosine in regulating GFR (Hall, 1985; Hall, 1986; Murray, 1984), controlling renin secretion (Churchill, 1985; 1987; Murray, 1984) and inducing mesangial cell contraction (Olivera, 1989). Although a large munber of studies have been performed to elucidate the role and function of adenosine receptors, the interaction between adenosine-receptors and intracellular signal transduction systems are still unclear. Recently, other second messenger systems such as IP_3-calcium interaction system have began to attract attention. It has been disclosed that adenosine receptors coupled not only to cAMP system but to a system which involves inositol phosphate production, leading to changes in cytosolic free calcium (Arend, 1989; Brunatoska, 1991). In summary, the results of the present study suggest that that both A_1 and A_2 receptors are present in rat glomeruli and that they possess different effects on the production of cAMP.

ACKNOWLEDGEMENTS

This study was supported in part by a Grant-in-Aid for Scientific Research (No. 02454260) from the Ministry of Education, Science and Culture, Japan.

REFERENCES

Abboud, M.E. & Dousa, T.P. (1983): Action of adenosine on cyclic 3', 5'-nucleotides in glomeruli. Am.J.Physiol. 244: F633-638.
Arend, L.T., et al. (1989): Adenosine-sensitive phosphoinositide turnover in a newly established renal cell line. Am.J.Physiol. 256: F1067-1074.
Arend, L.T., et al. (1987): A_1 and A_2 adenosine receptors in rabbit cortical collecting tubule cells-modulation of hormone-stimulated cAMP. J.Clin Invest. 79: 710-714.
Burnatowska-Mledin, M.A., & Spielman W.S. (1991): Effects of adenosine on cAMP production and cytosolic Ca^{2+} in cultured rabbit medullary thick limb cells. Am.J.Physiol.260: C143-150.
Churchill, P.C., & Bidani A. (1987): Renal effects of selective adenosine receptor agonists in anesthetized rats. Am.J.Physiol.252: F299-303.
Churchill, P.C. & Churehill M.C. (1985): A_1 and A_2 adenosine receptor activation inhibits and stimulates renin secretion of rat renal cortical slices. J. Pharmacol. & Exp. Ther. 232: 589-594.
Freissmuth, M., et al. (1987): Glomeruli and microvessels of the rabbit kidney contain both A_1 and A_2 adenosine receptors. Naunyn-Schmiedeberg's Areh Pharmacol.335: 438-444.
Hall, J. E. & Groangor J.P. (1986): Adenosine alters glomerular filtration control by angiotensin II. Am.J Physiol. 250; F917-923.
Hall, J.E., et al. (1985): Interactions between adenosine and angiogensin II in controlling glomerular filtration. Am.J.Physiol. 248: F340-346.
Murray, R.D., & Churchill P.C. (1984): Effects of adenosine receptor agonists in the isolated, perfused rat kidney. Am.J.Physiol. 247: 343-348.
Miyamoto, M., et al. (1988): Effects of intrarenal adenosine on renal function and medullary blood flow in the rat. Am.J.Physiol. 255: F1230-1234.
Olivera, A., et al. (1989): Adenosine induces mesangial cell contraction by A_1-type receptor. Kidney Int. 35: 1300-1305.
Palaci,O J.M., et al. (1987): Visualization of adenosine A_1 receptors in the human and the geinea-pig kidney. European J.of Pharmacol. 138: 273-276.
Weber, R.G., et al. (1990): Demonstration of A_1 adenosine receptors on rat medullary thick ascending limb tubules by radioligand binding. Kidney int. 37: 380.

Impaired natriuretic response to intermittent bilateral carotid artery traction in spontaneously hypertensive rats

Jean-Pierre Valentin, Sami A. Mazbar and Michael H. Humphreys

Division of Nephrology, San Francisco General Hospital and University of California San Francisco, San Francisco, CA, USA

INTRODUCTION

The carotid baroreflex is an important regulator of the cardiovascular system. Activation of the baroreflex leads to vasodepression [Abboud et al., 1976], one manifestation of which is a decrease in sympathetic efferent renal nerve activity (ERNA) [Wilson et al., 1971]; decreased ERNA can result in natriuresis [DiBona, 1982]. Some years ago, Keeler showed that traction on a carotid artery activated the carotid sinus baroreceptors on that side and initiated a reflex which led to natriuresis [Keeler, 1974]. Spontaneously hypertensive rats (SHR) have many abnormalities that could contribute to the development and/or maintenance of hypertension; among these are abnormalities in functioning of the sympathetic nervous system [Janssen and Smits, 1989]. Recently, we described a technique to evaluate the reflex control of renal function by repetitive activation of both carotid sinus baroreceptors in anesthetized, euvolemic Sprague-Dawley rats [Valentin et al., in press]. The present study sought to explore the effect of carotid sinus baroreceptor activation on renal function using this technique in anesthetized, euvolemic SHR and their normotensive control Wistar Kyoto rats (WKY).

METHODS

We studied 12 WKY and 13 SHR (Charles River Laboratory, Watick, MA) (age 12-14 weeks, wt 240-320 g). They were anesthetized with Inactin^R (110 mg/kg ip), placed on a heated table to maintain rectal temperature at 37±0.5°C, and tracheostomized to allow spontaneous breathing. Catheters were inserted into a femoral vein and the two femoral arteries for infusing solutions, sampling blood, and recording arterial pressure. A PE60 catheter was inserted into the dome of the urinary bladder via a midline suprapubic incision for urine collections. Both common carotid arteries were dissected free of surrounding fascia and a ligature was placed around them. The left ligature was tied securely while the right remained loose. These ligatures were then used for the subsequent application of traction. During the surgical preparation, a solution of 5% bovine serum albumin (Sigma Chemical, St. Louis, MO) was infused via a syringe pump until a total volume of 1% body weight was administered to replace estimated fluid losses. After completion of the surgery, albumin was discontinued and replaced by a 0.9% solution of sodium chloride containing meglumine iothalamate (Conray 60^R, Mallinkrodt Inc., St. Louis, MO), and infused at 2.4 ml/hr for the rest of the experiment. After a 45-60 minute stabilization period, three to four urine collections of 20 minutes each were obtained. At the end of this control period, manual traction on both carotid arteries was applied by pulling on the previously placed ligatures for the first minute of consecutive 15 min periods. Urine was collected for six such periods following the initiation of the first traction into preweighed plastic vials and urine volume determined gravimetrically. Urine sodium and potassium concentrations were determined by flame photometry, and urine and plasma iothalamate concentrations measured by fluorescence excitation. The urinary clearance of iothalamate was used as a measure of GFR. The results of three to four clearance measurements were averaged to provide a single value for the control period and of the last three clearance measurements for the experimental period for each rat. Data are expressed as mean ± SE. Repeated measures analysis of variance and Student's t test were used to assess significance within and between groups. A P value of 0.05 was considered the mininum level of significance.

RESULTS

In WKY, intermittent bilateral carotid artery traction (BilCAT) produced an immediate, transient (less than 2 minutes), and reproducible fall in mean arterial pressure (MAP) of 33±3 mmHg from a value of 120±6 mmHg (Fig. 1A). This maneuver led to a progressive natriuresis that was fully developed 45-90 min after the initial application of the traction (Fig. 1B). When the values of the last 3 periods were averaged, the increase in water, sodium and potassium were respectively 80±20, 132±31 and 85±68% (all $P<0.05$). BilCAT also increased GFR from 2.2±0.2 to 2.9±0.2 ml/min ($p<0.02$). There was no change in MAP (from 119±4 to 120±6 mmHg), except for the initial dip as a result of BilCAT. SHR had a significantly higher MAP (173±4 vs 119±4) compared to WKY. As shown in Fig 1A, BilCAT led to a significantly greater fall in MAP of 51±3 mmHg from this higher baseline. In contrast to WKY, and despite the greater dip in MAP, the SHR failed to exhibit diuretic (-47±26%), natriuretic (25±36%) or kaliuretic (-23±8%) responses to BilCAT ($P=NS$ for all). In addition, no significant change in GFR occurred in this group (2.1±0.1 to 1.8±0.1 ml/min, $P=NS$).

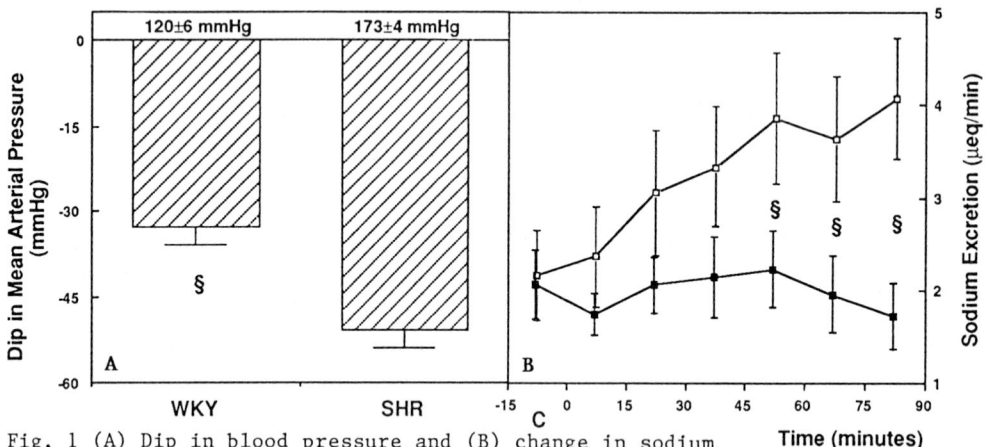

Fig. 1 (A) Dip in blood pressure and (B) change in sodium excretion after BilCAT. § significant difference between WKY and SHR, $p < .05$.

DISCUSSION

Activation of carotid sinus baroreceptors elicits reflex vasodepression mediated chiefly by a reduction in efferent sympathetic outflow [Abboud et al., 1976; Wilson et al., 1971]. In 1974, Keeler devised a model of unilateral CAT which allowed him to monitor electrolyte excretion in conscious rats. Unilateral traction led to a marked increase in sodium excretion that was abolished by carotid sinus denervation and that was still present although blunted in rats with bilateral renal denervation [Keeler, 1974]. Recently, we reported a technique to evaluate the reflex control of renal function and sodium excretion by repetitive activation of both carotid sinus baroreceptors [Valentin et al., in press]. In the present study, intermittent BilCAT in WKY resulted in a progressive natriuresis that was fully developed within 45 min and lasted at least for 90 min, the point at which we terminated our experiments. The time course and the magnitude of the natriuresis were similar to those observed in Sprague-Dawley rats [Valentin et al., in press] as well as after application of a constant traction to one carotid artery in a somewhat more hydropenic anesthetized rat preparation [Mazbar et al., 1990]. In contrast the SHR failed to exhibit a natriuresis in response to BilCAT despite an even greater reflex vasodepression caused by the maneuver. These results indicated that the reflex pathways mediating natriuresis after intermittent BilCAT are disrupted in SHR. With bilateral CAT

[Valentin et al., and present study] as well as with unilateral CAT [Mazbar et al., 1990] the fall in arterial pressure was brief; however the magnitude of the fall is greater after bilateral CAT than after unilateral CAT, presumably because of the stimulation of both carotid sinus baroreceptors as compared to only one after unilateral CAT. The increase in sodium excretion is associated with a parallel increase in GFR, in contrast to Keeler's observation, in which the natriuresis after CAT developed without change in renal hemodynamics [Keeler, 1974]. It is conceivable that a decrease in sympathetic ERNA resulting from BilCAT could participate in the natriuresis, since carotid baroreceptor activation is known to decrease ERNA [Wilson et al., 1971] and in a preliminary study we have shown that the renal nerves mediate this reflex natriuresis in Sprague-Dawley rats through a hemodynamic effect on GFR [Valentin et al., 1991]. SHR have alterations in baroreflex mechanisms, altered metabolism of catecholamines in vasoregulatory regions of the hypothalamus, and an increase in peripheral efferent nerve activity to various organ beds including the kidneys [Janssen and Smits, 1989]. SHR have also blunted neural renorenal reflex responses to renal mechanoreceptor and chemoreceptor activation [Kopp et al., 1987]. Thus, alteration in the sympathetic nervous system is a prominant aspect of the hypertension in this strain and may be responsable for the blunted reflex natriuresis to BilCAT we observed. Treatment with angiotensin converting enzyme inhibitors normalizes blood pressure in SHR and corrects several of the sympathetic nervous system abnormalities [Kopp and Smith, 1989]. Therefore, the possibility that treatment with an angiotensin converting enzyme inhibitor may restore this reflex natriuresis in the SHR is an attractive hypothesis for future study.

In summary, bilateral activation of the baroreceptors in the carotid sinus using a relatively simple technique resulted in a reproducible vasodepressor response and progressive reflex natriuresis in WKY rats. This reflex natriuresis did not occur in SHR despite exaggerated vasodepression caused by this maneuver. The mechanism of this blunted natriuretic response to activation of the baroreceptors in SHR will be of interest to identify, since it may relate to the pathogenesis of hypertension in this strain.

ACKNOWLEDGEMENTS

Supported by grant DK 31623 from the National Institutes of Health and grant-in-aid 891124 from the American Heart Association. J-P Valentin was the recipient of a fellowship from ICI-Pharma, Paris, France, and from the American Heart Association, California Affiliate.

REFERENCES

Abboud, F.M., Heistad, D.D., Mark, A.L. and Schmid P.G. (1976): Reflex control of the peripheral circulation. Prog. Cardiovasc. Dis. 18, 371-403.

Wilson, M.F., Ninomiya, I., Franz, G.N. and Judy, W.V. (1971): Hypothalamic stimulation and baroreceptor reflex interaction on renal nerve activity. Am. J. Physiol. 221, 1768-1773.

Keeler, R. (1974): Natriuresis after unilateral stimulation of carotid receptors in unanesthetized rats. Am. J. Physiol. 226, 507-511.

Valentin, J.P., Mazbar, S.A. and Humphreys, M.H.: Natriuretic effect of intermittent bilateral carotid artery traction in the rat. J. Hypertension (in press).

Mazbar, S.A., Wiedemann, E. and Humphreys, M.H. (1990): Mechanism of the natriuretic effect of unilateral carotid artery traction in the rat. J. Am. Soc. Nephrol. 1, 266-271.

Landgren, S., and Neil, E. (1951): The contribution of carotid chemoreceptor mechanisms to the rise of blood pressure caused by carotid occlusion. Acta Physiol. Scand., 23, 152-157.

Valentin, J.P., Mazbar, S.A. and Humphreys, M.H. (1991): Renal denervation prevents reflex natriuresis following bilateral carotid artery traction. FASEB J., 5, A1485.

Janssen, B.J.A., and Smits, J.F.M. (1989): Renal nerves in hypertension. Miner. Electrolyte Metab. 15:74-82.

Dibona, G.F. (1982): The functions of the renal nerves. Rev. Physiol. Biochem. Pharmacol. 94:75-181.

Kopp, U.C. and Smith, L.A. (1989): Renorenal reflexes present in young and captopril-treated adult spontaneously hypertensive rats. Hypertension 13:430-439.

Kopp, U.C., Olson, L.A., and DiBona, G.F. (1987): Impaired renorenal reflexes in spontaneously hypertensive rats. Hypertension 9:69-75.

Effects of one hour and one week ramipril treatment on plasma and renal brush border angiotensin converting enzyme in the rat

Bruno Michel [1], Michèle Grima, Corinne Welsch, Catherine Coquard, Mariette Barthelmebs [1] and Jean-Louis Imbs [1]

[1] Institut de Pharmacologie, URA DO 589 CNRS, Faculté de Médecine and Hypertension Clinique, CHR, Université Louis Pasteur, 67000 Strasbourg, France

INTRODUCTION

The role of tissue activity in the antihypertensive effect of angiotensin converting enzyme (ACE) inhibitors is still a subject of debate. It has now been clearly demonstrated that tissue ACE activity in rats is inhibited after acute treatment with ACE-inhibitors. The effects of prolonged treatment are less clear : tissue ACE activity measured during long term treatment with ACE-inhibitors probably results from both inhibition and induction, as described in rat plasma, lung or kidney (Fyhrquist et al., 1980; Song et al., 1988).

We compared renal and plasma ACE activity (in normotensive rats) measured one hour after a single dose of ramipril and 24 h after the last dose of a 7 day administration. Ramipril is an esterified precursor of ramiprilat, a potent diacid ACE-inhibitor. Enzyme activity in the kidney, and in particular in the ACE rich brush borders of the proximal tubules, was measured before and after elimination of the ramiprilat still in the tissue when the samples were taken. This made it possible to identify variations in tissue ACE activity resulting from prolonged treatment.

MATERIAL AND METHODS

Rat treatment

Forty eight Wistar rats were divided into four groups (n = 12 for each group). One control group received distilled water and three ramipril treated groups received respectively 0.1, 0.3 or 1 mg/kg of ramipril. In the first experiment, rats were tube-fed with a single dose of ramipril and were sacrificed one hour later. In the second experiment, rats were tube-fed daily with ramipril for 7 days and were killed 24 hours after the last dose.

Plasma and brush border membranes preparation

Blood was collected in a heparinised tube and centrifuged at 2000 g x 10 min to separate the plasma. Brush border membranes were isolated from the renal cortex according to the method of Malathi et al. (1979).

ACE activity measurement

ACE activity was measured in the plasma, renal cortex homogenates and brush border membranes with a fluorimetric assay using carbobenzoxy Phe-His-Leu as an artificial substrate for ACE. To ensure that a linear relationship was maintained between ACE activity and protein content (Welsch et al., 1989), the protein concentration, established using the method of Lowry et al. (1951), was maintained in the assay at 1 mg/ml (tissue) or 20 mg/ml (plasma).

Elimination of ramiprilat in the brush border membranes

The presence of Zn^{2+} at the active site of ACE is necessary for inhibitor binding. Brush borders were therefore treated with EGTA which, by chelating the Zn^{2+} of ACE, promoted the dissociation of the ACE-inhibitor complex. Ramiprilat and EGTA were then eliminated by a washing of the membranes and ACE activity was restored by the addition of Zn^{2+}. We had established in previous experiments that 80% inhibition of ACE activity in the renal cortex due to 10^{-7} M of ramiprilat was completely eliminated in the brush borders after EGTA treatment.

Statistics

The results are expressed as the mean ± SEM and compared with an analysis of variance followed by the application of Scheffe's test. Values of $p < 0.05$ were considered to be significant.

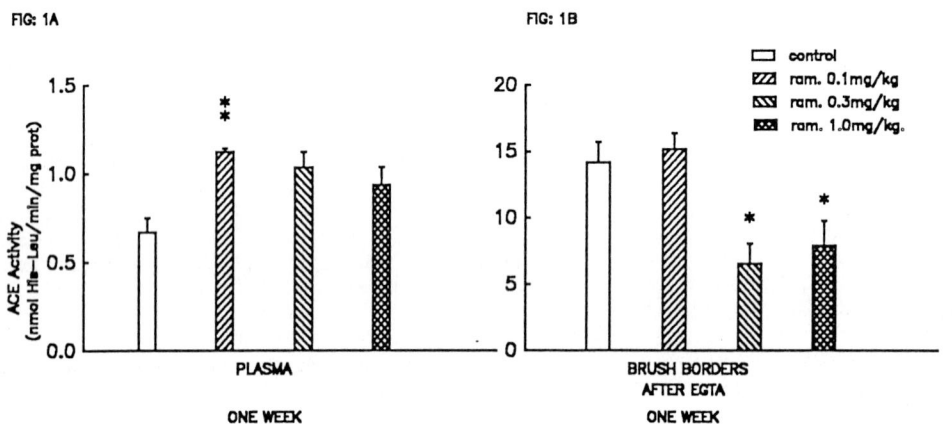

Fig. 1. Effects of one week treatment with ramipril on angiotensin converting enzyme (ACE) activity in plasma (1A) and in EGTA treated brush border membranes (1B). m ± SEM; n = 6, only comparison to control values; $*p < 0.05$, $**p < 0.01$.

RESULTS

Effects of ramipril on plasma ACE activity

The one hour treatment with ramipril brought about a dose-dependent decrease in plasma ACE activity with 22% inhibition at the dose of 0.1 mg/kg, 51% at 0.3 mg/kg and 72% at 1 mg/kg. In contrast, the one week treatment with ramipril induced an increase in plasma ACE activities : 67% at 0.1 mg/kg, 49% at 0.3 mg/kg and 40% at 1 mg/kg (fig. 1A).

Effects of ramipril on renal cortex ACE activity

At the dose of 0.1 mg/kg of ramipril, the one hour and one week treatments did not affect the renal cortex ACE activity. At doses of 0.3 mg/kg and 1 mg/kg of ramipril, the one hour and one week treatments brought about a decrease in renal cortex ACE activity. The one hour treatment produced a decrease of 40% at 0.3 mg/kg and 72% at 1 mg/kg. The one week treatment elicited a decrease of 38% at 0.3 mg/kg and 34% at 1 mg/kg.

Effects of ramipril on brush borders ACE activity after EGTA treatment

The decrease in renal cortex ACE activities could be linked to the presence of ramiprilat in the tissue samples. Therefore, during the preparation of brush borders, which were isolated from the renal cortex, the residual ACE-inhibitor was eliminated by applying the EGTA treatment. In such conditions, after the one hour treatment, no decrease could be measured in brush borders ACE activity, indicating that the decrease in renal cortex ACE activity was an inhibition due to the presence of ramiprilat. In contrast, after the one week treatment, a marked decrease in brush borders ACE activity persisted after EGTA treatment (Fig. 1B) with a 55% decrease at 0.3 mg/kg and 44% at 1 mg/kg, indicating that the decrease observed in the renal cortex was not due to the presence of residual ramiprilat.

CONCLUSION

These results show a clear dissociation between the effects of one week ramipril treatment on plasma and renal ACE activities. This suggests that plasma and renal ACE may have specific regulatory factors.

The increase in rat plasma ACE activity after this prolonged administration of ramipril has already been described for other ACE-inhibitors (Fyhrquist et al., 1980).

The persistence of the decrease in brush borders ACE activity after EGTA treatment suggests that during prolonged ramipril treatment two effects may appear successively in the renal cortex : immediate inhibition due to the presence of the ACE-inhibitor, followed by a decrease in ACE concentration which participates in the development of a stronger and sustained decrease in renal ACE activity.

Acknowledgement

We acknowledge the support of the Groupe d'Etude du Système Rénine Angiotensine Tissulaire (GESRAT).

REFERENCES

Fyhrquist, F., Forslund, T., Tikkanen, I. and Grönhagen-Riska C (1980): Induction of angiotensin I-converting enzyme in rat lung with captopril (SQ 14225). Eur. J. Pharmacol. 67: 473-475.

Lowry, OH., Rosebrough, NM., Lewis Farr, A. and Randall, RJ. (1951): Protein measurement with the phenol reagent. J. Biol. Chem. 193: 265-275.

Malathi, P., Preiser, H., Fairclough, P., Mallett, P. and Crane, RK. (1979) A rapid method for the isolation of kidney brush border membranes. Biochimical et Biophysica Acta 554: 259-263.

Song, G.B., Tominaga, M., Kanayama, Y., Ikemoto, F. and Yamamoto, K. (1988): Enhancement of angiotensin-converting enzyme activity in the inner cortex of rat kidney by captopril. Renal Physiol. Biochem. 11: 43-49.

Welsch, C., Grima, M., Giesen, EM., Helwig, JJ., Barthelmebs, M., Coquard, C. and Imbs, JL. (1989) Assay of tissue angiotensin converting enzyme. J. Cardiovasc. Pharmacol. 14(suppl. 4): S26-S31.

Rat prorenin is activable at acidic pH

Fumiaki Suzuki, Akihiko Takahashi, Kazuo Murakami *
and Yukio Nakamura

*Department of Biotechnology, Gifu University, 501-11, Gifu, Japan and * Institute of Applied Biochemistry Tsukuba University, 305, Tsukuba, Japan*

Prorenin is an inactive precursor of renin which plays an important role in control of blood pressure and electrolyte balance. More than half amount of total renins circulates in the bloodstream as prorenin. As several strains of rats are most widely used as a model animal in the studies on blood pressure regulation and hypertension, rat prorenin has attracted the attention of many investigators. However, little information is currently available for the source and activation mechanisms of rat prorenin, because it has been difficult to obtain pure prorenin from the rat plasma and organs. Recently, rat preprorenin cDNA was isolated (Burnham, 1987; Tada, 1988), so that we succeeded in expressing recombinant rat prorenin to use sufficient quantities of it for detailed biochemical and physiological studies (Hosoi, 1991). In this study, we investigated whether rat prorenin was reversibly activable *in vitro* at acidic pH using rat recombinant prorenin as a model of plasma prorenin.

Chinese hamster ovary cells (CHO cells, DXB-11 strain) were transfected with an expression vector (pSVRRn1) containing rat preprorenin cDNA sequence (Tada, 1988). The expression vector was prepared by substituting the rat cDNA sequence for human renin cDNA inserted at a *Bam* HI site of an expression plasmid (pSVDPRnPA33, Poorman, 1986). The CHO cells screened as highest prorenin-secreting colonies were cultured in the Dulbecco's modified Eagle medium containing 11.5 mg/l proline and 10 per cent of dialyzed fetal calf serum for 5 days and in a serum-free medium, S-Clone SF-O (Sanko Pure Chemical, Japan) including 11.5 mg/l proline for successive 5 days. As described previously, the CHO cells have been observed to secrete into the medium inactive prorenin with similar properties to that of plasma prorenin for physicochemical aspects (Hosoi, 1991). The serum-free culture medium was accordingly used as a rat prorenin fraction in this study. The prorenin fraction was acidified at 4° or 25°C by dialysis against 0.1M acetate, pH 3.3, including 5 mM ethylendiamine tetraacetatic acid and 0.02 per cent of sodium azide. The renin activity of the acid-activated prorenin was analyzed by the standard assay system (Murakami, 1980) including angiotensin I-enzyme-linked immunosorbent assay (Suzuki, 1990). The renin activity in each dialyzed medium was presented by the percentage to the activity of fully activated prorenin by a treatment with 50 μg/ml trypsin (Sigma) at 25°C for 20 min. The activity of the trypsinized prorenin was 50 μg angiotensin I/ml medium/h.

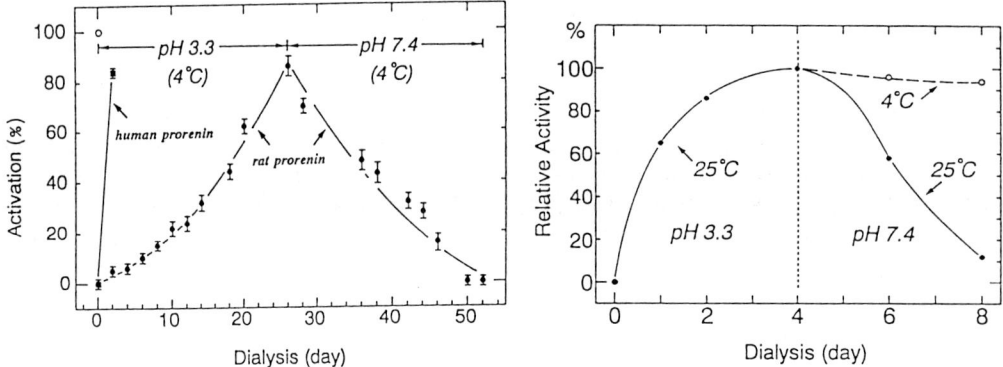

Fig. 1. (Left panel) Reversible acid-activation of rat prorenin at low temperature. The rat prorenin fraction (●) was dialyzed at pH 3.3 and 4°C for 25 days, and then at pH 7.4 and 4°C for another 25 days. The human prorenin fraction (■) was obtained from the culture medium for the CHO cells transfected with the pSVDPRnPA33 containing human preprorenin cDNA (Poorman, 1986). The percentage of activation for prorenin was represented as mean±S.D.(n=4). The 100% of activation (o) was defined as the renin activity in the rat prorenin fraction after the trypsinization. **Fig. 2.** (Right panel) Acid-activation and re-inactivation of rat prorenin at room temperature. The renin activity (≈25 μg angiotensin I/ml/h) in the prorenin fraction dialyzed for 4 days at pH 3.3 was represented as 100%.

Rat prorenin was little activated by dialysis for 2 days at pH 3.3 at 4°C, although more than 80 percent of human prorenin was activated under these conditions. However, the activation of rat prorenin was found to reach at the same level as that of human prorenin by dialyzing for 25 days, as shown in **Fig. 1**. The activated-prorenin was completely re-inactivated by dialysis at pH 7.4 and 4°C for 25 days, which was the same days as that taken for the acid-activation step. The activation was accelerated with increasing the temperature for the dialysis (**Fig. 2**). Addition of sodium chloride (0.1 M) stimulated the activation of prorenin at acidic pH. The acid-activated prorenin adsorbed to affinity columns with potent renin inhibitors, octapeptide H77 (Szelke, 1982), and pepstatin A (Murakami, 1975) as ligands at pH 7.4 and 3.3, respectively. The active prorenin was eluted from these columns by 0.1 M acetate, pH 3.0 and 0.1 M acetate, pH 5.5 containing 0.1 M sodium chloride, respectively. On the contrary, non-treated and re-inactivated prorenin could not adsorb to these columns. These results suggest that the acid-activated prorenin has the similar enzymatic properties to those of renal renin (Murakami, 1972; Kim, 1991).

We also investigated whether the re-inactivation process for rat prorenin was expedited by increasing the temperature. The acid-activated prorenin, obtained by dialyzing for 4 days at 25°C, was re-inactivated by dialyzing for 4 days at 25° and pH 7.4 (**Fig. 2**). This result confirmed the observation for human prorenin (Heinrikson, 1989). On the other hand, the re-inactivation process for rat prorenin was retarded by addition of 0.1 M sodium chloride. These results indicate that re-inactivation as well as acid-activation of **rat prorenin** depends on the temperature under the constant ionic strength.

The first-order rate constant for the activation was dependent on the protonation of polar group(s) with pK 3.0–3.5. This value was similar to that of human prorenin (Derkx, 1987), although the activation speed of rat prorenin was about 6 times slower than that of human prorenin. Additionally, sodium chloride stimulated the acid-activation of rat prorenin. These results suggest that an ionic bond(s) between a negatively charged residue(s) and a positively charged residue(s) in the prosegment sequence and the other sequence of prorenin plays an important role for sustaining the structure of inactive prorenin, although these groups could not be pointed out in the amino acid sequence of rat prorenin. It has been also unclear for human prorenin which ionic bond(s) in the molecule contributes to the inactivation, although it was examined which basic amino acid residues in the prosegment had its potentiality, using a technique of site-directed mutagenesis (Yamauchi, 1990). Accordingly, the difference between human and rat prorenin for activation and re-inactivation speeds may not be explained by only differences of the quantities and properties of acid, basic and hydrophobic amino acid residues in the prosegments of their prorenin molecules.

In this study, we found that rat prorenin was reversibly activable at acidic pH. It was, therefore, speculated that rat prorenin possibly opened the gate, the prosegment, when it was locally exposed to a low pH during the circulation.

ACKNOWLEDGEMENTS

This work was supported by Grants-in-Aid for Scientific Research (02806016) from Ministry of Education, Science and Culture of Japan, Naito Foundation (89-126), and Chichibu Cement Co.

REFERENCES

Burnham, C.E., Hawelu-Johnson, C.L., Frank, B.M., and Lynch, K.R. (1987): Molecular cloning of rat renin cDNA and its gene. *Proc. Natl. Acad. Sci. USA* 84: 5605-5609.

Derkx, F.M., Schalekamp, M.P.A., and Schalekamp, M.A.D.H. (1987): Two-step prorenin-renin conversion. Isolation of an intermediary form of activated prorenin. *J. Biol. Chem.* 262: 2472-2477.

Heinrikson, R.L., Hui, J., Zürcher-Neely, H., and Poorman, R.A. (1989): A structure model to explain the partial catalytic activity of human prorenin. *Am. J. Hypertension* 2: 367-380

Hosoi, M., Kim, S., Yamauchi, T., Watanabe, T., Murakami, K., Suzuki, F., Takahashi, A., Nakamura, Y., and Yamamoto, K. (1991): Similarity between physicochemical properties of recombinant rat prorenin and native inactive renin. *Biochem. J.* 275: 727-731.

Kim, S., Hosoi, M., Kikuchi, N., and Yamamoto, K. (1991): Amino-terminal amino acid sequence and heterogeneity in glycosylation of rat renal renin. *J. Biol. Chem.* 266: 7044-7050

Murakami, K., and Inagami, T. (1975): Isolation of pure and stable renin from hog kidney. *Biochem. Biophys. Res. Commun.* 62: 757-763.

Murakami, K., Suzuki, F., Morita, N., Ito, H., Okamoto, K., Hirose, S., and Inagami, T. (1980): High molecular weight renin in stroke-prone spontaneously hypertensive rats. *Biochim. Biophys. Acta* 622: 115-122.

Poorman, R.A., Palermo, D.P., Post, L.E., Murakami, K., Kinner, J.H., Smith, C.W., Readon, I., and Heinrikson, R.L. (1986): Isolation and characterization of native human renin derived from chinese hamster ovary cells. *Proteins* 1: 139-145.

Suzuki, F., Yamashita, S., Takahashi, A., Ito, M., Miyazaki, S., Nagata, Y., and Nakamura, Y. (1990): Highly sensitive microplate-ELISA for angiotensin I using 3,3',5,5'-tetramethylbenzidine. *Clin. Exper. Hyper. A(12):* 83-95.

Szelke, M., Leckie, B.J., Tree, M., Brown, A., Grant, J., Hallet, A., Huges, A., Jones, D.M., and Lever, A.F. (1982): A potent new renin inhibitor. In vivo and in vitro studies. *Hypertension* 4(Suppl2): 59-69

Tada, M., Fukamizu, A., Seo, M.S., Takahashi, S., and Murakami, K. (1988): Nucleotide sequence of rat renin cDNA. *Nucl. Acid. Res.* 16: 3576.

Yamauchi., T., Nakagawa, M., Watanabe, M., Ishizuka, Y., Hori, H., and Murakami, K. (1990): Site-directed mutagenesis of human prorenin. Substitution of three arginine residues in the propeptide with glutamine residues yields active prorenin. *J. Biochem.* 107: 27-31.

Angiotensin converting enzyme in the spontaneously hypertensive rat

Masahiro Kohzuki, Bing-Zhong Chen, Vincent Mooser, Karin Jandeleit and Colin I. Johnston

University of Melbourne, Department of Medicine, Austin Hospital, Heidelberg 3084, Victoria, Australia

Angiotensin converting enzyme (ACE) is the last step in the renin-enzymatic cascade and is one of the most important factors controlling blood pressure. Changes in plasma and tissue ACE have been reported in the spontaneously hypertensive rat (SHR) (Rosenthal et al., 1984, Nakamura et al., 1987). However the difference between SHR and WKY in ACE in various tissues and whether ACE inhibitors have different effects in the SHR compared to the WKY have not been evaluated.

The purpose of the present study was to compare the location and concentration of ACE between the SHR and WKY control rats and to compare the acute effect of increasing doses of perindopril on inhibition of ACE in the heart, aorta and kidney in SHR compared to WKY rats using quantitative in vitro autoradiography.

METHODS

SHR and WKY were purchased from the Biological Research Laboratory, Austin Hospital. 11 week old SHR and age matched normotensive WKY were decapitated 4 hours after perindopril (1, 4, 16 mg/kg, p.o.) or vehicle and heart, aorta and kidneys were taken for in vitro autoradiography. Plasma perindoprilat was measured by radioinhibitor binding assay (Jackson et al., 1987, Johnston et al., 1988). ACE was quantitated by in vitro autoradiography using 125I-351A, a lisinopril derivative, as the radioligand. The autoradiograms were quantitated by computerized densitometry as previously described (Sakaguchi et al., 1988, Kohzuki et al., 1991).

Three sections from each tissue from each rat were fixed on to one slide and six slides were taken from each tissue. Slides 1 and 3 were preincubated with EDTA to dissociate the drug from the enzyme in the tissue section and to measure total ACE. Slides 2 and 4 were not preincubated with EDTA and gave a measure of free ACE or the amount of ACE inhibited by the drug. Further slides were used for nonspecific binding by adding 1 mM EDTA. All slides were then incubated with the radioligand for one hour at 20°C. ACE concentration in the various tissues of the SHR and WKY were calculated from the "total ACE" measured after dissociation with EDTA. Inhibition of ACE in each tissue was calculated as (Kohzuki et al., 1991):

$$\% \text{ inhibition} = 100 \times \frac{\text{(free ACE (-EDTA))dpm/mm}^2}{\text{(total ACE (+EDTA))dpm/mm}^2}$$

RESULTS AND DISCUSSION

There were no significant differences in the concentration of ACE in the kidney (1335 ± 33 v 1138 ± 27 dpm/mm^2), heart (272 ± 12 v 220 ± 15.7 dpm/mm^2) or the aorta (1425 ± 72 v 1443 ± 72 dpm/mm^2 between WKY and SHR animals.

There were dose dependent increases in plasma perindoprilat levels with increasing oral doses of the drug. The plasma levels of perindoprilat achieved were comparable in SHR to WKY (SHR vs. WKY: 4 mg/kg; 145 ± 28 vs 177 ± 49 ng/ml). The degree of inhibition by 1, 4 and 16 mg/kg perindopril in the kidney, heart and aorta of WKY and SHR is shown in Fig. 1. There was dose related inhibition of ACE in the kidney, heart and aorta following 1, 4 and 16 mg/kg of perindoprilat in both WKY and SHR. Inhibition of ACE in all tissues was comparable in WKY and SHR rats.

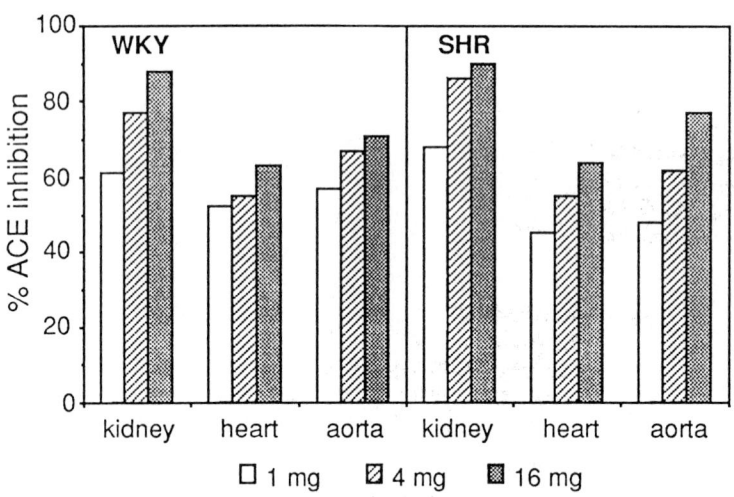

Fig. 1. Comparison of ACE activity in the kidney, heart and aorta 4 hours after perindopril (1, 4, 16 mg/kg, p.o.) administration to WKY and the SHR rats.

Previous studies have reported higher ACE activity in the aorta of the SHR compared to the WKY rat (Rosenthal et al., 1984, Nakamura et al., 1987). In our study, however, no differences in the concentration of ACE in the heart, aorta or kidney could be demonstrated between SHR and WKY rats. The reason for this discrepancy is not clear although different, less specific methods were used in these previous studies to measure tissue ACE. ACE is known to be highly localized in specialized structures. The previous studies, using tissue homogenates of aorta, were unable to take into account the localization of ACE to discrete areas and structures compared with our in vitro autoradiography technique. Furthermore, in our study, acute administration of perindopril inhibited ACE in the tissue to an equivalent degree in SHR and WKY. In conclusion no qualitative or quantitative difference in ACE could be demonstrated in the SHR compared to the WKY rat in this study.

REFERENCES

Jackson, B. et al. (1987): Angiotensin converting enzyme inhibitors: measurement of relative inhibitory potency and serum drug levels by radioinhibitor binding displacement assay. J. Cardiovasc. Pharmacol. 9, 699-704.

Johnston, C.I. et al. (1988): Inhibition of angiotensin converting enzyme (ACE) in plasma and tissues: studies ex vivo after administration of ACE inhibitors. J. Hypertens. 6(Suppl 3), 17-22.

Kohzuki, M. et al. (1991): Measurement of angiotensin converting enzyme induction and inhibition using quantitative in vitro autoradiography: Tissue selective induction after chronic lisinopril treatment. J. Hypertens. 9, 579-587.

Mendelsohn, F.A.O. et al. (1984): In vitro autoradiographic localization of angiotensin-converting enzyme in rat brain using 125I-labelled MK351A. J. Hypertens. 2(Suppl 3), 41-44.

Nakamura, Y. et al. (1987): Difference in response of vascular angiotensin converting enzyme activity to cilazapril in SHR. Clin. and Exper. Hypert. A9, 351-355.

Rosenthal, J.H. et al. (1984): Investigations of components of the renin-angiotensin system in rat vascular tissue. Hypertension 6, 383-390.

Sakaguchi, K. et al. (1988): Inhibition of tissue angiotensin converting enzyme: quantitation by autoradiography. Hypertension 11, 230-238.

Long-term blood pressure effects of angiotensin in SHR are developmental stage-specific

Stephen B. Harrap and Austin E. Doyle

Genetic Physiology Unit, Department of Medicine, Austin Hospital, Heidelberg, Victoria 3084, Australia

Introduction:

The tracking of blood pressure in spontaneously hypertensive rats (SHR) depends on an orderly but pathogenic series of events. It is possible to alter this track and reduce blood pressure in the long-term by treating young SHR with a brief course of angiotensin converting enzyme (ACE) inhibitors (Harrap *et al* 1986, 1990) or non-peptide angiotensin antagonists (Lever *et al* 1991). These persistent effects are not seen after treatment of young SHR with other classes of antihypertensive drugs (Giudicelli *et al* 1980, Smeda *et al* 1988, Christensen *et al* 1989), after ACE inhibitor treatment in old SHR (Unger *et al* 1986, Harrap *et al* 1990) or after ACE inhibitor treatment in young rats of other genetically hypertensive strains (Mulvany *et al* 1991). These observations suggest that angiotensin plays a strain- and developmental stage-specific role in the genesis of SHR hypertension, possibly through effects on the kidney (Harrap 1991) and vascular hypertrophy (Harrap & Lever 1989). This hypothesis is supported by the restoration of blood pressure tracking in young ACE inhibitor-treated SHR by the concomitant administration of angiotensin II. If, in SHR, angiotensin exerts its greatest effects on blood pressure tracking during youth, then if administered in later life, its long-term effects may not be as great. This study addresses this hypothesis.

Methods:

Male SHR were used in this study and were derived from direct descendants of NIH SHR that are maintained as an inbred colony maintained in the Genetic Physiology Unit. All experiments were approved by the Austin Hospital Animal Welfare Committee.

Two groups of SHR were studied. Both were treated with the ACE inhibitor perindopril (3mg/kg/d by gavage) from 6 to 10 weeks of age. Systolic blood pressure was measured each week by the indirect tail-cuff technique (Narco Biosystems). At 28 weeks of age, rats were anaesthetised briefly with methohexitone (40mg/kg, intraperitoneally) for the insertion of subcutaneous osmotic minipumps (Alzet model 2002, Alza, Palo Alto, California, USA) in the interscapular region. In one group (n=8) these minipumps contained angiotensin II (Hypertensin, Ciba Geigy Ltd., Basel, Switzerland) at a concentration that resulted in a delivery rate of 200ng/kg/min. In the other group (n=7) the minipumps contained vehicle only. Fresh minipumps were substituted at 30 weeks of age and all pumps were removed two weeks later. Blood pressure was measured for a further 3 weeks after angiotensin treatment. The statistical analysis of longitudinal blood pressure data was performed using SPSS/PC+ MANOVA program for repeated measures analysis of variance.

Results:

Figure 1 shows the systolic blood pressures of the two experimental groups, and those of a separate group of untreated male SHR for comparison. The blood pressures of the groups were well-matched before the commencement of perindopril treatment (Fig. 1). During treatment from 6 to 10 weeks of age, the blood pressure of both perindopril groups fell to a similar degree (Fig. 1). When treatment was stopped, blood pressure in both groups rose and plateaued at about 187 mmHg, which was approximately 25-30mmHg less than the blood pressure of untreated SHR of the same age (Fig. 1). During adulthood, the blood pressures of SHR that had received perindopril were not significantly different (MANOVA: $F_{1,13}=1.21$, $P=0.29$).

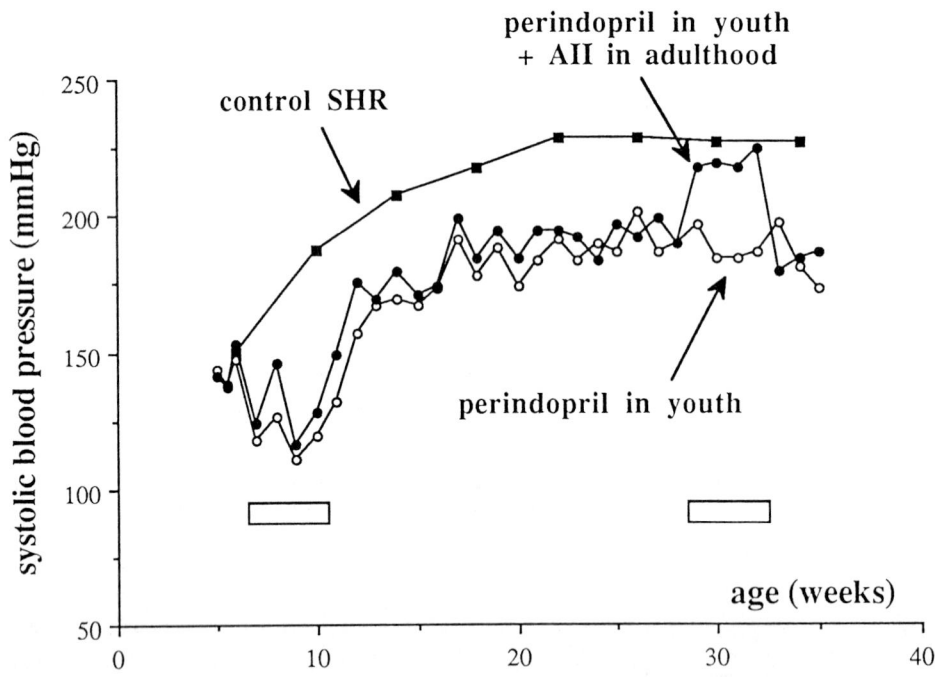

Fig. 1: Systolic blood pressure of male SHR. ○ = SHR that received perindopril from 6 to 10 weeks of age and vehicle from 28 to 32 weeks of age, ● = SHR that received perindopril from 6 to 10 weeks of age and angiotensin II (AII) from 28 to 32 weeks of age, ■ = data from control untreated SHR for comparison. Error bars have been omitted for clarity. See text for statistical comparisons.

The blood pressure of SHR that received angiotensin II rose significantly by about 30mmHg between 28 and 32 weeks of age (MANOVA: $F_{1,13}=14.9$, $P=0.002$), and was roughly equivalent to untreated SHR. There were no significant changes in the blood pressure of SHR that received vehicle by minipump during this period. After removal of the minipumps, the blood pressure of vehicle-treated SHR remained stable, but that of the SHR that had received angiotensin fell by about 30mmHg, returning to levels seen before the infusion of angiotensin. During the last three weeks of the study the blood pressure of the angiotensin- and vehicle-treated SHR were not significantly different (MANOVA: $F_{1,13}=0.08$, $P=0.78$).

Discussion:

In young, but not old SHR, ACE inhibitor treatment is associated with a persistent effect on blood pressure. This difference may reflect a change in the response of the SHR cardiovascular system to angiotensin with increasing age. This suggestion is supported by the findings of this study, in which w have demonstrated that the effect of angiotensin in perindopril-treated SHR is developmental stage-specific. In young SHR, a 4 week administration of angiotensin restores the track of blood pressure to that seen in untreated SHR (Harrap et al 1990). A similar 4 week course of angiotensin in adult SHR was associated with transient return of blood pressure to levels seen in untreated SHR, but did not reset blood pressure levels in the long-term.

These studies provide further evidence of differences in the control of blood pressure in young and adult SHR and emphasise the importance of angiotensin during the development of hypertension. A major difference in the effects of converting enzyme inhibitors in young and mature SHR occurs in their renal hemodynamic responses. In young animals, ACE inhibition appears to have a selective action on renal vascular resistance, which has disappeared by the time that the raised blood pressure has become established (Harrap 1991). Furthermore, ACE inhibitor treatment is followed not only by a long-term reduction in blood pressure, but also by a persistent reduction in renal vascular resistance (Harrap et al 1986).

The idea that the effects of angiotensin II on renal vascular resistance are particularly important in the pathogenesis of the rise in blood pressure in SHR is reinforced by the finding that increased renal vascular resistance co-segregates with blood pressure in F2 rats formed by cross-breeding SHR and Wistar Kyoto rats (Harrap & Doyle 1988), and that in the F2 rats renal vascular resistance and plasma renin activity are closely correlated. We suggest that the renovascular effects of angiotensin in young SHR, which have largely disappeared in older rats, may be one important triggering mechanism for the subsequent development of hypertension in this model.

References:

Christensen KL, Jespersen LT, Mulvany MJ (1989): Development of blood pressure in spontaneously hypertensive rats after withdrawal of long-term treatment related to vascular structure. J Hypertens 7: 83-90

Giudicelli J-F, Freslon JL, Glasson S, Richer C (1980): Captopril and hypertension development in the SHR. Clin Exp Hypertens 2A: 1083-1096

Harrap SB, Nicolaci J, Doyle AE (1986): Persistent effects on blood pressure and renal hemodynamics following chronic angiotensin converting enzyme inhibition with perindopril. Clin Exp Pharmacol Physiol 13: 753-765

Harrap SB, Doyle AE (1988): Genetic co-segregation of renal hemodynamics and blood pressure in the spontaneously hypertensive rat. Clin Sci 74: 63-69

Harrap SB, Lever AF (1989): The long-term effects after ACE inhibitor treatment in young spontaneously hypertensive rats - Clues to the pathogenesis of high blood pressure, in Sever P, MacGregor (eds): Current Advances in ACE Inhibition. Edinburgh, Churchill Livingstone, pp 69-77

Harrap SB, Van der Merwe WM, Griffin SA, Macpherson F, Lever AF (1990): Brief angiotensin converting enzyme inhibitor treatment in young spontaneously hypertensive rats reduces blood pressure long-term. Hypertension 16: 603-614

Harrap SB (1991): Angiotensin converting enzyme inhibitors, regional vascular hemodynamics, and the development and prevention of experimental genetic hypertension. Am J Hypertens 4: 212S-216S

Lever AF, Beattie E, Brown W, Folkow B, Griffin SA, Harrap SB, Macpherson F, Morton JJ, Mulvany M (1991): Effects of angiotensin II, growth factors and inhibitors of the renin-angiotensin system on arterial pressure and cardiovascular structure, in Sever P, MacGregor (eds): Current Advances in ACE Inhibition II. Edinburgh, Churchill Livingstone, in press.

Mulvany MJ, Persson AEG, Andersen J (1991): No persistent effect of angiotensin converting enzyme inhibitor treatment in Milan hypertensive rats despite regression of vascular structure J Hypertens 9: 589-594

Smeda JS, Lee RMKW Forrest JB (1988): Prenatal and postnatal hydralazine treatment does not prevent renal vessel wall thickening in SHR despite the absence of hypertension. Circ Res 63: 534-542

Unger T, Morusi M, Ganten D, Herman K, Lang RE (1986): Antihypertensive action of the converting enzyme inhibitor perindopril (S9490-3) in spontaneously hypertensive rats: Comparison with enalapril (MK421) and ramipril (HOE498). J Cardiovasc Pharmacol 8: 276-285

Adaptation to sodium restriction in enalapril-treated spontaneously hypertensive rats

Bernard Jover, Kamel Wahba, Albert Mimran

Groupe Rein et Hypertension, Centre Hospitalier Universitaire, Hôpital Saint-Charles, 34059 Montpellier Cedex, France

In spontaneously hypertensive rats (SHR), chronic or acute blockade of angiotensin-converting enzyme reduces hypertension (Bengis et al, 1978; Levy et al, 1988) and prevents development of hypertension when treatment is initiated during the prehypertensive phase (Richer et al, 1981). In addition, chronic immunization against renin lowers blood pressure in SHR (Lo et al, 1990), thus suggesting that arterial pressure regulation is dependent upon the renin-angiotensin system in this model of hypertension.

The role of the renin-angiotensin system becomes crucial in the control of arterial pressure, renal function and sodium homeostasis in states associated with a consistent activation of the system such as volume depletion and unilateral renal artery stenosis. When dietary sodium is abruptly reduced, urinary excretion of sodium rapidly falls and a new steady state is achieved within 3 to 5 days whereas plasma renin activity and circulating angiotensin II increase. In sodium-restricted normotensive rats, chronic treatment by angiotensin-converting enzyme inhibitors (CEI) was associated with a fall in arterial pressure and an inability to achieve sodium balance leading to a sodium-wasting state (Jover & Mimran, 1984; Mimran et al, 1988). In a recent study conducted in SHR and WKY rats, renin immunization impaired the systemic but not the renal adaptation to sodium restriction (Jover et al, in press). As discrepancies may be related to the way used to achieve renin-angiotensin system blockade, the present work was undertaken in order to assess the influence of the CEI, enalapril, on systemic and renal adaptation to dietary sodium removal in spontaneously hypertensive rats and their normotensive controls, Wistar Kyoto rats.

MATERIAL AND METHODS

Twelve male SHR and 12 normotensive Wistar-Kyoto (WKY) rats weighing 270-320 g were used in these experiments. Rats were housed individually in metabolic cages and fed a normal sodium diet for 6 days (low sodium chow containing less than 5 mmoles of sodium per kg chow and distilled water containing 77 mmol Na+/l as drinking fluid). Then, sodium was abruptly and totally removed from the drinking fluid for the 6 following days. Six animals of each strain received the converting enzyme inhibitor, enalapril, in the drinking fluid at a concentration of 10 mg/100 ml (WKY-CEI and SHR-CEI groups) whereas 6 WKY and 6 SHR received no treatment (WKY-Vehicle and SHR-Vehicle groups). Enalapril was given 3 days prior to and during the 6-day period of the low sodium diet. Urinary excretion of water, sodium, potassium and creatinine were measured daily. In addition, systolic arterial pressure was measured in conscious rats (tail-cuff method) before any treatment (day -4) and during enalapril administration on normal sodium intake (day -1) and low sodium intake (days 2, 4 and 6).

At the end of the low sodium period, catheters were inserted under light ether anesthesia into the left ventricule and abdominal aorta. Arterial pressure response to angiotensin I bolus (100 ng i.v.) was evaluated in all animals. At least 4 hours later, catheters were connected to a pressure transducer (Statham P23dB) and arterial pressure and heart rate continuously recorded. After a 10-minute stabilization period, renal blood flow (RBF) was assessed using the radioactive microsphere technique in awake, freely moving animals. Blood was sampled for determination of angiotensin-converting enzyme activity (ACE activity) and plasma sodium concentration. Kidneys were removed for radioactivity counting.

Results are expressed as mean ± SEM. Statistical analysis used one-way analysis of variance followed by a multiple comparisons of means using Dunnett's t test. Values of $p < 0.05$ were considered statistically significant.

RESULTS

Efficiency of ACE inhibition

As reported in Table 1, enalapril treatment was associated with a complete inhibition of ACE activity in both strains that was confirmed by the total inhibition of arterial pressure response to angiotensin I injection.

Influence of CEI on the systemic and renal adaptation to sodium restriction.

In untreated groups, renal adaptation to dietary sodium removal was similar in WKY and SHR. In enalapril-pretreated WKY and SHR, a sodium loss was observed in response to sodium restriction as clearly shown by the enhanced cumulative sodium excretion (UNaV) from day 1 to 6 of low sodium diet (Table 1). Cumulative sodium excretion was similar in CEI-treated WKY and SHR.

Table 1 : Influence of enalapril (CEI) pretreatment on renal and systemic adaptation to sodium restriction in WKY and SHR.

Groups	MAP mmHg	Cumulative UNaV μmol/6 days	RBF ml/min/g	PACE nmol/ml/h	ANG I ΔmmHg
WKY-Vehicle	116 ± 4	572 ± 108	8.7 ± 0.5	68 ± 5	18 ± 3
WKY-CEI	85 ± 8*	1709 ± 107*	10.7 ± 1.1*	1 ± 1*	1 ± 1*
SHR-Vehicle	160 ± 4	810 ± 52	7.1 ± 0.5	31 ± 3	17 ± 4
SHR-CEI	125 ± 7*	1262 ± 117*	11.1 ± 1.0*	2 ± 1*	1 ± 1*

* indicates P<0.05 (Vehicle versus CEI).

Arterial pressure (AP) was not affected by dietary sodium restriction in both vehicle-treated WKY and SHR. In contrast, AP gradually fell in WKY-CEI and SHR-CEI in response to sodium restriction. At the end of the low sodium period, the fall in arterial pressure corresponds to a 21 ± 8 % and 28 ± 3 % reduction in the pre-depletion value, respectively in WKY-CEI and SHR-CEI. Mean arterial pressure measured directly in conscious animals was similar in WKY-Vehicle and SHR-CEI (Table 1) thus showing that enalapril treatment combined with sodium restriction lead to normalization of arterial pressure in SHR.

As expected, renal vascular resistance was significantly higher in SHR-Vehicle (23.3 ± 1.7 mmHg.min.g/ml) than in WKY-Vehicle (13.3 ± 0.6 mmHg.min.g/ml). Blood flow to the kidneys was lower but not significantly different in untreated SHR and WKY rats. In CEI-treated sodium-depleted groups, renal vascular resistance decreased (8.1 ± 0.8 and 11.5 ± 0.9 mmHg.min.g/ml in WKY-CEI and SHR-CEI respectively) whereas and renal blood flow increased in both strain of rats.

DISCUSSION

In the present investigation, it is clearly shown that renal and systemic adaptation to sodium restriction was not altered in spontaneously hypertensive rats when compared to age-matched normotensive animals. Inhibition of angiotensin converting enzyme was associated with an impairment in the systemic and renal adaptation to sodium restriction in both strains. In addition, combination of volume depletion with ACE inhibition induced a normalization of arterial pressure in SHR.

During dietary sodium restriction, inhibition of angiotensin-converting enzyme was associated with a consistent decrease in arterial pressure in both strain of rats. Of interest, at the end of the 6-day period of low sodium intake, arterial pressure was normalized in enalapril-treated SHR when compared to untreated WKY. These findings are in agreement with those obtained in sodium-depleted SHR chronically immunized against renin (Jover et al, in press), and thus confirmed the key role of the renin-angiotensin system in arterial pressure regulation.

Pretreatment by enalapril was associated with an excessive urinary loss of sodium during the 6-day period of low sodium intake in both WKY and SHR strains. The sodium-wasting state occured despite the fall in arterial pressure which was directly correlated to the amount of sodium lost during sodium restriction. Analogous findings have been found in normotensive sodium-depleted rats treated by CEIs (Jover & Mimran, 1984; Mimran et al, 1988). In contrast, the renal adaptation to sodium restriction was not affected in SHR chronically immunized against renin (Jover et al, in press). The discrepancy between renin-immunization and enalapril treatment may be related to a better blockade of intrarenal angiotensin II generation by enalapril or to a non renin-mediated renal effect of converting enzyme inhibition. Such a possibility was suggested by the correction of sodium wasting and renal vasodilatation obtained with a prostaglandin-synthetase inhibitor in sodium-depleted normotensive rats pretreated by enalapril (Mimran et al, 1988). In the same experiments, enalapril was associated with a drastic reduction in aldosterone response to sodium restriction. In the absence of data on the effect of renin immunization on aldosterone response to sodium restriction, the possibility remains that sufficient stimulation of aldosterone release by a non renin-mediated mechanism (direct effect of potassium retention on adrenal glomerular cells) may have occured.

In conclusion, the present observations demonstrate that an efficient renin-angiotensin system is required in the systemic and renal adaptation to sodium restriction in normotensive as well as in spontaneously hypertensive rats. The sodium wasting induced by enalapril but not by renin-immunization suggests that converting enzyme inhibitors may act through a non renin-mediated effects or efficiently inhibits the angiotensin II-stimulated tubular sodium transport.

REFERENCES

Bengis R.G., Coleman T.G., Young D.B., McCaa R.E. (1978): Long-term blockade of angiotensin formation in various normotensive and hypertensive rat model using converting enzyme inhibitor (SQ 14225). *Circ. Res.* 43 (Suppl.1), 45-53.

Jover B & Mimran A. (1984): Effect of converting enzyme inhibition by enalapril on sodium homeostasis in the rat. *Br. J. Clin. Pharmacol.* 18, 209S-214S.

Jover B., Michel J.B., Dupont M., Corvol P., Mimran A. (in press): Adaptation to sodium restriction in renin-immunized spontaneously hypertensive and normotensive rats. *Am. J. Physiol.* (Heart Circ. Physiol.).

Levy B., Michel J.B., Salzmann J.L. et al (1988): Arterial effects of angiotensin converting enzyme inhibition in renovascular and hypertensive rat. *J. Hypertension* 6 (Suppl.3), 23-25.

Lo M., Julien C., Michel J.B. et al (1990): Antirenin immunization versus angiotensin converting enzyme inhibition in rats. *Hypertension* 16, 80-88.

Mimran A., Jover B., Dupont M. (1988): Enalapril-induced disturbance in the renal adaptation to sodium restriction in the rat. *Kidney Int.* 34 (Suppl 25), 28-32.

Richer C., Doussau M.P., Giudicelli J.F. (1981): MK 421 and prevention of genetic development in young spontaneously hypertensive rats. *Eur. J. Pharmacol.* 79, 23-29.

Chronic dopaminergic system impairment induces hypertension and hyperaldosteronism in rats

Agostinho Tavares, Davilson Bossolan, Maria T. Zanella, Artur B. Ribeiro and Osvaldo Kohlmann Jr

Nephrology Division, Escola Paulista de Medicina, Rua Botucatu, 740 04023 São Paulo, Brazil

INTRODUCTION

A possible role for dopamine in blood pressure regulation through its central and/or peripheral actions (Goldberg, 1976) has been suggested in the literature. Dopamine has the ability to produce a variety of cardiovascular and renal effects either by acting directly on its specific receptors at vessels wall, nervous endings (Goldberg, 1976) and kidney (Bass & Murphy, 1990) or indirectly through effects upon secretion or action of many vasoative hormones, such as aldosterone (Carey & Drake, 1986), renin-angiotensin (Carey & Drake, 1986), vasopressin (Hatzinikolaou et al, 1984), atrial natriuretic factor (Coruzzi et al, 1990), prolactin (Horrobin et al, 1979) and prostaglandins (Horton et al, 1990). However, the role of the dopaminergic system in the development of hypertension remains unclear. Therefore, the present study was designed to investigate: 1- whether chronic dopaminergic system impairment with metoclopramide, a non specific dopamine receptor blocker, associated or not with salt overload increases blood pressure of normotensive rats and 2- possible mechanisms that would be involved in this experimental model.

METHODS

Male normotensive, 10-12 weeks old Wistar rats were used in these experiments. All animals were submitted to uninephrectomy at the left side, and were kept on regular Purina rat chow. One week later, metoclopramide started to be administered every 12 hours through subcutaneous injections, at dosages of either 4mg/kg/day or 8mg/kg/day during 6 consecutive weeks. According to groups distribution, animals treated with both metoclopramide dosage drank either water (groups Me4,n=20 and Me8, n=20; groups without salt overload) or saline 1% (groups Me4S1, n=26 and Me8S1,n=17; groups with salt overload) ad libitum. Another 18 uninephrectomized animals treated with subcutaneous injections of vehicle instead of metoclopramide, but receiving saline 1% to drink were used as control (group Me0S1). Tail arterial pressure (TAP), through an microphonic method was recorded twice/week, in awaked animals from all studied groups. After 6 weeks of follow-up, in some animals of each group, mean blood pressure response to acute pharmacologic blockade of either sympathetic nervous system with propranolol 2mg/Kg+ phentolamine 10mg/Kg, or arginine-vasopressin with a specific V1-receptor antagonist 20mcg/rat were obtained. In the remaining animals, blood samples were collected for serum prolactine and aldosterone levels determinations by radioimmunoassay methods. Data is presented as Mean $\pm$ SEM. Two-way analyses of variance; Student's t-test and Mann-Witney test were used for the appropriate statistical analyses.

RESULTS

Chronic metoclopramide administration blocked effectively and in a dose-dependent manner the dopaminergic system since prolactin levels that were 8.7$\pm$0.6 ng/ml in the group Me0s1 rose to 57.6$\pm$6.1 and 114.4$\pm$15.2 ng/ml in groups Me4 and Me8 respectively. Also chronic metoclopramide administration at both dosage (4mg/Kg/day and 8mg/Kg/day) induced similar, progressive and sustained increases in tail arterial pressure of normotensive uninephrectomized Wistar rats. In animals treated with 4 mg/kg/day (group Me4) TAP rose from 114$\pm$1 mmHg in the baseline period to 133$\pm$1 mmHg after 6 weeks of treatment, and in group Me8 from 116$\pm$1 mmHg to 132$\pm$1 mmHg. Salt overload did not modified the hypertensive state induced by metoclopramide 4 mg/Kg (TAP from 121$\pm$1 mmHg at baseline to 135$\pm$1 mmHg after 6 weeks, change in TAP of +14$\pm$1 mmHg). However saline 1% significantly enhanced the rise in blood pressure induced by metoclopramide 8mg/Kg/day (TAP from 112$\pm$1 mmHg to 142$\pm$1 mmHg, change in TAP of +30$\pm$2 mmHg). Acute sympathetic nervous system blockade induced significant falls in blood pressure of all groups treated with metoclopramide specially in those with salt overload (Me4= -8$\pm$1.7 mmHg; Me8= -15$\pm$2.4 mmHg; Me4S1= -25$\pm$4.6 mmHg and Me8S1= -26.4$\pm$10.2 mmHg), pointing to a role for the sympathetic nervous system in this hypertension. On the other hand arginine vasopressin blockade did not cause any significant change in blood pressure of those animals (Me4= -1$\pm$2 mmHg; Me8= -4$\pm$2 mmHg; Me4s1= 0$\pm$2 mmHg and Me8S1= 0$\pm$2 mmHg). Plasma Aldosterone levels were normal in groups Me4 e Me8 (13.3$\pm$1.3 ng/dl e 14.6$\pm$1.2 ng/dl respectively), but was significantly supressed as expected in the control group (Me0S1) by the sodium overload (5.5$\pm$1.1 ng/dl). However in the animals from group Me8S1 and therefore also with sodium overload plasma aldosterone was at normal levels (11.4±1.2 ng/dl) meaning a high aldosterone level for that sodium balance state and therefore pointing to a relative hyperaldostronism induced by chronic dopaminergic system blockade.

We conclude that chronic dopaminergic system impairment with metoclopramide induces hypertension in Wistar rats. This hypertension is enhanced by sodium overload. A relative hyperaldosteronism and an augmented sympathetic nervous activity play role in this hypertension.

REFERENCES

Bass, A.S. & Murphy,M.B. (1990)- Role of endogeneous dopamine in the natriuresis accompaning various sodium challenges. Am J. Hypertens.,3 :90S- 92S

Carey, R.M. & Drake,C.R (1986)- Dopamine selectively inhibts aldosterone response to angiotensin II in humans. Hypertension, 8 :399-406

Corruzzi, P.; Musiari,L; Biggi,A.; Carra, N.;Ravanetti,C.; Minuz,P; Montanari,A. & Novarini,A- (1990) Sodium homeostasis and hormonal responses during dopaminergic blockade in normal humans. Am J. Hypertens, 3 : 87S-89S

Goldberg,L.I. (1976)- Cardiovascular and renal actions of dopamine : potential clinical applications. Pharmacol. Rev. , 24 : 1-29

Hatzinikolaou, P. Gavras H, North,W.G.; Kohlmannm, O. & Gavras,I (1984)- Evidence for dopaminergic regulation of vasopressin release in the anephric rat. J. Hypertens., 2: 311-315

Horton R.; Bughi,S; Jost-Vu,E.; Antonipillai,I.& Nadler,J. (1990)- Effect of dopamine on renal blood flow, prostaglandins renin and electrolyte excretion in normal and hypertensive humans. Am. J. Hypertens., 3: 108S- 111S

Horrobin D.F.; Manku,M.S.& Burstyn,P.G. (1973) - Effect of intraveneous prolactin infusion on arterial blood pressure in rabbits. Cardiovasc Res., 7: 585-587

Renal dopamine excretion and vasodilatation in spontaneously hypertensive rats (SHR)

Mariette Barthelmebs [1], Michèle Grima, Dominique Stephan and Jean-Louis Imbs [1]

[1] Institut de Pharmacologie, URA DO 589 CNRS, Université Louis Pasteur, 11, rue Humann and Service d'Hypertension artérielle et maladies vasculaires, CHRU, 67000 Strasbourg, France

Dopamine (DA) is synthesized in the kidney from circulating L-dopa. It acts as a paracrine substance which regulates renal hemodynamics (Barthelmebs et al., 1990) and contributes to the regulation of sodium excretion (Imbs et al., 1984; Siragy et al., 1989). DA-induced renal effects, vasodilatation and natriuresis are the opposite of those of noradrenaline. Since the activation of the sympathetic nervous system contributes to the development of hypertension in spontaneously hypertensive rats (SHR) of the Okamoto-Aoki strain, it has been suggested that there is an imbalance between the renal effects of dopamine and noradrenaline (Lee, 1989; Kuchel, 1990).

To test the kidney dopaminergic defect in SHR, we considered the possibility of a a disturbance of renal extraneuronal DA synthesis. Basal and L-dopa stimulated urinary DA excretions were therefore compared in SHR and WKY rats, both at the start of (7 wk) and after (12 wk) established hypertension . We also looked for a defect in renal vascular DA-induced vasodilatation. Indeed, this effect involves vascular DA1 receptors (Schmidt et al., 1987) and a defect in transduction of the tubular DA1 receptor signal has been associated with the decrease in the natriuretic effect of DA in SHR (Felder et al., 1990).

MATERIALS AND METHODS

Male SHR and control WKY rats (Iffa Credo) were maintained on a standard rat chow (0.4% sodium) with ad libitum access to water.

Twelve rats of both SH and WKY strains were used for studies in metabolic cages. They underwent two times a similar set of experiments, at 7 and 12 weeks of age. After their systolic blood pressure (SBP) has been measured (Sphygmomanometric measurement in conscious animals, Physiograph, Narco Bio Systems Inc), they were given two days to become accustomed to metabolic cages. The first day enabled us to measure basal parameters; on the second day, L-dopa (10 mg/kg, s.c., Sigma) was randomly allocated to half the animals of each of the SH and WKY strains, the other half receiving L-dopa solvent (2 ml/kg s.c.); the same animals received L-dopa at 7 and 12 weeks of age. Urine sodium (flame photometer), creatinine (Technicon) and free DA concentrations (HPLC with electrochemical detection, Waters) were measured, together with plasma creatinine concentration (rat tail blood).

Five SHR and WKY rats were used for in vitro studies; their kidneys were perfused in an open circuit, at constant flow according to Schmidt et al. (1987) with a Krebs-Henseleit solution supplemented with polygeline (Behringwerke). Perfusion pressure was adjusted at the beginning of experiment to the diastolic blood pressure level of each rat. Perfusion pressure was continuously recorded (Statham P23 Db). Having restablished a vascular tone (PGF_2alpha perfusion to increase renal vascular resistance by 20%) and blocked the alpha- and beta-adrenoceptors (phenoxybenzamine and sotalol, 10^{-5} M), DA was perfused at increasing concentrations (0.3 to 30 pmol/l). Results are given as means ± SEM. The BMDP statistical analysis program (Statistical solftware Ltd) was used to carry out the statistical analysis.

RESULTS

A decrease in the glomerular filtration rate and water and sodium excretions was observed as reported earlier in 7 week-old SHR (table 1). Conversely, basal urinary free DA excretion was higher in the future hypertensive animals. This increase persisted at 12 weeks, albeit at a lower level, whereas the other basal renal parameters had returned to a level similar to that in WKY rats.

Table 1. Basal parameters measured in 7 and 12 week-old SHR and WKY rats

Mean±SEM	n	SBP mm Hg	BW g	UV ml/day	UVNa mmol/day	UVDA pmol/day	GFR ml/min
7 week-old rats							
WKY	(12)	117±3	180±4	8.3±0.7	1.8±0.1	6±2	0.60±0.04
SHR	(12)	145±5**	172±4	4.8±0.4**	1.4±0.1*	16±4*	0.44±0.04**
12 week-old rats							
WKY	(12)	125±3	279±5	7.5±0.8	1.5±0.1	6±1	0.71±0.08
SHR	(12)	190±2**	277±6	7.8±0.7	1.7±0.1	10±1**	0.83±0.10

* $p < 0.05$, ** $p < 0.01$ Student's t test SHR vs WKY rats at 7 or 12 weeks of age.

A single L-dopa injection (10 mg/kg) induced a marked increase in the 24 h urinary DA excretion of 7 week-old rats, whatever the strain (table 2). This increase was also observed in 12 week-old rats; its magnitude however was half that of 7 week old rats, a difference nearly significant in SHR ($p = 0.053$). L-dopa treatment did not modify any of the other renal parameters.

Table 2. L-dopa induced increase and spontaneous evolution in urinary dopamine excretion (UVDA) in 7 and 12 week-old SHR and WKY rats.

Mean±SEM	n	Treatment	Increase in UVDA pmol/day/100 g body weight	ANOVA
7 week-old rats				
WKY	(6)	solvent	4±2	<0.001
WKY	(6)	L-dopa	1101±342*	
SHR	(6)	solvent	5±4	
SHR	(6)	L-dopa	1132±290*	
12 week-old rats				
WKY	(6)	solvent	12±6	<0.001
WKY	(6)	L-dopa	645±135**	
SHR	(6)	solvent	4±2	
SHR	(6)	L-dopa	493±53**	

* $p < 0.05$, ** $p < 0.01$ Scheffé's test, L-dopa vs solvent treated group.

The isolated kidneys from 12 week-old SHR and WKY rats were perfused respectively at a pressure of 133 ± 14 and 83 ± 3 mm Hg, after adjustement of renal flow to 27 ± 2 and 18 ± 3 ml/min.g of kidney. On these isolated (and denervated) kidneys, there was no difference between the two strains in basal renal vascular resistance (5.6 ± 0.2 vs 5.6 ± 0.7 mm Hg.min/ml) nor in DA-induced renal vasodilatation ($EC_{50} = 0.66 \pm 0.11$ and 1.75 ± 4.7 µmol/l; Emax = 100 ± 2 and 91.5 ± 5% suppression in PGF_2alpha-induced increase in renal vascular tone).

DISCUSSION

These results show that renal extraneuronal DA synthesis, as reflected in urinary dopamine excretion, is not impaired in SHR. This is true whatever basal or L-dopa stimulated DA synthesis is considered and applies to 7 week and 12 week-old rats. Moreover, a paradoxical increase in basal urinary DA excretion was found during the development of hypertension in SHR. A similar observation was previously reported in young Okamoto genetic hypertensive rats (Kuchel et al., 1987). Our concomitant observation of an increase in urinary DA excretion and sodium retention and glomerular hypofiltration underlines the impaired DA renal paracrine function. A defect in the tubular DA1 receptor-second messenger coupling mechanism has been found in 3 week-old rats (Kinoshita et al., 1989). At 12 weeks, we found no difference in the responsiveness of vascular DA1 receptors. Although this point has to be confirmed in younger rats, it is likely that the renal DA defect in SHR is not linked to an abnormal renal DA synthesis or vasodilatation.

These results show that renal extraneuronal dopamine synthesis is enhanced during the development of hypertension in SHR. Despite normal renal dopamine vascular effects, hypertension occurred in these animals. Abnormal renal sodium handling in the proximal tubula may be involved.

REFERENCES

Barthelmebs, M., Caillette, A., Ehrhardt, JD., Velly, J. and Imbs, JL. (1990): Metabolism and vascular effects of gamma-L-glutamyl-L-dopa on the isolated rat kidney. Kidney Int. 37: 1414-1422.
Felder, RA., Seikaly, MG., Cody, P., Eisner, GM. and Jose, PA. (1990): Attenuated renal response to dopaminergic drugs in spontaneously hypertensive rats. Hypertension 15: 560-569.
Imbs, JL., Schmidt, M., Ehrhardt, JD. and Schwartz, J. (1984): The sympathetic nervous system and renal sodium handling : Is dopamine involved ? J. Cardiovasc. Pharmacol. 6: S171-S175.
Kinoshita, S., Sidhu, A. and Felder, RA. (1989): Defective dopamine-1 receptor adenylate cyclase coupling in the proximal convoluted tubule from the spontaneously hypertensive rat. J. Clin. Invest. 84: 1849-1856.
Kuchel, O., Racz, K., Debinski, W., Falardeau, P. and Buu, NT. (1987): Contrasting dopaminergic patterns in two forms of genetic hypertension. Clin. and Exper. Theory and Practice, A9(5&6): 987-1008.
Kuchel, O. (1990): Dopamine and hypertension. Current Opinion in Cardiology 5: 594-600.
Lee, MR. (1989): Dopamine, the kidney and essential hypertension. Clin. Exp. Hypertens. A11(suppl. 1): 149-158.
Schmidt, M., Krieger, JP., Giesen-Crouse, EM. and Imbs, JL. (1987): Vascular effects of selective dopamine receptor agonists and antagonists in the rat kidney. Arch. Int. Pharmacodyn. 286: 195-205.
Siragy, HM., Felder, RA., Howell NL., Chevalier, RL., Peach MJ. and Carey RM. (1989): Evidence that intrarenal dopamine acts as a paracrine substance at the renal tubule. Am. J. Physiol. 257: F469-F477.

SHRsp response to high salt diet

Judith M. Lange [1] [2], Brian P. Brockway [2] and Mario F. Sylvestri [3]

[1] University of Minnesota, Minneapolis, MN 55455; [2] Data Sciences International, 2678 Patton Road, St. Paul, MN 55113; [3] University of Oklahoma, Oklahoma City, OK 73019, USA

SHRsp rats implanted with a telemetric monitoring device, maintained in 12:12 lighting, and fed a high 4% NaCl diet showed significantly higher systolic arterial pressures (SAP) and diastolic arterial pressures (DAP) than rats fed a normal salt diet (SAP: 244.2 vs 208.3 mmHg and DAP: 168.8 vs vs 156.2 mmHg, respectively) when these pressures were viewed at 10 Hours After Lights Off (HALO). At 22 HALO, no difference was seen in SAPs or DAPs when comparing the high to normal salt groups (SAP: 195.7 vs 188.9 mmHg and DAP: 135.4 vs 141.2 mmHg, respectively). Heart rate did not significantly differ between groups at either time.

It is well documented in the literature and generally accepted in the scientific community that high salt diets produce or exacerbate hypertension in hypertension-prone strains of rats, including spontaneously hypertensive rats (SHR). Notable exceptions have been offered by Chen et al. (1988) who have identified a substrain of SHR rats resistant to salt in their diet (SHR-R) and by Ganguli and Tobian (1990) who have shown the protective effect of dietary potassium.

Typically, pressure measurements are obtained using conventional techniques such as tail-cuff plethysmography, intra-arterial catheterization under anesthesia, or tethers. Each of these methods can produce measurement errors introduced by artifacts associated with restraint, handling, anesthesia, and/or sympathetic nervous system stimulation (Proceedings.., 1977; Adams, et al., 1988). These artifacts limit the predictive value of the data.

Wireless telemetry allows pressure measurements to be taken from conscious animals while they remain undisturbed in their home environment (Brockway, et al., 1991). This telemetric system allowed us to show that blood pressures taken at night when rats are normally active showed a pressure response to high NaCl diets, but pressures taken during certain times of the day did not.

MATERIALS AND METHODS: Nine-week-old male stroke-prone SHR rats were obtained from Dr. Brody, University of Iowa and were individually housed in plastic 23 X 45 X 20 cm cages with food and water ad lib. Fluorescent lighting was kept on for 12 hours beginning at 7:00 AM and off for 12 hours beginning at 7:00 PM.

Rats were surgically implanted with radio-telemetric devices (Data Sciences International) capable of transmitting blood pressure waveforms. Receivers were placed under the cages and connected to the Dataquest data acquisition and analysis system, which allowed each animal to be sequentially sampled for 10 seconds every 10 minutes. Systolic arterial pressure (SAP), diastolic arterial pressure (DAP), and heart rate (HR) were extracted from the waveforms.

Twelve days post-surgery, rats were divided into two groups whose blood pressure and body weight (BW) were not significantly different. Group I (n=3, SAP=172.7 mm Hg, BW=244 gm) continued eating normal 0.5% NaCl diet; Group II (n=3, SAP=164.3 mmHg, BW=231 gm) was changed to high 4% NaCl diet (Zeigler Brothers, Gardners, PA).

Animals continued to be monitored for 15 weeks. The last three days of observation, two data points for each group were compared: 10 Hours After Lights Off (10 HALO) when the room was dark and the rats were active, and 22 HALO when the room was light and the rats were inactive.

The telemetric implants were validated against an intra-arterial cannula threaded via the carotid to within 1 cm of the implant catheter in the aorta. Simultaneous tracings of the two pressures were taken and compared. The implant devices were surgically removed and gross examination of the peritoneal cavity was performed.

RESULTS: Circadian rhythms were evident for systolic and diastolic pressures (Figures 1 and 2) and for heart rate (not shown).

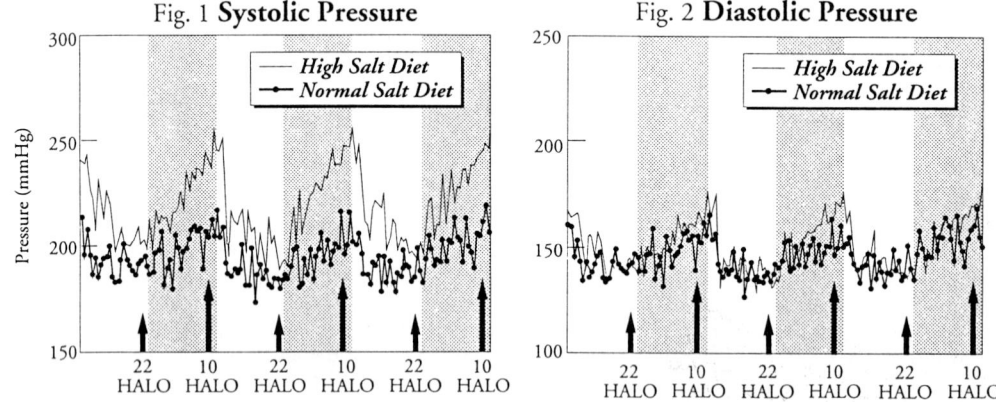

At 10 HALO, normal salt Group I had a systolic pressure of 208.3 +/- 8.0 mmHg (1 SD unit) whereas high salt Group II had a systolic pressure of 244.2 +/- 12.1 mmHg. Systole of Group II was significantly higher (p<.001) than Group I. Diastolic pressure for Group I was 156.2 +/- 16.8 mmHg, while Group II was significantly higher (p<.001) at 168.8 +/- 8.5 mmHg. There was no significant difference in the HR (Group I =350.5 +/- 26.0 and Group II =343.7 +/- 19.6 beats per minute).

At 22 HALO, when the lights were on, systolic pressure for Group I was 188.9 +/- 12.0 mmHg, while systole for high salt Group II was 195.7 +/- 10.1 mmHg. These pressures were not significantly different. Diastolic pressure for Group I was 141.2 +/- 16.2 mmHg, while for Group II was 135.4 +/- 16.0 mmHg (no significant difference). Heart rates for both groups were lower at 22 HALO (Group I=242.0 +/- 50.7; Group II=260.4 +/- 17.0 beats per minute) but there was no significant difference between the two groups. Results are summarized below in Table 1.

Validation showed the telemetric pressures agreed well (within 5% on average) with values simultaneously obtained using a calibrated transducer system. Average offset drift for 16 weeks was -8.1 mmHg. No tissue or anatomical changes were seen in the peritoneum (no bleeding, hematomae, intestinal obstructions, or infections). Explantation results are summarized in Table 2.

Table 1

Systolic Arterial Pressure (mmHg)

22 Halo (Daylight)

	I (NS)	II (HS)
Mean	188.9	195.7
SD	12.0	10.1
p	NS	

10 Halo (Nighttime)

	I (NS)	II (HS)
Mean	208.3	244.2
SD	8.0	12.1
p	<.001	

Diastolic Arterial Pressure (mmHg)

22 Halo (Daylight)

	I (NS)	II (HS)
Mean	141.2	135.4
SD	16.2	16.0
p	NS	

10 Halo (Nighttime)

	I (NS)	II (HS)
Mean	156.2	168.8
SD	16.8	8.5
p	<.001	

Heart Rate (beats/minute)

22 Halo (Daylight)

	I (NS)	II (HS)
Mean	242.0	260.4
SD	50.7	17.0
p	NS	

10 Halo (Nighttime)

	I (NS)	II (HS)
Mean	350.5	343.7
SD	26.0	19.6
p	NS	

Table 2
Explantation Results

Rat #	Diet	16 Wk Drift	Pressure Validation TELEMETRY	Pressure Validation INTERARTERIAL	% DIFFERENCE
002	HS	-7.5	195/145	195/150	0 / 3.4
005	NS	-8.4	209/165	198/155	5.2 / 6.0
010	HS	-15.7	190/160	198/160	4.2 / 0
011	NS	-17.3	180/138	198/158	10.0 / 12.6
013	NS	-7.1	192/157	199/168	3.6 / 7.0
016	HS	+7.5	246/178	249/182	1.2 / 2.2

N=6 Mean Drift - 8.1   Systolic Difference 4.0%   Diastolic Difference 5.2%

DISCUSSION: The data presented clearly indicate that SHRsp rats on a high salt diet have higher blood pressures than SHRsp rats on a normal salt diet during the night but do not have significantly higher pressures during certain periods of the day. Rats are nocturnal, sleeping the least at the 10th hour of dark (10 HALO) and the most during light periods, beginning at the 2nd hour (Trachsel, et al., 1986).

Neural activity in rats follows a circadian pattern. Ono, et al (1987) have found higher ventromedial hypothalamic (VMH) and lateral hypothalamic area (LHA) activity during the dark. It is well known that circadian rhythms exist for adrenal steroids, pituitary LH, plasma and adrenal corticosterone, and plasma and pituitary ACTH. Vasopressin, vasoactive intestinal polypeptides, and prostaglandin D2 (Hayaishi, 1991) are higher during light cycles.

The results of the present study suggest: (1) telemetry offers a viable alternative to conventional techniques of monitoring blood pressure and heart rate; and (2) additional studies using telemetric technology may further elucidate the connection between circadian rhythms of certain substances and blood pressure, in the presence or absence of a high salt diet.

REFERENCES:
Adams M, Kaplan J, Manuck S, Uberseder B, and Larkin K. (1988): Persistent sympathetic nervous system arousal associated with tethering in Cynomolgus Macaques. Laboratory Animal Science, Vol 38, No 3: 279-281.

Brockway B, Mills P, and Azar S. (1991): A new method for continuous chronic measurement and recording of blood pressure, heart rate and activity in the rat via radio-telemetry. Clinical & Experimental Hypertension, in press.

Chen Y, Meng Q, Wyss J, Jin H, Oparil S. (1988): High NaCl diet reduces hypothalamic norepinephrine turnover in hypertensive rats. Hypertension Dallas 11: 55-62.

Ganguli M and Tobian L. (1990): Dietary K determines NaCl sensitivity in NaCl-induced rises of blood pressure in spontaneously hypertensive rats. American Journal of Hypertension, Vol 3, No 6, Part 1: 482-484.

Hayaishi O. (1991): Molecular mechanisms of sleep-wake regulation: roles of prostaglandins D2 and E2. FASEB Journal, Vol 5, No 11: 2575-2581.

Ono, T, Sasaki K, and Shibata R. (1987): Diurnal- and behaviour-related activity of ventromedial hypothalamic neurones in freely behaving rats. Journal of Physiology, Vol 394: 201-220.

Proceedings of a Workshop on Blood Pressure Measurement in Hypertensive Animals Models. (1977): DHEW Publication No (NIH) 78-1473.

Trachsel L, Tobler I, and Borbely A. (1986): Sleep regulation in rats: effects of sleep deprivation, light, and circadian phase. American Journal of Physiology, Vol 251, No 6, Part 2: R1037-R1044.

Hyperoxia alters salt intake in spontaneously hypertensive rats (SHR) but not in normotensive Wistar-Kyoto rats (WKY)

Reinhard Behm, Hanko Dewitz and Hartmut Mewes

Department of Physiology, University of Rostock, 9 Gertrudenstrasse, D-2500 Rostock, Germany

Little is known about the central nervous regulation of salt appetite in rats. SHR exhibit an exaggerated salt appetite. Various humoral factors have been postulated to contribute to this phenomenon (Fregly & Rowland, 1985; Weiss et al. 1986). Evidence has cumulated that salt appetite is closely linked to chemoreceptor activity and that this relationship is particularly tight in SHR (Honig 1989). Both physiological and pharmacological stimulation of the arterial chemoreceptors alters salt intake in SHR (Behm et al. 1984, Behm et al. 1989). Recently, we were able to demonstrate that exposure of SHR to hyperoxia results in an increase in salt intake (Behm et al. 1991). Similar experiments conducted in WKY rats are lacking. To further clarify the role of peripheral arterial chemoreceptors in sodium intake we investigated the effects of normobaric hyperoxia on voluntary salt intake in conscious SHR and WKY.

METHODS

Experiments were carried out in 16 male SHR (Okamoto-Aoki strain) and 8 male WKY rats weighing 250-350 g. Animals were housed individually in metabolic cages which were placed in a large chamber. During the experiments, rats were given a permanent two-bottle choice between a 2.5 % saline solution (435 mmol/l) and tap water. Standard laboratory chow was available ad libitum. Fluid intake and body weight were measured daily. Normobaric air stream was circulated through the chamber and adjusted to approximately 20 l/h. Carbon dioxide was absorbed by potassium hydroxide. After a 3-day acclimatization period, rats were subjected to consecutive periods of normoxia (5 days), hyperoxia (4 days) and again normoxia (5 days). The hyperoxic gas was adjusted to 50 % oxygen in nitrogen.
Results are expressed as means ± S.E.M. The differences between basic normoxic levels and those recorded on subsequent days were checked for statistical significance with Student's t-test for paired data. They were considered significant if $p<0.05$.

RESULTS

As shown in Fig. 1, exposure of conscious SHR and WKY to normobaric hyperoxia increased 2.5 % saline intake significantly only in the SHR group. In contrast, no significant alterations in salt intake was observed in WKY during exposure to hyperoxia. Table 1 summarizes body weight, water intake and salt preference in SHR and WKY exposed to hyperoxia. Moderate normobaric hyperoxia had a small but significant negative effect on body weight in WKY which persisted also during the postnormoxic period. There was a significant difference in water intake between SHR and WKY during the normoxic control period (10.5 ± 0.3 vs. 5.1 ± 0.3 ml/100g.d) In both groups a significant increase in water intake was observed during the hyperoxic period. Salt preference (calculated as percentage of saline solution from the total fluid) differed markedly in both groups during the normoxic control period (21.7 ± 3.0 vs. 62.2 ± 7.2 %). Only SHR showed a significant increase in salt preference during exposure to normobaric hyperoxia.

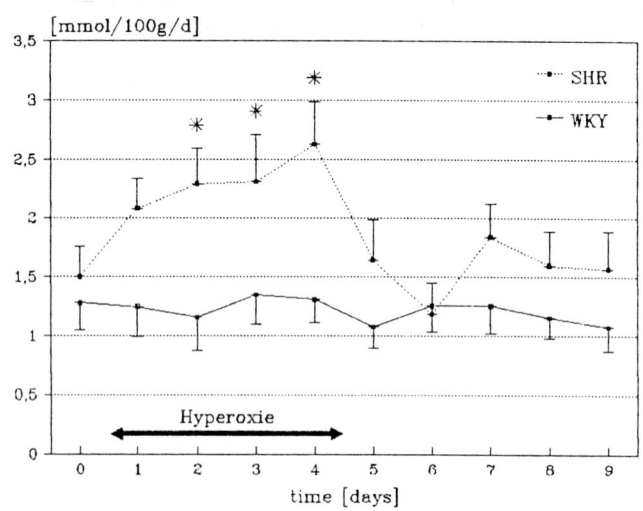

Fig.1: Effect of hyperoxia on salt intake in SHR and WKY. Values are means ± S.E.M. (* Significant differences from the normoxic control period at p<0.05.)

Table 1: Effect of normobaric hyperoxia on body weight, water intake and salt preference in SHR and WKY. Values are means ± S.E.M., * significant differences from the control period at p<0.05.

	Body Weight [g]		Water Intake [ml/100g d]		Salt Preference [%]	
	SHR	WKY	SHR	WKY	SHR	WKY
0	274 ± 4	330 ± 5	10.5 ± 0.3	5.1 ± 0.3	21.7 ± 3.0	62.2 ± 7.2
1	279 ± 5 *	334 ± 6	12.5 ± 0.6 *	6.0 ± 0.3 *	29.6 ± 4.6	67.2 ± 9.1
2	279 ± 5 *	332 ± 6	12.4 ± 0.8 *	5.8 ± 0.8 *	28.7 ± 2.6 *	68.4 ± 8.3
3	282 ± 5 *	329 ± 5	12.2 ± 0.7 *	5.4 ± 0.2	28.1 ± 3.3 *	63.1 ± 7.1
4	284 ± 6 *	328 ± 6 *	11.8 ± 0.8 *	5.8 ± 0.3 *	32.3 ± 3.0 *	65.2 ± 7.9
5	284 ± 5 *	326 ± 5 *	11.1 ± 0.9	5.4 ± 0.4	24.1 ± 3.4	67.9 ± 8.1
6	287 ± 4 *	323 ± 6 *	10.3 ± 0.6	5.4 ± 0.6	19.1 ± 3.1	64.9 ± 8.5
7	290 ± 5 *	323 ± 5 *	9.9 ± 0.5	5.1 ± 0.3	28.4 ± 2.9 *	63.3 ± 7.6
8	287 ± 5 *	321 ± 5 *	8.6 ± 0.6 *	4.8 ± 0.4	27.7 ± 4.2	62.7 ± 7.1
9	290 ± 4 *	321 ± 7 *	9.3 ± 0.4 *	5.2 ± 0.6	25.9 ± 3.7	67.0 ± 7.2

DISCUSSION

Exposure of conscious SHR and WKY to moderate normobaric hyperoxia resulted in a sustained enhancement of salt intake only in SHR. These results support our hypothesis that a link exists between chemoreceptor activity and voluntary salt intake in SHR. At least two different mechanisms may explain our results. HONIG (1989) speculated that SHR need a high chemoreceptor drive to keep their sodium appetite on a certain level. Hypoxia increases chemoreceptor discharge and thus leads to a sustained suppression of salt intake whereas hyperoxia lowers chemoreceptor activity and thereby increases salt appetite. In normotensive rats this "drive" is much less pronounced compared to SHR as documented by lower ventilation (Pfeiffer et al. 1984, Fukuda et al 1987). This mechanism could explain why no effect of hyperoxia on salt intake has been noted in WKY. This assumption is supported by previous results obtained with carotid body denervated SHR. The increase in salt intake due to hyperoxia was at least partially abolished by denervation of the peripheral arterial chemoreceptors (Behm et al. 1991).

On the other hand it is well documented that various hormonal systems play a substantial role in the regulation of sodium intake or sodium homeostasis respectively. It has been shown that hormones such as angiotensin II and aldosterone play an important role in salt appetite in rats (Weiss et al 1986; Fregly & Rowland, 1985). However, to our knowledge no data exist on electrolyte and fluid balance in conscious hyperoxic rats or the implication of the renin-angiotensin-aldosterone system in this behaviour. Recently, were able to show that chronic exposure (3 weeks) of SHR and WKY to moderate hyperoxia resulted in similar changes in plasma angiotensin-converting enzyme activity and dopamine concentration in both groups, whereas plasma norepinephrine was increased in SHR and decreased in WKY (unpublished observation). This fits well with observations by others (Koepke & DiBona, 1985, Lundin & and Thoren 1982)that stressful environmental stimulation is more effective in SHR than in normotensive WKY rats. As a consequence, the higher sensitivity of SHR to such stimuli may result in increased renal nerve activity and thereby increased renal tubular sodium reabsorption. Whether or not such mechanisms play any role in salt intake in SHR remains to be elucidated.

REFERENCES:

Behm, R., Gerber, B., Habeck, J.-O., Huckstorf, C., and Rückborn, K. (1989): Effect of hypobaric hypoxia and almitrine on voluntary salt and water intake in carotid body denervated spontaneously hypertensive rats. Biomed. Biochim. Acta 48, 689-695.

Behm, R., Rückborn, K., and Franz, U. (1991): Hyperoxia increases salt intake in spontaneously hypertensive rats (SHR). Physiol. Behav. 49, 165-167.

Fregly, M.J., and Rowland, N.E. (1985): Role of renin-angiotensin-aldosterone-system in NaCl-appetite of rats. Am. J. Physiol. 248, R1-R11.

Fukuda, Y., Sato, A., and Trzebski,A. (1987): Carotid chemoreceptor discharge responses to hypoxia and hypercapnia in normotensive and spontaneously hypertensive rats. J. Autonom. Nerv. Syst. 19, 1-11.

Honig, A. (1989): Peripheral arterial chemoreceptors and reflex control of sodium and water homeostasis. Am. J. Physiol 257, R1282-R1302.

Koepke, J.P., and DiBona, G.F. (1985): High sodium intake enhances renal nerve and antinatriuretic responses to stress in spontaneously hypertensive rats. Hypertension 7, 357-363.

Lundin, S., and Thoren,P. (1982): Renal function and sympathetic activity during mental stress in normotensive and spontaneously hypertensive rats. Acta Physiol. Scand. 115, 115-124.

Pfeiffer, C., Habeck, J.-O., Rotter, H., Behm, R., Schmidt, M. and Honig, H, (1984): Influence of age on carotid body size and arterial chemoreflex effects in spontaneously hypertensive rats (SHR) and normotensive rats. Biomed. Biochim. Acta 43, 207-215.

Weiss, M.L., Moe, K.E., and Epstein A.N. (1986): Interference with central actions of angiotensin II suppresses sodium appetite. Am. J. Physiol. 250, R250-R259.

Suppressed hepatointestinal reflex in spontaneously hypertensive rats

Hironobu Morita, Tsunenori Matsuda, Takao Horiba, Keisuke Miyake, Hideo Yamanouchi, Hideo Ohyama, Masanobu Hagiike, Hiroshi Hosomi, Katsumi Ikeda*, Yasuo Nara* and Yukio Yamori*

Department of Physiology, Kagawa Medical School, Kagawa 761-07, Japan and * Department of Pathology, Shimane Medical University, Izumo 693, Japan

Accumulating experimental data in spontaneously hypertensive rats (SHR) indicates that dietary salt intake is important in the development of hypertension and that SHR is more sensitive to oral salt load in comparison with normotensive Wistar-Kyoto rats (WKY). A recent study from our laboratory demonstrated that net NaCl absorption in the intestine is reflexively regulated by the NaCl receptor in the liver (Morita et al., 1990). Accordingly, the purpose of the present study was to examine whether hepatointestinal reflex was impair in SHR.

Male WKY (n=7), stroke-resistant SHR (SHRSR, n=7), and stroke-prone SHR (SHRSP, n=7) in Shimane Institute of Health Science, Izumo, Japan were obtained at 8-9 wk of age. 3-5 days before experiments, systolic arterial blood pressure and heart rate were measured by an indirect tailcuff method. Rats were deprived of food 24 h before experiments. Water remained available throughout the food-deprivation period. Rats were anesthetized with pentobarbital sodium (30 mg/kg, i.p.). Then a venous catheter was inserted into the superior vena cava via the external jugular vein for the infusion of hypertonic NaCl. A tracheostomy tube was inserted. Through the central laparotomy, the jejunal loop was made, which was 20 cm long and started 3 cm distal to the ligament of Treitz. The loop was washed with Ringer's solution and flushed with air, and intubated in both ends of the loop. The proximal tube was for the administration of the solution, and the distal tube was for the collection of the solution. A non-occlusive portal catheter for the infusion of hypertonic NaCl was inserted. The intestine was returned to the abdominal cavity. The tubes and catheter were exteriorized, and the incision was closed.

A 30-60 min equilibration period was observed before the experiment. To examine the jejunal electrolyte absorption, warmed Ringer's solution was perfused through the jejunal loop with a syringe infusion pump at the rate of 0.3 ml/min during four 30-min periods. Ringer's solution had the following composition (in mEq/l): Na 147; K 4; Ca 4.5; Cl 155.5. Phenol red was added to Ringer's solution for a nonabsorbable volume marker. Na and Cl concentrations of the administered and collected fluid were measured by a flame photometer and Cl counter. Phenol red concentration was determined by a spectrophotometer (558 nm, pH 8.4). The volume of the collected fluid was also measured. Water and electrolyte net absorption were calculated as the difference between the absolute values of the perfused solution and the absolute values of the collected solution. During the second and third perfusion period, jejunal net absorption was measured with the infusion of 9% NaCl at a rate of 5 1/100g b.w./min via the portal vein or the superior vena cava. During the first and fourth perfusion periods, jejunal net absorption was measured without any infusion via the portal vein or the superior vena cava. Because there was no significant difference in net absorption between the first and the fourth perfusion period, average values of these two periods was used for statistical analysis. A 30-min equilibration period was observed between each perfusion period.

Systolic arterial blood pressure in SHRSR (190 ± 4 mmHg) and SHRSP (204 ± 4 mmHg) was significantly higher than that in WKY (135 ± 2 mmHg). A precision of collected volume was examined by phenol red. When the yield of phenol red was less than 95%, data was not included in the text. During no infusion period, there was no significant difference in net fluid and NaCl absorption among WKY, SHRSR, and SHRSP. In WKY, net fluid and NaCl absorption were not influenced by the superior vena caval infusion of 9% NaCl, although it was significantly depressed by the portal infusion of 9% NaCl (Fig. 1). That is, net fluid, Na, and Cl absorption were depressed from 1.0 ± 0.1 ml/30 min, 135 ± 27, and 145 ± 13 Eq/30 min to 0.7 ± 0.1 ml/30 min, 70 ± 17, and 83 ± 13 Eq/30 min, respectively. Conversely, in SHRSR and SHRSP, the portal infusion of 9% NaCl did not have any significant effects in net absorption.

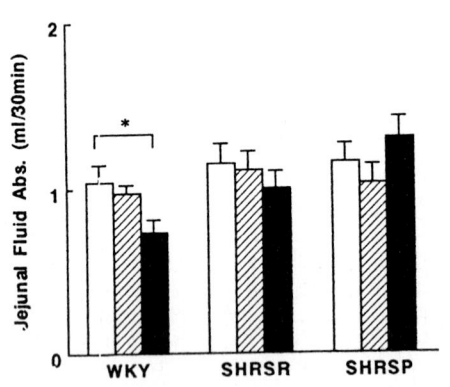

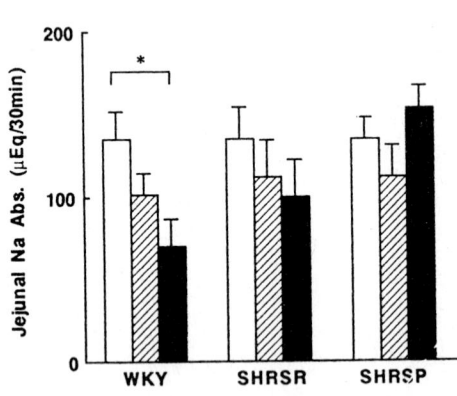

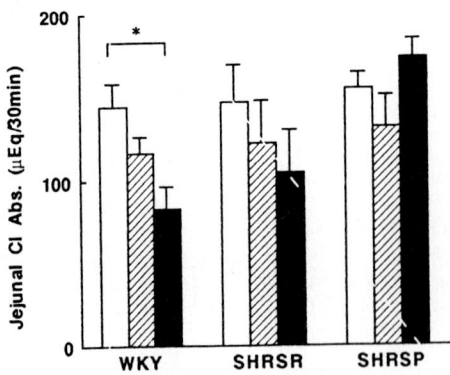

☐ No infusion
▨ SVC 9% NaCl infusion
■ PV 9% NaCl infusion

Fig. 1. Effects of 9% NaCl infusion via the superior vena cava (SVC) or the portal vein (PV) on net fluid absorption (Abs.), net Na absorption, and net Cl absorption. All values presented here are reported as means ± SE. * $P<0.05$.

The major findings of this study are 1) in WKY, the portal infusion of hypertonic NaCl decreases the jejunal net absorption of fluid, Na, and Cl (hepatointestinal reflex) and 2) hepatointestinal reflex is impaired in SHRSR and SHRSP.

The quantity of intestinal absorption of fluid and electrolytes are controlled by neural and humoral mechanisms and the intestine, as well as the kidney, plays an important role in controlling body fluid homeostasis by means of controlling the input of the body. It has been reported that SHR has a disorder in NaCl and water homeostasis, and high sympathetic (Thoren and Ricksten, 1979) and renin-angiotensin (Trippodo and Frohlich, 1981) activities, both of which are known to influence intestinal absorption process (Levens et al., 1981). Thus, the rate of fluid and NaCl absorption in SHR may be augmented. However, during no infusion period, the jejunal loops of WKY, SHRSR, and SHRSP absorbed fluid and NaCl at similar rates. This finding agrees with the previous report by Sjovall et al. (1986), who demonstrated that there was no significant difference in intestinal fluid transport rate between WKY and SHR, although the sympathetic nervous system had a tonic influence on fluid transport in SHR but not in WKY. These result suggests that when they intake normal NaCl food, SHR absorbs fluid and NaCl at similar rate to WKY, even though SHR has high sympathetic tone in the intestine.

A recent study from our laboratory has demonstrated that an increased NaCl concentration in the hepatic portal circulation reflexively depresses jejunal absorption of NaCl (Morita et al., 1990) This suggests that the quantity of NaCl absorbed in the jejunum is regulated by a postabsorptive mechanism. In WKY, jejunal NaCl absorption was depressed by the portal infusion of hypertonic NaCl. Conversely, the depression of jejunal NaCl absorption in response to the portal hypertonic NaCl infusion did not occurred in SHRSR and SHRSP. These results suggest that when they intake high NaCl food, WKY absorbs less NaCl than SHR by means of inhibition of hepatointestinal reflex. This mechanism may be partly involved in the high sodium sensitivity in SHR.

In conclusion: 1) the quantity of salt absorbed in the jejunum is regulated by a postabsorptive mechanism that is probably located in the liver (hepatointestinal reflex) 2) hepatointestinal reflex is impaired in SHRSR and SHRSP and 3) the lack of hepatointestinal reflex in SHRSR and SHRSP may contribute in part to salt sensitivity in these rats.

REFERENCES

Levens, N.R., Peach, M.J., and Carey, R.M. (1981): Interactions between angiotensin peptides and the sympathetic nervous system mediating intestinal sodium and water absorption in the rat. J. Clin. Invest. 67: 1197-1207.

Morita, H., Ohyama, H., Hagiike, M., Horiba, T., Miyake, K., Yamanouchi, H., Matsushita, K., and Hosomi, H. (1990): Effects of portal infusion of hypertonic solution on jejunal electrolyte transport in anesthetized dogs. Am. J. Physiol. 259: R1289-R1294.

Sjovall, H., Ely, D., Westlander, G., Kohlin, T., Jodal, M., and Lundgren, O. (1986): The adrenergic nervous control of fluid transport in the small intestine of normotensive and spontaneously hypertensive rats. Acta. Physiol. Scand. 126: 557-564.

Thoren, P. and Ricksten, S.E. (1979): Recordings of renal and splanchnic sympathetic nervous activity in normotensive and spontaneously hypertensive rats. Clin. Sci. 57: 197s-199s.

Trippodo, N.C. and Frohlich, E.D. (1981): Similarities of genetic (spontaneous) hypertension. Man and Rat. Circ. Res. 48: 309-319.

Sabra salt-sensitive (SBH) rats are deleted in one α_2-adrenoceptor subtype in renal cortex when compared with Sabra salt-resistant (SBN)

Jean-Pierre Dausse, Jean-François Cloix, Wen Qing and Drori Ben-Ishay

Groupe de Signalisation, UFR Biomédicale, 45, rue des Saints-Pères, 75270 Paris, France

INTRODUCTION

Adrenergic receptors are implicated in at least three renal functions involved in the control of blood pressure : glomerular filtration (Strandhoy, 1985), renin secretion (Insel and Snavely, 1981) and tubular sodium reabsorption (DiBona, 1982). Modifications of renal $alpha_2$-adrenergic receptors properties have been detected between hypertensive (SBH) and normotensive (SBN) Sabra rats (Parini et al., 1983). These last years, reports have shown pharmacological evidence that $alpha_2$-adrenoceptors were not a homogeneous population but might be subclassified into the subtypes $alpha_{2A}$, $alpha_{2B}$ and $alpha_{2C}$ (Bylund, 1985; Bylund, 1988). The pharmacological definition of these subtypes is based on the differential potencies of the ligand prazosin, oxymetazoline, ARC 239, and WB 4101. It is conceivable that an abnormality in distribution of these $alpha_2$-adrenoceptor subtypes might be involved in sodium-induced hypertension. In the present study we determined $alpha_2$-adrenoceptor subtypes present in renal cortex of salt-sensitive (SBH) and salt-resistant (SBN) Sabra rats, using (^{3}H)-yohimbine binding and the five $alpha_{2A}$- or $alpha_{2B}$- selective drugs rauwolscine, prazosin, oxymetazoline, ARC 239, and WB 4101.

METHODS

We used male Sabra rats (aged 8 to 10 weeks), bred at C.S.E.A.L. (Orléans, France). Preparation of reno-cortical membranes and the (^{3}H)-yohimbine binding assay were carried out as previously described (Parini et al., 1988). Briefly, the membranes were incubated with 5 nM (^{3}H)-yohimbine and 20 concentrations of the competing agents for 30 min. at 25°C. Non-specific binding was defined as binding in the presence of 25 uM phentolamine. For the experiments with oxymetazoline, 100 uM Gpp(NH)p was used in the incubation mixture. The resulting competition curves were analysed using a non-linear least-squares curve-fitting program (GraphPad Inplot, San Diego, CA) for calculating Ki and Hill slope values. The stastistical analysis used the F-ratio test to measure the goodness of fit of the competition curves for either one or two sites. All data are given as means+/-s.e.m..

RESULTS

In renal membranes of SBH rats all drugs inhibited (^{3}H)-yohimbine binding with steep, monophasic competition curves with Hill values near 1 (not shown) and the following order of potency: rauwolscine > ARC239> prazosin> WB4101> oxymetazoline (Table 1). Curves were best fitted for the interaction with a single class of alpha$_{2B}$-adrenoceptors (i.e. high affinity for ARC239 and prazosin, low affinity for oxymetazoline).

Table 1. Ki values for adrenergic drugs on alpha$_{2A}$- and alpha$_{2B}$-adrenoceptors in renal cortex of SBH and SBN rats.

	SBH	SBN	
	alpha$_{2B}$	alpha$_{2B}$	alpha$_{2A}$
Rauwolscine	5+/-1		7+/-0.4
ARC239	15+/-3	7+/-2 (70+/-5%)	851+/-70 (30+/-4%)
Prazosin	45+/-5	8+/-1 (64+/-15%)	1288+/-71 (36+/-14%)
WB4101	105+/-8	270+/-40 (74+/-4%)	3+/-1 (26+/-4%)
Oxymetazoline	270+/-40	741+/-40 (60+/-3%)	3+/-1 (40+/-3%)

Means+/-s.e.m., n=6, Ki values (nM) were determined from competition curves by the iterative curve-fitting program and numbers in parentheses show the relative amount (%) of alpha$_{2A}$- and alpha$_{2B}$-adrenoceptors.

In renal membranes of SBN rats, however, only the competition curve for rauwolscine was monophasic, while those for the other drugs were shallow with Hill coefficients near 0.5 (not shown) suggesting interaction with a heterogeneous population of alpha$_2$-adrenoceptors. Analysis of these competition curves using the iterative curve-fitting program revealed that in these renal membranes about 60-74% of alpha$_2$-adrenoceptors were of the alpha$_{2B}$-subtype, while 24-40% were of the alpha$_{2A}$-subtype (i.e. high affinity for oxymetazoline low affinity for prazosin and ARC239 (Table 1).

DISCUSSION

The alpha$_{2A}$- and alpha$_{2B}$-adrenergic selective drugs oxymetazoline, WB4101, ARC239 and prazosin have been used for the characterization of these receptor subtypes in renal cortex of salt-sensitive and salt-resistant Sabra rats. In SBH rat, these drugs inhibited binding of (^{3}H)-yohimbine with competition curves that were best fitted to interaction with a single class of binding sites. The order of potency for these drugs was ARC239> prazosin> WB4101> oxymetazoline. These results confirm previously reported data that kidney of normotensive Sprague-Dawley rats contain a homogeneous class of alpha$_{2B}$-adrenoceptors (Cheung et al., 1986). In SBN rats, however, these drugs inhibited (^{3}H)-yohimbine binding with competition curves that were significantly better fitted to interaction with two classes of binding sites indicating the coexistence of alpha$_{2A}$- and alpha$_{2B}$-

adrenoceptors. These results show a striking difference in distribution of $alpha_2$-adrenoceptor subtypes between SBH and SBN rats in renal cortex. The difference between SBH and SBN rats might represent a genetically mediated change responsible for the sensibility ot the resistance to the development of salt-induced hypertension. From the absence of $alpha_{2A}$-adrenoceptor subtype might result altered renal functions in SBH rats and by consequence responsible for high blood pressure after high sodium intake. Conversely, the presence of the $alpha_{2A}$-adrenoceptor subtype in SBN rats might account for the resistance to salt-induced hypertension.

REFERENCES

Bylund, D.B. (1985): Heterogeneity of $alpha_2$-adrenergic receptors. Pharmacol.Biochem.Behav. 22, 835-843.

Bylund, D.B. (1988): Subtypes of $alpha_2$-adrenoceptors: pharmacological and molecular biological evidence converge. Trends Pharmacol.Sci. 9, 356-361.

Cheung, Y.D., Barnett, D.B., and Nahorski, S.R. (1986): Heterogeneous properties of $alpha_2$-adrenoceptors in particulat and soluble preparations of human platelet and rat and rabbit kidney. Biochem. Pharmacol. 35, 3767-3775.

DiBona, G.F. (1982): The functions of renal nerves. Rev. Physiol. Biochem.Pharmacol. 94, 75-181.

Insel, P.A., and Snavely, M.D. (1981): Catecholamines and the kidney: receptors and renal functions. Ann.Rev.Physiol. 43, 625-636.

Parini, A., Diop, L., Dausse, J.P., Meyer, P., and Ben-Ishay, D. (1983): Alpha-adrenoceptors in Sabra hypertensive (SBH) and normotensive (SBN) rats: effect of sodium. J.Hypertension 1(Suppl. 2, 204-206.

Parini, A., Coupry, I., Laude, D., Diop, L., Vincent, M., Sassard, J. and Dausse, J.P. (1988): Noradrenaline content and adrenergic receptors in kidney and heart of the prehypertensive and hypertensive Lyon rat strain. Am.J.Hypertens. 1, 140-145.

Strandhoy, J.W. (1985): Role of $alpha_2$-receptors in the regulation of renal functions. J.Cardiovasc.Pharmacol. 7(Suppl.8), S28-S33.

Decreased alpha$_2$-adrenoceptor function in spontaneously hypertensive (SH) rats is secondary to an attenuated renal action of vasopressin

Ping Li, S. Brian Penner and Donald S. Smyth *

Departments of Internal Medicine and Pharmacology and Therapeutics, University of Manitoba, 770 Bannatyne Avenue, Winnipeg, Manitoba, R3E OW3, Canada

Summary: In the present study, the renal function of α_2-adrenoceptors and vasopressin was determined in SH rats by the infusion of an α_2-adrenoceptor agonist, clonidine, and the V2 vasopressin receptor antagonist, ([d(CH$_2$)$_5$,D-Ile^2,Ile^4]AVP), respectively. Although clonidine produced a dose related increase in urine flow rate, the response in SH rats was significantly attenuated as compared to the two normotensive strains of rat (SD, WKY). The V2 vasopressin receptor antagonist also produced a dose related increase in urine flow rate and sodium excretion in the three strains of rats, however, a decreased response in SH rats was observed. This decreased response in SH rats to clonidine and the V2 antagonist was associated with an attenuation of the increase in free water clearance. Together, the decreased response to both an α_2-adrenoceptor agonist and a V2 receptor antagonist in SH rats would be consistent with a decreased renal action of vasopressin and not necessarily a defect in the α_2-adrenoceptor.

INTRODUCTION

In recent years, the physiological effects of α_2-adrenoceptor stimulation in the kidney have been investigated (Stanton et al., 1987; Blandford and Smyth, 1988). These, and similar studies, documented a dose related increase in urine flow rate and solute excretion. This increase in urine flow rate seen at low doses was primarily due to an increase in free water clearance (Blandford and Smyth, 1988), most conceivably mediated through the inhibition of the renal effects of vasopressin (Blandford and Smyth, 1990; Gellai, 1990).

In rats genetically predisposed to the development of high blood pressure, the density of α_2-adrenoceptors in the kidney has been found to be elevated (Michel, et al., 1990). This has been documented in the Spontaneously Hypertensive rat (Sanchez and Pettinger, 1981), the Dahl Salt Sensitive rat (Pettinger et al., 1982), the Sabra Hypertensive rat (Diop et al., 1984) and the New Zealand Genetically Hypertensive rat (Smyth et al., In Press). The significance of this increase in renal α_2-adrenoceptor density in these different strains of rats has not been determined.

In the present study, we determined the effects of a direct intrarenal infusion of clonidine, an α_2-adrenoceptor agonist, on urine flow rate and solute excretion. Since these effects have been previously attributed to the antagonism of the renal effect of vasopressin, we also determined the effects of a V2 antagonist. The decreased response to clonidine as well as a V2 antagonist in the SH rats suggests that the altered response to the α_2-adrenoceptor agonist may be secondary to a decreased renal activity of vasopressin in these animals.

METHODS

The methods utilized have previously been

reported from our laboratory (Blandford and Smyth 1988; 1990). Sprague-Dawley (SD), Wistar Kyoto (WKY) and Spontaneously Hypertensive (SH) rats, which have been previously uninephrectomized (right kidney and adrenal gland, ether anesthesia) 7 to 10 days earlier, were anesthetized with Nembutal (50 mg/kg, I.P.) and placed on a thermostatically controlled table to maintain body temperature at 37°C. A tracheotomy was performed and the animal allowed to breathe spontaneously. The carotid artery was cannulated (PE60) for recording of blood pressure with a Statham pressure transducer (Model P23DC), recorded on a Grass Model V polygraph. The jugular vein was cannulated to allow administration of saline (97 ul/min), anesthetic or a V2 antagonist ([d(CH$_2$)$_5$,D-Ile^2,Ile^4]AVP, 30 nmol/kg, 0.2 ml bolus). The remaining kidney was exposed by a left flank incision and the left ureter cannulated (PE50) for collection of urine. A 31 gauge needle was inserted into the aorta advanced into the renal artery for the later infusion of clonidine (3 ug/kg/min, at 3.4 ul/min). Following a 45 minute stabilization period, 5 urine collections of 15 minutes each were obtained. Immediately following the first urine collection, the experimental intervention was undertaken. The subsequent urine collections were used to determine the effects of these interventions on urine flow rate and solute excretion. Urine flow rate is the sum of water excretion (free water clearance) and solute excretion (osmolar clearance) and these data are presented. The data represent the mean ± standard error of the mean of at least 6 animals per group. Data from the third collection period, which is representative of the changes observed, has been presented.

RESULTS

The experimental interventions used in this study failed to alter blood pressure and creatinine clearance except clonidine which produced an increase in blood pressure in the Sprague-Dawley (~10 mmHg) and WKY (~30 mmHg) rats.

Clonidine (3 ug/kg/min) produced a significant increase in urine flow rate in SD and WKY rats but not in SH rats (Fig. 1). The increase in urine flow rate in the SD and WKY rats was due to an increase in free water clearance. Osmolar clearance was only increased in the WKY rats as compared to the control group which may have been secondary to the increase in blood pressure observed in this group.

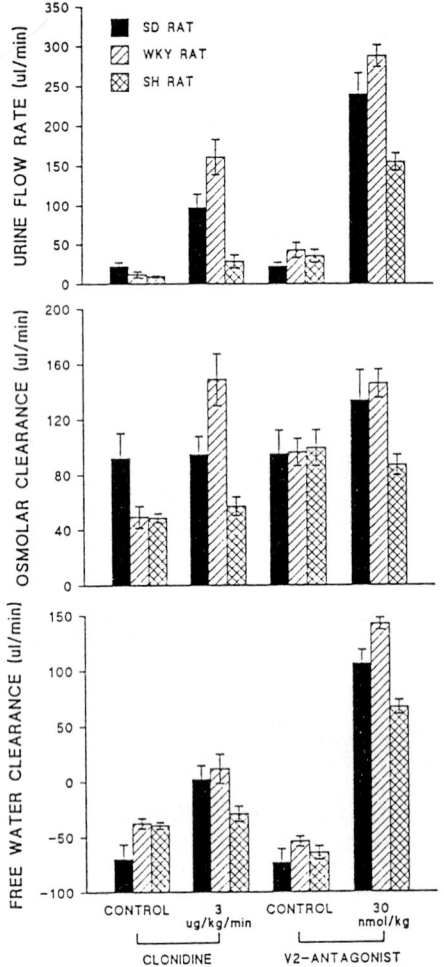

Fig. 1. The effects of saline vehicle (control), clonidine (3 ug/kg/min) and a V2 antagonist (30 nmol/kg) on urine flow rate and free water and osmolar clearance.

The V2 antagonist increased urine flow rate in all three strains of rats, however, the response in the SH rats was significantly less than that of the SD and WKY rats (Fig.1). Similarly, the increase in urine flow rate was associated with an increase in free water clearance, again with the response in the SH rats being less than that observed with the other two strains. This increase in free water clearance was the primary mechanism for the increase in urine flow rate. Osmolar clearance was also slightly increased in SD and WKY rats but not SH rats.

DISCUSSION

Previous studies have determined that the renal effects of α_2-adrenoceptor stimulation were mediated through the inhibition of the renal effects of vasopressin (Blandford and Smyth, 1988; Gellai, 1990). In fact, blockade of renal tubular vasopressin receptors with a specific V2 antagonist completely attenuated the effects of α_2-adrenoceptor stimulation (Blandford and Smyth, 1990). The function of increased α_2-adrenoceptors in kidneys of genetically hypertensive rats has not been determined. In the present study, the decreased response to an α_2-adrenoceptor agonist in SH rats, despite increased receptor density, may indicate a defect in this receptor. Alternatively, since the effects of this receptor are dependent on the renal effects of vasopressin, a change in the renal activity of vasopressin in these rats may explain the difference.

The response to a V2 antagonist was decreased in SH rats as compared to the two normotensive strains of rat. A plausible explanation is that the decreased response to an α_2-adrenoceptor agonist is not related to a defect in this receptor per se but rather an alteration in the activity of vasopressin in these rats. The reason for this decreased response is not clear. Other laboratories have demonstrated that vasopressin levels are unaltered or only slightly elevated in these 12 week SH rats. We have also failed to observe a change in vasopressin receptors in kidneys from SH rats as compared to SD and WKY rats (unpublished observation). Thus, the decreased response cannot be attributed to a change in agonist levels or receptor density. Similarly, the significance of a decreased response to vasopressin in the pathogenesis and/or maintenance of high blood pressure in SH rats remains to be determined.

Acknowledgements: This work was supported by a grant from the Medical Research Council of Canada. PL is a recipient of the Nordic Fellowship from the Canadian Hypertension Society and DDS is a recipient of a Scholarship from the Heart and Stroke Foundation of Canada.

REFERENCES

Blandford, D.E. and Smyth, D.D. (1988): Dose selective dissociation of water and solute excretion after renal α_2-adrenoceptor stimulation. J. Pharmacol. Exp. Ther. 247: 1181-1186.

Blandford, D.E. and Smyth, D.D. (1990): Role of vasopressin in response to intrarenal infusions of α_2-adrenoceptor agonists. J. Pharmacol. Exp. Ther. 255: 264-270.

Diop, L., Parini, A., Dausse, J.P. and Ben-Ishay, D. (1984): Cerebral and renal α-adrenoceptors in Sabra Hypertensive and normotensive rats. J. Cardiovasc. Pharmacol. 6: S742-S747.

Gellai, M. (1990): Modulation of vasopressin antidiuretic action by renal α_2-adrenoceptors. Am. J. Physiol. 259: F1-F8.

Michel, M., Brodde, O.E. and Insel, P.A. (1990): Peripheral adrenergic receptors in hypertension. Hypertension 16:107-120.

Pettinger, W.A., Sanchez, A., Saavedra, J. et al., (1982): Altered renal α_2-adrenergic receptor regulation in genetically hypertensive rats. Hypertension 4: II-188-II-192.

Sanchez, A. and Pettinger, W.A. (1981): Dietary regulation of blood pressure and renal α_1- and α_2-receptors in WKY and SHR. Life Sci. 29: 2795-2802.

Smyth, D.D., Stanko, C. and Phelan, E.L. (in press). Renal α_2-adrenoceptors in New Zealand Genetically Hypertensive rats. J. Autonom. Pharmacol.

Stanton, B., Puglisi, E. and Gellai, M. (1987): Localization of α_2-adrenoceptor mediated increase in Na^+, K^+ and water excretion. Am. J. Physiol. 248:F1016-F1021.

The hypertensinogenic activity of 18,21-anhydroaldosterone in adrenalectomized rats

S. Fragman, M. Harnik, E. Peleg, N. Zamir and T. Rosenthal *

* *The Chorley Hypertension Institute, Chaim Sheba Medical Center, Tel Hashomer (SF, EP and TR), Department of Physiology and Phamacology, Sackler Faculty of Medicine (NZ), and Department of Biotechnology, George S. Wise Faculty of Life Sciences (MH), Tel Aviv University, Tel Aviv, Israel*

18,21-anhydroaldosterone, a product of decomposition of aldosterone under acidic conditions, has not yet been found in urine, though no serious attempt has been made to locate it in biological fluids. Harnik and Kashman's (Harnick, Kashman et al., 1990) finding that this compound has a low relative binding affinity to the mineralocorticoid receptor in human mononuclear leukocytes, despite its resemblance to aldosterone, prompted us to investigate its hypertensinogenic properties in SHR.

The adrenalectomized rat model used for screening potentially hypertensinogenic steroids (Kenyon, DeConti, et al., 1981) was used to examine the hypertensinogenic activity of 18,21-anhydroaldosterone, synthesized by us (Harnik, Kashman, et al., 1989).

SUBJECTS AND METHODS

Six-week-old male SHR weighing 140-160 g underwent bilateral adrenalectomy. Constant 2-week Alzet miniosomotic pumps, model 2002 (Alza Corp., Palo Alto, CA) were implanted in the dorsal cervical subcutaneous tissue. Rats were randomly divided into six groups according to the steroid examined. Pumps were loaded with steroid compounds, dissolved in propylene glycol, with or without aldosterone, as follows:

Group I:	18,21-anhydroaldosterone	5 µg/day	n=13
Group II:	18,21-anhydroaldosterone	10 µg/day	n=12
Group III:	aldosterone	5 µg/day	n=13
Group IV:	aldosterone	10 µg/day	n=13
Group V:	18,21-anhydroaldosterone + aldosterone	5 µg each/day	n=19
Group VI:	vehicle (propylene glycol) only		n= 6

Animals were allowed free access to Purina rat chow and tap water during the week of acclimatization. Following adrenalectomy 0.9% NaCl was given ad libitum. Prior to surgery and every 3 days thereafter for 2 weeks rats were weighed and systolic blood pressure (SBP) was measured in conscious animals, by indirect tail cuff method using an electrosphygmomanometer and pneumatic pulse transducer (Narco Biosystems, Inc., Houston, TX). The mean of three measurements was recorded as the representative blood pressure for each rat. Data were compared by Student's t test.

RESULTS

Continuous infusion of 18,21-anhydroaldosterone alone (Group I) did not result in a rise in blood pressure, even when given in 10 µg/day dosage, and in fact lowered it: from 162.6±7.4 mmHg to 145.5±6.1 mmHg after adrenalectomy (Fig. 1). Aldosterone in 10 µg/day dose increased blood pressure by 30 mmHg, from 154.2±6 to 184.4±14.3 mmHg (p<0.001) (Group III). In 5 µg/day dose the blood pressure changed very slightly: from 152.3±7.7 to 149.8±7.6 mmHg (P=0.812) (Group IV) (Fig. 2). Aldosterone combined with 18,21-anhydroaldosterone, 5 µg of each, increased blood pressure by 25 mmHg: from 154.6±7.4 mmHg to 178.4±19.7 mmHg (P<0.001) (Fig. 1). Plasma renin concentration (PRC) decreased from 32.1±8.1 before operation to 6.9±4.8 ng/ml/h 2 weeks post surgery. Rats that did not receive any steroid compound (Group VI) showed a 28 mmHg decrease in blood pressure.

Thus, in adrenalectomized SHR rats, 18,21-anhydroaldosterone potentiated the hypertensinogenic effect of simultaneously administered aldosterone. When the compounds were administered alone, 18,21-anhydroaldosterone was much less effective than the same dose (10 µg/day) of aldosterone.

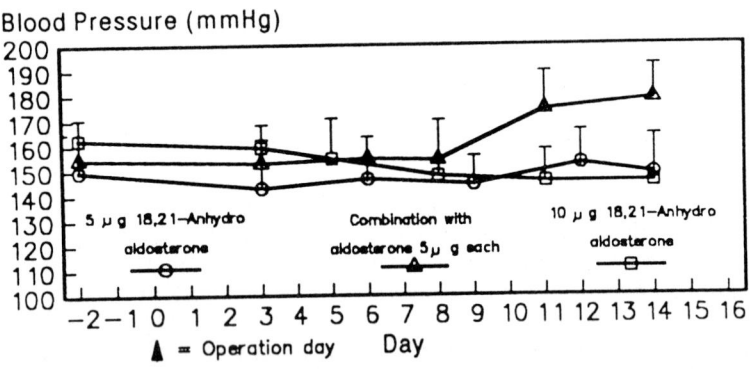

Fig. 1: Hypertensinogenic effect of 18,21-anhydroaldosterone combined with adlosterone, 5 µg each, compared to lack of effect of 18,21-anhydroaldosterone alone, in adrenalectomized SHR.

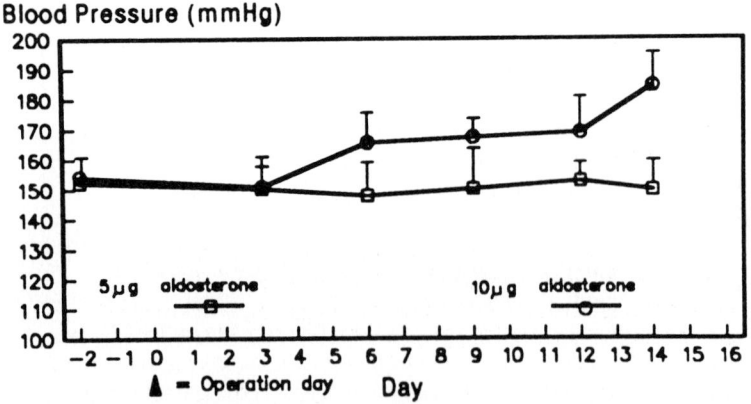

Fig. 2: Hypertensinogenic effect of adlosterone, 10 µg, in adrenalectomized SHR.

DISCUSSION

The present study shows that 18,21-anhydroaldosterone, inactive by itself in adrenalectomized SHR, has synergistic hypertensinogenic activity with a small amount (5 µg) of aldosterone which is inactive by itself at this dosage. Aldosterone activity was amplified by 16µ, 18-dihydroxy-DOC (Dale and Melby 1974), and by 5µ- dihydrocortisol (Adam et al., 1978). The same was observed with 19-OH-androstenedione (Sekihara, 1983), but this could not be confirmed by Gomez-Sanchez and Gomez-Sanchez (1986) and by Murase et al. (1991).

Amplification of aldosterone by 18-hydroxy-19-nor-corticosterone and by 18,19 dihydroxycorticosterone was found by us in two previous studies (Rosenthal, Shani, et al., 1988; Fragman, Harnik, et al., 1991): neither 18-hydroxy-19-nor-corticosterone (10 µg/day) nor 18,19 dihydroxycorticosterone increased blood pressure in SHR when given alone, but when administered together with aldosterone (5 µg/day inactive by itself) resulted in a significant increase in blood pressure.

Our present findings and those reported in the literature are also supported by the significant drop in plasma renin concentration (PRC). They reconfirm the thesis that small amounts of mineralocorticoids, which are inactive by themselves, may in the presence of aldosterone under physiological conditions be an important etiological factor in hypertension.

REFERENCES

Adam, W.R., Funder, J.W., Mercer, J. & Ulick, S. (1978): Amplification of the action of aldosterone by 5 alpha-dihydrocortisol. *Endocrinology* 103, 465-471.

Dale, S.L. & Melby, J.C. (1974): Altered adrenal steroidogenesis in "low-renin" essential hypertension. *Trans. Assoc. Am. Physicians* 87, 248-257.

Fragman, S., Harnik, M., Peleg, E., Zamir, N. & Rosenthal, T. (1991): The hypertensinogenic activity of 18,19-dihydroxycorticosterone in adrenalectomized rats. *Am. J. Hyper.* 4:118A.

Gomez-Sanchez, E.P. & Gomez-Sanchez, C.E. (1986): A reevaluation of the mineralocorticoid and hypertensinogenic potential of 19- hydroxyandrostenedione. *Endocrinology* 118, 2582-2587.

Harnik, M., Kashman, Y, Cojocaru, M., Lewicka, S. & Vescei, P. (1989): 18,21-Anhydroaldosterone and derivatives. *Steroids* 54, 11-19.

Harnik, M., Kashman, Y., Cojocaru, M., Bauer, H., Laux, M., Lewicka, S. & Vescei, P. (1990): Synthesis of 4,19-di substituted derivatives of DOC. Radioreceptor assay of some corticosteroid derivatives in human mononuclear leukocytes. *J. Steroid Biochem. & Molec. Biol.* 87, 261-267.

Kenyon, C.J., DeConti G.A., Cupolo N.A. & Morris D.J. (1981): The role of aldosterone in the development of hypertension in spontaneously hypertensive rats. *Endocrinology* 109, 1841-1845.

Murase, H., Yasuda, K., Mercado-Asis, L., Mori, A., Shimada, T., Mune, T., Morita, H., Noritake, N., Yamakita, N. & Miura, K. (1991): 19-Hydroxyandrostenedione does not modulate [3H] aldosterone binding to human mononuclear leukocytes and rat renal cytosol. *J. Steroid Biochem. Mol. Biol.* 38, 331-337.

Rosenthal, T., Shani, M., Peleg, E. & Harnik, M. (1988): The hypertensinogenic activity of 18-Hydroxy-19-Norcorticosterone in the adrenalectomized rat. *Amer J. Hyper.* 1, 49S-52S.

Sekihara, H. (1983): 19-Hydroxyandrosterone-dione. Evidence of a new class of sodium-retaining and hypertensinogenic steroid. *Endocrinology* 113, 1141-1148.

The acute antihypertensive action of cicletanine is mediated by muscarinic receptor stimulation

Oliver Chung, Peter Rohmeiss, Thomas Schips, Sabine Rohmeiss and Thomas Unger

Department of Pharmacology and German Institute for High Blood Pressure Research, University of Heidelberg, Im Neuenheimer Feld 366, W-6900 Heidelberg, Germany

Introduction:

Cicletanine (Cic) is a novel antihypertensive belonging to the furopyridine class of drugs. The mechanisms responsible for the blood pressure lowering effect of Cic have not yet been clarified. It has been speculated that the blood pressure lowering effect of Cic might be due to a direct interaction with vascular smooth muscle cells via a stimulation of endogenous prostaglandin synthesis (Dorian et al. 1984) and interaction with agents mobilizing intercellular calcium. Furthermore, interactions with alpha-1 receptors and histaminergic receptors have been described as well as diuretic effects at higher doses.
However, the profound bradycardic effects that accompany the depressor responses to bolus injections suggest a vagal contribution to the antihypertensive actions of Cic.
In the present study we investigated the influence of unspecific and specific muscarinergic receptor blockade on the cardiovascular responses to intravenous bolus injections of Cic in conscious, chronically instrumented spontaneously hypertensive rats (SHR).

Materials and methods:

Cicletanine hydrochloride was provided by IHB-IPSEN research laboratories (Le Plessis Robinson, France). Cic was dissolved in dimethyl sulfoxide at a concentration of 50 mg / 250 ul. Methylscopolamine and acetylcholine (ACh) were obtained from SIGMA (Munich, Germany) and dissolved in isotonic saline solution (0.9% NaCl). Pirenzepine, AF-DX 116 and hexocyclium were generous gifts from Prof. G. Lambrecht (Frankfurt, Germany) and were each dissolved in 0.9% NaCl.

All experiments were performed in conscious male SHR weighing between 250 and 350 g. The animals were kept under controlled conditions with respect to temperature, humidity and day-night cycle. Chronic catheters were implanted in the femoral vein and femoral artery 2 days before commencing of the acute experiments. During the experiments, mean arterial blood pressure (MAP) and heart rate (HR) were recorded. Details of these methods have been published previously (Unger at al. 1984).

Statistics:

Results are reported as means ±S.E.M. Student's two-tailed t-test for unpaired observations was used when appropriate to evaluate differences between groups. A significance level of $P < 0.05$ was accepted.

Blood pressure and heart rate responses to acute intravenous injections of Cic under unspecific muscarinergic receptor blockade with methylscopolamine:

The rats were divided into two groups of 7 animals. Group 1 served as control and received intravenous bolus injections of 0.9% NaCl instead of metylscopolamine. Group 2 received an intravenous bolus injection of methylscopolamine (20 ug), followed by 10 ug each 20 minutes to guarantee an adequate receptor blockade during the experiment (Veelken et al., 1989). Both groups received intravenous bolus injections of increasing doses of Cic (0.5/ 0.75/ 1.0/ 1.5 mg). Between injections at least 30 minutes were allowed for recovery of baseline values of MAP and HR.

Blood pressure and heart rate responses to acute intravenous injections of Cic and ACh under a M1, M2 and M3 specific muscarinergic receptor blockade:

The rats were divided into 8 groups of 7 animals. Groups 3 and 4 were pretreated with 1 mg iv of the M1-receptor antagonist pirenzepine (Doods et al., 1987); groups 5 and 6 were pretreated with 0.5 mg iv of the M2-receptor antagonist AF-DX 116 (Doods et al., 1987); groups 7 and 8 were pretreated with 1.43 mg iv the M3-receptor antagonist hexocyclium (Waelbroeck et al., 1989). Groups 9 and 10 were pretreated with all 3 antagonists (M1, M2, M3) at the above doses. Twenty minutes after this pretreatment injections groups 3, 5, 7 and 9 received Cic (1 mg iv) while groups 4, 6, 8 and 10 received equidepressor doses of ACh (0.8 g iv) instead. Pilot experiments had shown that the vehicles of ACh and Cic had no effects on MAP and HR.

Results:

Pretreatment with methylscopolamine completely prevented the effects of iv injections of Cic on MAP and HR (Fig. 1)

Selective pretreatment with the more specific muscarinergic antagonists yielded the results given in Table 1:

Table 1: Percent inhibition by muscarinergic antagonists of maximal decrease of MAP and HR in response to intravenous Cic and ACh

	Cicletanine		Acetylcholine	
	MAP	HR	MAP	HR
Pirenzepine (1 mg iv)	34%	19%	19%	70%
AF-DX 116 (0.5 mg iv)	27%	38%	12%	92%
Hexocyclium (1.43 mg iv)	34%	44%	89%	88%

Pretreatment of the animals with all 3 muscarinergic receptor antagonists almost completely prevented the Cic-induced decrease in MAP (85% inhibition / $P < 0.001$) and HR (90% / $P < 0.001$). The ACh-induced changes in MAP and HR were completly abolished by the combined blockade (Fig. 2)

Discussion:

The present study demonstrates, that Cic is a potent antihypertensive drug when applied as an iv bolus. The dose-dependent decreases in MAP after Cic were accompanied by dose-dependent HR reductions suggesting a direct vagal stimulation. The fact that pretreatment with methylscopolamine completely prevented the antihypertensive as well as the bradycardiac effects of acute injections of Cic gives rise to the hypothesis that the acute antihypertensive action of Cic is mediated through muscarinergic receptors.
Pretreatment of the animals with either pirenzepine AF-DX 116 or hexocyclium partially inhibited the antihypertensive and bradycardiac effects of Cic. In contrast to ACh, the acute cardiovascular effects of Cic appear to be mediated via M1, M2 and M3 receptors to a similar extent. Whether there is a direct interaction of Cic with muscarinergic receptors or a Cic-mediated enhanced release of endogenous ACh remains to be explored
Combined receptor blockade (M1-M3) completely blocked the cardiovascular effects of Cic and was

qualitativly comparable with that of methylscopolamine. These results suggest that three muscarinergic receptorsubtypes (M1-M3) are involved in the acute cardiovascular effects of Cic.

Fig. 1:   Fig. 2:

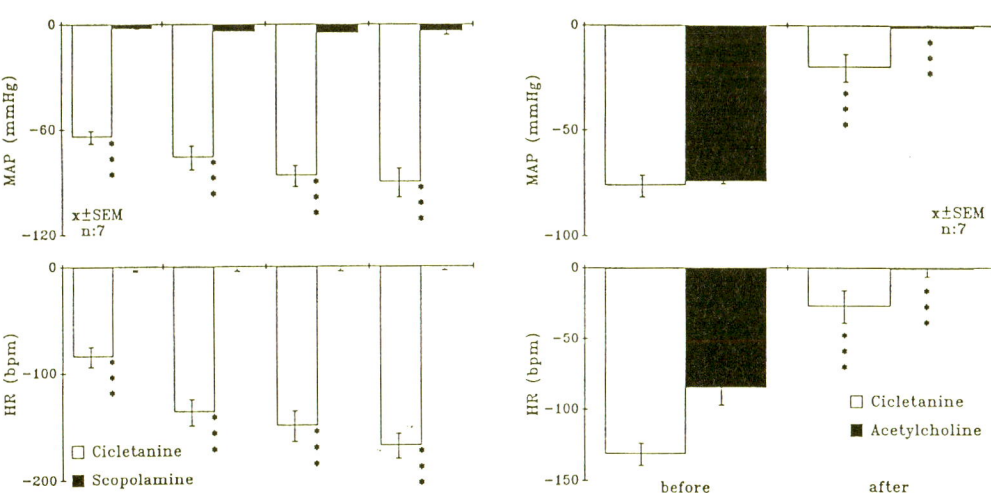

Fig 1. Influence of a muscarinergic receptor blockade with methylscopolamine on the maximal response of MAP and HR to Cic (0.5/ 0.75/ 1.0/ 1.5 mg iv: black bars). Control group: white bars.

Fig2. Influence of a combined muscarinergic (M1, M2, M3) receptor blockade on the maximal response of MAP and HR to Cic (1 mg iv) and ACh (0.8 ug iv). Before: control response before pretreatment. After: response after pretreatment with combined muscarinergic blockade.

References:

Doods H. N., Mathy M.-J., Davidesko D., Van Charldorp K. J., de Jong A., van Zwieten P. a. (1987): Selectivity of muscarinic antagonists in radioligand and in vivo experiments for the putative M1- M2- and M3- receptors. J. Pharmacol. Exp. Ther. 242: 257-262.

Dorian B., Larrue J., DeFeudis F.V., Salari H., Borgeat P. (1984): Activation of prostacyclin synthesis in cultured aortic smooth muscle cells by "diuretic-antihypertensive" drugs. Biochem. Pharmacol. 33, 2265-2269.

Unger Th., Becker H., Dietz R., Ganten D., Lang R. E., Rettig R., Schömig A., Schwab N. A. (1984): Antihypertensive effect of the GABA receptor antagonist muscimol in spontaneously hypertensive rats: role of the sympathoadrenal axis. Circ. Res. 54, 30-37.

Veelken R., Danckwart L., Rohmeiss P., Unger Th. (1989): Effects of intravenous AVP on cardiac output, mesenteric hemodynamics and splanchnic nerve activity. Am. J. Physiol. 255: H, 11206-1210.

Waelbroeck M., Tastenoy M., Camus J., Christophe J., Strohman C., Linoh H., Zilch H., Tacke R., Mutschler E., Lambrecht G. (1989): Binding and functional properties of antimuscarinics of the hexocyclium/sila-hexocyclium and hexahydro-diphenidol/hexahydro-sila-diphenidol type to muscarinic receptor subtypes. Br. J. Pharmacol. 98: 197-205.

Calcium

Calcium

Decreased expression of inhibitory guanine nucleotide regulatory proteins and adenylate cyclase activity in rat platelets in spontaneously hypertensive rats

Madhu B. Anand-Srivastava and Christelle Thibault

Department of Physiology, Faculty of Medicine, University of Montreal, CP 6128, succursale A, Montreal, Quebec, H3C 3J7, Canada

INTRODUCTION

The elevation of blood pressure in essential hypertension is due to a general increase in the resistance of peripheral vessels (Ferrario and Page, 1978). A part of this heightened peripheral resistance has been attributed to structural changes in the vessels, abnormalities in calcium movement and aberration in cyclic nucleotide metabolism (see review by Postnov and Orlov, 1983). It has been suggested that the adenylate cyclase/cAMP system is one of the biochemical system implicated in the regulation of arterial tone and reactivity (Triner *et al*, 1972). Several anomalies in adenylate cyclase activities and cAMP levels, in cardiovascular tissues of Spontaneously Hypertensive Rats (SHR), have been implicated in the pathogenesis of hypertension (Triner *et al*, 1972; Anand-Srivastava, 1988).

The adenylate cyclase system is composed of three components: extracellular receptor, catalytic subunit and guanine nucleotide regulatory proteins (G proteins). The hormonal stimulation and inhibition of adenylate cyclase are mediated via two different G proteins, Gs and Gi respectively (Gilman, 1984). We have previously reported an enhanced expression of Gi in heart and aorta from SHR as compared to their normotensive Wistar Kyoto control (WKY) (Anand-Srivastava *et al*, 1991a). This alteration in Gi levels was associated with an increased inhibition of adenylate cyclase by inhibitory hormones and a decreased stimulation by stimulatory hormones (Anand-Srivastava, 1990). We have extended our studies in rat platelets, a model easily accessible, with an eventual purpose of utilizing this model system in human essential hypertension. We have determined the levels of G proteins by bacterial toxin catalyzed ADP-ribosylation and immunoblotting techniques using specific antibodies against G proteins. In addition, we have also examined the adenylate cyclase activity and its responsiveness to stimulatory and inhibitory hormones.

METHODS

Rat platelet membranes from SHR and age matched WKY rats (12 weeks) were prepared as described previously (Anand-Srivastava *et al*, 1991b). The determination of adenylate cyclase activity and the ADP-ribosylation studies using pertussis toxin (PT) or cholera toxin (CT) were performed as previously described by Anand Srivastava *et al* (1991a). The immunoblotting experiments using specific antibodies against Gi (AS/7) and Gs (RM/1) (Dupont, Canada) were performed as described by Anand-Srivastava *et al* (1991a).

RESULTS AND DISCUSSION

We have recently reported an enhanced expression of Gi and an increased inhibition of adenylate cyclase by inhibitory hormones in heart and aorta from SHR as compared to WKY rats (Anand-Srivastava, 1990). In order to investigate if a similar alteration is also observed in platelets, we have determined the levels of Giα in platelets from SHR and WKY by PT-catalyzed ADP-ribosylation and immunoblotting techniques using a specific antibody (AS/7) against Gi. PT, in the presence of $[\alpha^{32}P]$-NAD, catalyzed the ADP-ribosylation of only one protein band of approximately 40,000 Da in both WKY and SHR platelets (fig.1A), however, the labeling of this band was significantly lower in SHR platelets as compared to WKY. Similarly, AS/7 antibody recognized a single protein of 40-41,000 Da and the relative amount of the immunodetectable Giα was significantly decreased in SHR as compared to WKY (fig.1B). An alteration in Gi protein levels correlated with an altered function has also been reported in other pathophysiological conditions (Bristow et al, 1990).

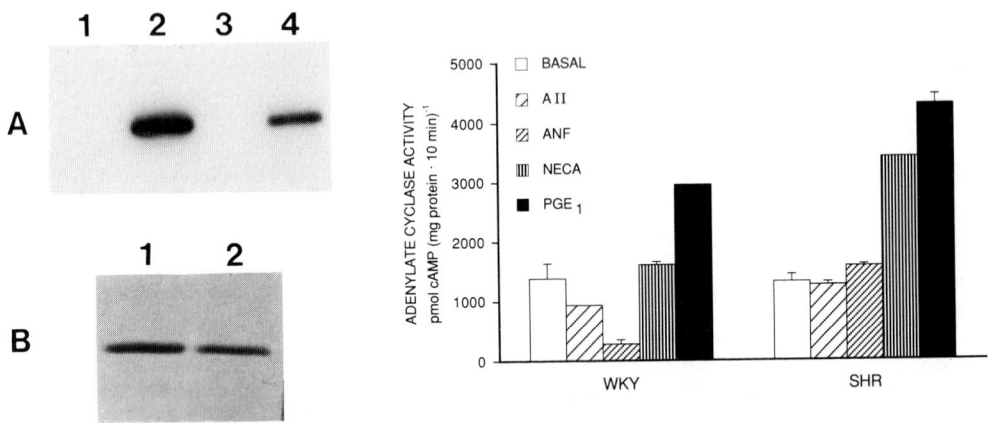

Fig. 1: A, PT-catalyzed ADP-ribosylation in rat platelets from WKY (lanes 1 and 2) and SHR (lanes 3 and 4) in the absence (lanes 1 and 3) or in the presence of PT (lanes 2 and 4).
B, quantitative immunodetection of Giα subunits in rat platelets from WKY (1) and SHR (2) by specific antibody AS/7.

Fig. 2 Effect of hormones on adenylate cyclase activity in rat platelets from WKY and SHR. Values are the means ± S.E.M. of three separate experiments.

Since the dual regulation of adenylate cyclase implicates both, Gi and Gs proteins, we also examined the levels of Gsα by CT-catalyzed ADP-ribosylation and immunoblotting techniques using a specific antibody agaisnt Gs (RM/1). By these techniques, no alteration in Gsα levels was observed in SHR platelets (data not shown). An altered or unaltered Gs protein levels associated with or without altered functions have been demonstrated in congestive heart failure by several investigators (Bristow et al, 1990).

Since G proteins mediate the hormonal stimulation and inhibition of adenylate cyclase, it was of interest to examine if the altered/unaltered expression of Gi/Gs could be reflected in the hormonal regulation of adenylate cyclase. To investigate this, we studied the effects of some hormones which inhibit or stimulate the adenylate cyclase activity through Gi and Gs respectively in platelets. As shown in fig.2, the inhibitory effect of atrial natriuretic factor

(ANF) and angiotensin II (AII) on adenylate cyclase was completely abolished in SHR platelets. This attenuation of ANF and AII-mediated inhibition of adenylate cyclase in SHR may be due to a decrease in the hormone receptors in SHR, or an impairment of the post-receptor events. From the present results, it is clear that the decreased expression of Gi may partly be responsible for such an attenuated response of AII and ANF on adenylate cyclase. On the other hand, the stimulations of adenylate cyclase, exerted by N-ethylcarboxamide adenosine (NECA) and prostaglandin (PGE1) were augmented in SHR. The potentiation of the stimulatory effect of PGE1 on adenylate cyclase in platelets has also been reported previously (Hamet et al, 1980). The increased sensitivity of adenylate cyclase to stimulatory hormones may not be due to an increased level of Gs, because the Gs levels, as shown by CT-catalyzed ADP-ribosylation and immunological studies were not different in SHR as compared to WKY. It may be possible that the hormone receptors for NECA and PGE1 are upregulated in SHR platelets and thereby result in the hyperresponsiveness to adenylate cyclase stimulation. The other possibility may be that the decreased levels of Gi in SHR, shown in the present studies may be responsible for the increased sensitivity of adenylate cyclase to stimulatory hormones in SHR. The increased responsiveness of adenylate cyclase to stimulatory hormones has also been reported in splenocytes from SHR, however the mechanism responsible for an enhanced sensitivity was not elucidated (Zeng et al, 1991).

In conclusion, we have shown that the rat platelets from SHR have decreased levels of Gi associated with attenuated responses of inhibitory hormones to adenylate cyclase inhibition and hypersensitivity of stimulatory hormones to adenylate cyclase stimulation. It may thus be suggested that the decreased expression of Gi may partly be responsible for the altered function of platelets in hypertension.

REFERENCES

Anand-Srivastava, M.B. (1988): Altered responsiveness of adenylate cyclase to adenosine and other agents in the myocardial sarcolemma and aorta of spontaneously hypertensive rats. Biochem.Pharmacol. 37,3017-3022

Anand-Srivastava, M.B. (1990): Enhanced expression of inhibitory guanine nucleotide regulatory protein in spontaneously hypertensive rats: relationship with adenylate cyclase. Eur. J. Pharmacol. 183,2069

Anand-Srivastava, M.B. et al (1991a): Altered expression of inhibitory guanine nucleotide regulatory proteins (Giα) in spontaneously hypertensive rats. Am. J. Hypertension (In press)

Anand-Srivastava, M.B. et al (1991b): The presence of atrial natriuretic factor receptors of ANF-R2 subtype in rat platelets. Biochem.J. 278, 211-217

Bristow, M.R. et al (1990): β-adrenergic pathways in nonfailing and failing human ventricular myocardium. Circulation 82(suppl I),I-12-I-25

Ferrario, C.M. and Page, I.H. (1978): Current views concerning cardiac output in the genesis of experimental hypertension. Circulation Res. 43,821-831

Gilman, A.G.(1984): G protein and dual control of adenylate cyclase. Cell 36,577-579

Hamet, P. et al (1980): Cyclic nucleotides in hypertension. Adv.Cyclic Nucleotide Res. 12,11-23

Postnov, Y.V and Orlov, S.N. (1983): Alteration of cell membranes in primary hypertension in "Hypertension" 2nd edition, editors Genest, J., Kuchel, O., Hamet, P. and Cantin, M. pp. 95-108

Triner, L. et al (1972): Adenylate cyclase-phosphodiesterase system in arterial smooth muscle. Life Sci. 11,817-824

Zeng, Y.Y. et al (1991): Increased responsiveness of the adenylate cyclase (AC) signalling system in splenocytic membranes from spontaneously hypertensive rats (SHR).Faseb J.5,A1597

Ca-induced and IP3-induced Ca-release in vascular smooth muscle of SHRSP and WKY observed by Ca-indicator Fura 2

Satoru Sunano, Kenzo Moriyama and Keiichi Shimamura

Research Institute of Hypertension, Kinki University, Osaka-Sayama, and Factory of Pharmacy, Kinki University, Higashi-Osaka, Japan

A Number of experiments have been performed to investigate the changes in Ca-influx, which have found that both the voltage-dependent and receptor operated Ca channels are increased in the vascular smooth muscle of hypertensive rats (Cauvin et al., 1989). On the other hand, little has been known of the changes in the release of Ca from sarcoplasmic reticulum. In addition, some discrepant results have been presented. It has been reported that the contractile proteins and the regulatory proteins are unaltered in the vascular smooth muscle of hypertensive rats (Mrwa et al., 1986). The present experiment was performed to investigate the changes in the release of Ca from sarcoplasmic reticulum. It has been proposed that the Ca is released from two Ca-release sites, Ca- and IP3-induced sites, and the former being initiated by caffeine and the latter by agonists. In the present study, the contraction and increase in intracellular Ca concentration induced by caffeine or noradrenaline were observed. Those in the vascular smooth muscles of stroke-prone spontaneously hypertensive rats (SHRSP) and of control normotensive Wistar Kyoto rats (WKY) were compared using mesenteric arteries from these rats.

METHODS

Mesenteric arteries were excised and spirally cut preparations were made from second branches of the mesenteric arteries. The preparations were incubated in a modified Tyrode's solution and changes in tension (contractions) were measured isometrically. Prior to the initiation of caffeine- or noradrenaline-induced contraction, the preparations were loaded with Ca immersing the preparations in high-K-Tyrode's solution for 5 minutes and then immersed in Ca free Tyrode's solution to remove extracellular Ca for 10 minutes. Changes in the intracellular free Ca concentration were observed by means of Fura 2 method.

RESULTS AND DISCUSSION

1. Blood pressure of rats
The blood pressure of SHRSP and WKY at 16 weeks was 244 ± 3.3 mmHg (n = 20) and 134 ± 1.0 mmHg (n = 20), respectively. The blood pressure of SHRSP was thus significantly higher than that of WKY ($p < 0.001$).

2. Caffeine-induced contraction in the absence of extracellular Ca.
Caffeine induces contraction in smooth muscle of the mesenteric artery both by

increasing Ca influx and releasing Ca from sarcoplasmic reticulum (Moriyama et al., 1989). In the present experiment, the contraction was initiated in the absence of extracellular Ca, applying caffeine 10 minutes after the removal of extracellular Ca. Caffeine of the concentration higher than 0.1 mM induced a transient phasic contraction. The contraction was initiated noncumulatively with the refilling of sarcoplasmic reticulum Ca before each initiation as described in the Methods. The maximum contraction was observed with caffeine of 30 mM. Since we have observed that the high-K-induced contraction of mesenteric artery was completely abolished within 8 minutes, the possibility of the contraction due to the influx of extracellular Ca can be excluded. Caffeine-induced contraction of the smooth muscle of the mesenteric artery in the absence of extracellular Ca was significantly greater in the preparation from SHRSP. Caffeine has been known to release Ca from the Ca-induced Ca-release site of the sarcoplasmic reticulum (Iino et al., 1988). Therefore, it can be considered that the release of Ca from this site is increased in the smooth muscle of the mesenteric artery of SHRSP when compared with that of WKY.

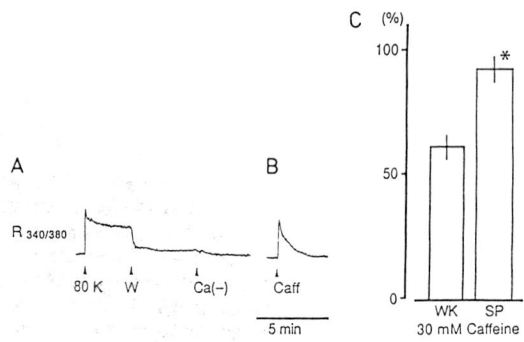

Fig. 1. Caffeine-induced increase in intracellular free Ca concentration as observed by Fura 2 method. B was taken 10min after Ca removal (Ca (-)) in A. Since the experiment was performed in the absence of extracellular Ca, the increase in Ca signal is thought to be due to the Ca release from sarcoplasmic reticulum. The increase by caffeine was expressed as percentages of the increase by 80 mM K (C). Note the difference in the size of Ca signal between WKY and SHRSP preparations.

The increase in the Ca release was proved by the experiment with intracellular free Ca indicator, Fura 2. The caffeine-induced increase of Fura 2 - Ca signal observed in the absence of extracellular Ca was greater in the preparation from SHRSP. The reduction time-course of the caffeine-induced contraction after the removal of extracellular Ca indicated that the greater amount of stored Ca in the sarcoplasmic reticulum is the cause of the increased release of Ca (Moriyama, 1989).

2. Noradrenaline-induced contraction in the absence of extracellular Ca.
Noradrenaline induced a transient phasic contraction in the absence of extracellular Ca. Each contraction was initiated after refilling the sarcoplasmic reticulum with Ca as described in the Methods. The contraction induced by noradrenaline was significantly greater in the preparation from SHRSP when compared with that of WKY. As the contraction was initiated after the high K-induced contraction was abolished in Ca-free Tyrode's solution, the involvement of Ca-influx through receptor-operated and/or voltage-dependent Ca

channels can be excluded. It has been established that noradrenaline stimulates the production of IP3 and IP3 releases Ca from the IP3-sensitive site of sarcoplasmic reticulum. The result then suggests that the release of Ca from this site is also greater in the smooth muscle of the mesenteric artery of SHRSP than that of WKY, although the changes in the sensitivity of contractile proteins to Ca under the same level of free Ca can still not be excluded.

The results of the experiment with Ca-indicator (Fura 2) proved the increased Ca-release in the smooth muscle of mesenteric artery of SHRSP, thus showing that the Fura 2 - Ca signal induced by noradrenaline was significantly greater in the preparation from SHRSP when compared with that of WKY (Fig. 1).

The mechanisms of the increase in Ca release is still unknown. The increased Ca content in the sarcoplasmic reticulum is the most likely explanation as in the case of the increased caffeine-induced contraction (Moriyama et al., 1989). However, the possibility of the changes in receptors, in the IP3 formation or in the sensitivity of sarcoplasmic reticulum to IP3 can still not be disregarded.

Conclusion

It was demonstrated in the present experiment that both the caffeine- and noradrenaline-induced contractions of the smooth muscle of the mesenteric artery in the absence of extracellular Ca were greater in the preparation from SHRSP when compared with those of WKY. The experiment with intracellular free Ca indicator revealed that the increased contractions are due to the increased release of Ca from sarcoplasmic reticulum. The increased Ca content in sarcoplasmic reticulum is thought to be the most probable cause of the increase in Ca release. Finally, these changes may contribute to the increase in the tone of resistant blood vessels and thus to the elevation of blood pressure.

References

Cauvin, C., Johns, A., Yamamoto, M., Hwang, O., Gelband, C., & Van Breemen, C. (1989): Ca^{2+} movements in vascular smooth muscle and their alteration in hypertension. In: Kwan, C. Y. (ed) *Membrane abnormalities in hyper-tension Vol. I Boca Raton,* pp. 145-179. Florida: CRC Press.

Iino, M., Kobayashi, T., & Endo, M. (1988): Use of ryanodine for functional removal of the calcium store in smooth muscle cells of the guinea-pig. *Biochem. Biophys. Res. Commun.* 152: 417-422.

Moriyama, K., Osugi, S., Shimamura, K., & Sunano, S. (1989): Caffeine-induced contraction in arteries from stroke-prone spontaneously hypertensive rats. *Blood Vessels* 26: 280-289.

Mrwa, U., Guth, K., Haist, C., Troschka, M., Herrmann, R., Wojciechowski, R., & Gagelmann, M. (1986): Calcium-requirement for activation of skinned vas-cular smooth muscle from spontaneously hypertensive (SHRSP) and normo-tensive control rats. *Life Sci.* 38: 191-196.

Altered calcium-dependent calcium release from intracellular sites of perfused heart in spontaneously hypertensive rats

Hitoshi Ebata, Yukihiro Houjoh, Uichi Ikeda, Yoshio Tsuruya, Takashi Natsume and Kazuyuki Shimada

Department of Cardiology, Jichi Medical School, Minamikawachi-machi, 3 29-04 Tochigi, Japan

This work was supported in part by grants-in-aid from the Ministeries of Education and Culture, and Health and Welfare of Japan

Abstract

The effluents from the perfused heart were collected. After labeling of the heart with $^{45}Ca^{2+}$ (100μM), the uptake of $^{45}Ca^{2+}$ was found to be saturated and washing with calcium (Ca)-free perfusion showed two exponential curves for dissociation of Ca^{2+}, indicating a fast (α) and a slow (β) phase. The half-life of β phase for both 4-, and 8-week-old SHR was significantly shorter than that for WKY. Further, a significant reduction in the amount of Ca-dependent $^{45}Ca^{2+}$ release in β phase was observed in both 4-, and 8-week-old SHR in comparison with age-matched WKY. Lanthanum, caffeine, ionomycin and treatment of the heart with EGTA did not alter this Ca-dependent $^{45}Ca^{2+}$ release, suggesting that the $^{45}Ca^{2+}$ is released from intracellular pool of Ca^{2+}, and not from extracellular site or sarcoplasmic reticulum (SR). These findings provided the evidence for Ca-handling defect in SHR under physiological conditions.

Introduction

Reduced Ca binding to isolated vesicles from many tissues from SHR has been reported in comparison with those from WKY (1-2), and this decrease seems to cause the excess increase of cytosolic free Ca^{2+} in SHR. However, it is uncertain whether the obtained results represent true *in situ* binding, because the preparation method can produce artifacts, e.g. reversed vesicles and/or alteration of the physicochemical characteristics of the biomembrane, leading to differences from the situation *in vivo*. To clarify further details of Ca-handling in SHR by preserving the physiological environment of the cell membrane, therefore, we used whole hearts for comparison of Ca flux between SHR and WKY.

Experimental Procedures

Using the Langendorff technique, the aorta was cannulated and perfused with modified Krebs-Henseleit solution (KHS), containing 118 mM NaCl, 25 mM $NaHCO_3$, 4.7 mM KCl, 1.2 mM KH_2PO_4, 1.2 mM $MgSO_4$, 11 mM glucose, 50 mM 3-(N-morpholino) propane sulfonic acid (MOPS pH 7.4). The solution was bubbled with 95% O_2 and 5% CO_2 and warmed to 37 °C.
KHS with 100 μM $CaCl_2$ containing $^{45}Ca^{2+}$ (2x10,000 cpm/ml) was perfused at a constant flow rate (0.8ml/min) with a syringe pump at 37°C, and the heart was labeled with $^{45}Ca^{2+}$ for 21 min. The labeled heart was then perfused with Ca-free KHS to wash out the bound $^{45}Ca^{2+}$. The effluent was collected every 3 min and the radioactivity was measured. The amount of labeled $^{45}Ca^{2+}$ released in each fraction was then calculated. To monitor myocardial destruction, CPK activity was assayed in

the eluent. Elution curves were analyzed as described by Greenblatt (3) with the aid of a microcomputer. The statistical significance of differences between two age-matched groups was analyzed by unpaired Student's t test.

Results

A: Comparison of $^{45}Ca^{2+}$ elution curves between SHR and WKY

Figure 1 shows representative $^{45}Ca^{2+}$ elution curves from 4-week-old SHR (Fig. 1A) and WKY (Fig. 1B). Both curves exhibited a summation of two exponential lines (α and β phases). In this case, the half-life of the β phase was decreased in 4-week SHR as compared with age-matched WKY. In slow phase, perfusion with 2 mM Ca^{2+} caused a transient release of $^{45}Ca^{2+}$ from the heart. This release was induced in Ca-dependent manner (Kd 0.5 for Ca^{2+} = 0.5 mM data not shown). Table 1 shows the half-lives of the α and β phases, and Ca-dependent $^{45}Ca^{2+}$ release from 4- and 8-week-old SHR and WKY. Both the half life of the β phase and the amount of $^{45}Ca^{2+}$ released from SHR were significantly (p<0.01) lower in SHR than in WKY at both 4, and 8 weeks of age. To examine whether Ca perfusion on β phase causes Ca-paradox(4), we measured CPK activity in all fractions. But perfusion of 2 mM Ca^{2+} after Ca-free KHS caused no significant CPK release, indicating no myocardial injury throughout the experimental period and suggesting that the membrane of the heart is preserved intact. It was also clarified that the $^{45}Ca^{2+}$ release induced by Ca^{2+} was not due to the Ca-paradox, which results from membrane damage and leads to leakage of $^{45}Ca^{2+}$ from the intracellular Ca pool.

B: Effect of lanthanum (La^{3+}), caffeine, ionomycin and EGTA

1) Effect of La^{3+}: In β phase, La^{3+} caused a transient release of $^{45}Ca^{2+}$, presumably due to release of $^{45}Ca^{2+}$ bound to the extracellular membrane of the heart. After perfusion with La^{3+}, 2 mM Ca^{2+} perfusion also caused transient $^{45}Ca^{2+}$ release, and the amount of $^{45}Ca^{2+}$ released was unchanged.
2) Effect of caffeine:
    10 mM caffeine increased $^{45}Ca^{2+}$ transiently, but did not alter the $^{45}Ca^{2+}$ release induced by 2 mM Ca^{2+}. This might have been caused by the release of Ca^{2+} from the SR (Ca-induced Ca release).
3) Effect of Ca ionophore, ionomycin:
    Infusion of ionomycin (1 µM) during the β phase caused a transient release of $^{45}Ca^{2+}$, perhaps due to $^{45}Ca^{2+}$ leakage from the intracellular Ca pool, but ionomycin did not affect the $^{45}Ca^{2+}$ release induced by 2 mM Ca^{2+} perfusion. CPK activity measurement revealed that perfusion with La^{3+}, caffeine and ionomycin did not cause severe myocardial damage by this method.
4) Effect of EGTA:
    To remove the extracellular Ca^{2+} and to study this experimental system using accurate Ca^{2+} con-

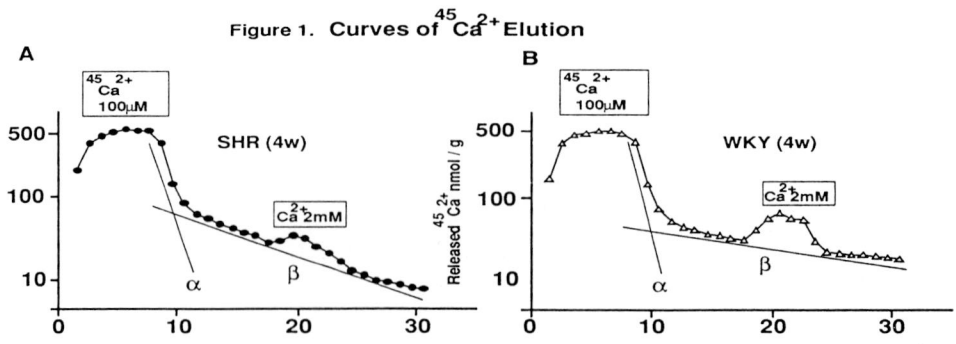

Figure 1. Curves of $^{45}Ca^{2+}$ Elution

centrations, EGTA buffer was used. Perfusion with 2 mM Ca^{2+} caused a transient release of $^{45}Ca^{2+}$ (unaccompanied by an increase of CPK release.). After 2 mM Ca^{2+} perfusion, CPK activity was slightly increased, along with a slight increase of $^{45}Ca^{2+}$ release (perhaps due to $^{45}Ca^{2+}$ leakage resulting from membrane injury).

The above results indicate that $^{45}Ca^{2+}$ is not displaced from extracellular sites, but from the intracellular pool of Ca^{2+}. Furthermore, this $^{45}Ca^{2+}$ release is independent of the caffeine-sensitive releasing pool (presumably the SR), and distinct from it.

		BP	HW	HW/BWx100	T(α)	T(β)	Released $^{45}Ca^{2+}$
4wk	SHR	119±8	340±32	575±34*	2.3±0.1	21±4.2*	29±4.6*
	WKY	117±12	377±22	500±20	2.2±0.1	38±2.9	43±6.2
8wk	SHR	177±7*	1023±130*	494±36*	2.8±0.2	25±3.3*	26±5.4*
	WKY	138±6	727±119	430±34	2.6±0.1	41±2.9	51±3.6
	(n=12)	(mmHg)	(mg)	(g/body wt)	half life(min)		(nmol/g)

Table 1. (mean±SD, *p<0.01 vs WKY   HW&BW: heart & body weight)

Discussion

The elution curves from both SHR and WKY exhibited a summation of two exponential lines (fast (α) phase and slow (β) phase), indicating the presence of two kinds of binding site in the heart. The half-life of the β phase in SHR was significantly shorter than that of WKY, reflecting more rapid dissociation of membrane-bound Ca from the SHR heart as a result of loose binding. In both 4- and 8-week-old SHR, the amount of Ca-depedent $^{45}Ca^{2+}$ release (induced by 2 mM Ca^{2+}) was only about half of that for the age-matched WKY. These significances (half-life of β and $^{45}Ca^{2+}$ release) might reflect a primary alteration of Ca-handling in this rat strain. Perfusion with La^{3+}, caffeine, ionomycin and EGTA did not affect the $^{45}Ca^{2+}$ release, suggesting that $^{45}Ca^{2+}$ binds specifically to intracellular rather than extracellular sites, and that the $^{45}Ca^{2+}$ release from the heart is not caused by leaky membranes. Furthermore, these intracellular sites seemed to be Ca-binding pools other than the SR. Kowarski et al reported a lower content of Ca-binding protein in tissues from SHR including heart membranes (5). Therefore, it is likely that $^{45}Ca^{2+}$ binded specifically to a Ca-binding protein such as calmodulin and that in SHR the content of this Ca-binding protein might be significantly reduced.

Although we used an indirect approach (efflux study) to estimate $^{45}Ca^{2+}$ flux in whole hearts from SHR and WKY, these results first provided the evidence for a Ca-handling defect in SHR under physiological conditions and appeared to confirm the results obtained from binding studies on isolated cardiac sarcolemma (1).

Acknowledgements

We are grateful for the excellent secretarial assistance of Ms Sachiko Tanaka, Ms Etsuko Chiku and Ms Mitsuko Sugimoto.

References

1. Pernollet MG, Devynck MA, Meyer P: Clin Sci, 1981; 61:45s
2. Devynik MA, Pernollet MG, Nunez AM, Meyer P: Clin Exp Hypertension, 1981;3(4):797
3. Greenblatt JD, Weser JK: N Eng J Med,1975;293:702
4. Zimmerman ANE, Hulsmann WC: Nature, 1966; 211:646
5. Kowarski S, Cowen L, Schachter D: Proc Natl Acad Sci USA, 1986;83:1097.

Cytoplasmic free calcium concentration in isolated vascular smooth muscle cells from spontaneous hypertensive rats

B. Schüssler [*], W. Völker [**], K.H. Rahn [*], W. Zidek [*]

[*] Medizinische Poliklinik Albert-Schweitzer-Strasse 33 and [**] Institut für Arterioskleroseforschung, D4400 Münster, Germany

Introduction:
Though the pathophysiological mechanism of essential hypertension is still unknown, there is strong evidence for some dysregulation of the calcium metabolism (Hermsmeyer et al., 1989), which could be the primary disturbance in this disease. While cytoplasmic free calcium $[Ca^{2+}]_i$ was studied extensively in blood cells from spontaneous hypertensive rats (SHR)(Postnov et al., 1979), only few studies exist on $[Ca^{2+}]_i$ in vascular smooth muscle cells (VSMC). We examined $[Ca^{2+}]_i$ in aortic VSMC from SHR and normotensive Wistar-Kyoto-rats (WKY) at pH of 7.0, 7.25, and 7.4 using the intracellular fluorescent dye Quin-2 (Grynkiewicz et al., 1985). Cells were isolated either enzymatically or by tissue explantation.

Material and methods:
Three months old male Wistar-Kyoto-rats (WKY) and their spontaneous hypertensive equivalents from the Münster-strain with systolic blood pressure of at least 180 mmHg were killed by neck dissection. The aorta was taken out and its medial layer prepared according to Ross (1971). Smooth muscle cells were isolated in two different ways:

a) Explantation:
The pieces of tissue were explanted into culture flasks and, after one hour, carefully covered with Dulbecco's Modification of Eagle's Medium (DMEM) containing 10 per cent fetal calf serum (FCS). After three days, smooth muscle cells grew out. The explants were removed four days later.
b) Enzymatic Isolation:
The pieces of tissue were incubated in a solution of 0,05 per cent trypsin-EDTA at 37°C for 30 min. Cells were washed and incubated in 50 U elastase in DMEM without FCS, but with 15 mM HEPES. Another washing was followed by incubation in 2000 U collagenase in DMEM with 10 per cent FCS and 15 mM HEPES. The enzymatic activity was stopped with 25 per cent FCS. The suspension of cells was washed and brought into culture flasks covered with DMEM with 10 per cent FCS .
In both methods, cells were removed from flasks by trypsinisation after about one week, centrifuged and resuspended in physiological saline solution (PSS), which contained 135 mM NaCl, 5 mM KCl, 1mM $CaCl_2$, 1mM $MgSO_4$, 5,5 mM glucose, 10mM HEPES and had an acidity of pH 7.00, 7.25, or 7.40.
Incubation with Quin-2:
2,5 µM Quin-2-acetoxymethylester from a 1mM stem solution in DMSO was added to this cellular suspension. After incubation for 60 min at 37°C, the cells were washed and resuspended, resulting in a concentration of 100 000 cells/ml. The vitality, tested with trypan blue, always showed at least 95 per cent vital cells, else the sample was rejected.

Measuring of free cytoplasmic calcium:
In a 1cm^2 quartz cuvet, the fluorescence F of the stained cells was measured at 492 nm wavelength for emission and excitation at 339 nm. We used a Kontron spectrofluorimeter SFM 23/B. Maximal and minimal fluorescence were achieved by addition of 1 per cent Triton-X-100. $[Ca^{2+}]_i$ resulted from the formula of Grynkiewicz (4), where K_d of
58 nM was inserted according to the room temperature.

Data were statistically analysed with the student-t-test and the Wilcoxon-rank-sum-test.

Results:
Table 1 shows mean values and s.e.m. of $[Ca^{2+}]_i$ (nmol/l, *:p<0,05, number of animals in brackets) in VSMC isolated by tissue explantation. Table 2 compares the figures of explanted and enzymatically isolated cells of the two strains at pH 7.25.

Tab.1:

pH	7,0	7,25	7,4
WKY	280 ± 38 (9) *	103 ± 10 (10)	100 ± 4 (10)
SHR	265 ± 33 (9)	130 ± 16 (10)	124 ± 14 (10)

Tab.2:

	enzym. isol.	explant isol.
WKY	198 ± 78 (15) *	103 ± 10 (10)
SHR	232 ± 47 (15) *	130 ± 16 (10)

The results show that $[Ca^{2+}]_i$ was elevated in VSMC of SHR compared to WKY at pH 7.25 and 7.4. With rising acidity of the medium, $[Ca^{2+}]_i$ continuously increased. Enzymatic isolation of VSMC was associated with markedly elevated $[Ca^{2+}]_i$ in comparison to explanted cells.

Discussion:
In agreement with previous studies (Spieker et al., 1982), our examinations reveal that VSMC from SHR have a higher $[Ca^{2+}]_i$ than cells from WKY, no matter which way of isolation was used. This is remarkable, because at the time of examination the cultured cells had already been living under the same standardized conditions for eight days. Thus all external blood or tissue factors were excluded. These findings are consistent with the results of previous studies showing significant differences in calcium metabolism (Hermsmeyer et al., 1989, Postnov et al., 1979), that could be fixed genetically. But we must also consider the possibility that an in vivo acting agent, e.g. a hypertension inducing circulating factor, causes cellular changes, which are maintained under culture conditions. Studies by Zidek et al. give strong evidence into that direction (Zidek et al., 1983).

The effect of acidity on $[Ca^{2+}]_i$ may be due to voltage dependent changes in permeability of plasma membrane calcium channels, such as the Na^+-Ca^{2+}-exchange (Ashida et al., 1989).

$[Ca^{2+}]_i$ is significantly higher in enzymatically isolated cells. Since the viability examined with trypan blue is the same using both ways of isolation, the results suggest that different cellular populations are obtained. This is in good agreement with the observation of Grünwald & Wischer (1985) that the vascular medial layer consists of morphologically and metabolicly different populations of smooth muscle cells.

Surprisingly, this seems to be connected with a difference in calcium metabolism. Another possibility is a denaturation of membrane proteins secondary to the enzymatic activity during the isolation process that could result in a higher level of $[Ca^{2+}]_i$.

References:

1.) Ashida, T., Kuramochi, M. & Omae, T.(1989): Increased sodium-calcium exchange in arterial smooth muscle of spontaneously hypertensive rats. Hypertension 13, 890-895.

2.) Grünwald, J. & Wischer, W. (1985): Ultrastructural morphometry of cultivated smooth muscle cells from normotensive and hypertensive rats. Exp. Path. 27, 91-98

3.) Grynkiewicz, G., Poenie, M. & Tsien, R. (1985): A new generation of Ca^{2+}- indicators with greatly improved fluorescence properties. J. Biol. Chem. 260, 3440-3450

4.) Hermsmeyer, K. & Rusch, N.J. (1989): Calcium channel alterations in genetic hypertension. Hypertension 14, 453-456

5.) Postnov, Y.V., Orlov, S.N.& Podukin, N.I. (1979): Decrease in calcium binding by the red blood cell membranes in spontaneously hypertensive rats and in essential hypertension. Pfluegers Arch. 379, 191-195

6.) Ross R (1971): The smooth muscle cell. J. Cell.Biol. 50, 172- 186

7.) Spieker, C., Heck, D., Zidek, W., Kerenyi, G., Losse, H. & Vetter H. (1982): The evaluation of tissue Ca^{2+} by proton-induced X-ray emission in the arteries of spontaneous hypertensive and normotensive rats. Klinische Wochenschrift 63 (suppl.3), 74-77

8.) Zidek, W., Kerenyi, T., Losse, H. & Vetter, H. (1983): Intracellular sodium and calcium in aortic smooth muscle cells after enzymatic isolation in spontanously hypertensive rats. Res. Exp. Med. 183, 129-132

Cytosolic Ca²⁺ and pH in cultured cardiac myocytes and fibroblasts from newborn hypertensive rats of the Okamoto strain

M. David-Dufilho, E. Millanvoye-Van Brussel, M. Freyss-Béguin,
C. Astarie and M.A. Devynck

Département de Pharmacologie, CNRS 6167, CHU Necker, 156, rue de Vaugirard, 75015 Paris, France

The intracellular Ca^{2+} concentration ($[Ca^{2+}]_i$) is a cellular messenger directly involved in cell excitability, growth and proliferation. $[Ca^{2+}]_i$ results from the balance of the activities of Ca^{2+}-channels, Na^+-Ca^{2+} exchange and Ca^{2+}-pumps with the participation of membrane and cytosolic Ca^{2+}-binding protein as an intracellular Ca^{2+} buffer. Intracellular pH (pHi) is also a critical feature of cell activation, growth and proliferation. pHi is controlled by H^+ influx, release and/or production by cellular metabolism, the intracellular buffer capacity and by various direct and indirect membrane extrusion systems.

The genetic hypertension of the Okamoto rat (SHR) is associated in particular with hypertrophy and hyperplasia of vascular smooth muscle cells (Mulvany, 1983; Scott-Burden *et al.*, 1989) and with cardiac hypertrophy (Fröhlich, 1986). This cardiac hypertrophy evaluated by the heart weight to body weight ratio appeared early in the hypertensive process (Clubb *et al.*, 1987; Engelmann & Gerrity, 1988). It has been proposed to proceed from an increase in both number and volume of cardiac cells. In heart sarcolemmal membranes, many abnormalities in Ca^{2+} transport mechanisms have been observed in SHR, but results are controversial (David-Dufilho *et al.*, 1984; Sharma *et al.*; 1986; Dillon *et al.*, 1989). As far as we know, pHi and its regulatory mechanisms has not been investigated in cardiac cells from SHR.

This study was designed to investigate $[Ca^{2+}]_i$ and pHi in heart myocytes and fibroblasts from SHR and their normotensive control Wistar-Kyoto rats (WKY), before the rise in blood pressure.

METHODS

<u>Animals</u>: 3-4 day-old pups were taken from SHR and WKY females supplied by Janvier (Le Genest Saint-Isles,France). At this age, the ratio of heart to body weight was already greater in SHR than in WKY rats (7.6 ± 0.1 vs 6.0 ± 0.1 mg/g, n=10 and 7 groups of 20-40 animals each, p<0.001).

<u>Culture of cardiac cells</u>: Cell cultures were performed as previously described (Freyss-Beguin et al., 1989). Cells were isolated by trypsinization and myocytes separated from fibroblasts by a differential attachment method. The purity of myocyte cultures was maintained by addition of ß-D arabino-furanosyl-cytosine. Under these conditions, myocytes displayed a spontaneous contractile activity which became synchronous at the fourth day in culture. Cells were cultured on coverslips.

<u>Measurements of $[Ca^{2+}]_i$ and pHi</u>: Cytosolic free Ca^{2+} concentration and pHi were determined using the fluorescent Ca^{2+} chelator, fura-2, and the fluorescent pH indicator, BCECF. Thirty minutes before each experiment, culture medium was replaced by a buffer containing in mM: NaCl 108, KCl 5.4, $CaCl_2$ 1.8, NaH_2PO_4 0.8, $MgSO_4$ 0.8, $NaHCO_3$ 4, glucose 5.5, Hepes 25 (pH 7.4 at 37°C), a mixture of amino acids, glutamine and 10% new born calf serum. Cells were then incubated at 37°C with 2µM fura-2AM or BCECF-AM for 30 minutes. The presence of fura-2 inside the myocytes decreased their beating activity from 65% on average in both SHR and WKY whereas BCECF did not affect it.

For fluorescence measurements, cells were rinced twice with the loading buffer containing only 1% new born calf serum. The fluorescence signals were recorded on a spectrofluorimeter SPEX CM111 with a quartz-suprasil cuvette thermostated at 37°C and specially designed to allow frontal fluorescence measurements. The intrinsic fluorescence intensities of cells was systematically substracted from loaded cell recordings.

$[Ca^{2+}]_i$ was calculated from the ratio of excitation fluorescence intensities measured at 335 and 385 nm with an emission wavelength of 510 nm according to the equation established by Poenie et al., 1985. Calibration of fura-2 intracellular fluorescence intensities was performed using the Ca^{2+}-ionophore, ionomycin (10µM) and the K^+-ionophore, nigericin (1µM) on ATP-depleted cells incubated in a K^+-rich medium. pHi was directly calculated from the ratio of excitation fluorescence intensities measured at 440 nm and 503 nm with an emission wavelength of 531 nm. Calibration of pHi versus BCECF fluorescence intensities was performed using nigericin (1µM), as described by Thomas et al., 1979. The intracellular calibration parameters of fura-2 and BCECF did not differ between myocytes and fibroblasts or between SHR and WKY rats thereby allowing the use of the same parameters whatever the cell type or the rat strain was.

RESULTS AND DISCUSSION

After fura-2 loading, part of myocytes stopped beating. The present $[Ca^{2+}]_i$ data have been determined on these cells. In SHR and WKY, the ratios of fluorescence intensities at 335 and 385 nm, reflecting the mean $[Ca^{2+}]_i$ values, progressively increased from the 1st to the 3th day in culture (Fig.1A). From this day, it reached stable values up to the end of culture in SHR, but it decreased after the 4th day and reached stable values from the 6th to 9th in WKY.

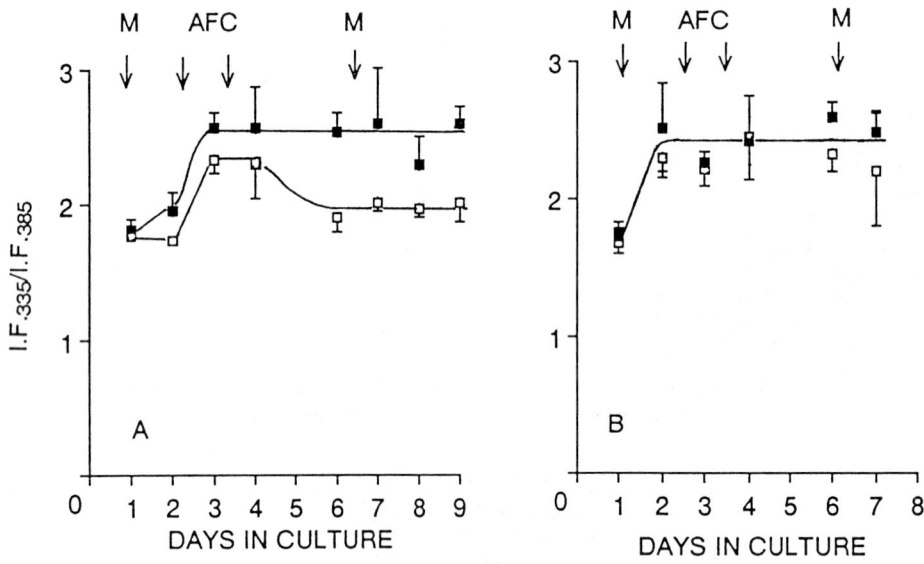

Fig. 1. Influence of culture age on the ratio of fluorescence intensities measured at 335 and 385 nm in myocytes (A) and fibroblasts (B) from SHR (■) and WKY (□).
The arrows indicated the medium reniewal (M) or the addition of ß-D-arabinofuranosyl-cytosine(AFC). Results are expressed as means from 4 independent experiments.

At the beginning of culture, no difference in the ratios of fluorescence intensities was observed between SHR and WKY. $[Ca^{2+}]_i$ values became significantly higher in SHR than in WKY myocytes from the 6th day in culture. Under our conditions, myocyte cultures became confluent on and after the 4th day in culture. The lack of difference during the first days of culture may be due to the remanent effects of trypsine in sarcolemmal membranes. At the end of this period, the in vivo membrane

organization is probably reestablished. In fibroblasts, we similarly observed low values of the fluorescence intensity ratios on the first days in culture (Fig. 1B). The perturbation of transmembrane Ca^{2+} movements by trypsine, resulting in a decreased cytosolic Ca^{2+} concentration is highly probable. On and after the second day in culture, the ratio of fluorescence intensities remained stable. It did not differ between SHR and WKY indicating similar $[Ca^{2+}]_i$ values in the two strains.
In confluent non beating myocytes loaded with fura-2, the mean $[Ca^{2+}]_i$ value was significantly higher in SHR than in WKY (157±8 and 118±8 nM, n=18 and 23, respectively, p<0.01) whereas in confluent fibroblasts, it did not differ.

Whatever the cell type or the rat strain studied, pHi remained stable between the 6th and the 8th day in culture. pHi data obtained during these days were thus pooled. Under these conditions, the cytosol of myocytes was more alkaline in SHR than in WKY (7.19±0.03 and 7.13±0.02 u.pH, respectively, n=26 for both, p=0.05). In contrast, no difference was observed between fibroblasts from SHR and WKY (7.21±0.03 and 7.19±0.02, respectively, n=15 for each).

These $[Ca^{2+}]_i$ and pHi alterations were found in myocytes and not in fibroblasts from 3-4 day-old SHR suggesting that they are expressed early in excitable cells only. The cytosolic alkalization and the increase in $[Ca^{2+}]_i$ observed in SHR myocytes, if present *in vivo*, may contribute to the development of cardiac hypertrophy. This observation in cardiomyocytes from newborn SHR in the absence of neurohumoral regulation and haemodynamic stress suggests that these alterations are genetically determined.

REFERENCES
Clubb, F.J., Bell, P.D., Krisman and J.D., Bishop, S.P. (1987): Myocardial cell growth and blood pressure. Development in neonatal spontaneously hypertensive rats. *Lab. Investigation* 56, 189-196.
David-Dufilho, M., Devynck, M.A., Kazda, S. and Meyer, P. (1984): Stimulation by nifedipine of calcium transport by cardiac sarcolemmal vesicles from spontaneously hypertensive rats. *Eur. J. Pharmacol.* 97, 121-127.
Dillon, J.S., GU, X.H. and Nayler, W.G. (1989): Effect of age and hypertrophy on cardiac Ca2+ antagonist binding sites. *J. Cardiovasc. Pharmacol.* 14, 233-240.
Engelmann, G. and Gerrity, R. (1988): Biochemical characterization of neonatal cardiomyocyte development in normotensive and hypertensive rats. *J. Mol. Cell. Cardiol.* 20, 169-177.
Freyss-Beguin, M., Millanvoye-Van-Brussel, E. and Duval, D. (1989): Effect of oxygen deprivation on metabolism of arachidonic acid by cultures of newborn rat heart cells. *Amer. J. Physiol.* 247, H444-H451.
Fröhlich, E. (1986) Is the spontaneously hypertensive a model for human hypertension. *J. Hypertension* 4, S15-S19.
Mulvany, M.J. (1983): Do resistance vessel abnormalities contribute to the elevated nblood pressure of spontaneously hypertensive rats? A review of some of the evidence. *Blood Vessels* 20, 1-22.
Poenie, M., Alderton, J., Tsien, R.Y. and Steinhardt, R.A. (1985): Changes of free calcium levels with stages of the cell division cycle. *Nature* 315, 147_149.
Thomas, J.A., Buchsbaum, R.N., Zimniak, A. and Raker, E. (1979): Intracellular pH measurements in Erlich ascites tumor cells utilizing spectroscopic probes generated in situ. *Biochemistry* 18, 2210-2218.
Scott-Burden, T., Resink, T.J. and Bühler, F.R. (1989): Enhanced growth and growth factor responsiveness of vascular smooth muscle cells from hypertensive rats. *J. Cardiovasc. Pharmacol.* 14, S16-S21.
Sharma, R.V., Dutters, C.A. and Bhalla, R.C. (1986): Alterations in the plasma membrane properties of the myocardium of spontaneously hypertensive rats. *Hypertension* 8, 583-591.

Chronic treatment with captopril plus hydrochlorothiazide and intracellular free calcium in the tail artery of the adult SHR

Nathalie Thorin-Trescases, Laurence Oster, Jeffrey Atkinson and Christine Capdeville-Atkinson

Laboratoire de Pharmacologie cardio-vasculaire, Faculté de Pharmacie, 5, rue Albert Lebrun, 54000 Nancy, France

Although several reports show that in hypertension the intracellular free calcium concentration $[Ca^{2+}]_i$ is increased in several blood cell types such as platelets, it is far less certain that a similar increase occurs in vascular smooth muscle cells. The first objective of the present experiment was, therefore, to determine whether $[Ca^{2+}]_i$ is increased in a small muscular artery, the tail artery, removed from adult SHR. The second objective was to determine whether changes in $[Ca^{2+}]_i$ - vasoreactivity coupling mechanisms are involved in the antihypertensive effect of chronic treatment with a combination of the angiotensin I converting enzyme (ACE) inhibitor, captopril, and the diuretic, hydrochlorothiazide. Although this combination is thought to acutely lower blood pressure via diuretic stimulation of the renin angiotensin system then blockade of this latter system by the ACE inhibitor, the mechanism behind its chronic antihypertensive effect is less well documented.

Experiments were performed in 22 adult, male SHR and 14 age-matched, male WKY rats. Thirteen of the SHR were given a specially prepared diet containing captopril (CAP, 44 mg/kg per day) and hydrochlorothiazide (HCTZ, 22 mg/kg per day) for 10 weeks. At the end of the 10 weeks' treatment period, systolic arterial pressure was measured in awake, prewarmed rats using the tail cuff method. A segment (1 cm) of the proximal tail artery was then dissected free and the endothelium removed using a metallic wire. The segment was mounted in a specially constructed perfusion system placed in a spectrofluorimetric cuvette (4 ml), and perfused (1.5 ml/min) with physiological saline solution (PSS, for details see Thorin-Trescases, et al., 1990). PSS was switched to PSS plus fura-2/AM (5 µM, Sigma Co., Saint Louis, MO, USA) for 90 min then back to PSS alone for 15 min. Segments were then illuminated with a xenon lamp at excitation wavelengths of 340 nm and 380 nm with a change in wavelength every second, and fluorescence measured at 510 nm using a photomultiplier system (Shimadzu RF-5000, Kyoto, Japan, see figure).

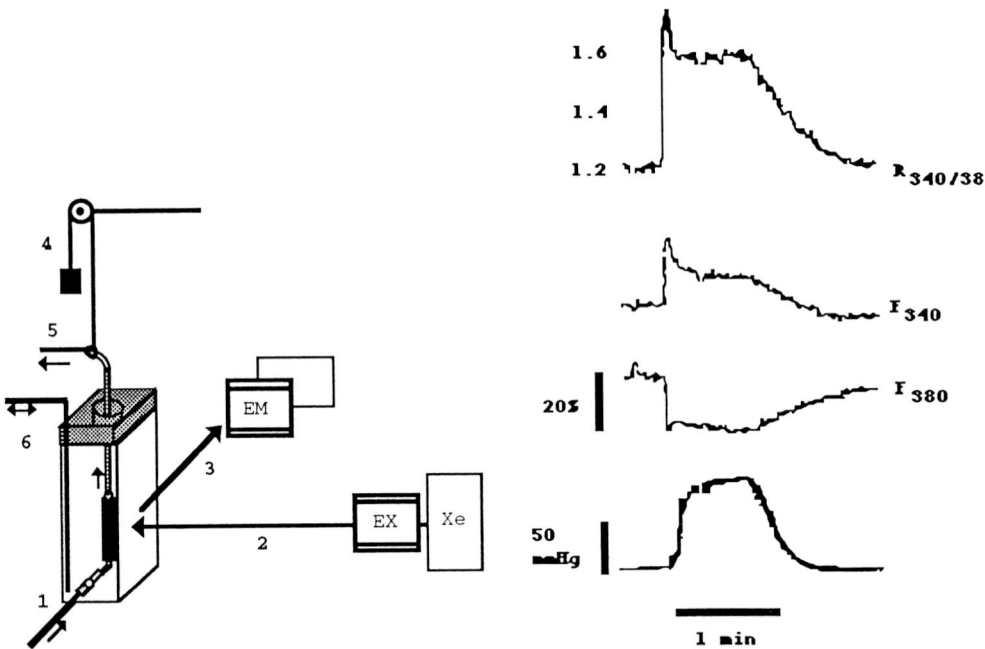

Left: Schematic diagram of the perfusion system of the tail artery segment: 1 = PSS, 2 = excitation, 3 = emission, 4 = 0.5 g, 5 = PSS, 6 = cuvette wash out. Right: Ratio of fluorescence and fluorescence (arbitrary units) measured at 510 nm following excitation at 340 or 380 nm, and change in perfusion pressure following noradrenaline.

Basal perfusion resistance was measured and then segments were vasoconstricted with noradrenaline (1 µM for 1 min). The maximum increase in the ratio of the two emissions ($R_{340/380}$) was used as an estimation of the relative change in $[Ca^{2+}]_i$ following perfusion with noradrenaline. The maximum increase in perfusion pressure measured simultaneously was taken as an estimation of the vasoconstrictor response to noradrenaline. Following return to base-line, basal $[Ca^{2+}]_i$ was calculated according to the following formula (Grynkiewicz et al., 1985 as modified by Scanlon et al., 1987):

$$[Ca^{2+}]_i = ((R_{340/380} - R'_{min}) \times K_D \times ß)/(R'_{max} - R_{340/380})$$

where R'_{min} was determined in the presence of EGTA (10 mM) plus ionomycin (10 µM) and R'_{max} was determined in the presence of $CaCl_2$ (4 mM) plus ionomycin (10 µM). The K_D for fura-2 was taken as being 224 nM (Grynkiewicz et al., 1985) and ß was estimated from the value for F_{380} measured under "R'_{min}" conditions, divided by the value for F_{380} measured under "R'_{max}" conditions (see above). Treatment with CAP + HCTZ lowered systolic arterial pressure to a level (160 ± 5 mmHg, n = 12) not significantly different from that of WKY rats (145 ± 2 mmHg, n = 10; SHR controls: 237 ± 9, n = 11). In vitro basal perfusion resistance and $[Ca^{2+}]_i$ of tail arteries from SHR were higher than those of WKY and treatment with CAP + HCTZ produced a fall in these values back to the same as those of WKY rats (Table 1). Increases in perfusion pressure and in calcium mobilisation following perfusion with noradrenaline were also increased in SHR but treatment with CAP + HCTZ had no effect on these parameters (Table 1).

Table 2. Basal perfusion resistance (mmHg/ml/min) and ($[Ca^{2+}]_i$ nM) and increase in perfusion pressure (Δ mmHg) and relative $[Ca^{2+}]_i$ ($\Delta R_{340/380}$ %) following perfusion with noradrenaline (1 μM, 1 min) (m ± SEM) in tail arteries from SHR treated with captopril (CAP 44 mg/kg per day) plus hydrochlorothiazide (HCTZ, 22 mg/kg per day), control SHR and WKY.

		mmHg/ml/min	nM	ΔmmHg	$\Delta R_{340/380}$%
SHR/ CAP + HCTZ	12	23 ± 3*	137 ± 13*	68 ± 12¶	18.3 ± 2.2¶
SHR	11	31 ± 4	290 ± 45	63 ± 13¶	19.5 ± 2.8¶
WKY	10	23 ± 3*	171 ± 20*	16 ± 4	11.0 ± 1.4

* = P < 0.05 versus SHR. ¶= P < 0.05 versus WKY.

In conclusion our results suggest that hypertension is accompanied in the SHR tail artery in vitro preparation, by an increase in basal and noradrenaline - stimulated vasoreactivity and calcium mobilisation and that treatment with CAP + HCTZ, which lowers systolic arterial pressure to normotensive levels, modifies the basal parameters but does not change the sensitivity to noradrenaline.

REFERENCES.

Grynkiewicz, G., Poenie M. and Tsien, R.Y. (1985): A new generation of Ca^{2+} indicators with greatly improved fluorescence properties. J. Biol. Chem. 260: 3440-3450.

Scanlon, M., Williams, D.A. and Fay, F.S. (1987): A Ca^{2+} - insensitive form of fura-2 associated with polymorphonuclear leukocytes. J. Biol. Chem. 262: 6308-6312.

Thorin-Trescases, N., Oster, L., Atkinson, J. and Capdeville, C. (1990): Norepinephrine and serotonin increase the vasoconstrictor response of the perfused rat tail artery to changes in cytosolic Ca^{2+}. Eur. J. Pharmacol. 179: 469-471.

The authors would like to acknowledge the financial assistance of Théraplix Laboratories, Paris and the helpful discussions with Joël Guillou from this laboratory.

Parathyroid transplantation in Lyon and Milan rat strains : preliminary results on blood pressure

Christophe Burkard, Madeleine Vincent *, Patrizia Ferrari **, Jean Sassard * and Alexis Gairard

*Faculté de Pharmacie and CNRS, URA 600, Pharmacologie Cellulaire et Moléculaire, Université Louis Pasteur, Strasbourg, France; * URA 606, Département de Physiologie et Pharmacologie Clinique, Université Claude Bernard, Lyon, France; ** Cellular Pharmacology, Prassis, Sigma-Tau, Settimo Milanese, Italy*

Parathyroidectomy (PTX) lessens the development of hypertension in SHR (Schleiffer et al., 1981) and LH rats (Pernot et al., 1990) Moreover a low calcium diet enhances the level of blood pressure and a high calcium diet lowers it (Schleiffer et al. , 1984; Pernot et al., 1990). On the other hand clinical studies show a high prevalence of hypertension in primary hyperparathyroidism (Christensson et al., 1977) and after PTX in the patients the blood pressure returns to normal values (Broulik et al. 1985). Mechanisms still remain unclear since parathyroid hormone (PTH) acutely administered display hypotensive effects in several species (Berthelot et Gairard, 1975, Pang et al., 1980). Recently a new hypertensive factor was described in SHR parathyroid glands (PT) and biologically characterized after transplantation by Pang et al.,1989 and by Neuser et al.,1990 in SHR/SP. Here we present similar results from 2 genetic hypertensive models which display altered calcium metabolism, the Lyon (LH) and the Milan (MHS) rats (Pernot et al.,1990; Ferrari et al.,1987; Cirillo et al., 1989).

METHODS
One parathyroid gland was obtained by surgical excision under ketamin-xylazin anesthesia from 5 week-old LH or MHS donor and immediately grafted within the neck muscles, above the thyroid in normotensive recipient of the same age. Control animals were either sham operated (C) or grafted with one PT from the corresponding normotensive strain. Body weight, serum calcium by fluorimetric technic and blood pressure (tail-cuff method on awake animals, Narco Biosystem ^{R}) are bimonthly measured from week 7 onwards. Commercial chow (ref: UAR, AO4 Ca .6%, Na .24%, VIT D_3 150 I.U.%) is freely offered with distilled water.

RESULTS
After PT transplantation serum calcium reestablishes to nearly normal values (2.4 mmol/l) between weeks 6-8 and growth is not impaired. In male LH/LN rats (parathyroid donor's strain/recipient's strain) blood pressure significantly increases compared to LN C (+8mmHg; mean increase for weeks 9-14, p<0.001 by variance analysis, 10 rats,Fig.1,top and left). A control experiment in normotensive LL strain show that after week 9, when serum calcium is reestablished to normal values blood pressure in LL/LL rats do not differ from sham LL rats (top and right). Moreover in female LH/LN a small increase during the same period is also present and statistical significant (+5 mmHg,mean increase,p<0.05, variance analysis weeks 9-28, 8 rats). In male MHS/MNS results obtained during weeks 7-14

Lyon Strain
Male

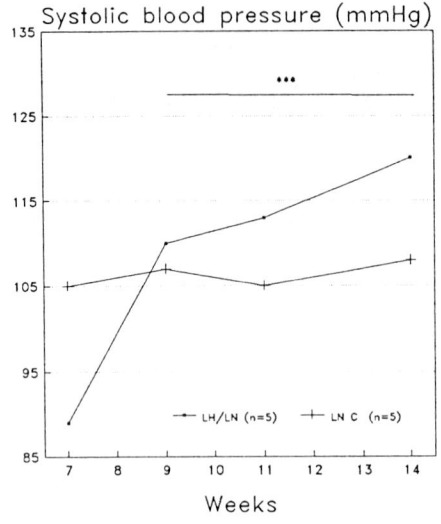

Lyon Strain
Female

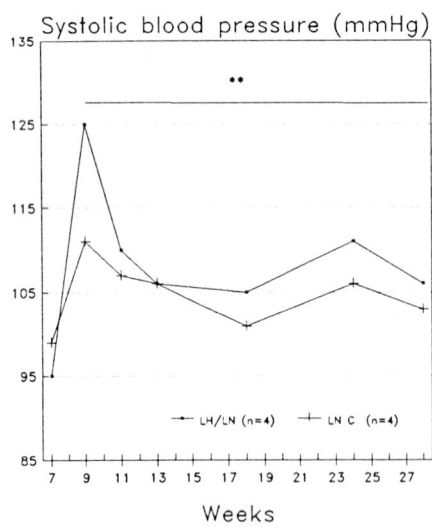

Milan Strain
Male

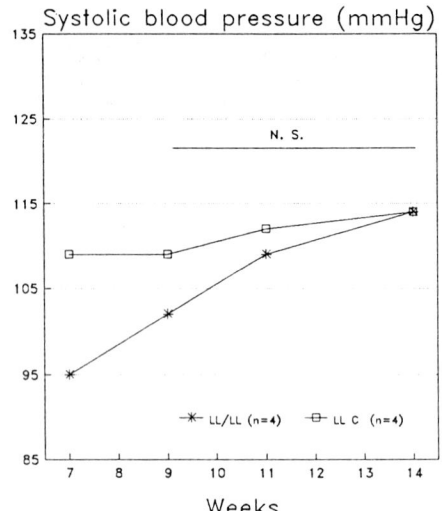
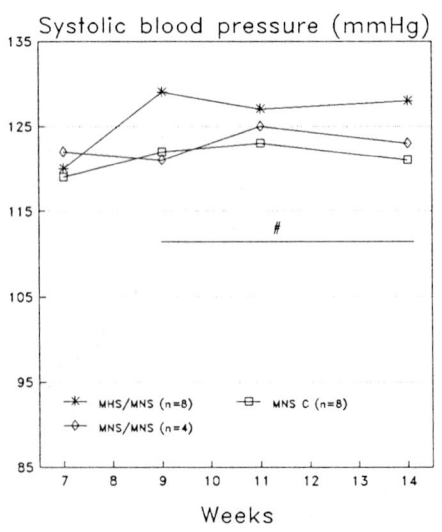

Fig.1 Evolution of systolic blood pressure after transplantation of one parathyroid gland in parathyroidectomized animal. LH/LN: donor gland strain / recepient rat strain; C: sham rat; n: number of rats; N.S., not significant; * or # $p<0.05$, (# MHS/MNS versus MNS C and MNS/MNS), ** $p<0.01$, *** $p<0.001$ by variance analysis.

show a significant increase (+8mmHg, mean increase, $p<0.05$, variance analysis weeks 9-14, 20 rats).

DISCUSSION

To further extend the importance of PT in genetic hypertension, it was important to verify that PT transplantation from two other genetic hypertensive strains was also able to increase blood pressure. Our results demonstrate that one PT from just weaned LH and MHS rats, transplanted in normotensive rat, PTX just before, is able to reestablish a normal serum calcium level and induces a sustained blood pressure enhancing effect. In addition blood pressure increasing effect of PT transplantation is also present in female LN rats but less important than in male LN rats. Recently a circulating hypertensive factor was described in SHR plasma which disappears after PTX (Pang and Lewanczuk, 1989). Morever essential hypertensive subjects present a circulating pressor factor with similar characteristics (Lewanczuk et al.,1990).

In conclusion PT transplantation from LH and MHS, both genetic hypertensive strains, induces a significant increase in blood pressure in their respective normotensive controls by mechanisms to be further delineated.

REFERENCES

Berthelot A.and Gairard A.(1975): Effet de la parathormone sur la pression artérielle et la contraction de l'aorte isolée de rat. Experientia 31:457-458.

Broulik P.D., Horky K., Pacovsky V.(1985): Blood pressure in patients with primary hyperparathyroidism after parathyroidectomy. Exp. Clin. Endocrinol. 86:346-52.

Cirillo M., Galletti F., Strazzullo P., Torielli L., and Melloni M.C.(1989):On the pathogenetic mechanism of hypercalciuria in genetically hypertensive rats of the Milan strain. Am. J Physiol. 2:741-746.

Christensson T., Helstrom K., Wengle B.(1977): Blood pressure in subjects with hypercalcemia and primary hyperparathyroidism detected in health screening program. Eur. J. Clin. Invest. 7: 109-113.

Ferrari.P., Barber B.R., Torielli B.L., Ferrandi M. ,Salardi S., and G.Bianchi(1987): The Milan hypertensive rat as a model for studying cation transport abnormality in genetic hypertension. Hypertension 10(suppl.I):I.32-I.36.

Lewanczuk R.Z., Resnick L.M., Blumenfeld J.D., Laragh J.H.and Pang P.K.T.(1990): A new circulating hypertensive factor in the plasma of essential hypertensive subjects. J. Hypertens. 8:105-108.

Neuser D,Schulte-Brinkmann R, Kazda S.(1989): Development of hypertension in WKY rats after transplantation of parathyroid glands from SHR/SP. J. Cardiovasc. Pharmacol. 6:971-974.

Pang P.K.T., Lewanczuk R.Z.(1989): Parathyroid origin of a new circulating hypertensive factor in spontaneously hypertensive rats. Am. J. Hypertens. 2:898-902.

Pang P.K.T., Tenner T.E., Yee J.A., Yang M.C.M., and Janssen H.F. (1980): Hypotensive action of parathyroid hormone preparations on rats and dogs. Proc. Natl. Acad. Sci. U.S.A. 77:675-678.

Pernot F., Schleiffer R., Vincent M., Sassard J., and Gairard A. (1990): Parathyroidectomy in the Lyon hypertensive rat: cardiovascular reactivity and aortic responsiveness. J. Hypertens. 8:111-1117.

Pernot F., Schleiffer R., Bergmann C., Vincent M., Sassard J., and Gairard (1990): Dietary calcium, vascular reactivity and genetic hypertension in the Lyon rat strain. Am. J. Hypertens. 3:846-853.

Schleiffer R., Berthelot A., Pernot F., and Gairard A.(1981): Parathyroidectomy, thyroid and development of hypertension in SHR. Jap. Circ. J. 45:1272-1279.

Schleiffer R., Pernot F., Berthelot A., and Gairard A.(1981): Low calcium diet enhances development of hypertension in the spontaneously hypertensive rat. Clin. Exp. Hypertens. 6:783-794.

Differing blood pressure responses to dietary calcium between male and female LH, LN and LL rats

Fanny Pernot, Madeleine Vincent *, Jean Sassard * and Alexis Gairard

*CNRS URA 600, Pharmacologie Moléculaire et Cellulaire, Faculté de Pharmacie, Université Louis Pasteur, Strasbourg, France and * CNRS URA 606, Département de Physiologie et Pharmacologie Clinique, Faculté de Pharmacie, Université Claude Bernard, Lyon, France*

A large amount of data is available on the relationships between hypertensive pathology, dietary calcium and calcium metabolism. Thus, in essential hypertension systolic blood pressure is often associated with decreased intestinal calcium absorption (McCarron and Morris, 1985) and with increased urinary calcium excretion (Strazzulo et al., 1983; Hvarfner et al., 1987). Some authors describe hypercalcemia in hypertension (Kesteloot, 1986) whereas others find no relation between these two parameters. Moreover systolic blood pressure is negatively correlated with ionized plasma calcium (McCarron , 1982; Folsom et al; 1986). In experimental hypertension disturbances of calcium metabolism have been reported in the SHR strain (Lau et al., 1984), the Milan strain (Cirillo et al., 1989), and the Lyon strain (Pernot et al., 1991). The aim of this work was to study the effect of hypo and hypercalcic diets on the evolution of systolic blood pressure, body weight and plasma calcium in male and female rats of the genetically hypertensive Lyon strain (LH) and their normotensive (LN) and low blood pressure (LL) controls.

Male and female LH, LN and LL rats born in Lyon were weaned at the age of three weeks. After on week of adaptation to our laboratory with a normal calcium diet (0.6%), they were randomly divided into three groups, drinking distilled water *ad libitum* and receiving different calcium diets (UAR, France) from 4 to 23 weeks of age : normocalcic diet containing 0.6% Ca (NCa), hypercalcic (2.5%, HCa) and low calcic (0.03%, LCa) diet. These diets are equilibrated in vitamins and other minerals. The rats were weighted and systolic blood pressure measured from 6 to 23 weeks of age on awake animals by the sphygmomanometric tail-cuff method (Narco Biosystem). Plasma total calcium was determined at the end of the experiment by fluorimetry (Corning 940). Data are expressed as means ± s.e.m.

In hypertensive 23 week-old LH male rats, hypercalcic and low calcic diets do not modify body weight (Fig. 1) but induce opposite effects on systolic blood pressure and plasma calcium : HCa decreases blood pressure and increases calcemia whereas LCa increases blood pressure and decreases calcemia. In hypertensive LH female animals, the two diets reduce body weight while HCa reduces blood pressure without

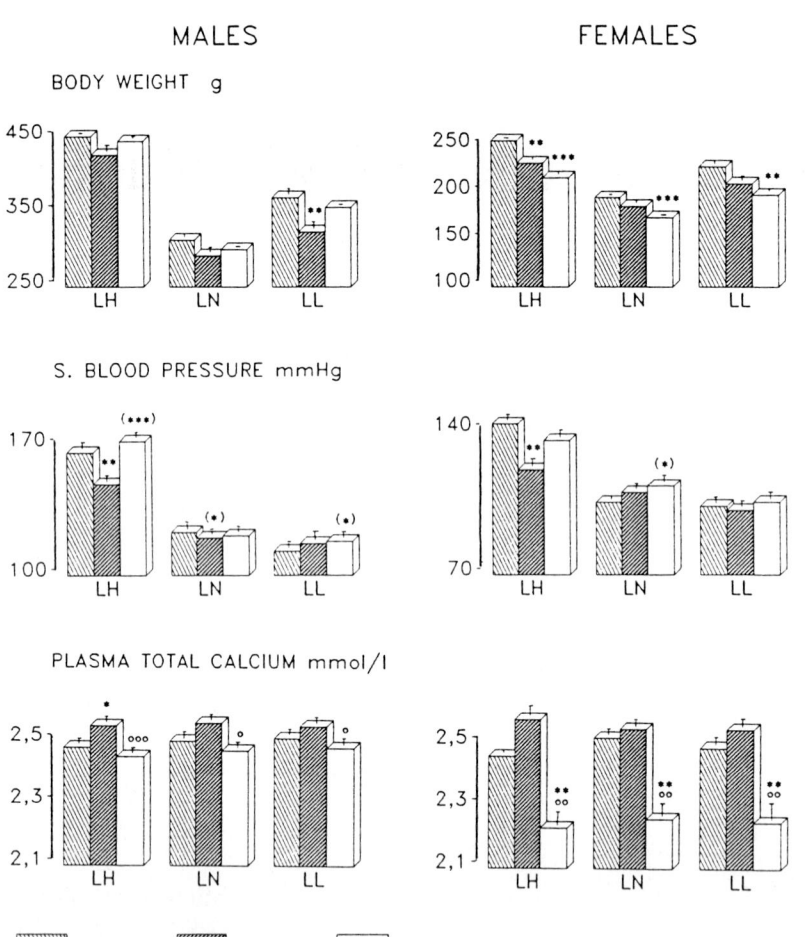

Fig. 1 : Effect of normocalcic (NCa), hypercalcic (HCa) and low calcic (LCa) diets on body weight, systolic blood pressure and total plasma calcium in the Lyon hypertensive (LH), normotensive (LN) and low blood pressure (LL) male or female 23 week-old rats. Groups of 7 to 12 rats. Statistical comparisons: * $p<0.05$; ** $p<0.01$; *** $p<0.001$, HCa or LCa versus NCa, ( ) two ways ANOVA including the measures from 6 to 23 weeks of age; ° $p<0.05$; °° $p<0.01$; °°° $p<0.001$, LCa versus HCa.

affecting calcemia and LCa has no effect on blood pressure but decreases high significantly calcemia. In control strains, in male as in female, the effects of diets on systolic blood pressure are less important. However, LCa diet decreases body weight and calcemia in female but display only a small increasing effect on blood pressure in LN with no significant effect in LL.

This experiment shows the importance of dietary calcium in the evolution of blood pressure in hypertensive rats of the Lyon strain. Recently we have demonstrated that HCa diet decreases cardiovascular reactivity and increases *in vitro* aortic response to norepinephrine in LH male rats (Pernot et al., 1990). Therefore HCa diet could interact with blood pressure regulation by modifications of cellular calcium repartition which is known to be disturbed in hypertension (Shibata et al., 1975). These results on peripheral events could also be explained by sodium diuresis, polypeptides synthesis like ANF or PHF, Parathyroid Hypertensive Factor (Lewanczuk et al., 1990) or by central effects recently observed on alpha$_2$ hypothalamic receptors (Yang et al., 1989).

REFERENCES

Ayachi S. (1979): Increased dietary calcium lowers blood pressure in the spontaneously hypertensive rat. Metabolism 28: 1234-1238.

Cirillo M., Galletti F., Strazzullo P., Torielli L. and Melloni M.C. (1989): On the pathogenic mechanism of hypercalciuria in genetically hypertensive rats of the Milan strain. Am. J. Hypertens. 2: 741-746.

Folsom A.R., Smith C.L., Prineas R.J. and Grimm R.H. (1986): Serum calcium fractions in essential hypertensive and matched normotensive subjects. Hypertension 8: 11-15.

Hvarfner A., Bergström R., Mörlin C., Wide F. and Ljunghall S. (1987): Relationship between calcium metabolic indices and blood pressure in patients with essential hypertension as compared with a healthy population. J. Hypertens. 5: 451-456.

Kesteloot H. (1986): Relationship between calcium and blood pressure. Am. J. Nephrol. 6(suppl. 1): 10-13.

Lau K., Zikos D., Spirnak J. and Eby B. (1984): Evidence for an intestinal mechanism in hypercalciuria of spontaneously hypertensive rats. Am. J. Physiol. 247: E625-E633.

Lewanczuk R.Z., Chen A. and Pang P.K.T. (1990): The effects of dietary calcium on blood pressure in spontaneously hypertensive rats may be mediated by parathyroid hypertensive factor. Am. J Hypertens. 3: 349-353.

McCarron D.A. (1982): Low serum concentrations of ionized calcium in patients with hypertension. N. Engl. J. Med. 307: 226-228.

McCarron D.A. and Morris C.D. (1985): Blood pressure response to oral calcium in persons with mild to moderate hypertension. Ann. Intern. Med. 103: 825-831.

Pernot F., Schleiffer R., Bergmann C., Vincent M., Sassard J. and Gairard A. (1990): Dietary calcium, vascular reactivity and genetic hypertension in the Lyon rat strain. Am. J. Hypertens. 3: 846-853.

Pernot F., Luthringer C., Vincent M., Sassard J., Berthelot A. and Gairard A. (1991): Calcium metabolism in the Lyon hypertensive rat. Ann. Nutr. Metab. 35: 45-52.

Schleiffer R., Pernot F., Berthelot A. and Gairard A. (1984): Low calcium diet enhances development of hypertension in the spontaneously hypertensive rat. Clin. Exp. Hypertens. A6: 783-793.

Strazzullo P., Nunziata V., Cirillo M., Giannattasio R., Ferrara L.A., Mattioli P.L. and Mancini M. (1983): Abnormalities of calcium metabolism in essential hypertension. Clin. Sci. 65: 137-141.

Yang R.H., Jin H., Chen Y.F., Oparil S. and Wyss J.M. (1989): Dietary calcium supplementation prevents the enhanced responsiveness of anterior hypothalamic alpha$_2$ adrenoceptors in NaCl-loaded spontaneously hypertensive rats. J. Cardiovasc. Pharmacol. 13: 162-167.

Acute effect of Ca deprivation on duodenal CaBP, CaBP mRNA, Ca transport and plasma calcitriol levels in spontaneously hypertensive (SHR) and WKY control rats

S. Chabanis, P. Duchambon, H. Banide *, D. Auchère *, A. Jardel *,
B. Lacour and T. Drüeke

*INSERM U.90, Hôpital Necker, Paris; * Physiologie, Faculté de Pharmacie, Châtenay-Malabry, France*

ABSTRACT : The vitamin D dependent intestinal calbindin 9K (CaBP 9K) has been shown to be decreased, and the intestinal adaptation to short-term Ca deprivation to be abnormal in the 12-week-old male SHR compared with the WKY. To determine the time course of intestinal response to Ca deprivation we performed a study in these rats fed a low (0.1%) Ca diet for 3, 6, 9 or 12 days compared with rats of either strain on normal (1.0%) Ca diet. For plasma calcitriol, duodenal CaBP 9K, CaBP 9K mRNA, alkaline phosphatase activity and active calcium transport, no significant difference between strains was observed with 1.0% Ca diet. In response to low-Ca diet, the WKY and SHR showed a similar increase in mean plasma calcitriol level (nearly 50 %) at day 6 of this diet. However, only the WKY had the expected adaptation at the intestinal level. The SHR showed only a transient, but not significant, increase of several intestinal parameters. Duodenal CaBP 9K concentration and Ca transport ratio were lower in SHR than WKY rats in response to low Ca diet. However, both strains had a similar increase of active calcium transport in response to a single injection of calcitriol. In conclusion, these experiments showed that the 12-week-old SHR was able to increase transiently calcitriol production in response to short-term Ca deprivation but failed to adapt significantly at the intestinal target level during the 12-day low-Ca diet. Our results suggest a relative intestinal resistance to endogenous calcitriol, which could be overcome with a high dose of exogenous calcitriol.

The vitamin D dependent intestinal calbindin 9K (CaBP 9K) has been shown to be decreased (1, 2), and the intestinal adaptation to calcium deprivation to be abnormal in the spontaneously hypertensive rat (SHR) compared with its genetic normotensive control, the Wistar Kyoto rat (WKY) (3). Although the intestinal response to a short-term (10 days) Ca deprivation appears to be normal in the young (6 week-old) prehypertensive SHR, the adult (12 week-old) hypertensive SHR lost the ability to adapt (3). Thus, a defect in the vitamin D endocrine system has been suggested to exist in the SHR, which may mainly reside in an intestinal resistance to calcitriol. Nevertheless, the CaBP 9K and Ca transport adaptations to long-term (8 weeks) Ca deprivation are identical in adult SHR and WKY (4, 5).
To further investigate the response pattern of cacitriol level and related intestinal adaptation in the SHR, we performed a time-course study of various parameters reflecting plasma hormone and target organ changes during a short-term low Ca diet. We also measured the response to exogenous calcitriol in SHR and WKY at this age.

METHODS

Time course study: twelve-week-old male SHR and WKY (Iffa Credo, France) fed a low (0.1 %) Ca diet were compared with rats of either strain on a normal (1 %) Ca diet. The dietary content of P was 0.46 % and that of vitamin D_2 2200 IU/kg.

Animals had free access to a french mineral water of low Ca content. They were killed between 9 and 10 a.m. in the non-fasted state.

Plasma calcitriol was measured by radiocompetition assay (6), duodenal CaBP 9K by radioimmunoassay (7), duodenal CaBP 9K mRNA by densitometric analysis of Northern blots using a specific cDNA probe (8) and normalized to actin mRNA. Cytosolic alkaline phosphatase of duodenal mucosa was assayed using para-nitrophenylphosphate as a substrate (9). Active calcium transport was measured in everted duodenal sacs (3 cm distal from pylorus) and expressed as the serosa-to-mucosa ratio at 90 min (10).

Response to exogenous calcitriol: twelve-week-old male SHR and WKY on standard laboratory diet were injected intraperitoneally with a single dose of calcitriol (600 ng in absolute ethanol) or with vehicle alone and calcium transport was measured 6 hr after dosing (10).

RESULTS

Expressed as mean ± SEM, n= 4-8 animals.
Statistical analysis by analysis of variance (ANOVA)

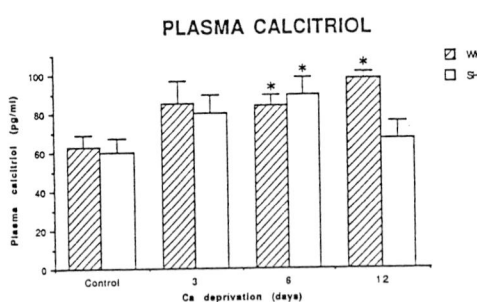

* : statistically different from control value of same strain (p<0.05), one-way ANOVA

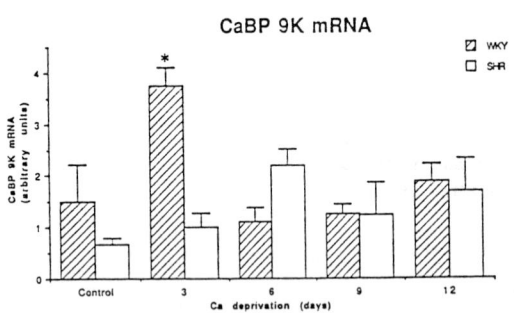

* : statistically different from control value of same strain (p<0.05), one-way ANOVA

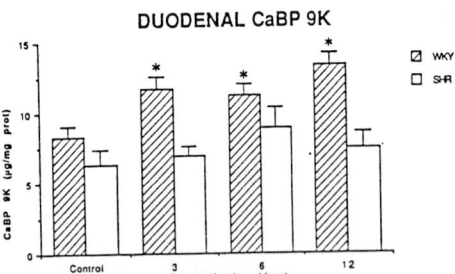

Statistical difference between strains : p<0.001, two-way ANOVA
* : statistically different from control value of same strain (p<0.05), one-way ANOVA

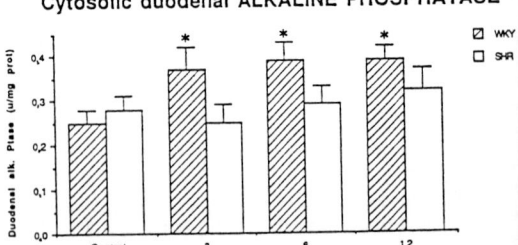

Statistical difference between strains : p<0.05, two-way ANOVA
* : statistically different from control value of same strain (p<0.05), one-way ANOVA

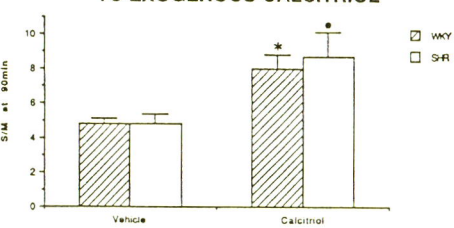

Statistical difference between strains : p<0.05, two-way ANOVA
* : statistically different from control value of same strain (p<0.05), one-way ANOVA

* : different from vehicle treated animals (p<0.01)
● : different from vehicle treated animals (p<0.05)

SUMMARY
1. The basal levels of all the parameters tested in the time course study were identical in the SHR and WKY (i.e. with the 1% Ca diet) and the two strains showed a similar increase (≈50%) of calcitriol level in response to six days of low Ca diet. However, the expected adaptation at the duodenal level occurred only in the normotensive rats, with an increase of CaBP 9K content, CaBP 9K mRNA abundance, alkaline phosphatase activity, and active Ca transport. The SHR showed a transient but not significant increase of CaBP 9K and CaBP 9K mRNA at day 6.
2. By contrast, the stimulation of active calcium transport by a single intraperitoneal administration of a high dose of calcitriol was the same in SHR and WKY.

CONCLUSION
The present study suggests that the SHR is able to increase his endogenous calcitriol production when fed a low Ca diet. However, he is unable to fully adapt in terms of duodenal Ca absorption during a time period of 12 days. The underlying defect could be a failure to generate sufficient amounts of CaBP 9K message and protein in response to the low-Ca regime and the subsequent physiological stimulation of calcitriol production.

REFERENCES
1 : Cloney D.L., Gray R.W., Bruns M.E., Burnett S.H., Smith M.L., Felder R.A. and Bruns D.E. (1991) : Intestinal vitamin D-dependent calbindin-D9K and alkaline phosphatase in spontaneously hypertensive rats. Am. J. Physiol. 260, G691-697.
2 : Roullet C.M., Roullet J.B., Duchambon P., Thomasset M., Lacour B., Mc Carron D.A. and Drüeke T. (1991) : Abnormal intestinal regulation of calbindin-D9K and calmodulin by dietary calcium in genetic hypertension. Am.J.Physiol. 261, F474-480,
3 : Cloney D.L., Burnett S.H., Bruns M.E. and Bruns D.E. (1990) : Adaptation of calbindin-D9K to a low Ca diet does not occur in the 14-week-old spontaneously hypertensive rats (SHR). Abst 760, ASBMR, Atlanta.
4 : Lucas P.A., Brown R.C., Drüeke T., Lacour B, Metz J.A. and Mc Carron D.A. (1986) : Abnormal vitamin D metabolism, intestinal Ca transport, and bone Ca status in the spontaneously hypertensive rat compared with its genetic control. J. Clin. Invest. 78, 221-227.
5 : Bourgouin P., Lucas P., Roullet C., Pointillart A., Thomasset M., Brami M., Comte L., Lacour B., Garabédian M., Mc Carron D.A. and Drüeke T. (1990) : Developmental changes of Ca, PO_4, and calcitriol metabolism in spontaneously hypertensive rats. Am.J.Physiol. 259, F104-110.
6 : Shepard R.M., Horst R.L., Hamstra A.J. and De Luca H.F. (1979) : Determination of vitamin D and its metabolites in plasma from normal and anephric man Biochem. J. 182, 55-69.
7 : Thomasset M., Parkes C.O. and Cuisinier-Gleizes P. (1982) : Rat calcium binding proteins : distribution, development, and vitamin D dependence. Am.J.Physiol. 243, E483-488.
8 : Desplan C., Thomasset M. and Moukhtar M. (1983) : Synthesis, molecular cloning and restriction analysis of DNA complementary to vitamin D dependent CaBP mRNA from rat duodenum. J.Biol.Chem. 258, 2762-2765.
9 : Bessey O.A., Lowry O.H. and Brock M.J. (1946) : Method for determination of alkaline phosphatase with 5 mm^3 of serum. J.Biol.Chem. 164, 321-329.
10 : Martin D.L. and De Luca H.F. (1969) : Influence of Na on Ca transport by the rat small intestine. Am.J.Physiol. 216, 1351-1359.

Treatment with vitamin D_3 reduces blood pressure of spontaneously hypertensive rats

Lucia M. Vianna, Antonio C. M. Paiva and Therezinha B. Paiva

Department of Biophysics, Escola Paulista de Medicina, Caixa Postal 20.388, 04034 São Paulo, São Paulo, Brazil

Previous studies have suggested that alterations in calcium metabolism may play a role in the mechanism of hypertension, both in humans and in SHR (for a review see McCarron, 1989). In SHR, plasma levels of calcium and of vitamin D_3 are reported to be decreased, and those of serum parathyroid hormone (PTH) are elevated, as compared to normotensive Wistar Kyoto (WKY) controls. In addition, an abnormal vitamin D metabolism in SHR (Lucas et al., 1986) suggests a link with the mechanism of hypertension in this model. To further understand this problem, we studied the effect of treatment with vitamin D_3 on the blood pressure of adult SHR and WKY rats.

METHODS

Female SHR and WKY rats (200 ± 5 g body weight), maintained in metabolic cages, were fed a standard diet (Labina rat chow, Purina) with 6,600 IU vitamin D_3/kg. After a basal period of ten days the animals received, by gavage, a daily supplementation with vitamin D_3 (Sigma, St. Louis, MO), dissolved in 0.35 ml of coconut oil. Control groups received only the vehicle. Body weight, food and water intake as well as urine output were recorded daily, and systolic blood pressure was recorded by a plethysmographic method. Serum calcium was measured by atomic absorption spectrometry, and serum PTH and urinary cAMP by radioimmunoassays. Hematological parameters were determined by Coulter analysis.

RESULTS AND DISCUSSION

Both SHR and WKY rats showed no significant changes in food and water intake, body weight and urine output during a 3-week period of treatment with three dose levels of vitamin D_3. SHR and WKY rats which received only the vehicle (controls) or 6.25 µg/100 g body weight per day showed no significant alteration of systolic blood pressure. However, at the dose levels of 12.5 or 50 µg/100 g/day, the SHR, but not the WKY rats, showed a significant decrease of their systolic blood pressure. This is shown in Fig. 1, where the dose dependence of the hypotensive effect may be seen (values for control

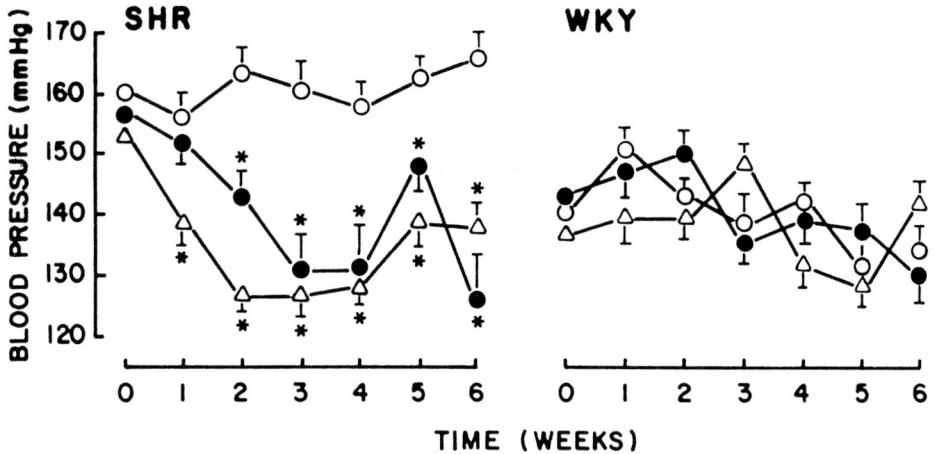

Fig. 1. Effect of oral supplementation with vitamin D_3 on the systolic blood pressure of SHR and WKY rats. O, control; ●, 12.5 μg/100 g body weight/day; Δ, 50 μg/100 g body weight/day.

animals are omitted from the figure, for clarity).

A group of male SHR ($n = 6$, 344 ± 6 g body weight) treated with 12.5 μg vitamin D_3/100 g/day also showed a significant decrease in BP from 170 ± 4 mmHg to 150 ± 3 mmHg already at the second week of treatment.

Since vitamin D_3 is closely implicated with calcium homeostasis, its hypotensive effect might be thought to be due to the increase of serum calcium levels. However, although an increase in serum calcium levels was observed in WKY, no changes were seen in SHR (Table 1). This is in agreement with previous reports (Schedl et al., 1984) on the unresponsiveness of the gut of SHR to vitamin D_3 and rules out the possibility that the hypotensive effect of vitamin D_3 may be linked to serum calcium levels.

Another explanation for the hypotensive effect of vitamin D_3 might be associated with the possible inhibition of PTH secretion due to the chronic supplementation with this vitamin. A hypertensive effect of PTH has been proposed, although this is a controversial subject (for a review see Kaplan et al., 1986). However we found that the treatment with vitamin D_3 did not change serum PTH levels in SHR, although a significant decrease was seen in WKY (Table 1). Treatment with vitamin D_3 did not alter urinary calcium nor serum calcium levels in SHR, but the WKY rats, which had lower basal values of serum calcium, had these values increased by the treatment (Table 1). Our results confirm a correlation between serum calcium and PTH levels and rule out the possibility of the hypotensive effect of vitamin D_3 being mediated by suppression of PTH secretion.

The fact that vitamin D_3 has an important effect on membrane lipid structure, increasing membrane fluidity, and the report of a reduced cell membrane fluidity in SHR (Devynck et al., 1982), led us to investigate whether vitamin D_3 supplementation would alter blood viscosity, which is known to depend on the physical state of the red

Table 1. Responses of SHR and WKY rats after 6 weeks of dietary supplementation with 12.5 µg of vitamin D_3/100 g body weight/day

Group	Serum calcium (mg/dl)	Serum PTH (pmoles/l)	Urinary Ca^{2+} (mEq/24h)	Hematocrit (%)
SHR				
Before	8.2 ± 0.2†	26.3 ± 1.5†	0.325 ± 0.08	42.8 ± 1.5
After	8.3 ± 0.3†	29.9 ± 3.4†	0.365 ± 0.06	20.9 ± 0.8*
WKY				
Before	9.6 ± 0.2	20.9 ± 1.2	0.235 ± 0.06	41.2 ± 1.1
After	10.7 ± 0.4*	15.5 ± 0.8*	0.290 ± 0.03	23.1 ± 0.5*

Values are means ± SEM of 6 animals. *Significantly different from value before treatment ($p < 0.05$). †Significantly different from WKY rats ($p < 0.05$).

blood cell membrane. The hematocrit is the major determinant of blood viscosity and its reduction is associated with decreases in blood pressure. Although we found no differences between WKY and SHR as to basal hematocrit, treatment with vitamin D_3 caused a significant reduction of the haematocrit in SHR (Table 1). Thus, the hypotensive effect of vitamin D_3 may be linked to its action on blood viscosity. On the other hand, the lack of blood pressure change on WKY rats, in spite of a decrease in their hematocrit (Table 1), might be due to a compensatory mechanism, since the two strains react differently to decreases in the hematocrit, whose hypotensive effect is more efficiently compensated in the normotensive animals (Susic et al., 1984).

REFERENCES

Devynck, M.A., Pernollet, M.G., and Nunez, A.M. (1982): Diffuse structural alterations in cell membranes of spontaneously hypertensive rats. *Proc. Natl. Acad. Sci.* 79, 5057-5060.
Kaplan, N.M., and Meese, R.B. (1986): The calcium deficiency hypothesis of hypertension: a critique. *Ann. Intern. Med.* 105, 947-955.
Lucas, P.A., Brown, R.C., Drüeke, T., Lacour, B., Metz, J.A., and McCarron, D.A. (1986): Abnormal vitamin D metabolism, intestinal calcium transport, and bone calcium status in the spontaneously hypertensive rat compared with its genetic control. *J. Clin. Invest.* 78, 221-227.
McCarron, D.A. (1989): Calcium metabolism and hypertension. *Kidney Int.* 35: 717-736.
Schedl, H.P., Miller, D.L., Pape, J.M., Horst, R.L., and Wilson, H.D. (1984): Calcium and sodium transport and vitamin D metabolism in the spontaneously hypertensive rat. *J. Clin. Invest.* 73, 980-986.
Susic, D., Mandal, A., and Kentera, D. (1984): Hemodynamic effects of chronic alteration in hematocrit in spontaneously hypertensive rats. *Hypertension* 6, 262-266.

Cerebral circulation
Circulation cérébrale

Manidipine, a new calcium antagonist, prevents the development and progression of cerebrovascular lesions in stroke-prone spontaneously hypertensive rats

Akinobu Nagaoka, Tetsuji Imamoto, Masahiro Sekiguchi, Keisuke Hirai, Yasuo Nagai and Akio Shino

Biology Research Laboratories, Research and Development Division, Takeda Chemical Industries, Ltd., Osaka 532, Japan

In previous studies, we demonstrated that the development and maintenance of hypertension in spontaneously hypertensive rats (SHR) are closely related to the lowered ability to excrete sodium and water, and vascular reactivity to vasoactive substances in the kidneys (Nagaoka et al. 1978;1982). Furthermore, the development of severe hypertension and its vascular complications in stroke-prone SHR (SHRSP) was implicated in renal vascular changes, especially sclerotic and proliferative changes in renal afferent arterioles, resulting in a decrease in renal perfusion pressure and renal ischemia (Nagaoka et al., 1980). From these findings, we speculated that antihypertensive agents that acted to improve renal hemodynamic alterations are therapeutically beneficial to hypertensive patients. The dihydropyridine derivative, manidipine, discovered on the basis of this speculation is a new calcium antagonist with a long-lasting antihypertensive action (Kakihana et al., 1988). The calcium antagonist shows little cardiodepressant action, but does exhibit a highly selective vasodilation effect (Nakaya et al., 1988). In SHRSP rats, manidipine dilates renal vascular bed, increases renal blood flow, and accelerates sodium and water excretion (Nagaoka et al., 1989; Nagaoka and Shibota, 1989). In the present study, prophylactic and therapeutic effects of manidipine on cerebrovascular lesions (stroke) are investigated in SHRSP.

METHODS <u>Prophylactic effect on onset of stroke:</u> In allocating SHRSP (male, 8 weeks old) to control and drug-treated groups, an equal number of rats from a litter were assigned to each group. The rats were fed a high-salt powdered diet (3% salt diet) during the experimental period to accelerate the onset of stroke. Systolic blood pressure was measured by a tail pulse pick-up method once a week. The onset of cerebrovascular lesions was predicted by stroke signs and confirmed by autopsy (Nagaoka et al., 1976). Calcium antagonists were admixed with the powdered diet.

<u>Therapeutic effect on cerebral and renal vascular changes:</u> Male SHRSP (10 weeks old) were kept in individual cages and given normal chow with a 1% NaCl solution as drinking water for 3 to 5 weeks to shorten the onset time of stroke. When the rats developed the first stroke symptom, they were divided into a control group and two manidipine-treated groups, and were observed for 3 weeks during which time the salt solution was exchanged for tap water. The severity of neurological deficits was recorded according to a scoring system (Nagaoka et al., 1989). At the experiment termination, the brains and kidneys were removed and fixed with a 10% formaldehyde solution for histological observations. After fixation, each brain was cut into 4 frontal sections at distance of 5 mm, and embedded in paraffin. Then, serial sections were made from whole brain at intervals of 100 μm. These were stained with hematoxylin-eosin and observed with a light microscope. The kidneys were

embedded in paraffin as usual, and made into thin sections. They were stained with hematoxylin-eosin and periodic acid Schiff. Manidipine suspended in a 0.5% arabic gum solution was administered orally in doses of 1 and 3 mg/kg once daily for 3 weeks of the observation period.

RESULTS AND DISCUSSION Prophylactic effect on onset of stroke: The effects of dihydropyridine-type calcium antagonists (manidipine, nifedipine, nimodipine and nicardipine) on the development of stroke were investigated in SHRSP. The changes in the blood pressure in all groups of rats are shown in Table 1. Although relatively small doses of the calcium antagonists were selected in the present experiments, the antagonists significantly inhibited elevation of blood pressure and this inhibition was dose-dependent. The highest blood pressure in all rats exceeded the critical blood pressure level known to develop stroke in SHRSP (Nagaoka et al., 1976). The final incidence of stroke was 100% in the control group. All calcium antagonists delayed the onset of stroke but the potency was clearly different among them (Table 1). Manidipine dose-dependently inhibited the onset of stroke. The inhibition of the high dose (3.5 mg/kg/day) was perfect, and no occurrence of stroke was observed. The effects of the high doses of nifedipine (3.5 mg/kg/day) and nimodipine (14 mg/kg/day) were also prominent, but the effect of nicardipine was not clear at least in the doses used. Stroke occurrence was significantly delayed in the two dose groups of manidipine and the high dose group of nifedipine and nimodipine (Wilcoxon's two-sample test, $p<0.05$).

Table 1. Systolic blood pressure and final incidence of stroke.

Groups	Dose (mg/kg/day)	n	Blood Pressure (mmHg)				Final Incidence of Stroke (%)
			0	2	5	10 (weeks)	
Control		20	172±2	209±2	244±3	—	100
Manidipine	(1.4)	10	171±3	204±4	238±5*	247±4 (n=4)	70
	(3.5)	20	172±2	197±3*	225±5*	234±4	0
Nifedipine	(1.4)	10	170±4	205±5	232±6*	246±7 (n=6)	80
	(3.5)	10	169±4	201±7*	226±8*	239±9 (n=8)	40
Nicardipine	(3.5)	10	172±2	205±3	240±4	248±3 (n=3)	90
	(8.8)	10	171±3	201±3*	234±3*	248±5 (n=4)	90
Nimodipine	(3.5)	10	174±4	208±2	231±6*	250±4 (n=4)	80
	(14.0)	10	173±6	193±4*	226±4*	249±7 (n=7)	40

Drugs are admixed with powder diet. * $p<0.05$ vs Control

Protective effects of manidipine on progression of cerebral and renal damages: As manidipine showed the most potent prophylactic effect on onset of stroke in SHRSP, the protective effects of the drug on progression of cerebral and renal damages were assessed by post-treatment which was initiated after development of the first stroke symptom. Histopathological observation indicated that manidipine markedly inhibited the progression or recurrence of hemorrhage, vascular necrosis and degenerative changes in the brain (Fig.1), and the progression of hemorrhagic and necrotic changes in the kidneys. In the kidneys, sclerosis and/or hyalinosis in the glomerulus and the hyalin cast, were inhibited by the manidipine treatment. Body weight gain was markedly depressed in the untreated control but not in the manidipine-treated groups, particularly in the high dose group of rats. The severity of neurological deficits was also ameliorated by the manidipine treatment, dose-dependently, and the ameliorating effect was statistically significant in the high dose group.

Hypertensive treatment with calcium antagonists was effectively delayed the onset of stroke in SHRSP. Blood pressure changes in the manidipine, nifedipine and nimodipine high dose groups were almost the same in the early stage of the experiment, but the rate of onset of cerebrovascular lesions was different among the groups treated with the antagonists. The prophylactic effect of manidipine was particularly prominent, and perfect. This effect of manidipine seems to be partly due to its action of improving renal hemodynamics because it is known that the stroke development in SHRSP is closely related to a decrease in renal blood flow (Nagaoka et al., 1980) and the calcium antagonist increases renal blood flow in the rats (Nagaoka et al., 1989). In addition, manidipine dose-dependently inhibited the progression of vascular changes in the brain and kidneys, although the low dose(1 mg/kg) of this drug showed no significant hypotensive action and the high dose (3 mg/kg) evinced a mild hypotensive action in SHRSP (Kakihana et al., 1988). These results suggest that manidipine may be useful for the treatment of patients with stroke and that may have beneficial vascular-effects other than antihypertensive and renal vascular dilating effects.

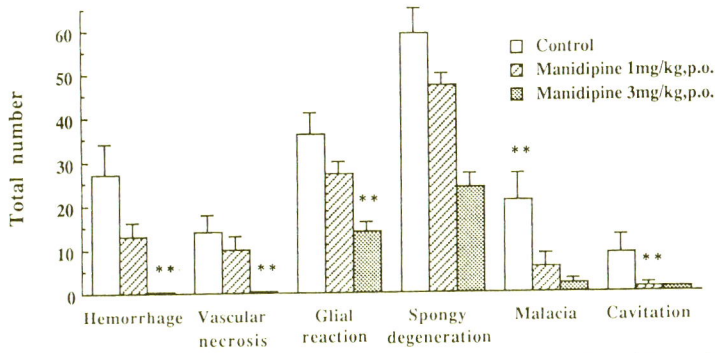

Fig.1. Effects of manidipine on cerebral lesions in SHRSP with stroke.
** $p<0.01$ vs control (Mann-Whitney test)

REFERENCES

Kakihana, M., Suno, M., and Nagaoka, A. (1988): Antihypertensive effect of CV-4093 · 2HCl, a new calcium antagonist, in three rat models of hypertension. Japan. J. Pharmacol. 48, 223-228.

Nakaya, H., Hattori, Y., Nakao, Y., and Kanno, M. (1988): Cardiac versus vascular effects of a new dihydropyridine derivative, CV-4093. In vitro comparison with other calcium antagonists. Europ. J. Pharmacol. 146, 35-43.

Nagaoka, A., Iwatsuka, H., Suzuoki, Z., and Okamoto, K. (1976): Genetic predisposition to stroke in spontaneously hypertensive rats. Am. J. Physiol. 230, 1354-1359.

Nagaoka, A., Toyoda, S., and Iwatsuka, H. (1978): Increased renal vascular reactivity to norepinephrine in stroke-prone spontaneously hypertensive rat (SHR). Life Sci. 23, 1159-1166.

Nagaoka, A., Shino, A., and Shibota, M. (1980): Implication of renal perfusion pressure in stroke of spontaneously hypertensive rats. Am. J. Physiol. 238, H317-H324.

Nagaoka, A., Kakihana, M., Shibota, M., and Fujiwara, K., and Shimakawa, K. (1982): Reduced sodium excretory ability in young spontaneously hypertensive rats. Japan. J. Pharmacol. 32, 839-844.

Nagaoka, A., and Shibota, M. (1989): Natriuretic action of manidipine hydrochloride, a new calcium channel blocker, in spontaneously hypertensive rats. Japan. J. Pharmacol. 51, 299-301.

Nagaoka, A., Shibota, M., and Hamajo, K. (1989): Effects of a new dihydropyridine derivative, CV-4093 · 2HCl, on renal hemodynamics in spontaneously hypertensive rats. Japan. J. Pharmacol. 51, 25-35.

Nagaoka, A., Kakihana, M., and Fujiwara, K. (1989): Effects of idebenone on neurological deficits following cerebrovascular lesions in stroke-prone spontaneously hypertensive rats. Arch. Gerantol. Geriatr. 8, 203-212.

The therapeutic effects of SQ 29,852 and manidipine on M-SHRSP and SHRSP with vascular lesions of brains and kidneys and other organs

Kozo Okamoto, Yoshio Ohta and Taka-Aki Chikugo

Department of Pathology, Kinki University School of Medicine, 377-2, Ohno-Higashi, Osaka-Sayama, Osaka 589, Japan

Introduction: Stroke-prone SHR (SHRSP), a strain established from SHR by Okamoto et al., in 1974, is considered a suitable model and is now being widely used in the study of human malignant hypertension. Malignant SHRSP (M-SHRSP), established from SHRSP in 1982, also by Okamoto et al., develop malignant hypertension, die at early stage of life. and appear to be a very useful animal model for the study of juvenile malignant hypertension (Okamoto et al., 1985). Previously, using SHRSP and M-SHRSP, we examined the effects of several antihypertensive drugs (Ohta et al., 1989; Chikugo et al., 1990). In this experiment, SHRSP and M-SHRSP already showing cerebrovascular lesions (brain hemorrhages and/or brain softenings) were selected, treated with an angiotensin converting enzyme inhibitor or calcium antagonist, and studied over the course of the treatment in order to see what effects these drugs have upon brain and vascular lesions, and especially upon angionecrosis in certain organs.

Materials and methods: Rats with abnormal symptoms or findings suggestive of hypertension and cerebrovascular lesions were selected from among 12-week-old and older male and 15-week-old and older female M-SHRSP, as well as from 20- to 23-week-old male and female SHRSP in accordance with the following primary criterion: (A) rats showing abnormal behaviors (hyperirritability, motion disturbance, etc.), and (B) rats showing enlarged heads. Drugs employed were orally an angiotensin converting enzyme inhibitor (SQ 29,852, Bristol-Myers Squibb K. K., Japan) and a calcium antagonist (manidipine, Takeda Chemical Industries Ltd., Japan), both mixed in food (Funabashi SF. powder), at dosages of 40 mg/kg/day. Blood pressures were measured using the tail-pulse pickup method without anesthesia. All of the animals were autopsied and examined pathologically for brain and vascular lesions, and especially for angionecrosis of the brains, kidneys, sex organs, and adrenal and thyroid glands following natural death or sacrifice after 1, 3, 6 and 12 months of observation.

Results: In almost all of the rats treated with either SQ 29,852 or manidipine abnormal symptoms disappeared within 5 days following the start of the study. After 6 months, the enlarged heads of some of the rats suffering this affliction had disappeared. The experimented rats, except for those which died early in the experiment, both with or without head enlargement, lived for longer periods, for this study at the most 365 days after treatment began. Blood pressures at the beginning were around 270 mmHg for M-SHRSP and around 290 mmHg for SHRSP. After treatment, blood pressures for M-SHRSP decreased without disregard to the presence of head enlargement. Blood pressures were around 250 mmHg for the SQ 29,852 group and around 210 mmHg for the manidipine group. The antihypertensive effect of manidipine was stronger than that of SQ 29,852. SHRSP blood pressures followed a course similar to those for M-SHRSP. At the beginning, M-SHRSP male and female body weights were about 180 g and 160 g respectively, for SHRSP they were about 280 g and 220 g respectively. These figures gradually increased for all groups following the start of the treatment. Histopathological examination revealed softenings and/or hemorrhages, and cyst formations, mostly in the cerebral anterior and posterior lobes. They also showed hemorrhages in parts of the midbrain of non-treated M-SHRSP and SHRSP, with or without accompanying head enlargement. Lesions in rats with enlarged heads were larger and ventricular expansions were observed in these groups. Arteriolar angionecrosis was detected in the kidneys of all of the animals, in about 70 per cent of the brains, hearts and testes, and in around 50 per cent or more of the ovaries, adrenal glands and thyroid glands. Fresh lesions, seen as softenings and hemorrhages, were found in rats treated with SQ 29,852 or manidipine during the first 14 days of treatment, but no such lesions were found after 14 days or more had passed. However, fat and/or iron granule cell aggregation, grial-mesenchymal scars and cyst formations, all seemingly part of the cerebral lesion healing process, were detected. These phenomena grew smaller or disappeared in rats without head enlargement after 12 months, but in rats with enlarged heads comparatively large brain cysts could still be found. Arteriolar angionecrosis of the kidneys and other organs disappeared within 10 days after treatment began in both groups of M-SHRSP. Further, proliferations of smooth muscle cells and arteriole hyalinizations were detected, and some of the arteriole even appeared to have been healed. After 6 months of treatment, intimal necrosis and fibrinoid substances were found in such large muscular arteries as the interlobar and arcuate arteries of the kidneys, as well as in some small arteries of the sex organs of a number of rats from both groups. Mesenteric arterial lesions were also found in 20 per cent or more of the rats suffering these problems. Arteriolar angionecrosis in SHRSP disappeared within 3 months. The healing effects (disappearance of arteriolar angionecrosis) were almost the same in both treatment groups for M-SHRSP or SHRSP.

Discussion: SHRSP and M-SHRSP suffer from malignant hypertension and a high frequency of brain, heart, kidney, sex organ, adrenal gland and thyroid glad arteriolar angionecrosis. We have previously reported that high frequencies of angionecrosis of their arteriole are also found whenever blood pressures were 210mmHg or more (Ohta et al., 1987). In particular, arteriolar angionecrosis in the kidneys, accompanied by severe hypertension, was detected in all 20-week-old or older SHRSP and 11-week-old or older M-SHRSP. From these groups, this study used rats which were already showing significant abnormal symptoms or evidencing head enlargements. Although the drugs used, an angiotensin converting enzyme inhibitor and a calcium antagonist, differed in function and degree of antihypertensive effect, similar results related to the disappearance of arteriolar angionecrosis and continued to exist in the treated rats for long periods of time. From these results, it seems that one or more factors other than the antihypertensive effects of SQ 29,852 or manidipine participate in healing cerebral lesions and arteriolar angionecrosis. After 6 months of treatment, findings of angionecrosis of muscular arteries are similar to those of arterioles at the start or at an early stage of treatment. Because angionecrosis in the muscular arteries appeares well after treatment with SQ 29,852 or manidipine had caused the arteriolar angionecrosis to disappears, as well as because the angionecrosis in the muscular arteries, did not respond to treatment at all, it appaers that the factors behind these angionecrosis in arterioles versus muscular arteries may be different.

REFERENCES

Chikugo, T., Ohta, Y., Shiokawa, H. and Okamoto, K. (1990): The effect of several antihyertensive drugs on vascular changes to organs on M-SHRSP and SHRSP. Jpn. Heart J. 31, 544.
Ohta, Y., Morita, N., Yamamoto, K., Shiokawa, H. and Okamoto, K. (1987): Studies on plasma aldosterone in M-SHRSP and SHR strains (1). Acta. Med. Kinki Univ. 10, 73-95.
Ohta, Y., Morita, N., Shiokawa, H., Hamada, Y., Chikugo, T. and Okamoto, K. (1989): The therapeutic effects of several anti-hypertensive drugs and diet on M-SHRSP. Jpn. Heart J. 30, 543.
Okamoto, K., Yamori, Y. and Nagaoka, A.(1974): Establishment of the stroke-prone spontaneously hypertensive rat(SHR). Cir. Res. 34, 35 (suppl) 143-153.
Okamoto, K., Yamamoto, K., Morita, N. and Ohta, Y.(1985): Establishment and characteristics of rat with precocious and severe hypertension (M-SHRSP). Acta. Med. Kinki Univ. 10, 73-95.
Okamoto, K., Yamamoto, K., Morita, N., Ohta, Y., Chikugo, T., Higashizawa, T. and Suzuki, T. (1986): Establishment and use of the M strain of stroke-prone spontaneously hypertensive rat. J. Hypertension 4 (suppl 3), S21-S24.

Examination of astrocytic functions in stroke-prone SHR applying co-culture techniques

Motoki Tagami, Kasuo Yamagata *, Yasuo Nara ** and Yukio Yamori **

*Department of Medicine, Sanraku Hospital, Chiyoda-Ku, Tokyo 101, * Biotechnology Section, Sumitomo Metal Industry, Sagamihara, Kanagawa 229 and ** Department of Pathology, Shimane Medical University, Izumo 693, Japan*

The basis for the blood-brain barrier in mammals is the selective transport properties of brain capillary endothelium, including the elaborate system of tight intercellular occluding junctions that occur between apposed membrane faces of these cells (Meresse et al, 1989).

The ability of brain endothelial cells to form the blood-brain barrier is not intrinsic to these cells but instead is induced by the environment of the central nervous system. In this study we maintained bovine aortic endothelial cells (BAECs) and astrocytes of Wister Kyoto rats (WKY) and stroke-prone SHR (SHRSP) in the same dish using co-culture techniques. We tried to provide direct evidence that astrocytes were capable of inducing blood-brain barrier properties in non-neural endothelial cells in vitro. Futhermore we compared the astrocytic functions of SHRSP with the ones present in WKY.

Materials and Methods

BAECs were isolated by standard techniques and used between passages 8 – 16. Astrocytes were prepared from the whole brains of fetal WKY as well as fetal SHRSP according to the method of Furukawa et al.(1986). Subcultured astrocytes were plated in the culture plate inserts (Millicell-CM ; pore size, $0.4 \mu m$: diameter, 30mm ; Millipore) which were coated with Type I or type IV collagen.

The culture plate inserts, in which astrocytes were maintained for 7-8 days, were settled within the dishes when the endothelial cells had become almost confluent. We maintained the endothelial cells simultaneously with the astrocytes in the same dishes for 4-6 days. The co-culture of BAECs and astrocytes was completed, and then the culture plate inserts, in which astrocytes grew, were removed. For tracer studies, 10mg/ml DMEM of horseradish peroxidase (HRP) was added in the dishes, where BAECs were maintained, for 1-7 minutes. Both of BAECs and astrocytes were fixed in 1% formaldehyde and 1.25% glutaraldehyde.

They were postfixed with 2% OsO₄, stained with uranyl acetate and embedded in Epon 812.

Results

Astrocytes, cultured in inserts coated with Type-I collagen, contained numerous intermediate filaments, endoplasmic reticula and mitochondria. The astrocytes, which were apposed to Type-I collagen on the surface of the inserts, consistently produced various amounts of collagenous substances and the cells adhered to Type-I collagen on the surface of the inserts. Astrocytes, cultured in inserts coated with Type-IV collagen, extended nemerous processes and were linked to one another by gap junctions. Numerous processes resulted in dense networks among the astrocytes. The astrocytes, apposed to Type-IV collagen on the surface of the inserts, produced considerable collagenous substances. The collagenous substances were clustered on the side facing Type-IV collagen in the insert, but not on the other sides of the astrocytes, indicating that the cells were polarized. BAECs in Type-I collagen, co-cultured with astrocytes of WKY and SHRSP, showed development in various degrees. Some cells were immature and had a lot of pseudo-podia like processes and plasmalemmal vasicles. In contrast some cells were well-matured. Tracer examinations revealed that reaction products of HRP were observed in the plasma membranes, plasmalemmal vesicles, intercellular junctions and subendothelial spaces as early as 1 minute after HRP was added. BAECs in Type-IV collagen, co-cultured with astrocytes of WKY, were consistently well-developed. The surfaces of the cells were smooth and the plasmalemmal vesicles decreased in number. Tracer experiments demonstrated that reaction products of HRP occasionally existed on the plasma membranes and within the

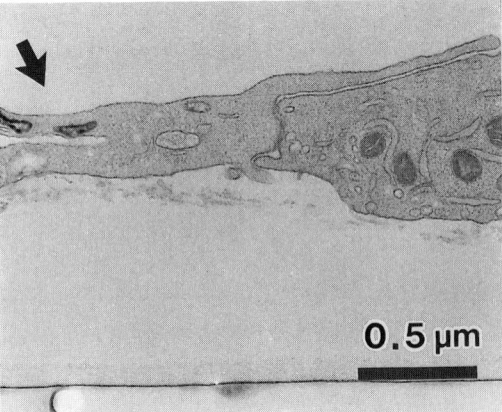

Fig. 1. BAECs in Type-IV collagen co-cultured with astrocytes of WKY. HRP detected within the plasmalemmal vesicles (arrow).

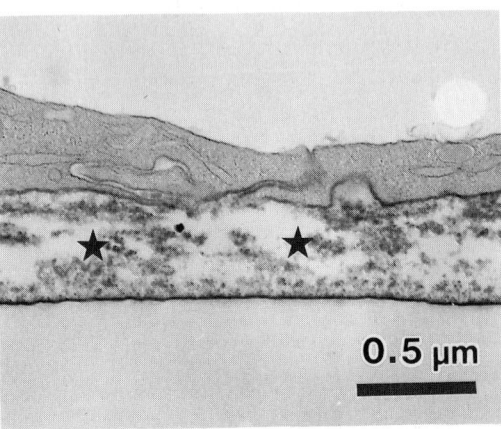

Fig. 2. BAECs in Type-IV collagen co-cultured with astrocytes of SHRSP. Large amounts of HRP are observed in the subendothelial space (stars).

plasmalemmal vesicles. HRP could not penetrate through the intercellular spaces. Reaction products of HRP were almost undetectable in the spaces between BAECs and Type-IV collagen coating dish at 7 minutes after HRP was added (Fig.1). Although BAECs in Type-IV collagen, co-cultured with astrocytes of SHRSP, developed more perfectly than BAECs in Type-I collagen, their barrier functions were not adequate. Therefore large amounts of HRP were observed in the spaces between BAECs and Type-IV collaten coating dish at 7 minutes after adding HRP (Fig.2).

Discussion

Several excellent studies indicated that astrocytes exerted a direct influence on the final developmental events of endothelial cells in the central nervous system (Arthur et al. 1987 ; Janzer and Raff 1987). In this study we demonstrate that Type-IV collagen is essential for the differentiation of BAECs as well as astrocytes. Furthermore the co-culture of BAECs and astrocytes of WKY, maintained in Type-IV collagen, demonstrates that BAEC-astrocyte interactions occur and BAECs reduce the number of plasmalemmal vesicles and construct tight junctions between interendothelial spaces. As a result both the vesicular and junctional transport of BAECs apparently decrease. In contrast the barrier functions of BAECs in Type-IV collagen, co-cultured with astrocytes of SHRSP, are not adequate. As a result large amounts of HRP are found in the subendothelial spaces at 7 minutes of HRP addition.

Conclusions

The local control of tight junction biogenesis depends on astrocyte-produced factors and Type-IV collagen. Astrocytes of SHRSP are weak in the production of these factors. Dysfunction of the astrocyte possibly causes the blood-brain barrier to break down which results in brain edema.

References

Arthur, F.E., Shivers, R.R., and Bowman, P.D. (1987) : Induction of tight junction formation in cultured brain microvessel endothelial cells : local control of cell specialization. Dev. Brain Res. 36 : 155-159

Furukawa, S, Furukawa, Y., Satoyoshi, E., and Hayashi, K.(1986) : Synthesis and secretion of nerve growth factor by mouse astroglial cells in culture. Biochem. Biophys. Res. Commun. 136 : 57-63

Janzer,.C., and Raff, M.C.(1987) : Astrocytes induce blood-brain barrier properties in endothelial cells. Nature 325 : 253-257

Meresse, S., Deheuck, M.P., Delerme, P., Bensaid, M., Touber, J.P., Derbart, C., Fruchart, J.C., and Cecchelli, R. (1989) : Bovine brain endothelial cells express tight junction and monoamine oxidase activity in long-term culture. J. Neurochem. 53 : 1363-1371

Acute administration of antihypertensive drugs produces different effects on cerebral blood flow in awake spontaneously hypertensive rats

Laure Bray-des Boscs, Isabelle Lartaud, Jeffrey Atkinson and Christine Capdeville-Atkinson

Laboratoire de Pharmacologie cardio-vasculaire, Faculté de Pharmacie, 5, rue Albert Lebrun, 54000 Nancy, France

Chronic hypertension shifts the lower limit of cerebral blood flow (CBF) autoregulation and it has been argued that at the onset of antihypertensive treatment there is a risk of cerebral ischaemia if blood pressure falls below the lower limit of CBF autoregulation (Zanchetti, 1989). As the adult spontaneously hypertensive rat (SHR) shows a similar shift in the lower limit of CBF autoregulation (Bray, et al., 1991), we investigated the acute effects of several antihypertensive drugs in this model.

We compared the acute effects of the angiotensin I converting enzyme inhibitor perindopril (PER), the alpha$_1$ adrenergic antagonist prazosin (PRAZ), the vasodilator hydralazine (HYD) and the calcium entry blocker isradipine (ISR) on mean arterial pressure (MAP) and CBF in awake SHR (Janian, et al., 1989). Cortical CBF was measured by the hydrogen clearance technique and MAP via a femoral artery cannula before and 15, 30, 60 min after an i.v. injection of PER (2 mg/kg, n = 6), PRAZ (1 mg/kg, n = 8), HYD (25 mg/kg, n = 8), ISR (0.5 mg/kg, n = 6) or NaCl (0.15 M, n = 6) in awake SHR. Following each CBF determination, blood gas parameters were measured.

Following NaCl, MAP and CBF did not change (Figures 1 and 2). All drugs except PER induced a rapid fall in MAP below 110 mmHg (Figure 1), the lower limit of CBF autoregulation (Janian et al., 1989). CBF fell following PRAZ, remained stable after PER and increased following HYD and ISR (Table 1, Figure 2).

Table 1. Effects in awake SHR of PER, PRAZ, HYD, ISR on CBF (ml/100g/min).

	PER	PRAZ	HYD	ISR
n	6	8	8	6
basal MAP (mmHg)	158 ± 5	148 ± 4	156 ± 4	157 ± 4
basal CBF	88 ± 2	104 ± 6	94 ± 6	95 ± 7
CBF (90-109 mmHg MAP)	90 ± 7	73 ± 9*	155 ± 4*	97 ± 2
CBF (70-89 mmHg MAP)	-	78 ± 8*	191 ± 12*	118 ± 13*

*: $P < 0.05$ versus basal value for same group (mean ± SEM). ANOVA/SCHEFFE.

Figure 1. Change in MAP (mmHg, m ± SEM) in awake SHR following saline (open squares, n = 6), PER (open triangles, n = 6), PRAZ (open circles, n = 8), HYD (full triangles, n = 8) or ISR (full squares, n = 6).

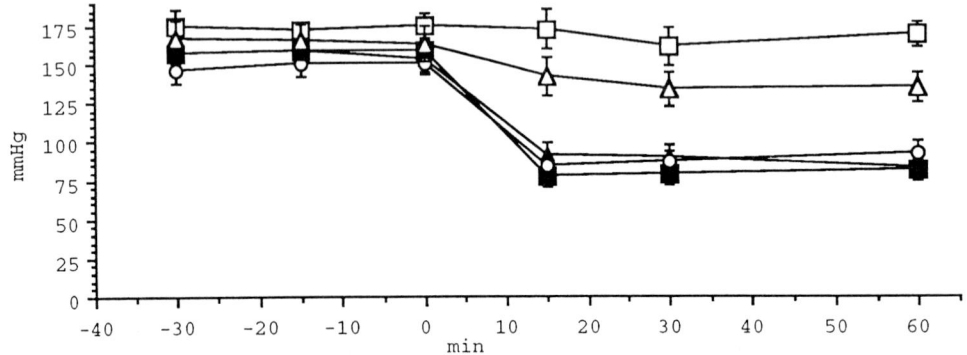

Figure 2. Change in CBF (ml/100g/min, m ± SEM) in awake SHR following saline (open squares, n = 6), PER (open triangles, n = 6), PRAZ (open circles, n = 8), HYD (full triangles, n = 8) or ISR (full squares, n = 6).

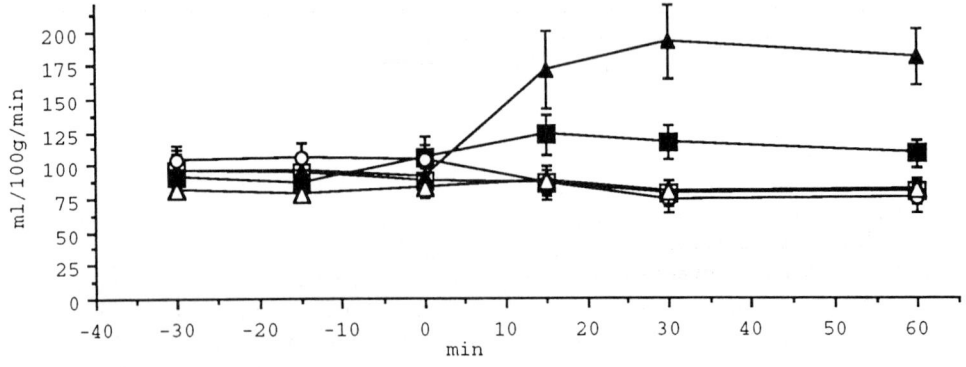

After PRAZ, HYD and ISR, PaO_2 increased but other blood gas parameters were stable (Figure 3).

Figure 3. Change in PaO$_2$ (mmHg, m ± SEM) in awake SHR following saline (open squares, n = 6), PER (open triangles, n = 6), PRAZ (open circles, n = 8), HYD (full triangles, n = 8) or ISR (full squares, n = 6).

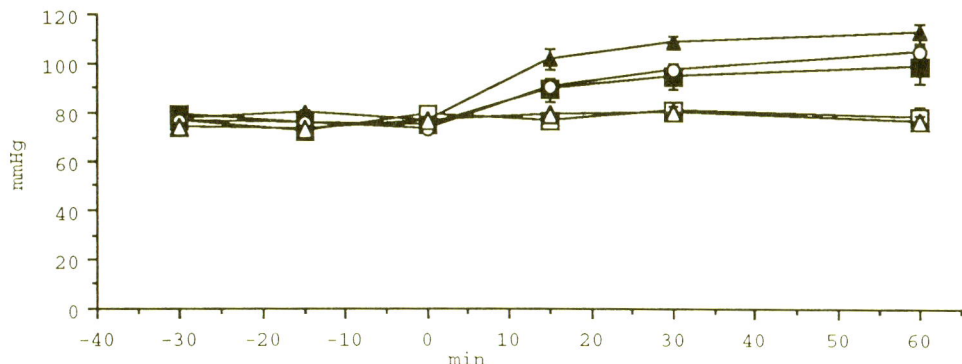

In conclusion, the change in CBF following a pharmacologically-induced fall in MAP is dependent upon the pharmacodynamic action of the antihypertensive drug used. Some drugs, such as HYD and ISR in our study, appear to produce an increase in CBF even though MAP falls to a level below the lower limit of CBF autoregulation. This effect appears to be unrelated to metabolic control of CBF as PRAZ increases PaO$_2$ in a fashion similar to that of ISR but the alpha adrenoceptor antagonist lowers CBF whilst the calcium entry blocker increases CBF. Finally, although hypertension is one of the most important risk factors for certain forms of stroke and clinical trials show that chronic antihypertensive treatment is beneficial, at the onset of treatment there may be a risk of cerebral ischaemia with drugs like PRAZ if blood pressure falls beyond the lower limit of CBF autoregulation, whereas with others like HYD the fall in blood pressure is accompanied by a substantial increase in CBF.

REFERENCES.

Bray, L., Lartaud I., Muller, F., Atkinson J. and Capdeville C. (1991). Effects of the angiotensin I converting enzyme inhibitor perindopril on cerebral blood flow in awake hypertensive rats. Am. J. Hypertens. 4: 246S-252S.
Janian, P., Lartaud, I., Muller, F., Atkinson, J. and Capdeville, C. (1989). Effect of chronic hypertension on the lower limit of autoregulation of cerebral blood flow in the awake rat. In "Neurotransmission and cerebrovascular function I". Edit. Seylaz, J. and MacKenzie, E.T., Elsevier, Amsterdam, pp. 185-188.
Zanchetti, A. (1989). How much should blood pressure be lowered ? The problem of the J-shaped curve. J. Hypertens. 7: S338-S348.

Author index
Index des auteurs

Abe M., 165
Agui T., 329
Akai S., 169
Akai T., 169
Allen T.J., 381
Anand-Srivastava M.B., 553
Astarie C., 569
Atherley R., 441
Atkinson J., 93, 573, 607
Auchère D., 585
Azar S.H., 437

Bachmann J., 81, 353
Bader M., 345, 359
Banide H., 585
Barouki F., 11
Barrès C., 27
Barthelmebs M., 475, 495, 519
Beach R.E., 463
Behm R., 527
Beilin L.J., 55
Ben-Ishay D., 385, 535
Benessiano J., 31
Benetos A., 273
Berrebi-Bertrand I., 265
Bertram J.F., 277
Bianchi G., 447
Bin Talib H.K., 317
Black M.J., 277
Blanc J., 181
Bobik A., 237
Boheler K.R., 401
Böhm M., 359
Bohuon C., 153
Bossolan D., 515
Bouaziz H., 273
Boucher F., 261
Bray-des Boscs L., 607
Brockway B.P., 523
Brunner H.R., 281
Bucher B., 7
Bühler F.R., 211
Buisson S., 145
Bunnemann B., 309
Burkard C., 577
Bursztyn M., 385

Campbell D.J., 467
Campbell J.H., 277
Cantor R., 321
Capdeville-Atkinson C., 93, 573, 607
Carlsen R.C., 441
Carrier L., 401

Castiglioni P., 185
Casto R., 321
Cerutti C., 189
Chabanis S., 585
Chaki S., 301
Chen B.Z., 503
Chen C.J., 463
Chen C.Y., 141
Chen L., 101
Cheng Y., 101, 149
Chikugo T.A., 393, 599
Chobanian A.V., 195
Chu Z., 55
Chung O., 547
Cloix J.F., 535
Cohen Y., 153
Cooper M.E., 381
Coquard C., 475, 495
Corbeil G., 305

Daffonchio A., 73, 105, 185
Dagher G., 479, 483
Dausse E., 223
Dausse J.P., 535
David-Dufilho M., 569
Davy M., 153
De Kloet E.R., 133
De Mey J.G.R., 85
Devynck M.A., 429, 569
Dewitz H., 527
Di Nicolantonio R., 177, 295
DiRienzo M., 185
DiBona G.F., 389
Djavidani B., 343
Doyle A.E., 381, 507
Drubaix I., 265
Drüeke T., 585
Dubar M., 157
Duchambon P., 585
Ducher M., 189

Ebata H., 561
Eerdmans P.H.A., 85
Eichberg J., 463
El Rawadi C., 153
El Fertak L., 11
Elghozi J.L., 181
Ernsberger P., 373
Endo J., 297

Ferracin F., 211
Ferrari A.U., 73, 105, 185
Ferrari P., 447, 577
Fior D.R., 117, 121

Fragman S., 543
Franzelli C., 73, 105, 185
Freslon J.L., 39
Freyss-Béguin M., 429, 569
Friberg P., 237
Fritsch S., 347
Fujimoto S., 245
Fujiwara T., 241
Fukamizu A., 295
Fukuda N., 227
Fukuda S., 417, 421
Fukumitu S., 35

Gairard A., 577, 581
Ganten D., 309, 313, 333, 345, 353, 359
Ganten U., 353
Garay R., 337
Georges M., 313
Gouzi L., 207
Gray S.D., 441
Grichois M.L., 181
Grima M., 475, 495, 519
Guerra P., 471
Guez D., 261, 285
Guicheney P., 223, 337
Gustin M.P., 189
Gutman A., 385

Habeck J.O., 97
Hackenthal E., 349
Hagiike M., 531
Hahn A.W.A., 211
Hamada M., 89, 219
Hamet P., 227, 305
Hanada H., 249
Hano T., 89
Hara K., 173
Harnik M., 543
Harrap S.B., 253, 341, 507
Harris E.L., 219
Hasegawa T., 35
Hashimoto T., 305
Hatano M., 173
Hattori K., 15, 51
Hayashi S., 487
Hayoz D., 281
Haywood J.R., 471,
Head G.A., 69
Heimburger M., 153
Henrotte J.G., 337
Hensleigh H., 437
Hilbert P., 313
Hirai K., 595

Hirawa N., 289, 487
Horiba T., 531
Hosoi M., 459
Hosomi H., 531
Houjoh Y., 561
Hsieh P.S., 77, 141
Huang W.C., 77, 141
Humphreys M.H., 491

Ida F., 65
Iida H., 417, 421
Ikeda K., 15, 23, 51, 295, 297, 325, 417, 421, 531
Ikeda T., 289
Ikeda U., 561
Ikemoto F., 43
Imai T., 295
Imamoto T., 595
Imbs J.L., 475, 495, 519
Inagami T., 301
Ishii M., 289, 487
Ito H., 257, 377
Ito S., 173
Itoh S., 113
Iwai N., 301
Iwamoto T., 487

Jamdeleit K., 503
Jandhyala B.S., 137
Janssen B.J.A., 133
Jardel A., 585
Jarott B., 157
Jerums G., 381
Jin J.S., 77, 141
Johnston C.I., 253, 503
Jones S.Y., 389
Jover B., 511
Julien C., 27
Junquéro D.C., 3

Kaling M., 309
Kaneko K., 47
Kassis N., 265
Kato Y., 289, 425
Katopothis A., 253
Kawamura H., 173
Kawamura K., 249
Kihara M., 487
Kim S., 459
Kimura S., 309, 409
Kisters K., 269
Kladis A., 467
Klir P., 305, 333
Kobayashi Y., 15, 51
Kohlmann Jr. O., 515
Kohzuki M., 503
Koletsky R.J., 373
Komatsu K., 173
Kondo M., 241

Kong D., 305
Kong X.B., 101, 149
Korner P.I., 237
Krefting E.R., 269
Kren V., 305, 317, 333
Kreutz R., 359
Krieger E.M., 65
Kubota J.N., 249
Kunes J., 305, 317, 333

Lacour B., 585
Lange J.M., 523
Lartaud I., 607
Lathrop M., 313
Lawrence A.C., 467
Leclercq Y., 265
Lee C.C., 109
Lee M.A., 345
Leiris J. (de), 261
Lelièvre L.G., 265
Lévy B.I., 11, 31, 233, 273, 285
Lewis S.J., 61
Li P., 539
Lindpaintner K., 313
Lindsey C.J., 117, 121
Liu Y., 487
Lokhandwala M.F., 463

Macrae I.M., 161
Maki M., 173
Malavaud B., 207
Mancia G., 105, 185
Markel A.L., 405
Martins D.T.O., 117, 121
Maser-Gluth C., 343
Masuyama Y., 89, 219
Matsubayashi K., 413
Matsuda T., 531
Matsumoto K., 329
Matsuyama S., 165, 409
Mazbar S.A., 491
Mc Auley M.A., 161
Mewes H., 527
Michel B., 475, 495
Millanvoye-Van Brussel E., 429, 569
Millar J.A., 219
Mimran A., 511
Minami N., 69
Mitchell G.A., 341
Miyake K., 531
Miyazaki T., 241
Mizushima S., 23
Molenaar P., 245
Mooser V., 253, 503
Moreira E.D., 65
Morita H., 531
Moriyama K., 557

Moukadiri H., 207
Mourlon-Le Grand M.C., 31
Mullins J.J., 309, 333, 345, 353
Münter K., 345, 349
Murakami K., 295, 499
Murakami S., 397

Nabika T., 297, 325
Nagai Y., 595
Nagaoka A., 595
Nakamura Y., 499
Nakanishi T., 35
Nara Y., 15, 23, 51, 295, 297, 325, 329, 397, 417, 421, 425, 531
Natori T., 329
Natsume T., 561
Nazaret C., 337
Nicolov N.A., 19
Niederberger M., 281
Nishikibe M., 43
Nishimura H., 249
Nishimura M. 35
Nishio I., 89, 219
Nishiyama S., 413
Noda K., 413
Norman T.L., 341

O'Brien R.C., 381
Oddie C., 237
Ogawa H., 169, 433
Ohta H., 61, 109
Ohta Y., 393, 599
Ohyama H., 531
Oka T., 249
Okada T., 413
Okamoto K., 377, 393, 599
Oliveira V.L.L., 65
Oster L., 573
Ottens E., 81
Ouedraogo S., 7

Pages N., 153
Paiva A.C.M., 589
Paiva T.B., 589
Pak H., 245
Paul M., 359
Paultre C.Z., 189
Paya D., 7
Peleg E., 543
Penner S.B., 539
Pequignot J.M., 97
Pernot F., 581
Peters J., 345
Pieddeloup C., 11
Plouët J., 207
Pourageaud F., 39
Pravenec M., 305, 317, 333
Printz M.P., 321
Pucheu S., 261

Qing W., 535
Qiu H.Y., 233, 285

Rahn K.H., 269, 565
Ramirez A.J., 185
Regenass S., 211
Reid J.L., 161
Resink T.J., 211
Ribeiro A.B., 515
Rohmeiss P., 547
Rohmeiss S., 547
Rong H.M., 215
Rosenthal T., 543
Rota R., 223, 337
Ruchoux M.M., 207
Rumble J.R., 381
Rustschmann B., 281

Safar M.E., 11, 273
Saito N., 413
Sakai T., 329
Sambhi M.P., 215
Sander M., 345
Sannajust F., 157
Santarromana M., 337
Sarhan S., 125
Sasagawa S., 169, 433
Sassard J., 97, 181, 577, 581
Sato T., 425
Sauterey C., 479
Sawamura M., 297, 325
Schatz C., 261, 285
Schini V.B., 3
Schips T., 547
Scholz U., 269
Schüssler B., 565
Schwartz K., 401
Scott-Burden T., 3
Sekigushi M., 595
Seiler N., 125
Shah J., 137
Shimada K., 561
Shimamura K., 47, 557
Shino A., 595
Shinozuka K., 51
Simon J., 429
Simpson F.O., 219
Skinner S.L., 177
Smyth D.D., 539
Soeda E., 295
Soukseun D., 245
Soussan K., 223

Spanos H.G., 177
Spence M.A., 321
Spieker C., 269
Stephan D., 519
Stock G., 353
Stoclet J.C., 7
Struyker-Boudier H.A.J., 85, 233
Su D.F., 101, 149
Sugimoto K., 289
Summers R.J., 245
Sun Y.L., 305
Sunano S., 47, 557
Suwa M., 249
Suzuki A., 19
Suzuki F., 499
Suzuki K., 173
Suzuki T., 257, 377
Swaminathan N., 215
Sylvestri M.F., 523

Tabeli R., 241
Tagami M., 23, 603
Takada T., 459
Takagi N., 289
Takahashi A., 499
Takahashi H., 35
Takahashi M., 169
Takeda K., 487
Takeshita H., 43
Talman W.T., 61, 109
Tanaka T., 169, 433
Tavares A., 515
Tepel M., 269
Terada M., 239
Thibault C., 553
Thomas S.R., 483
Thorin E., 93
Thorin-Trescases N., 573
Tokita Y., 289
Torii M., 257
Towrie A., 467
Toya Y., 289, 487
Tremblay J., 227, 305, 333
Tsuchikura S., 417, 421
Tsuruya Y., 561

Ueyama M., 249
Ueyama T., 89
Umemura S., 289, 487
Unger T., 547

Usui W., 173
Valentijn A.J., 467
Valentin J.P., 491
Valtier B., 233, 285
Van den Berg D.T.W.M., 133
Van den Buuse M., 113, 125, 129, 145
Vanhoutte P.M., 3
Vescei P., 345
Vianna L.M., 589
Vincent M., 97, 181, 577, 581
Völker W., 565
Voynikov T.I., 19
Voynikova I.N., 19
Vyas S.J., 463

Waeber B., 281
Wagner J., 357
Wahba K., 511
Wang H., 215
Watanabe Y., 241
Welsch C., 475, 495
Wisnewsky C., 401

Yamada T., 329
Yamagata K., 603
Yamaguchi M., 169
Yamamoto K., 459
Yamanishi Y., 19
Yamanouchi H., 531
Yamasaki Y., 413
Yamashita M., 397
Yamori Y., 15, 23, 51, 295, 297, 325, 329, 397, 417, 421, 425, 531, 603
Yang J., 149
Yano M., 43
Yasugi T., 173
Yin K., 55
Yoshimoto H., 165, 409
Yoshimura M., 35
Young S., 487

Zamir N., 543
Zanella M.T., 515
Zeh K., 357
Zhang Z.Q., 27
Zicha J., 317
Zidek W., 81, 269, 565
Zimmermann F., 309, 353

Colloques **INSERM**
ISSN 0768-3154

Other *Colloques* published as co-editions by John Libbey Eurotext and INSERM

153 Hormones and Cell Regulation (11th European Symposium). *Hormones et Régulation Cellulaire (11ᵉ Symposium Européen).*
Edited by J. Nunez and J.E. Dumont.
ISBN : John Libbey Eurotext 0 86196 104 8
   INSERM 2 85598 324 X

158 Biochemistry and Physiopathology of Platelet Membrane. *Biochimie et Physiopathologie de la Membrane Plaquettaire.*
Edited by G. Marguerie and R.F.A. Zwaal.
ISBN : John Libbey Eurotext 0 86196 114 5
   INSERM 2 85598 345 2

162 The Inhibitors of Hematopoiesis. *Les Inhibiteurs de l'Hématopoïèse.*
Edited by A. Najman, M. Guignon, N.C. Gorin and J.Y. Mary.
ISBN : John Libbey Eurotext 0 86196 125 0
   INSERM 2 85598 340 1

164 Liver Cells and Drugs. *Cellules Hépatiques et Médicaments.*
Edited by A. Guillouzo.
ISBN : John Libbey Eurotext 0 86196 128 5
   INSERM 2 85598 341 X

165 Hormones and Cell Regulation (12th European Symposium). *Hormones et Régulation Cellulaire (12ᵉ Symposium Européen).*
Edited by J. Nunez, J.E. Dumont and E. Carafoli.
ISBN : John Libbey Eurotext 0 86196 133 1
   INSERM 2 85598 347 9

167 Sleep Disorders and Respiration. *Les Evénements Respiratoires du Sommeil.*
Edited by P. Lévi-Valensi and D. Duron.
ISBN : John Libbey Eurotext 0 86196 127 7
   INSERM 2 85598 344 4

169 Neo-Adjuvant Chemotherapy. *Chimiothérapie Néo-Adjuvante.*
Edited by C. Jacquillat, M. Weil, D. Khayat.
ISBN : John Libbey Eurotext 0 86196 150 1
   INSERM 2 85598 349 5

171 Structure and Functions of the Cytoskeleton. *La Structure et les Fonctions du Cytosquelette.*
Edited by B.A.F. Rousset.
ISBN : John Libbey Eurotext 0 86196 149 8
   INSERM 2 85598 351 7

Colloques INSERM
ISSN 0768-3154

172 The Langerhans Cell. *La Cellule de Langerhans.*
Edited by J. Thivolet, D. Schmitt.
ISBN : John Libbey Eurotext 0 86196 181 1
INSERM 2 85598 352 5

173 Cellular and Molecular Aspects of Glucuronidation. *Aspects Cellulaires et Moléculaires de la Glucuronoconjugaison.*
Edited by G. Siest, J. Magdalou, B. Burchell
ISBN : John Libbey Eurotext 0 86196 182 X
INSERM 2 85598 353 3

174 Second Forum on Peptides. *Deuxième Forum Peptides.*
Edited by A. Aubry, M. Marraud, B. Vitoux
ISBN : John Libbey Eurotext 0 86196 151 X
INSERM 2 85598 354 1

176 Hormones and Cell Regulation (13th European Symposium). *Hormones et Régulation Cellulaire (13e Symposium Européen).*
Edited by J. Nunez, J.E. Dumont, R. Denton
ISBN : John Libbey Eurotext 0 86196 183 8
INSERM 2 85598 356 8

179 Lymphokine Receptors Interactions. *Interactions Lymphokines-récepteurs.*
Edited by D. Fradelizi, J. Bertoglio
ISBN : John Libbey Eurotext 0 86196 148 X
INSERM 2 85598 359 2

191 Anticancer Drugs (1st International Interface of Clinical and Laboratory responses to anticancer drugs). *Médicaments anticancéreux (1re Confrontation internationale des réponses cliniques et expérimentales aux médicaments anticancéreux).*
Edited by H. Tapiero, J. Robert, T.J. Lampidis
ISBN : John Libbey Eurotext 0 86196 223 0
INSERM 2 85598 393 2

193 Living in the Cold (2nd International Symposium). *La Vie au Froid (2e Symposium International).*
Edited by A. Malan, B. Canguilhem
ISBN : John Libbey Eurotext 0 86196 234 9
INSERM 2 85598 395 9

Colloques INSERM
ISSN 0768-3154

194 Progress in Hepatitis B Immunization. *La Vaccination contre l'épatite B.*
Edited by P. Coursaget, M.J. Tong
ISBN : John Libbey Eurotext 0 86196 249 4
INSERM 2 85598 396 7

196 Treatment Strategy in Hodgkin's Disease. *Stratégie dans la maladie de Hodgkin.*
Edited by P. Sommers, M. Henry-Amar,
J.H. Meezwaldt, P. Carde
ISBN : John Libbey Eurotext 0 86196 226 5
INSERM 2 85598 398 3

198 Hormones and Cell Regulation (14th European Symposium). *Hormones et Régulation Cellulaire (14ᵉ Symposium Européen).*
Edited by J. Nunez, J.E. Dumont
ISBN : John Libbey Eurotext 0 86196 229 X
INSERM 2 85598 400 9

199 Placental Communications : Biochemical, Morphological and Cellular Aspects. *Communications placentaires : aspects biochimique, morphologique et cellulaire.*
Edited by L. Cedard, E. Alsat, J.C. Challier,
G. Chaouat, A. Malassiné
ISBN : John Libbey Eurotext 0 86196 227 3
INSERM 2 85598 401 7

204 Pharmacologie Clinique : Actualités et Perspectives. (6ᵉ Rencontres Nationales de Pharmacologie clinique).
Edited by J.P. Boissel, C. Caulin, M. Teule
ISBN : John Libbey Eurotext 0 86196 225 7
INSERM 2 85598 454 8

205 Recent Trends in Clinical Pharmacology (6th National Meeting of Clinical Pharmacology).
Edited by J.P. Boissel, C. Caulin, M. Teule
ISBN : John Libbey Eurotext 0 86196 256 7
INSERM 2 85598 455 6

206 Platelet Immunology : Fundamental and Clinical Aspects. *Immunologie plaquettaire : aspects fondamentaux et cliniques.*
Edited by C. Kaplan-Gouet, N. Schlegel,
Ch. Salmon, J. McGregor
ISBN : John Libbey Eurotext 0 86196 285 0
INSERM 2 85598 439 4

Colloques INSERM
ISSN 0768-3154

207 Thyroperoxidase and Thyroid Autoimmunity. *Thyroperoxydase et auto-immunité thyroïdienne.*
Edited by P. Carayon, T. Ruf
ISBN : John Libbey Eurotext 0 86196 277 X
INSERM 2 85598 440 8

208 Vasopressin. *Vasopressine.*
Edited by S. Jard, R. Jamison
ISBN : John Libbey Eurotext 0 86196 288 5
INSERM 2 85598 441 6

210 Hormones and Cell Regulation (15th European Symposium). *Hormones et Régulation Cellulaire (15e Symposium Européen).*
Edited by J.E. Dumont, J. Nunez, R.J.B. King
ISBN : John Libbey Eurotext 0 86196 279 6
INSERM 2 85598 443 2

211 Medullary Thyroid Carcinoma. *Cancer Médullaire de la Thyroïde.*
Edited by C. Calmettes, J.M. Guliana
ISBN : John Libbey Eurotext 0 86196 287 7
INSERM 2 85598 440 0

212 Cellular and Molecular Biology of the Materno-Fetal Relationship. *Biologie cellulaire et moléculaire de la relation materno-fœtale.*
Edited by G. Chaouat, J. Mowbray
ISBN : John Libbey Eurotext 0 86196 909 1
INSERM 2 85598 445 9

215 Aldosterone. Fundamental Aspects. *Aspects fondamentaux.*
Edited by J.P. Bonvalet, N. Farman, M. Lombes, M.E. Rafestin-Oblin
ISBN : John Libbey Eurotext 0 86196 302 4
INSERM 2 85598 482 3

216 Cellular and Molecular Aspects of Cirrhosis. *Aspects cellulaires et moléculaires de la cirrhose.*
Edited by B. Clément, A. Guillouzo
ISBN : John Libbey Eurotext 0 86196 342 3
INSERM 2 85598 483 1

217 Sleep and Cardiorespiratory Control. *Sommeil et contrôle cardio-respiratoire.*
Edited by C. Gaultier, P. Escourrou, L. Curzi-Dascalora
ISBN : John Libbey Eurotext 0 86196 307 5
INSERM 2 85598 484 X

219 Human Gene Transfer. *Transfert de gènes chez l'homme.*
Edited by O. Cohen-Haguenauer, M. Boiron
ISBN : John Libbey Eurotext 0 86196 301 6
INSERM 2 85598 497 1

LOUIS-JEAN
avenue d'Embrun, 05003 GAP cedex

Dépôt légal : 229 — Mars 1992
Imprimé en France